Other Current Therapies

Brain and McCulloch:
    Current Therapy in Hematology-Oncology 1983-1984
Garcia, Mastroianni, Amelar, and Dubin:
    Current Therapy of Infertility 1982-1983
Gates:
    Current Therapy in Otolaryngology
    —Head and Neck Surgery 1982-1983
Kass and Platt:
    Current Therapy of Infectious Disease 1983-1984
Lichtenstein and Fauci:
    Current Therapy in Allergy and Immunology 1983-1984
Trunkey and Lewis:
    Current Therapy of Trauma 1983-1984

Forthcoming

Bayless:
    Current Therapy in Gastroenterology and Liver Disease 1984-1985
Cameron:
    Current Surgical Therapy 1984-1985
Cherniack:
    Current Therapy in Respiratory Medicine 1984-1985
Glassock:
    Current Therapy in Nephrology 1984-1985
Harrison:
    Current Therapy in Cardiology 1984-1985
Nelson:
    Current Therapy in Neonatology—Perinatology 1984-1985

CURRENT THERAPY IN ENDOCRINOLOGY 1983-1984

DOROTHY T. KRIEGER, M.D., D.Sc.
Professor of Medicine
Director, Division of Endocrinology
The Mount Sinai Medical Center of
the City University of New York
New York, New York

C. WAYNE BARDIN, M.D.
Director
Center for Biomedical Research
The Population Council
New York, New York

B.C. DECKER INC • Philadelphia • Toronto
The C.V. MOSBY COMPANY • Saint Louis • Toronto • London

Publisher: **B.C. Decker Inc.**
               3228 South Service Road
               Burlington, Ontario L7N 3H8

North American and worldwide sales and distribution:
               The C.V. Mosby Company
               11830 Westline Industrial Drive
               Saint Louis, Missouri 63141

In Canada: **The C.V. Mosby Company, Ltd**
               120 Melford Drive
               Toronto, Ontario M1B 2X5

Current Therapy in Endocrinology 1983–1984   ISBN 0-941158-04-7

Library of Congress catalog card number: 82-83695

               10   9   8   7   6   5   4   3   2   1

CONTRIBUTORS

CLAUDE D. ARNAUD, M.D.

Professor of Medicine and Physiology, University of California School of Medicine; Chief, Endocrine Section, Veterans Administration Medical Center, San Francisco, California
Primary Hyperparathyroidism

GERALD D. AURBACH, M.D.

Chief, Metabolic Diseases Branch, National Institute of Arthritis, Diabetes, and Digestive and Kidney Diseases, National Institutes of Health, Bethesda, Maryland
Pseudohypoparathyroidism

LOUIS V. AVIOLI, M.D.

Shoenberg Professor of Medicine, Washington University School of Medicine, St. Louis, Missouri
Hypocalcemia

H. W. G. BAKER, M.D., Ph.D.

Howard Florey Institute of Experimental Physiology and Medicine, University of Melbourne, Parkville, Victoria, Australia
Male Infertility of Undetermined Etiology

C. WAYNE BARDIN, M.D.

Director, Center for Biomedical Research, The Population Council, New York, New York
Impotence

FREDERIC C. BARTTER, M.D.

Associate Chief of Staff for Research, Audie L. Murphy Memorial Veterans Hospital, San Antonio, Texas; Professor of Medicine, University of Texas Health Science Center at San Antonio, San Antonio, Texas
Late-Onset Virilizing Congenital Adrenal Hyperplasia, Bartter's Syndrome

STEPHEN B. BAYLIN, M.D.

Associate Professor of Oncology and Medicine, The Johns Hopkins University School of Medicine, Baltimore, Maryland
Medullary Thyroid Carcinoma

NORMAN H. BELL, M.D.

Director, Division of Bone and Mineral Metabolism, Professor of Medicine and Pharmacology, Medical University of South Carolina; Clinical Investigator, Veterans Administration Medical Center, Charleston, South Carolina
Rickets

CHARLES L. BERGER, M.D.

Assistant in Medicine, Department of Medicine and Oncology, The Johns Hopkins University School of Medicine, Baltimore, Maryland
Medullary Thyroid Carcinoma

RICHARD E. BERGER, M.D.

Assistant Professor of Urology, University of Washington School of Medicine; Chief, Section of Urology, Seattle Veterans Administration Medical Center, Seattle, Washington
Infections of the Male Reproductive Tract

JOHN P. BILEZIKIAN, M.D.

Associate Professor of Medicine and Pharmacology, College of Physicians & Surgeons, Columbia University, New York, New York
Hypercalcemia

LEWIS E. BRAVERMAN, M.D.

Professor of Medicine and Physiology, Division of Endocrinology and Metabolism, University of Massachusetts Medical School, Worcester, Massachusetts
Thyroid Storm

STEVEN A. BRODY, M.D.

Clinical Associate, Developmental Endocrinology Branch, National Institute of Child Health and Human Development, National Institutes of Health, Bethesda, Maryland
Gynecomastia

W. VIRGIL BROWN, M.D.

Joe Low and Louis Price Professor of Medicine, Director, Division of Atherosclerosis and Metabolic Diseases, Mt. Sinai School of Medicine, New York, New York
Hyperlipoproteinemia

ROBERT E. CANFIELD, M.D.

Professor of Medicine, College of Physicians & Surgeons Columbia University; Director, General Clinical Research Center, The Presbyterian Hospital, New York, New York
Paget's Disease of Bone

NICHOLAS P. CHRISTY, M.D.

Chief of Staff, Brooklyn Veterans Administration Medical Center; Professor of Medicine, State University of New York Downstate, Brooklyn, New York; Lecturer in Medicine, Columbia University College of Physicians & Surgeons, New York, New York
Principles of Systemic Corticosteroid Therapy for Non-Endocrine Disease, Corticosteroid Withdrawal

v

ORLO H. CLARK, M.D.

Associate Professor of Surgery, University of California School of Medicine; Veterans Administration Medical Center, San Francisco, California
Primary Hyperparathyroidism

SARAH S. DONALDSON, M.D.

Associate Professor of Radiology, Stanford University School of Medicine, Stanford, California
Graves' Ophthalmopathy

STANLEY W. DZIEDZIC, M.D.

Instructor, Department of Medicine, Mt. Sinai School of Medicine, New York, New York
Pheochromocytoma

MAX ELLENBERG, M.D.

Clinical Professor of Medicine, Mt. Sinai School of Medicine; Attending Physician for Diabetes, Mt. Sinai Hospital, New York, New York
Diabetic Neuropathy

KARL ENGELMAN, M.D.

Associate Professor of Medicine and Pharmacology, Chief, Hypertension Section, University of Pennsylvania School of Medicine; Director, Clinical Research Center, Hospital of the University of Pennsylvania, Philadelphia, Pennsylvania
Carcinoid Syndrome

JOHN W. ENSINCK, M.D.

Professor of Medicine, University of Washington School of Medicine, Seattle, Washington; Program Director, Clinical Research Center University Hospital, University of Washington, Seattle, Washington
Postprandial Hypoglycemia

STEVENSON FLANIGAN, M.D.

Professor and Chairman, Department of Neurosurgery, University of Arkansas for Medical Sciences, Little Rock, Arkansas
Nonfunctioning Pituitary Tumors

JEFFREY S. FLIER, M.D.

Chief, Diabetes and Metabolism Unit, Beth Israel Hospital; Assistant Professor of Medicine, Harvard Medical School, Boston, Massachusetts
Insulin Resistance and Allergy

MICHAEL B. FOSTER, M.D.

Assistant Professor of Pediatrics, University of Louisville School of Medicine, Louisville, Kentucky
Delayed Puberty in Girls

BOY FRAME, M.D.

Head, Division of Bone and Mineral Metabolism, Henry Ford Hospital, Detroit, Michigan; Clinical Professor of Medicine, University of Michigan Medical School, Ann Arbor, Michigan
Osteomalacia

ANDREW G. FRANTZ, M.D.

Professor of Medicine, Chief, Division of Endocrinology, Columbia University College of Physicians & Surgeons, New York, New York
Hyperprolactinemia of Undefined Etiology

FRANK S. FRENCH, M.D.

Professor of Pediatrics, University of North Carolina School of Medicine, Chapel Hill, North Carolina
Delayed Puberty in Girls

JULIAN FRICK, M.D.

Professor and Chairman, Urological Department, General Hospital, Salzburg, Austria
Cryptorchidism

ELI A. FRIEDMAN, M.D.

Professor of Medicine, Director of Division of Nephrology, Downstate Medical Center, State University of New York, Brooklyn, New York
Diabetic Nephropathy

LAWRENCE A. FROHMAN, M.D.

Professor of Medicine, Director, Division of Endocrinology and Metabolism, University of Cincinnati College of Medicine, Cincinnati, Ohio
Hypopituitarism

KENNETH H. GABBAY, M.D.

Associate Professor of Pediatrics, Harvard Medical School; Director, Diabetes Unit, Children's Hospital Medical Center, Boston, Massachusetts
Childhood Diabetes Mellitus

EUGENE W. FRIEDMAN, M.D.

Clinical Professor of Surgery, Chief, Division of Head and Neck Surgery, Mt. Sinai School of Medicine, City University of New York, New York, New York
Well-Differentiated Thyroid Cancer,
Parathyroid Carcinoma

MARVIN C. GERSHENGORN, M.D.

Associate Professor, Department of Medicine, Division of Endocrinology, New York University Medical Center, New York, New York
Single Thyroid Nodule

EDMUND W. GIEGERICH, M.D.

Research Fellow, Department of Medicine, Division of Atherosclerosis and Metabolic Diseases, Mt. Sinai Medical Center, New York, New York
Diabetic Ketoacidosis

STANLEY E. GITLOW, M.D.

Clinical Professor of Medicine, Mt. Sinai School of Medicine, New York, New York
Pheochromocytoma

JAMES R. GIVENS, M.D.

Professor of Medicine and Head, Section of Reproductive Medicine, The University of Tennessee Center for the Health Sciences, Memphis, Tennessee
Hirsutism

ELI GLATSTEIN, M.D.

Chief, Radiation Oncology Branch, Division of Cancer Treatment, National Cancer Institute, National Institutes of Health, Bethesda, Maryland; Professor of Radiology, Uniformed Services University, Health Sciences, Bethesda, Maryland
Acromegaly

ROBERT B. GOLBEY, M.D.

Clinical Associate Professor, Department of Medicine, Cornell University Medical College; Attending Physician, Memorial Sloan-Kettering Cancer Center, New York, New York
Testicular Tumors

MARC GOLDSTEIN, M.D.

Director, The Male Reproduction and Urologic Microsurgery Unit; The New York Hospital-Cornell Medical Center; Associate Scientist, Center for Biomedical Research, The Population Council, New York
Impotence,
Vasectomy and Vasectomy Reversal

PHILLIP GORDEN, M.D.

Clinical Director, National Institute of Arthritis, Diabetes and Digestive and Kidney Diseases, Chief, Clinical and Cellular Biology Section, Diabetes Branch, National Institutes of Health, Bethesda, Maryland
Acromegaly

MONTE A. GREER, M.D.

Professor of Medicine, Head, Section of Endocrinology, Oregon Health Sciences University, School of Medicine, Portland, Oregon
Sporadic Nontoxic Goiters

JAMES E. GRIFFIN, M.D.

Associate Professor, Department of Internal Medicine, The University of Texas Southwestern Medical School, Dallas, Texas
Androgen Resistance Syndromes

GEORGE T. GRIFFING, M.D.

Assistant Professor of Medicine, Department of Medicine, University Hospital, Boston University School of Medicine, Boston, Massachusetts
Isolated Hypoaldosteronism

DAVID R. HALBERT, M.D.

Clinical Associate Professor of Medicine, Milton S. Hershey Medical Center, Hershey, Pennsylvania
Dysmenorrhea

JOHN W. HARE, M.D.

Physician, Joslin Clinic; Consultant in Medicine, Lying-In Unit, Brigham & Women's Hospital; Assistant Professor of Medicine, Harvard Medical School, Boston, Massachusetts
Diabetic Pregnancy

CHARLES S. HOLLANDER, M.D.

Professor of Medicine, New York University School of Medicine; Chief, Endocrine Division, Director, Clinical Research Center, New York University Medical Center, New York, New York
Hypothalamic Hypopituitarism

RICHARD HORTON, M.D.

Professor of Medicine, Chief, Section of Endocrinology, Unversity of Southern California School of Medicine, Los Angeles, California
Primary Aldosteronism

WILLA A. HSUEH, M.D.

Assistant Professor, Department of Medicine, Section of Endocrinology and Metabolism, University of Southern California School of Medicine, Los Angeles, California
Primary Aldosteronism

HOWARD L. JUDD, M.D.

Professor of Obstetrics and Gynecology, Chief, Division of Reproductive Endocrinology, UCLA School of Medicine, Los Angeles, California
Menopause

C. RONALD KAHN, M.D.

Director, Eliot P. Joslin Research Laboratory; Chief, Division of Diabetes and Metabolism, Brigham and Women's Hospital; Associate Professor of Medicine, Harvard Medical School, Boston, Massachusetts
Insulinoma and Non-Islet Tumors Producing Hypoglycemia

ELAINE M. KAPTEIN, M.D.

Assistant Professor, Department of Medicine, Division of Nephrology, University of Southern California School of Medicine, Los Angeles, California
Renal Osteodystrophy

MARVIN A. KIRSCHNER, M.D.

Professor of Medicine, New Jersey Medical School; Director of Medicine, Newark Beth Israel Medical Center, Newark, New Jersey
Polycystic and Sclerocystic Ovaries

PETER O. KOHLER, M.D.

Professor and Chairman, Department of Medicine, University of Arkansas for Medical Sciences, Little Rock, Arkansas
Nonfunctioning Pituitary Tumors

STANLEY G. KORENMAN, M.D.

Professor of Medicine, UCLA School of Medicine; Chairman, Department of Medicine, UCLA-San Fernando Valley Program, Chief, Medical Services, Sepulveda Veterans Administration Medical Center, Los Angeles, California
Principles of Estrogen Therapy

IONE A. KOURIDES, M.D.

Associate Professor of Medicine, Cornell University Medical College; Associate in Medicine, Memorial Sloan-Kettering Cancer Center, New York, New York
Inappropriate TSH Secretion

JOSEPH P. KRISS, M.D.

Professor of Medicine and Radiology, Chief, Division of Nuclear Medicine, Stanford University School of Medicine, Stanford, California
Graves' Ophthalmopathy

HOWARD E. KULIN, M.D.

Associate Professor of Pediatrics, Chief, Division of Pediatric Endocrinology, The Milton S. Hershey Medical Center, Hershey, Pennsylvania
Delayed Puberty in the Male

HAROLD E. LEBOVITZ, M.D.

Professor of Medicine, Department of Medicine, State University of New York, Downstate Medical Center, Brooklyn, New York
Empty Sella

MARK LESHIN, M.D.

Assistant Professor, Department of Internal Medicine, The University of Texas Southwestern Medical School, Dallas, Texas
Androgen Resistance Syndromes

LARRY I. LIPSHULTZ, M.D.

Professor of Urology, Baylor University College of Medicine, Houston, Texas
Varicocele

D. LYNN LORIAUX, M.D., Ph.D.

Chief, Developmental Endocrinology Branch, National Institute of Child Health and Human Development; Senior Investigator, National Institutes of Health, Bethesda, Maryland
Gynecomastia

MARGARET H. MacGILLIVRAY, M.D.

Professor of Pediatrics, State University of New York at Buffalo, School of Medicine; Co-Director, Division of Endocrinology, The Children's Hospital of Buffalo, Buffalo, New York
Short Stature

CHARLES M. MARCH, M.D.

Associate Professor, Chief, Section of Gynecology, Department of Obstetrics and Gynecology, University of Southern California School of Medicine, Los Angeles, California
Hypogonadotropism

GEOFFREY M. MAREL, M.D.

Assistant Physician, Division of Bone and Mineral Metabolism, Henry Ford Hospital, Detroit, Michigan
Osteomalacia

SHAUL G. MASSRY, M.D.

Professor of Medicine, Chief, Division of Nephrology, University of Southern California School of Medicine, Los Angeles, California
Renal Osteodystrophy

PIERRE MAUVAIS-JARVIS, M.D.

Professor of Medicine, Department of Reproductive Endocrinology, Necker Hospital, Paris, France
Hormonal Therapy of Benign Breast Disease

I. ROSS McDOUGALL, M.D.

Associate Professor of Medicine and Radiology, Stanford University School of Medicine, Stanford, California
Graves' Ophthalmopathy

WILLIAM L. McGUIRE, M.D.

Professor of Medicine, Department of Medicine, University of Texas Health Science Center, San Antonio, Texas
Endocrine Therapy of Metastatic Breast Cancer

J. WALLACE McMEEL, M.D.

Clinical Researcher, Eye Research Institute of the Retina Foundation, Boston, Massachusetts
Diabetic Retinopathy

JAMES C. MELBY, M.D.

Director, Evans Memorial Department of Clinical Research, University Hospital; Professor of Medicine, Bos-

ton University School of Medicine, Boston, Massachusetts
Isolated Hypoaldosteronism

GEOFFREY MENDELSOHN, M.D.

Assistant Professor of Pathology, The Johns Hopkins University School of Medicine, Baltimore, Maryland
Medullary Thyroid Carcinoma

CLAUDE J. MIGEON, M.D.

Professor of Pediatrics, The Johns Hopkins University School of Medicine; Director, Pediatric Endocrine Clinic, Johns Hopkins Hospital, Baltimore, Maryland
Congenital Adrenal Hyperplasia

ANTHONY D. MORRISON, M.D.

Associate Professor of Medicine, University of South Florida Medical Center; Director, Endocrinology, J. A. Haley Veterans Administration Medical Center, Tampa, Florida
Hyperosmolar Coma and Lactic Acidosis

RODRIGUE MORTEL, M.D.

Professor of Obstetrics and Gynecology, The Milton S. Hershey Medical Center, Hershey, Pennsylvania
Endocrine Treatment of Endometrial Malignancy

PATRICK J. MULROW, M.D.

Professor and Chairman, Department of Medicine, Medical College of Ohio, Toledo, Ohio
Adrenocortical Insufficiency

FREDERICK NAFTOLIN, M.D., Ph.D.

Professor and Chairman, Department of Obstetrics and Gynecology, Yale University School of Medicine, New Haven, Connecticut
Ovarian Tumors with Endocrine Manifestations

HARRIS M. NAGLER, M.D.

Assistant Professor of Urology, Columbia University College of Physicians & Surgeons; Co-Director, New York Male Reproductive Center, Columbia-Presbyterian Medical Center, New York, New York
Varicocele

WILLIAM A. NAHHAS, M.D.

Associate Professor Obstetrics and Gynecology, The Milton S. Hershey Medical Center, Hershey, Pennsylvania
Endocrine Treatment of Endometrial Malignancy

FRANCIS A. NEELON, M.D.

Associate Professor of Medicine, Department of Medicine, Duke University School of Medicine, Durham, North Carolina
Empty Sella

MARIA I. NEW, M.D.

Professor and Chairman, Department of Pediatrics, The New York Hospital-Cornell University Medical Center, New York, New York
Precocious Puberty

DAVID N. ORTH, M.D.

Professor of Medicine, Division of Endocrinology, Department of Medicine, Vanderbilt University Medical Center, Nashville, Tennessee
Cushing's Syndrome

C. KENT OSBORNE, M.D.

Associate Professor, Department of Medicine, University of Texas Health Science Center, San Antonio, Texas
Endocrine Therapy of Metastatic Breast Cancer

CHARLES Y. C. PAK, M.D.

Professor of Medicine, Department of Internal Medicine, Southwestern Medical School, University of Texas Health Science Center, Dallas, Texas
Urolithiasis

DAVID F. PAULSON, M.D.

Professor and Chairman, Department of Urology, Duke University School of Medicine, Durham, North Carolina
Carcinoma of the Prostate

DEMETRIUS PERTSEMLIDIS, M.D.

Clinical Professor of Surgery, Mt. Sinai School of Medicine, New York, New York
Pheochromocytoma

JOSEPH RANSOHOFF, M.D.

Chairman, Department of Neurosurgery, New York University Medical Center, New York, New York
Surgical Management of Craniopharyngiomas

BASIL RAPOPORT, M.D.

Associate Professor of Medicine, University of California, San Francisco, California
Myxedema Coma

ELLIOT J. RAYFIELD, M.D.

Associate Professor of Medicine, Division of Atherosclerosis and Metabolic Diseases, Mt. Sinai School of Medicine, New York, New York
Diabetic Ketoacidosis

SAMUEL REFETOFF, M.D.

Professor of Medicine, Division of Endocrinology, Department of Medicine, The Pritzker School of Medicine, University of Chicago, Chicago, Illinois
Primary Hypothyroidism

GEORGE RICCABONA, M.D.

Chirurgische Professor of Surgery, Universitats Klinik, Innsbruck, Austria
Endemic Goiter and Cretinism

B. LAWRENCE RIGGS, M.D.

Professor of Medicine, Chairman, Division of Endocrinology and Metabolism, Mayo Medical School, Rochester, Minnesota
Osteoporosis

ALAN G. ROBINSON, M.D.

Professor of Medicine, Chief, Division of Endocrinology and Metabolism, Department of Medicine, University of Pittsburgh School of Medicine, Pittsburgh, Pennsylvania
Hypothalamic Diabetes Insipidus

JESSE ROTH, M.D.

Chief, Diabetes Branch, National Institute of Arthritis, Diabetes, and Digestive and Kidney Diseases, National Institutes of Health, Bethesda, Maryland
Acromegaly

SUBIR ROY, M.D.

Associate Professor, Department of Obstetrics and Gynecology, University of Southern California School of Medicine, Los Angeles, California
Hormonal Contraception: Oral Contraceptives

LESTER B. SALANS, M.D.

Director, National Institute of Arthritis, Diabetes, and Digestive and Kidney Diseases, National Institutes of Health, Bethesda, Maryland
Obesity

DAVID H. SARNE, M.D.

Fellow, Division of Endocrinology, Department of Medicine, The Pritzker School of Medicine, University of Chicago, Chicago, Illinois
Primary Hypothyroidism

ARTHUR E. SCHWARTZ, M.D.

Associate Clinical Professor of Surgery, Mt. Sinai School of Medicine, New York, New York
Well-Differentiated Thyroid Cancer,
Parathyroid Carcinoma

PETER E. SCHWARTZ, M.D.

Associate Professor and Director, Gynecologic Oncology, Department of Obstetrics and Gynecology, Yale University School of Medicine, New Haven, Connecticut
Ovarian Tumors with Endocrine Manifestations

CHARLES F. SHARP, Jr., M.D.

Assistant Professor of Medicine, University of Southern California School of Medicine, Los Angeles, California
Hypoparathyroidism

RICHARD J. SHERINS, M.D.

Senior Investigator, Developmental Endocrinology Branch, National Institute of Child Health and Human Development, National Institutes of Health, Bethesda, Maryland
Hypogonadotropic Hypogonadism in Men

CHARLES R. SHUMAN, M.D.

Professor of Medicine, Temple University School of Medicine, Philadelphia, Pennsylvania
The Adult Diabetic Patient

FREDERICK R. SINGER, M.D.

Professor of Medicine, Section of Endocrinology, University of Southern California School of Medicine, Los Angeles, California
Hypoparathyroidism

ETHEL S. SIRIS, M.D.

Assistant Professor of Medicine, Columbia University College of Physicians & Surgeons, New York, New York
Paget's Disease of Bone

PETER J. SNYDER, M.D.

Associate Professor of Medicine, University of Pennsylvania School of Medicine, Philadelphia, Pennsylvania
FSH-Secreting Pituitary Adonomas

REBECCA Z. SOKOL, M.D.

Assistant Professor of Medicine, Division of Endocrinology, Department of Medicine, Harbor-UCLA Medical Center, UCLA School of Medicine, Torrance, California
Hypogonadism: Androgen Therapy

JOHN B. STANBURY, M.D.

Professor Emeritus, Department of Nutrition, Massachusetts Institute of Technology, Unit of Experimental Medicine, Cambridge, Massachusetts
Endemic Goiter and Cretinism

DAVID H. P. STREETEN, M.D., D.Phil.

Professor of Medicine, Head, Section of Endocrinology, State University of New York, Syracuse, New York
Idiopathic Edema

MARTIN I. SURKS, M.D.

Head, Division of Endocrinology and Metabolism, Montefiore Hospital and Medical Center; Professor of Medicine, Albert Einstein College of Medicine, Bronx, New York
Hyperthyroidism

RONALD S. SWERDLOFF, M.D.

Professor and Chief, Division of Endocrinology, Department of Medicine, Harbor-UCLA Medical Center, UCLA School of Medicine, Torrance, California
Hypogonadism: Androgen Therapy

MICHAEL O. THORNER, M.D.

Associate Professor, Department of Internal Medicine, University of Virginia Medical Center, Charlottesville, Virginia
Prolactinoma

HUGH D. TILDESLEY, M.D.

Instructor in Medicine, Division of Endocrinology, Department of Medicine, University of Alberta, Edmonton, Alberta, Canada
Hyperosmolar Coma and Lactic Acidosis

GEORGE TOLIS, M.Sc., M.D.

Associate Professor of Medicine, Obstetrics and Gynecology; Director, Clinical Investigation in Reproductive Endocrinology, McGill University, Montreal, Quebec, Canada
Galactorrhea

ROBERT D. UTIGER, M.D.

Professor of Medicine, Department of Medicine, University of North Carolina School of Medicine, Chapel Hill, North Carolina
Goitrous Autoimmune Thyroiditis (Hashimoto's Disease)

JOSEPH G. VERBALIS, M.D.

Assistant Professor, Department of Medicine, University of Pittsburgh School of Medicine, Pittsburgh, Pennsylvania
Hypothalamic Diabetes Insipidus

ROBERT A. VIGERSKY, M.D.

Assistant Chief, Kyle Metabolic Unit, Walter Reed Army Medical Center, Washington, District of Columbia; Associate Professor of Medicine, Uniformed Services University of Health Sciences, Bethesda, Maryland
Anorexia Nervosa

SAMUEL A. WELLS, Jr., M.D.

Professor and Chairman, Department of Surgery, Washington University School of Medicine, St. Louis, Missouri
Medullary Thyroid Carcinoma

FRANK C. WHEELOCK, Jr., M.D.

Surgeon, New England Deaconess Hospital; Clinical Assistant Professor of Surgery, Harvard Medical School, Boston, Massachusetts
Diabetic Peripheral Vascular Disease: Ulcer

JEAN D. WILSON, M.D.

Professor of Medicine, Department of Internal Medicine, The University of Texas Southwestern Medical School, Dallas, Texas
Androgen Resistance Syndromes

TERENCE D. WINGERT, M.D.

Assistant Professor of Medicine, Division of Endocrinology and Metabolism, Medical College of Ohio, Toledo, Ohio
Adrenocortical Insufficiency

PREFACE

The advances over the past decade in the understanding of the pathophysiology of endocrine disorders, as well as in the laboratory and roentgen diagnosis of endocrine disease, have been accompanied by an explosive increase in therapeutic approaches to individual disorders. Although there are a number of excellent textbooks of endocrinology, these deal primarily with physiology, pathophysiology, and differential diagnosis. There appears to be a dearth of material regarding specific therapeutic approaches to endocrine disease. These realizations have led to the preparation of this book.

Each chapter deals with an individual disorder or clinical entity. The authors were chosen because of their extensive knowledge of the field. It is assumed that in each instance the reader has made the correct diagnosis, so that the major discussion is devoted to rationales of treatment, preferred therapeutic plans, alternative approaches, and potential side effects. The common dosage forms are given and the end points of treatment are emphasized.

It should be stressed that the therapeutic approaches are those of individual authors. It was our intent that each contributor should give the type of personal opinion that would be provided if called upon as a consultant to see a patient. In this regard, however, the editors and the authors acknowledge that there are honest differences of opinion as to how a given disease might be managed. In a few areas in this volume these differences are evident. In other instances, the preferred drugs must be used under an IND (in the United States); in each such instance an alternative is recommended. It is further acknowledged that many of the modes of therapy will change over the next several years as new drugs are developed and new clinical trials published. It is anticipated that such changes will be incorporated into subsequent editions.

In a recent critique of a standard endocrinology text with regard to therapeutic considerations, Rossini (New Eng J Med 306:1184, 1982) implied that "young physicians" were in need of guidance with regard to endocrine therapy. If it is only the young who need help, then in this context the editors are certainly among that group. One of the great pleasures and benefits of editing this volume has been how much we have learned from the multiple colleagues who have provided the eighty-eight chapters which follow.

Dorothy T. Krieger, M.D., D.Sc.
C. Wayne Bardin, M.D.

June, 1982

CONTENTS

DISEASES OF THE BREAST

HYPOTHALAMIC DISEASE

HYPOTHALAMIC DIABETES INSIPIDUS

JOSEPH G. VERBALIS, M.D.
and ALAN G. ROBINSON, M.D.

GOALS OF THERAPY

Allow the Patient to Maintain a Normal Life Style

Most patients with diabetes insipidus have an intact thirst mechanism, and in most situations are able to drink enough water to maintain a relatively normal state of metabolic balance. Since diabetes insipidus itself does not cause progressive morbidity, nor does it cause secondary complications in other vital systems, in many cases the major manifestation is the inconvenience of thirst and frequent urination. Therapeutic agents should therefore be convenient in terms of the patient's life style and easy for the patient to administer and monitor, as well as effective in the prevention of polyuria and nocturia. The patient should know enough about the mechanism of the therapeutic agent to be able to exercise judgment and flexibility in its use, depending upon activities at any given time. Finally, because of the benign course of the disorder, the safety of any therapy must be an overriding consideration. Even with the use of safe and effective therapy, overtreatment should be avoided, because the side effects from this are often more detrimental than undertreatment.

Control of Potentially Life-threatening Situations

The benign nature of diabetes insipidus is predicated upon the ability of the patient to respond appropriately to an intact thirst center. Any situation in which the patient is either unable to sense thirst or unable to respond by drinking water is potentially life-threatening. After an auto accident, a surgical procedure, or any time that the patient is unconscious, no abnormality may be noted when the person is first seen by a physician because of the persistent effect of therapy. However, as the therapeutic agent reaches the end of its normal effective duration, diabetes insipidus may recur, resulting in the production of large volumes of urine in just a few hours with the potential for severe dehydration and cardiovascular collapse. To avoid this, every patient with diabetes insipidus should carry a medical card indicating that he or she has this disorder and also should wear a Medic-Alert tag. Diabetes insipidus is rare, and in an emergency the patient may be seen by a physician who is not familiar with the disorder, so the Medic-Alert tag and card should indicate that vasopressin may have to be administered and should also contain the name and telephone number of a physician who is familiar with the disorder, has been involved in therapy of the patient, and can be contacted during an emergency.

AGENTS AVAILABLE FOR THERAPY OF DIABETES INSIPIDUS

Water

Water is listed as a treatment to emphasize that water alone taken in sufficient quantity will correct any metabolic abnormality secondary to diabetes insipidus. All of the therapies described below are designed to reduce the necessary amount of water intake to tolerable levels. The tolerable level of water intake will vary from patient to patient and from day to day in any given patient. The physician (and a knowledgeable patient) should not be disturbed that occasional lapses in pharmacologic treatment require temporary increases in water ingestion. In fact, such lapses are at times beneficial to avoid overtreatment and subsequent water intoxication.

Antidiuretic Hormones

L-arginine Vasopressin. L-arginine vasopressin is the natural vasopressin of man and all mammals, with the exception of the pig.

1

Aqueous vasopressin is a buffered solution of L-arginine vasopressin which can be given parenterally. The product may be either purified bovine pituitary vasopressin or synthetic arginine vasopressin. It is provided in 1-ml snap-top vials at a concentration of 20 U/ml. It is usually given subcutaneously and has an onset of action within 1 to 2 hours and duration of effect from 4 to 8 hours. Intravenous bolus administration should be avoided, both because of an even shorter duration of action and because of potential significant pressor effects (hypertension, angina). Pitressin tannate in oil is a relatively crude extract of bovine posterior pituitary containing arginine vasopressin in a suspension of peanut oil. It also comes in snap-top vials at a concentration of 5 U/ml. Because this is a suspension, the active principle will sediment during storage, and sometimes the sediment will be in the hollow snap-top. Prior to administration the vial must be examined to locate this brown pellet and then warmed and vigorously shaken until the pellet is completely suspended. This preparation can be used only as an intramuscular injection. A single dose of 5–10 U will usually provide a 24- to 72-hour duration of effect if administered properly. The delayed absorption is due to the oily suspension.

Lysine Vasopressin. Lysine vasopressin is the naturally occurring vasopressin of the pig and is available commercially as a purified vasopressin in an aqueous buffer of 50 U/ml to be used as a nasal spray. The agent comes in a plastic atomizer bottle and can be sprayed directly into each nostril. Absorption of the vasopressin occurs rapidly across the nasal mucosa. The duration of effect is quite variable, but at most lasts 4 to 6 hours.

1-desamino-D-arginine Vasopressin (dDAVP). dDAVP is a synthetic analogue of L-arginine vasopressin in which the terminal amino group on the cystine has been removed and D-arginine has been substituted for L-arginine in position 8. Removal of the terminal amine prolongs the half-life of the drug in plasma, and substitution of D for L-arginine in position 8 reduces the pressor activity of the molecule. The agent is approximately 2000 times more specific for prolonged antidiuresis than is natural L-arginine vasopressin. dDAVP is available in a buffered aqueous solution containing 100 μg/ml. Fifty to 200 μl can be loaded into a soft plastic tube and administered by blowing into the nose. The onset of action is rapid and the duration of effect may vary from 6 to 24 hours. Despite this large variation among individuals, in a given patient the effect of similarly administered doses is quite reproducible. Although not yet approved in the United States, dDAVP is also available in 2 ml vials of 4 μg/ml for parenteral injection. When administered parenterally, about one-fifth the dose of dDAVP will produce an effect similar to dDAVP administered intranasally.

Orally Administered Pharmacologic Agents

Chlorpropamide. Chlorpropamide was serendipitously discovered to decrease free water excretion in patients with diabetes insipidus. The major action is to enhance the effect of vasopressin to stimulate cyclic AMP in the renal tubule and hence to increase the hydro-osmotic action of vasopressin. Some vasopressin is necessary for chlorpropamide to exert its antidiuretic effect, and the drug is of no use in treatment of diabetes insipidus in the complete absence of vasopressin. Chlorpropamide will cause a reduction of urine volume in patients with partial diabetes insipidus and some ability to secrete vasopressin. The usual dose is 100–500 mg orally per day, and maximum antidiuresis is observed after 4 days of administration of the drug. One must always be cautious of the development of hypoglycemia when treating diabetes insipidus, especially in cases of hypopituitarism in which normal counter-regulatory mechanisms may be absent.

Carbamazepine. This drug has been shown to cause release of antidiuretic hormone in patients with partial diabetes insipidus. As with chlorpropamide, the agent is of no use in patients with complete diabetes insipidus. The dosage used is 200–600 mg per day. Before prescribing this drug the physician should be thoroughly familiar with the potential toxicity, especially involving CNS, hemopoietic, cardiovascular, skin, and hepatic systems.

Clofibrate. This agent has also been shown to stimulate release of endogenous arginine vasopressin. Patients with partial diabetes insipidus may respond to 500 mg every 6 hours with a decreased urinary volume. However, because of the possibility of an increased incidence of gallbladder disease and carcinoma in patients taking clofibrate, the agent cannot be recommended for routine treatment of diabetes insipidus.

Thiazide Diuretics. Thiazides are usually thought of as diuretic rather than antidiuretic agents, but they will decrease urine volumes in patients with both hypothalamic and nephrogenic diabetes insipidus. Since this effect is seen even with complete diabetes insipidus, the mechanism is clearly different from that of the other oral agents and probably is secondary to primary natriuresis with subsequent volume contraction, decreased ultrafiltrate, and increased proximal tubular resorption of salt and water. Hydrochlorthiazide in a dosage of 50–100 mg per day is usually sufficient. Potassium replacement should be given as necessary to prevent hypokalemia.

Indomethacin. Prostaglandin E in the renal medulla is thought to inhibit the action of vasopressin. Indomethacin, which decreases the concentration of medullary prostaglandin E, results in an increased responsiveness of the distal tubule to vasopressin and enhances the effect of administered antidiuretic hormones. While this should not be considered a primary therapy for diabetes insipidus, it is important to be aware of this action for those patients with diabetes insipidus taking the drug for other reasons.

CLINICAL SITUATIONS

Acute Postsurgical Diabetes Insipidus

This occurs frequently following surgery in the hypothalamic pituitary area. Often the patient is receiving high doses of glucocorticoids, which may cause hyperglycemia and glycosuria, thus confusing the initial diagnosis of diabetes insipidus. Once the diagnosis is ascertained the only pharmacologic therapy for this acute condition is an antidiuretic hormone. However, since many neurosurgeons fear water overload and brain edema after this type of surgery, the patient is sometimes treated with intravenous water replacement for a considerable time prior to the use of antidiuretic agents. If the patient is awake and able to respond to thirst, one can treat with an antidiuretic hormone and allow the patient's thirst to be the guide for water replacement. If the patient is not able to respond to thirst, either because of a decreased level of consciousness or because of hypothalamic damage to the thirst center, he may continue to be thirsty even though water has been adequately replaced or may not sense thirst even with severe dehydration. Fluid balance will have to be maintained by intravenous fluid in either case. It is imperative that urine osmolality and serum sodium levels be checked every several hours during the initial therapy and then at least daily until stabilization or resolution of the diabetes insipidus.

The serum sodium level is an excellent guide to adequate replacement with antidiuretic hormone and water. Aqueous vasopressin will most often be the initial mode of therapy, though dDAVP may be used in cases in which it can be administered intranasally. Usually the patient will be hypernatremic when therapy is begun, thus establishing the diagnosis of diabetes insipidus in the face of hypotonic urine. The serum sodium level should be rechecked after the initial doses of vasopressin to be sure that there has been some improvement in the hypernatremia. If not, or if it is insufficient, it may be necessary to increase the water replacement in addition to continuing treatment with vasopressin. Once the serum sodium level has been corrected, input and output can be balanced by intravenous fluid therapy and administration of vasopressin. It is important to be careful with water replacement, because excess water during continued administration of vasopressin can create a syndrome of inappropriate antidiuresis and potentially severe hyponatremia. During the first several days after surgery at least one dose of vasopressin or dDAVP per day should be withheld until polyuria is re-established and the persistence of diabetes insipidus is confirmed.

In some cases of transient postsurgical diabetes insipidus, return of secretion of endogenous vasopressin may occur within hours. If this happens concurrently with continued intravenous replacement of large volumes of fluid, hyponatremia may develop. It can be avoided by withholding the vasopressin or dDAVP therapy each day until reestablishment of polyuria, and by careful monitoring of serum sodium levels. One must also recognize that secretion of endogenous vasopressin in the case of trauma to the posterior pituitary or stalk may not be under normal physiologic control. Rather, a "triphasic" resonse may occur, as seen with sectioning of the pituitary stalk. In this case, the secretion of vasopressin may not be suppressed by a water load, and water may have to be restricted in a patient who was encouraged to drink large volumes of water over the preceding days. Within the next several days diabetes insipidus may recur if the secretion of stored vasopressin in the axon terminals is depleted and normal recovery of the vasopressin neurons in the hypothalamus has not occurred. At this time complete or partial diabetes insipidus may occur, the third and final stage of the triphasic response.

In some situations it may be more appropriate to administer a dose of Pitressin tannate in oil. This will allow for a relatively steady control of polyuria for 24 to 48 hours in most patients, and if the thirst mechanism is intact and water intake is not excessive, there is little danger of water intoxication and hyponatremia. Further therapy need not be given until the dose has worn off and the persistence of diabetes insipidus has been demonstrated. This therapy may be especially valuable in patients who have had trans-sphenoidal hypophysectomy and in whom intranasal administration of dDAVP cannot be undertaken until the nasal packing is removed. In these cases Pitressin tannate in oil can provide stable control of diabetes insipidus over the few days prior to administration of dDAVP intranasally. It is also useful when the diabetes insipidus is severe and responds poorly to subcutaneous aqueous vasopressin because of this agent's short duration of effect.

While not yet available in this country, parenteral dDAVP is as efficacious as the intranasal preparation. Postoperatively this agent may be given in a dose of 4 μg subcutaneously or intramuscularly. Prompt reduction in urine output should occur, as described above under treatment with aqueous vasopressin. The same guidelines as for parenteral aqueous vasopressin should be followed for administration of subsequent doses of parenteral dDAVP. This agent will eventually be approved for administration in the United States, and when available it will become the primary form of therapy for the acute treatment of postsurgical diabetes insipidus.

Acute Traumatic Diabetes Insipidus

This can occur after an injury to the head, usually in an automobile accident. Diabetes insipidus is more common with injuries to the lateral skull which result in a shearing action on the pituitary stalk, cause hemorrhagic ischemia of the hypothalamus and posterior pituitary, or both. As in postsurgical diabetes insipidus, the condition is diagnosed by the presence of hypotonic polyuria in the face of an increased serum osmolality. Management is similar to that for postsurgical diabetes insipidus as outlined above, with the exception that the possibility of anterior pituitary insufficiency must be considered and the patient given stress doses of hydrocortisone until anterior pituitary function can be definitively evaluated.

Chronic Complete Diabetes Insipidus

Complete diabetes insipidus describes cases in which there is no vasopressin in the circulation and no ability to concentrate urine with a standard dehydration test. All of these patients will require replacement with some form of antidiuretic hormone. The treatment of choice is dDAVP. First, the patient must be taught to use the rhinyl catheter and to measure an appropriate dose of dDAVP. A solution of saline can be utilized to fill the tubing for practice. Once an appropriately measured dose is in the catheter, it can be held in a U-shape with both ends in a superior position, allowing the measured dose of hormone to drop to the dependent loop of the tube. The catheter is then raised to the mouth and about half an inch inserted into the nostril, being careful to maintain the other end above the nadir of the U. The patient than takes a moderate inspiration and holds his breath while placing the other end of the catheter in his mouth. Blowing through the catheter with a swift puff, as one might imagine doing to blow a ball out of a straw, will deliver hormone high into the nose. Either the physician or an assistant must be trained in the proper use of the rhinyl catheter to assist in teaching the patient. A patient who is not properly trained can waste some of the hormone by letting it drip out the end of the catheter, swallowing it, or blowing it into the external nares in a position too low to allow absorption.

In initiating treatment it is useful to have the patient test 50, 100, and 200 μl of the drug. This is best done in a controlled environment where each voided urine specimen can be measured for volume and osmolality. The next most desirable situation would be to measure volume and specific gravity, or, as a last resort, volume alone. In fact, measurement of urinary volume can provide a good index of duration of drug action. A baseline polyuria is established after all traces of previous medication disappear from the patient's system. This is not difficult in patients with complete diabetes insipidus. Once polyuria of about 4 ml/min is established, 50 μl of dDAVP are administered. A prompt decrease in urinary volume occurs 1 to 2 hours later. The effect of the dose will last 6 to 24 hours, usually around 12 hours. Establishing this duration of action in individual patients is helpful in planning therapy and in assuring the patient and the physician that early administration of a second dose of drug (which may be necessary as described below) will not lead to any adverse effect.

Having tested three doses of drug on the patient, the physician must decide the dosage and time of day to administer the drug. Individualization of this protocol cannot be overemphasized. Occasional patients will maintain satisfactory control of urinary output with a single dose per day, but most patients will require two doses per day. Two small doses per day (for example, 50 μl) will usually be more cost-effective than one large dose (for example, 200 μl). As the biologic half-life of dDAVP is about 4 hours, doubling the dose will extend the duration only by that amount of time. Many suggest that, when a single dose of drug per day is used, it be given at bedtime to allow the patient to sleep throughout the night. We find that many patients would rather have the drug administered in the morning to allow a full day of work or other activities without interruption for frequent voiding. A single episode of nocturia may be preferable to multiple interruptions during the work day. When two doses of dDAVP are necessary the time of administration should again be based upon the activity of that patient for that day. The first dose should almost always be given early in the morning to allow an uninterrupted work day. Timing of the second dose should be individualized. If the patient is home for the evening it is usually best to delay the administration of the second dose until late in the evening to allow a full night's sleep. If the patient is going out for the evening and knows from experience that polyuria will occur prior to returning home, it is best to administer the second dose of medication in the late afternoon or early evening. If this dose is not sufficient to allow an adequate night's sleep, a third dose of medication may be taken on that particular day just prior to bedtime. Three 50 μl doses taken in this manner will be readily accepted by a patient who has already tolerated 200 μl as a single dose during the initiation of therapy.

The obvious danger of a flexible program is the possibility that the patient will take repeated doses of dDAVP to maintain urine volume at a low output and will then become volume expanded, natriuretic, and hyponatremic. To avoid this complication, at least once and preferably two to three times a week, the patient should withhold dDAVP until pronounced polyuria recurs with excessive thirst. This guards against hyponatremia from overzealous use of dDAVP and provides ongoing documentation that diabetes insipidus persists. The latter is especially useful in cases of postsurgical or post-traumatic diabetes insipidus, in which renewed ability to secrete vasopressin may occur within the first several years after the initial insult.

Treatment with Pitressin tannate in oil provided satisfactory therapy for many years, but intramuscular injections are so distasteful to most patients that therapy with this agent is no longer recommended.

The only disadvantage of dDAVP is expense. Becuase of this some physicians prescribe a combination of an oral agent with dDAVP to prolong the action of dDAVP, thus decreasing the expense. Both chlorpropamide and indomethacin will prolong the effect of an administered dose of dDAVP. However, it is our feeling that potential complications from drugs that are not otherwise indicated make this attempt to decrease the cost of therapy undesirable. It is important to recognize that when any of the drugs described in the section on orally administered pharmacologic agents are given for routine medical indications, they may augment the effect of dDAVP and predispose the patient to water retention and hyponatremia. Thus the dose of dDAVP may have to be altered if one of these agents is utilized for treatment of another disease.

Partial Diabetes Insipidus

"Partial" diabetes insipidus refers to the condition of patients who have some endogenous secretion of vasopressin but not in sufficient amounts to achieve maximum urinary concentration or remain free of polyuria and thirst. Most patients will not become hypernatremic but will complain of excessive thirst and polyuria. Probably the safest form of therapy for these patients is dDAVP. The guidelines for initiating and maintaining therapy in partial diabetes insipidus are essentially identical to those described above for the treatment of complete diabetes insipidus, with the exception that these patients often tolerate a somewhat less frequent administration of the drug because the polyuria and the thirst are not so severe.

In some of these patients administration of pharmacologic agents may be indicated (see the section orally administered pharmacologic agents). In an occasional patient who suffers from both diabetes insipidus and either diabetes mellitus or congestive heart failure, it may be appropriate to treat both diseases with a single agent—chlorpropamide for the former and thiazide diuretics for the latter. The agent is prescribed as necessary to treat the primary disease, for example, diabetes mellitus or congestive heart failure, and the effect upon the diabetes insipidus is observed. The need for further therapy with an antidiuretic hormone will depend upon the response to these agents.

If a patient with partial diabetes insipidus is unable to utilize dDAVP because of poor vision or for economic reasons, chlorpropamide may be an acceptable alternative. Therapy can be initiated with 100 mg per day and increased every 4 days until appropriate antidiuresis is obtained. Usually little additional antidiuresis is obtained with dosages above 500 mg per day. When beginning treatment with an oral agent, the appropriate index of therapeutic effectiveness is the 24-hour urine volume and the patient's symptomatic response in terms of thirst. In patients with coexistent panhypopituitarism and lack of ACTH and growth hormone, the increased potential for hypoglycemia during treatment with chlorpropamide must be recognized, and frequent feedings given and routine blood sugar measurements obtained. In mild cases of partial diabetes insipidus a trial of thiazide diuretics may be undertaken. Some patients will have sufficient reduction of urine output and decrease of thirst on this agent alone to be satisfactorily controlled.

We do not use clofibrate, carbamazepine, or indomethacin for the treatment of partial diabetes insipidus. In our opinion the side effects of each of these agents are too great to justify the use to treat a disease for which other acceptable forms of therapy are available. Furthermore, patients with partial diabetes insipidus who will respond to treatment with any oral agents will respond to either chlorpropamide or thiazides.

Diabetes Insipidus in Pregnancy

A number of cases of adult onset diabetes insipidus have begun during pregnancy and have been reported because the diabetes insipidus has generally not interfered with the progress of parturition and lactation. The agent of choice to treat diabetes insipidus in pregnancy is again dDAVP. This agent has 4 to 75 times less oxytocic activity than does arginine vasopressin or lysine vasopressin, so that one is able to obtain potent antidiuresis with minimal uterotonic action.

When diabetes insipidus occurs in pregnancy it may be especially severe because increased serum oxytocinase activity tends to decrease the effectiveness of endogenously secreted vasopressin. Similarly, in patients with diabetes insipidus who become pregnant, the dose of dDAVP may have to be increased during the pregnancy because of oxytocinase. In women whose diabetes insipidus begins during pregnancy the same protocol for initiation of therapy as in complete diabetes insipidus can be undertaken. Many of these patients may require administration of dDAVP three times

a day. At parturition the patient will usually be alert enough to take intermittent doses of dDAVP intranasally. The only caution is that excessive amounts of fluids should not be administered, as this may cause water intoxication and hyponatremia. After parturition the dosage of dDAVP often has to be adjusted downward because of decreased serum oxytocinase activity.

It should be noted that dDAVP does not have specific approval for use in pregnancy but would logically be the most appropriate agent if some therapy must be given. Any of the oral agents described above are potentially teratogenic. Lysine vasopressin results in unacceptable levels of control in most normal subjects and this is magnified in pregnant women. Arginine vasopressin has the potential for inducing uterine cramps and must be given by injection. Since dDAVP is the closest to a natural hormone, has no known teratogenic effects, and will provide adequate control of antidiuresis, it is the best drug to prescribe.

Diabetes Insipidus with Inadequate Thirst

This constitutes the most difficult management problem of patients with diabetes insipidus. Some patients may secrete some vasopressin under certain circumstances but do not respond normally with either thirst or secretion of vasopressin in response to increases of serum osmolality within the normal physiologic range. These cases represent a variant of partial diabetes insipidus, and they have the potential to respond to oral agents. A trial of chlorpropamide, up to 500 mg per day, is indicated because in some cases it will not only decrease the urine volume but increase the recognition of thirst. If chlorpropamide is not effective, dDAVP is the drug of choice.

To determine the duration of action of dDAVP it may be necessary to give a water load either orally or intravenously to bring the sodium into the normal range and to assure a good urine output. dDAVP can then be administered as described in the section on chronic complete diabetes insipidus, with the difference that voided urine is matched volume for volume by administered fluid until the antidiuresis is terminated. At this point a second dose of dDAVP is administered. Once the duration of effect of dDAVP is established, the patient must be put on a rigid regimen of dDAVP and water intake. It is usually necessary to measure volumes of fluid to be administered over a given length of time each day. Even with this careful monitoring of dDAVP and water, regular measurement of serum sodium levels is necessary, because these patients are prone to develop water intoxication with hyponatremia or, alternatively, recurrent dehydration with hypernatremia.

Influence of Diabetes Insipidus on Other Therapeutic Decisions

Routine Surgical Procedures in Patients with Diabetes Insipidus. It is necessary for the physician caring for the patient with diabetes insipidus to contact the surgeon and the anesthesiologist to discuss specific management during surgery. For most surgical procedures, dDAVP intranasally the morning of surgery and then careful administration of intravenous fluids during surgery will adequately control fluid balance. During long procedures serum sodium levels should be checked, and in all cases they should be checked at the end of surgery. If the patient is unable to administer dDAVP before or after the surgical procedure, the next choice of therapy (when approved in this country) would be parenteral dDAVP. Otherwise, one of the treatment regimens with injectable vasopressin can be used.

Diabetes Insipidus with Panhypopituitarism. Because its etiologic agent is frequently a sellar or suprasellar tumor, diabetes insipidus is commonly accompanied by panhypopituitarism. In these cases either hypoadrenalism or hypothyroidism causes an inability to excrete a water load. In a patient with diabetes insipidus there may be no polyuria when hypoadrenalism and/or hypothyroidism is present, and the diagnosis of diabetes insipidus may not be suspected during initial evaluation. As the patient is treated with thyroid and (more dramatically) with hydrocortisone, there will be a prompt increase in urine output and obvious manifestations of diabetes insipidus. At this time the patient requires evaluation as to the presence of either complete or partial diabetes insipidus and initiation of therapy as outlined above.

Maintenance therapy for patients with diabetes insipidus, hypoadrenalism, and hypothyroidism must be continued. Patients who continue treatment for diabetes insipidus but interrupt the treatment of adrenal or thyroid deficiency are extremely prone to water intoxication and hyponatremia.

Craniopharyngioma. In patients with craniopharyngioma or other suprasellar lesions treated by transfrontal cranial surgery, there is great danger of damaging the neurohypophyseal system and causing permanent diabetes insipidus (see Chapter 7). This is an almost invariable outcome of attempts at radical complete removal of a craniopharyngioma. The possibility of a patient developing lifelong diabetes insipidus should spur us on to develop safer modes of therapy for craniopharyngioma, such as stereotaxic implantation of radioisotopes into cystic lesions.

Granulomatous Diseases. Diabetes insipidus in these cases may be partial or complete and may require specific therapy as described above. In some cases there has been remission of the diabetes insipidus with appropriate therapy for the underlying condition, but this is so rare that attempts to tailor therapy for the granulomatous disease specifically to try to cure diabetes insipidus—for example, by radiotherapy to the hypothalamic area—are probably not indicated.

Diabetes Insipidus in Patients with Cardiovascular Disease. A few patients with coronary vascular disease may experience angina pectoris after LVP or injected AVP. This problem has been eliminated by dDAVP because of the markedly reduced pressor activity in the dosage used to produce antidiuresis.

Information for this chapter was based on research supported by NIH AM 16166 and CRC NIH Grant RR-0056.

PRECOCIOUS PUBERTY

MARIA I. NEW, M.D.

Sexual precocity has fascinated physicians for centuries. There is a 1658 report by Mandeslo (quoted by Lenz, 1913) of a girl whose menarche occurred at 3 years of age and who gave birth to a son at 6 years of age. Another famous case is that described by Escomel of a precocious child, Lina Medina, who at 5 years of age gave birth to a son by cesarean section. The case best described among the older case reports is that of Anna Mummenthaler, described by Haller in 1751 (quoted by Ahlfeld, 1898). Anna Mummenthaler first menstruated at age 2, has a stillborn infant at age 9, menopause at age 52, and died at age 75. This early description answers a common question posed by parents of sexually precocious children: "Does early sexual development mean early menopause?" The answer is, it does not.

Although children with sexual precocity rarely demonstrate precocious sexual behavior, there are dubious old reports of sexually precocious boys who may have fathered children. Stone in 1852 cites a patient seen by Craterus who was "infant, youth, adult, father, old man, and corpse in seven years." The only other report is that recorded by Klause (quoted by Nobecourt and Babonneix, 1936), in which the boy was a father at 9 years of age. No details are given.

These old reports emphasize an attitude that views sexually precocious children as interesting experiments of nature, and point out the risk these children suffer as a result of misinformed adults. This risk is not diminished today.

The onset of puberty in most normal children is usually after age 8 years in girls and after age 9 years in boys. The first sign of puberty in girls in most instances in the appearance of breast "buds" and, in some cases, pubic or labial hair. In boys, testicular enlargement and changes in scrotal skin texture are the first signs of puberty, and pubic hair growth follows these changes.

Sexual precocity is the condition in which the onset of signs of puberty occurs at an earlier stage than expected from the genetic and environmental background of the child. As a useful guide, sexual development before age 8 years in girls and age 9 years in boys is generally regarded as precocious.

The conditions of precocious thelarche and precocious adrenarche must be distinguished from true precocious puberty.

PRECOCIOUS THELARCHE

Precocious, or premature, thelarche refers to isolated bilateral (or rarely, unilateral) breast tissue development in girls without any other signs of puberty and without progress in the size of the breast until pubertal age. Numerous cases have been reported indicating that girls with precocious thelarche are normal with respect to further sexual and statural development. No treatment is indicated; however, continued follow-up of girls with precocious thelarche, with monitoring of other pubertal events and linear and skeletal growth (every six months), is advised to confirm the diagnosis of precocious thelarche, since it may be the first sign of true puberty. Breast biopsy is not indicated.

PRECOCIOUS ADRENARCHE

Precocious adrenarche has been defined as the development of sexual hair growth (labial and/or pubic, with or without axillary hair) without any other signs of puberty or other signs of excess androgenization in girls under age 8 and in boys under age 9. In these cases adrenarche is usually either nonprogressive or slowly progressive. Thus precocious adrenarche is considered to be a benign condition of isolated premature sexual hair growth.

In children with precocious adrenarche normal sexual development and growth ultimately occur, and thus no treatment is indicated. However, in these cases it is best to continue to evaluate growth, development of secondary sex characteristics, and hormonal maturation by measurement of androgens until the patient has experienced the normal events of puberty. Unlike precocious thelarche, precocious adrenarche is frequently accompanied by central nervous system disorders, such as mental retardation, abnormal EEG, epilepsy, and spastic palsy. These associated abnormalities must be managed with conventional therapy for the specific condition.

TRUE SEXUAL PRECOCITY

True sexual precocity is defined as early sexual development as a result of early maturation of the hypothalamic-pituitary-gonadal axis. This may occur as an abnormality at the time of the onset of puberty without demonstrable organic pathology, or it may result from a cerebral lesion that stimulates LHRH secretion or prevents normal inhibitory influences on LH/LHRH secretion. Pathologic causes of true (gonadotropin mediated) sexual precocity include the following:

1. Oncongenic, for example, tumors near the posterior region of the hypothalamus, such as pinealomas

2. Following infection, for example, following meningitis

3. Neurofibromatosis, McCune-Albright syndrome (polyostotic fibrous dysplasia). (Recently, however, this latter syndrome has been attributed to ovarian causes.)

4. Congenital abnormalities of the hypothalamus, for example, hamartomas

5. Endocrinopathies: (a) hypothyroidism; (b) congenital adrenal hyperplasia in which treatment is begun after bone age is advanced.

When no organic lesion can be established in the etiology of sexual precocity, it is referred to as cryptogenic or idiopathic, sexual precocity, which is the commonest form of true sexual precocity. In this form fertility may be present in childhood.

Sexual precocity with stimulation of the gonads from a gonadotropin producing tumor, for example, chorionepithelioma, hepatoma, and teratoma, may be difficult to distinguish from LHRH mediated true precocious puberty. Specific tests for the stimulating hormone (either LH or HCG) and its regulation may help in the differential diagnosis and localization of the lesion.

True sexual precocity, in which either LH or LHRH is secreted precociously, must be differentiated from precocious pseudopuberty, in which steroidal sex hormones are secreted in excess by the gonad or adrenal, or are administered from exogenous sources. The latter condition is treated either by removal of the source of the hormone, as in drug ingestion or tumor, or by suppression of the excessive sex hormone secretion, as in males with untreated congenital adrenal hyperplasia due to 21-hydroxylase deficiency or to 11β-hydroxylase deficiency (see Chapter 31). In girls, ovarian follicular cysts are a common cause of rapid onset of breast development and menstrual bleeding. Ovarian cysts are treated by watchful waiting to see if the cyst resolves, or by surgical removal of the cyst.

TREATMENT OF CRYPTOGENIC TRUE SEXUAL PRECOCITY

Since this is the commonest cause of sexual precocity, the goals of the treatment should be clearly established. These are:

1. to arrest further sexual maturation until the normal pubertal age;

2. to reverse the secondary sexual characteristics already present;

3. to achieve normal final height by preventing accelerated epiphyseal maturation;

4. to preserve fertility in adulthood (and prevent pregnancy in childhood); and

5. to prevent emotional disturbances resulting from sexual precocity.

Medical and Surgical Management

In discussing modes of treatment, it is regrettable that the words of Morse (1897) still apply: "The medical treatment of this condition is absolute abstinence of therapeutic measures. The psychological treatment, however, is important."

Most drugs have proven ineffective in achieving all the above goals. Only treatment with LHRH analogues, still in the experimental stage, may provide the outcome desired. Preliminary reports of LHRH analogues in the treatment of sexual precocity are promising, but sufficient time has not elapsed to evaluate ultimate fertility and stature.

Drugs that have been approved for treatment in the United States are medroxyprogesterone acetate and danazol. Both drugs act as progestational agents to suppress gonadotropin secretion. Both are generally effective in suppressing menstruation; however, neither drug reverses secondary sexual characteristics or stops the acceleration of skeletal maturation. The complication of short stature in the untreated patient is not prevented by treatment with medroxyprogesterone acetate or danazol. Further, medroxyprogesterone acetate produces undesirable cushingoid features. Thus we do not recommend either drug for the treatment of sexual precocity unless menstruation per se is causing such psychologic damage as to outweigh the risk of the drug. In these cases, we administer medroxyprogesterone acetate orally in doses of 5–15 mg per day. If this fails, intramuscular administration is tried in doses of 100–200 mg once monthly. The dosage must be individualized. The presence of cushingoid features must be monitored and the lowest dosage possible to prevent menstruation should be aimed for. A complication derived largely from animal data is the potential for development of mammary tumors. Chromosomal abnormalities noted during meiosis in testicular biopsies have been observed.

Cyproterone acetate has been used in Europe. Though it acts to suppress gonadotropins and to block androgen action at the target cell, it has not proved effective in preventing acceleration of skeletal maturation.

Analogues of LHRH which surpass the native molecule in potency and duration of effect have been synthesized. Although there is an initial stimulation of LH secretion, chronic administration of these LHRH analogues leads to refractoriness of the pituitary LH secreting cell to LHRH stimulation. Thus chronic administration of the LHRH analogues results in decreased LH secretion. This decreased LH secretion has been utilized as a therapeutic tool for treatment of idiopathic precocious puberty by investigators granted permission to use the LHRH analogues experimentally. One of the treatment protocols utilizes a dose of 100 μg sub. cu. of long-acting LHRH agonist (D-Trp^6-Pro^9-NEt-LHRH) on the first day and 4 μg/kg daily thereafter for 8 weeks. In a 2-year-old girl with sexual precocity, the LH and FSH levels, as well as the pulsatile discharge of the gonadotropins, was suppressed during treatment with the analogue for 8 weeks. Following discontinuation of therapy for two months, the gonadotropin returned to pretreatment levels and the pulsatile battery of secretion was restored. The treatment period was associated with decreased estradiol levels and decreased estrogenization of the vaginal mucosa. Both these parameters returned to the pretreatment condition following a two-month period during which therapy with the LHRH analogue was halted. Although this treatment is promising in that it suppresses LH secretion without apparent side effects, it is too early to know if this experimental treatment will fulfill all the goals of therapy outlined above.

TREATMENT OF TRUE SEXUAL PRECOCITY DUE TO ORGANIC CAUSES

When precocious puberty results from an organic lesion, removal of the cause should be accomplished whenever possible. HCG producing tumors may be treated with radiation or chemotherapy. Neurosurgical procedures for brain tumors carry high risks because the lesions producing sexual precocity occur near vital centers. Therefore only highly experienced neurosurgeons and radiotherapists should attempt treatment of central nervous system lesions causing sexual precocity.

If the sexual precocity is associated with hypothyroidism, thyroid treatment with L-thyroxine is indicated. In congenital adrenal hyperplasia, if the treatment begins when the bone age is advanced well beyond the chronologic age, hypothalamic-pituitary-gonadal maturation may ensue at an early chronologic age. In this case, the sexual pseudoprecocity becomes true sexual precocity. The treatment is then the same as for true sexual precocity.

PSYCHOLOGIC MANAGEMENT

Psychologic counseling is the keystone of treatment for sexual precocity. With regard to psychologic consequences, the etiologic agent of the sexual precocity is not as important as the increased emotional burden the sexual precocity places on the child. Thus attention must be given to the psychologic factors in all children with sexual precocity, whatever its cause.

Precocious Puberty in Girls

The girl with sexual precocity must deal with several factors. The most important are increased physical size and appearance of the secondary sexual characteristics. Adults will tend to relate to her based more on her physique than her chronologic age and will tend to make more demands upon her as well as delegate greater responsibilities. The child will also have to cope with the fact that although she is a tall child, she will be a short adult.

School acceleration may be an effective means of treatment, provided mental function and IQ permit this. Advancing to the next grade will decrease the disparity in size and physical development between the child and her classmates. The method has been tried with success. Precocious girls were able to hold their own with children one to two years older and were able to catch up socially and academically.

School acceleration helps prevent or at least ameliorates the difficulty of being different from one's peers. Further, since precocious children chose playmates among older children similar in physical size and appearance, school placement with an older group helps to develop psychosocial behavior that is more appropriate to the physical and biologic age.

Parents must be assured that the sexually precocious girl will have normal gender role behavior and normal sexual and maternal behavior. Fears about early sexual interest, excessive masturbation, and unusually frequent premarital intercourse must be allayed. These activities in sexually precocious girls remain related to chronologic, not biologic, age.

The girl with sexual precocity may become a victim of sexual abuse, and physicians should be alert for this problem. Further, since pregnancy, though rare, is possible in cases of true sexual precocity, the sexually precocious girl may not only suffer sexual abuse but also become pregnant.

Finally, sex education for the sexually precocious child and her family is imperative. Parents need to be advised on how to explain breast development and menstruation. Frank and explicit communication with the child is essential because the sexually precocious girl is deprived of this means of education through the usual peer exchange, since her prepubertal peers are usually not themselves interested or informed on sexual development. Should parents feel unable to give this counseling, the pediatrician or a psychiatrist should consider this as an important therapeutic responsibility. Should these counseling and educational measures fail, more intense psychotherapy is indicated.

Precocious Puberty in Boys

Precocious puberty in boys is associated with the same problems as in girls, except that parental fear that sexual behavior may become a problem at an early age is even greater for boys than it is for girls. This fear is unwarranted. Although erotic fantasies and masturbation may occur earlier than usual, overt sexual behavior is typically not in advance of the chronologic age. Boys will have more trouble than girls in bathrooms and locker rooms and may be teased because of the size of the penis or presence of sexual hair. The boy does not consider his large build and sexual precocity as an asset in childhood, and the ultimate short stature of adulthood caused by early epiphyseal fusion is seen as a detriment. More than girls, boys will require a radical reorientation of ambitions and expectations and revision of idealized body image in adolescence when classmates accelerate in growth and they do not.

The therapeutic plan to manage the disparity between chronologic and physical age, according to John Money, is to attempt to accelerate social age and "thus close the gap between social age and physical age, leaving only chronologic age discrepant." If IQ and school achievement permit, the boy should be advanced in grade. Lapses in the behavior, in which the child acts his chronologic age, are to be expected. However, the advantages of school acceleration far outweigh the disadvantages. The physician must explain to the boy the effect that the difference in chronologic, social, and physical age will have on adults and other children, so that he understands it. Teaching the child "wisecracks" and "quips" as responses to teasing is often helpful.

The sexually precocious boy is more boisterous and overactive. In the preteen years, age-mates are less competent in sports while physique-mates are more advanced socially and in physical coordination. Aggression is not a problem, but physical strength compared to peers may be interpreted as aggression.

Sexually precocious boys are not exhibitionistic or voyeuristic. Sexual play is normal, but in the context of precocious sexual development it becomes an item of concern for parents. Parents and physicians should counsel the boy to be more private in his sexual play, and this usually solves the problem.

In careful studies of precocious boys, advanced psychosexual development was not the automatic byproduct of precocious hormonal secretion. Only erotic imagery and masturbation were more frequent, a result of early androgen secretion. To quote Jonn Money: "metaphorically, the erotic flame burned higher, when androgen fuelled it, but the content of erotic imagery and the type of sexual practice remained qualitatively anchored to a boy's chronologic and/or social age."

Straightforward sexual education from an early age is necessary and more important in the sexually precocious boy than in the normal boy to ensure that moral standards and restraints are taught by parents rather than by classmates who are not well informed. Sexually precocious children are capable of learning restraints in presenting their bodies and in sexual conduct.

In summary, sexually precocious children can be managed according to the following guidelines:

Parents and teachers should be advised to be tolerant of increased physical energy and strength. Provide time and space for energy expenditure.

Educate children factually about their condition. This will prevent them from thinking of themselves as freaks and will increase confidence and self-esteem.

Early sex education is important for behavioral restraint, and for encouragement of privacy in sexual activities.

Accelerate children in school by one or two years so that they are associating with children closer to their physical size if cognitive development permits.

Intensive psychotherapy is necessary for children who are withdrawn, hostile, or otherwise disturbed, if simple measures are ineffective.

Parents, friends, and teachers must be constantly reminded that expectations from the child must be related to age and not to the child's size and physical development.

ANOREXIA NERVOSA

ROBERT A. VIGERSKY, M.D.

Anorexia nervosa (AN) has become a widespread disorder that has been estimated to affect 1 percent of teenage women in both Europe and the United States. Young men represent only about 10 percent of all cases. Because of the large number of affected individuals and the protean manifestations of this disorder, many physicians may have primary care or consultative encounters or both with AN patients. The principles of treatment are described in this chapter, but the foundations for treatment are based on the ability to make the proper diagnosis. Several research groups have used strict criteria to exclude patients with "nonclassic" AN. The advantage of using such strict criteria is that patients with underlying organic or other psychiatric disorders will be discovered and offered the appropriate treatment. On the other hand, the use of such rigid criteria does not allow the inclusion of patients with more mild disease or atypical cases. Criteria for diagnosis of AN which

Note: the opinions or assertions contained herein are the private views of the author and are not to be construed as official or reflecting the views of the Department of the Army or the Department of Defense.

allow for the inclusion of a wider range of patients are listed in Table 1. Adherence to these diagnostic criteria should prevent multiple referrals for evaluation of isolated aspects of the disorder and promote earlier treatment.

Treatment of AN should be a multidisciplinary endeavor. The effort should be led by a psychiatrist who has experience with such patients and who enlists the aid of an internist, pediatrician, or endocrinologist to assist with the nonpsychiatric manifestations of the disorder. Since AN may have protean symptoms, knowledge of what to anticipate and the use of appropriate consultation may not only assist in the recovery of the patient but, more importantly, may prevent unnecessary morbidity and mortality. While the published mortality rate of up to 10 percent may be an overestimation now that there are more mild cases and the syndrome is recognized earlier, AN is still a potentially lethal disease if not diagnosed early and treated vigorously. From the medical consultant's viewpoint, AN, while at the present time it must be considered a psychiatric disease, encompasses numerous problems associated with inanition of any origin as well as some features unique to AN.

ENDOCRINE TREATMENT

While numerous abnormalities of the endocrine system have been demonstrated, most are corrected with weight gain and require no specific therapy. The well-informed physician will recognize these abnormalities as secondary to the weight

TABLE 1 Diagnostic Criteria for Anorexia Nervosa

Standard Criteria	Modifying Features
Age of onset before 25	Patients may present at a later age but have had earlier eating behavior abnormalities that had remitted.
Weight loss of at least 25 percent of original body weight	Patients' weight may fluctuate widely, particularly in a bulimic phase. Weight may be close to "ideal body weight" at the time of first visit.
A distorted, implacable attitude toward eating food, or weight that overrides hunger, admonitions, reassurances, and threats	This feature may be vigorously denied by the patient and may require evidence from family or friends.
No known medical illness that could account for the weight loss	Patients may have numerous and real symptoms. However, all are correctable with weight gain. The syndrome is rare in patients from low socioeconomic groups.
No other known psychiatric disorder	Patients may be depressed and even suicidal. This does not exclude them from the diagnosis.
At least two of the following: amenorrhea, lanugo hair, bradycardia, periods of overactivity, episodes of bulimia, vomiting (usually self-induced)	Some patients may have only one of the standard criteria features. Additional features should be: (1) diuretic and/or laxative abuse, (2) hypothermia, (3) hypercarotenemia. Amenorrhea may be primary or secondary. Exercise may often be excessive and surreptitious.

loss per se and not be tempted to intervene unnecessarily. However, documentation of these abnormalities may be helpful in following improvement and in educating the patient as to the medical seriousness of the weight loss.

Thyroid

Patients with AN have many clinical features of hypothyroidism, including bradycardia, dry skin, constipation, and hypothermia. In fact, one of the more common complaints of patients with AN is that of feeling cold all the time. Routine thyroid function tests may be misleading. Low or low normal serum thyroxine (T_4) levels are not uncommon. Resin T_3 uptake (RT_3U) may be at the upper end of the normal range or frankly high. However, direct measurement of "free" T_4 by dialysis or calculation of the "free" thyroxine index ($T_4 \times RT_3U$) are generally normal. AN patients do have profoundly low serum triiodothyronine (T_3) levels, which are directly correlated to the severity of weight loss and result from altered peripheral deiodination of T_4. This constellation of laboratory studies is similar to the low T_3 levels seen in numerous other chronic illnesses, making AN an example of the "euthyroid sick syndrome." Patients with AN have a normal response of thyroid stimulating hormone (TSH) to thyrotropin releasing hormone (TRH). Since there is no way of determining the cellular thyroid status of peripheral tissues, it remains unclear whether or not AN patients have "peripheral hypothyroidism." Therefore, treatment with thyroid hormone replacement is *not* indicated at the present time. Rarely, a patient with AN will have true primary or secondary hypothyroidism, in which case treatment does not differ from that in a patient without AN.

Pituitary-Gonadal Axis

Women with AN are profoundly hypoestrogenic. The origin of the hypogonadism is hypogonadotropism, which is in turn a result of the failure of the hypothalamus to produce normal amounts of gonadotropin releasing hormone (GNRH) to stimulate the pituitary gonadotrophs. Several studies have demonstrated that the administration of GNRH acutely and chronically produces normal serum LH and FSH responses. Indeed, ovulation and pregnancies have been achieved with the chronic administration of GNRH. In addition, the administration of human menopausal gonadotropin with human chorionic gonadotropin will induce ovulation in patients with AN, suggesting normal ovarian function under the appropriate stimulus. However, pregnancy is contraindicated in patients with AN because of the high risk to the fetus of intrauterine growth retardation. In the 30 percent of AN patients who have recovered their weight but are still amenorrheic, one or two courses of clomiphene citrate (Clomid), 50–100 mg a day for 7 days, will often stimulate ovulation. This should not be attempted until the patient's weight has been stable for four to six months and it is certain that she is not maintaining a borderline weight by engaging in vigorous exercise.

Ultimately, weight gain will restore the hypothalamic-pituitary-ovarian axis to normal in most, but not all, patients. Whether or not patients with AN should be treated in the interim with estrogens is not clear. This depends to a large extent on the chronicity of the disorder and the patient's prognosis. The evolving evidence that the hypoestrogenic state in amenorrheic runners and postmenopausal women is associated with accelerated bone loss suggests that, if for no other reason, estrogen replacement should be given to preserve bone mineral. In addition, sexually active patients may have improvement in their dyspareunia. Thus, patients who have had amenorrhea for more than one year or who have been primary treatment failures or both should be given estrogen replacement. This may be in the form of oral contraceptives, although these may not be psychologically acceptable to some patients because of monthly menstrual flow. The alternative is to use daily conjugated estrogens (Premarin, 0.625–1.25 mg) for 4 to 6 months with the addition of medroxyprogesterone acetate (Provera, 10 mg per day) for 5 days at the end of each 4- to 6-month time period. This regimen may not be acceptable to some patients because of breast enlargement and weight gain due to fluid retention. The physician should emphasize the medical desirability of estrogen replacement to the patient.

Though there have been many fewer studies about the pituitary-gonadal axis in men with AN, it appears that they also suffer from hypogonadotropic hypogonadism. The major clinical manifestation of this is decreased libido and potency, and occasionally decreased frequency of shaving. Treatment of these symptoms is administration of parenteral testosterone in the form of testosterone enanthate, 200 mg i.m. every 2 weeks. This will produce testosterone levels that remain within the normal range for the entire two-week interval.

Other Hormones

Of the other hormonal abnormalities associated with AN, none should be specifically treated. Many patients with AN have laboratory evidence of adrenocortical hyperfunction as documented by an increased cortisol production rate and increased urinary "free" cortisol or urinary 17-hydroxycorticosteroid levels. In addition, there are abnormalities in the diurnal rhythm of serum cortisol which may be due to increased production and/or abnormal binding of cortisol to cortisol binding globulin. All of these abnormalities are nonspecific for AN and may merely represent a nonspecific stress response, as seen in patients with depression. Alternatively, the elevation in cortisol secretion may be a counter-regulatory response to the intermittent hypoglycemia occasionally seen in patients with AN. A few patients with AN have had low cortisol levels in serum and urine and poor response of serum cortisol to exogenous ACTH administration. This may reflect the nonspecific adrenocortical hypofunction associated with hypothermia.

Serum growth hormone (GH) levels are often elevated in patients with AN and may be "inappropriately" stimulated by TRH. Obviously these patients are not acromegalic, probably because somatomedin-C levels are very low. As with elevated adrenocortical function, the high serum GH levels may be an attempt to defend against hypoglycemia and require no specific therapy.

A few studies have suggested that patients with AN have abnormalities of serum levels of testosterone. This is not a constant finding and does not require any specific therapy. The lanugo hair that AN patients often have is more likely due to the elevated levels of serum cortisol than to any testosterone abnormalities.

Patients with AN may have partial diabetes insipidus. This is usually asymptomatic and requires no specific therapy. Indeed, if symptomatic, complete diabetes insipidus is found, a hypothalamic disorder (such as tumor, sarcoid, and so on) should be suspected.

METABOLIC TREATMENT

The most serious metabolic abnormality is hypokalemia. This and the often attendant alkalosis are usually seen in patients who have abused diuretics or laxatives or both to achieve weight loss, or in those who are chronic vomiters. Bulimic patients often present with hypokalemic alkalosis. This finding requires prompt hospitalization so that potassium replacement can be accomplished. This should be done by the intravenous route, since surreptitious vomiting or the use of hidden diuretics may undermine this therapeutic intervention. Serum electrolytes should be monitored daily until they return to normal. Oral potassium supplements should then be used, since the patients are still total body potassium depleted.

Hypophosphatemia may be present prior to the initiation of primary therapy. Even if initially normal, total body phosphate stores are undoubtedly low. Serum phosphate levels may become precipitously lower during nutritional rehabilitation, causing intracellular adenosine triphosphate (ATP) depletion and cellular hypoxia. Clinically this may manifest itself as respiratory or heart failure, seizures, altered mental status, or myoneuropathy. Intravenous or oral phosphate supplements should be administered, depending on the severity of the hypophosphatemia and the overall clinical status. Daily measurement of serum phosphorus levels is advisable during the initiation of nutritional rehabilitation.

Prerenal azotemia is common in AN and will reverse with nutritional rehabilitation. However, some patients may develop permanent renal damage resulting in poor renal concentrating ability. The cause of the permanent impairment is unclear, but it may be due to chronic hypokalemia, thus providing another rationale for vigorous treatment of hypokalemic AN patients.

PRIMARY TREATMENT OF AN

Patients with AN are often resistant to being entered into any type of treatment program. Indeed, the initial role of the physician is the education and counseling of such patients to convince them to cooperate with a treatment plan. Reassurances that the patient will not be permitted to become obese and that many somatic complaints will improve with weight gain are often helpful approaches.

The initial approach to primary therapy depends to a large extent on the severity of the weight loss and the method by which it has been achieved. Upon presentation to the physician, all patients should have a complete physical examination, electrocardiogram, chest x-ray, urinalysis, and determination of electrolyte, renal, and hepatic function. If the weight loss is moderate, the duration is relatively short (four months or less), and no severe metabolic abnormalities are present, treatment may be initiated on an outpatient basis. The initial aim of therapy, whether inpatient or outpatient, is nutritional rehabilitation. Patients with AN suffer from the nonspecific symptoms of starvation, such as insomnia, depression, and irritability, which are easily reversible with weight gain. Improvement in body image and the patient's overestimation of an object's size will also improve with weight gain. On the other hand, programs focusing on weight gain only are doomed to failure. Patients will quickly learn to escape from the medical care system by rapidly gaining weight only to lose it shortly thereafter. Moreover, rapid weight gain may be dangerous in that it may stimulate suicidal thoughts and suicide attempts or convert the AN patient into a bulimic one. Behavioral therapy must therefore be combined with psychiatric treatment.

The psychiatrist attempts to uncover the underlying psychologic factors that have initiated and perpetuated the situation. This may involve traditional psychotherapy, but the education, counseling, and involvement of the family in therapy are critical components that pave the road to recovery. Numerous self-help groups have arisen in large cities which may provide emotional and educational support for selected patients, though the therapeutic efficacy of such a milieu remains to be proven. The Anorexia Nervosa Aid Society (133 Cedar Lane, Teaneck, NJ 07666) is one such organization.

Outpatient treatment should also include a behavior modification plan, which should be established and followed by the internist, pediatrician, or endocrinologist. This has the advantage of permitting frequent assessment of the patient's medical status and of isolating the psychiatrist from the anger that a patient may have toward the director of the weight gain program. A behavior modification program can only be adopted with help from the patient's family, who have local control of the positive reinforcements for weight gain. Reinforcements should be for weight gain, since surreptitious vomiting or diuretic and/or laxative abuse may subvert a program based on eating behavior. A written schedule or contract should be established at the beginning of a therapeutic program which outlines the specific goals and time schedule. Table 2 lists factors frequently used in a behavior modification program, whether outpatient or inpatient. This should be drawn up with

TABLE 2 Factors Used in the Development of a Behavior Modification Program

Positive Reinforcement for Weight Gain	Negative Reinforcement for Failure to Gain Weight
Return of privileges:	Tube feeding
Television or radio	Intravenous feeding
Smoking	Isolation
Access to money	Withdrawal of bathroom
Activity	privileges
Visitors	Bed rest
Phone calls	
Mail	

the cooperation of the patient and family and signed by the patient. This provides reassurance to the patient that weight gain will be slow (approximately 2 pounds per week) and limited to achieving a weight within 5 percent ideal body weight. Since the fear of obesity and loss of control are frequently major issues with which the patient is wrestling, this approach reassures the patient about the fear of too much weight gain and allows the patient to be an active participant in recovery. Under such an arrangement, weekly follow-up visits, preferably occurring at the same time of day, are necessary. The patient urinates, puts on a gown, and is weighed. This procedure avoids the pitfalls of a falsely elevated weight being recorded as a result of a patient placing weighty objects in pockets.

The help of a dietitian is useful at the outset, provided that the patient has accepted the diagnosis. The dietitian can provide an accurate calorie count using a one- or two-day diet recall. With an activity history, the dietitian can then give the patient a balanced diet that will provide an additional 1000 calories per day. Patients with AN have diminished gastric emptying and increased gastric volume following a meal. Therefore they may complain of abdominal discomfort or pain if the diet is increased precipitously. Gradual build-up to the additional 1000 calories per day over 1 to 2 weeks and the use of metoclopramide (Reglan) as an adjunct may prevent or improve these symptoms.

Hospitalization of a newly diagnosed AN patient is based on the discovery of severe, acute weight loss, or the presence of severe metabolic changes, such as hypokalemia with or without alkalosis (Table 3), or both. Patients with established, longstanding AN may be hospitalized for

TABLE 3 Indications for Hospitalization of Patients with Anorexia Nervosa

Rapid and severe weight loss
  to less than 75 percent of *ideal* body weight
  of more than 25 percent of *initial* weight in less than 3 months
Hypokalemia with or without alkalosis
Azotemia
Hypophosphatemia
Development of lethargy and listlessness
Suicidal thoughts
Lack of family involvement or pathologic family environment
Failure of an outpatient program

the same reasons or because of the failure of an outpatient treatment program. Suicidal thoughts or preoccupation should stimulate hospitalization in either type of patient. While the specific cause of death in AN is generally unknown because of the rarity of published autopsy reports in this group of patients, it is not unlikely that the combination of the severe sinus bradycardia (as low as 28 beats/minute), hypotension, and hypokalemic alkalosis predispose the patient to potential lethal abnormalities of cardiac rhythm. Ventricular ectopy, nodal escape rhythms, and ectopic atrial rhythms are not uncommon in AN. While nutritional rehabilitation will correct these abnormalities, patients should be treated with specific agents in a bed equipped with telemetry until they are stable and weight gain has begun.

AN patients rarely need oral or parenteral hyperalimentation. Behavior modification programs similar to that described for outpatient therapy can reverse weight loss and induce weight gain in most patients. It may take one to two weeks of observation of a new AN patient before enough information can be gathered to design a successful behavior modification program. However, the development of (1) cardiac arrhythmias, particularly in the presence of normokalemia; (2) lethargy in a patient who is usually hyperactive; or (3) a severe febrile illness (while patients with AN have abnormal phagocytic function of their leukocytes, hypocomplementemia, and leukopenia, they rarely develop infections) in a patient with severe and rapid weight loss are indications for initiation of oral hyperalimentation via a nasogastric tube with a nutritionally complete formula, such as Sustacal. Serum phosphorus levels should be monitored daily, as life-threatening hypophosphatemia may occur in these circumstances (see above).

PHARMACOTHERAPY

Drugs of several classes have been used to treat AN with little documented success. Few double-blind trials of any drugs have been completed. Among the drugs that have been used, cyproheptadine would appear to be the most effective and least harmful. Cyproheptadine (Periactin) is a serotonin and histamine antagonist which produces weight gain in animals, in children, and in geriatric patients. It may also enhance weight gain in patients with AN if used in doses of 4 to 8 mg 4 times per day. Drowsiness is the most commonly encountered side effect of cyproheptadine and may preclude its use in some outpatients. Phenothiazines, tricyclic antidepressants, L-dopa, and analeptics have all had anecdotal success but may produce multiple adverse effects. Of these, amitriptyline, beginning at 25 mg per day and increasing to 75–150 mg per day, may be the most effective, particularly if depression is a major component of the patient's illness.

HYPOTHALAMIC HYPOPITUITARISM

CHARLES S. HOLLANDER, M.D.

Hypopituitarism can be divided into two general categories: primary and secondary. Primary hypopituitarism, caused by the absence or destruction of hormone secreting cells of the pituitary, is discussed elsewhere in Chapter 5. Deficient pituitary hormone secretion may also be due to a lack of stimulation resulting from disorders of the vascular and/or neural connections with the brain at the level of the pituitary stalk, hypothalamus, or extrahypothalamic central nervous system. Historically, in light of its unique role in neuroendocrine regulation, attention was initially focused on the hypothalamus. Hypothalamic functions associated with the regulation of anterior pituitary secretion, whose deficiency constitutes the subject matter of this chapter, cannot be attributed to a specific nucleus and are more widely distributed in regions of the hypothalamus. In recent years it has become apparent that the pathogenesis of disorders of this kind is considerably more complex than was initially contemplated. For one thing, it is now recognized that diseases of brain loci outside of the hypothalamus and even nonlocalized disorders of the central nervous system may produce endocrine disorders whose clinical manifestations may be very similar to those of hypothalamic disease. This is not too surprising because these endocrine disturbances are mediated via altered neural input to the secretory hypothalamic neurons. Moreover, the pathogenesis of these neuroendocrine disorders is not necessarily limited to anatomic lesions in the hypothalamus and/or other interconnecting brain areas.

There are other more subtle derangements that may underlie identical clinical manifestations of secondary hypopituitarism. These include disordered neurotransmitter systems, which modulate releasing factor secretion, or more generally pathologic or iatrogenic alterations in peripheral vascular signals that modify the secretion or action of releasing factors. Conceivably, there might even be clinical disorders of anterior pituitary function on the basis of the secretion of abnormal hypothalamic hormones. In light of these complex interrelationships it is not surprising that in most of the examples of clinically recognized syndromes of secondary anterior pituitary hormone deficiency which will be described in this chapter, evidence of releasing factor dysfunction, specific hypothalamic disease, or both is indirect and inferential. Finally, abnormalities in endocrine dysfunction are frequently manifested in subtle ways, such as alterations in feedback, in stress-induced release, or in circadian periodicity rather than by an effect on basal levels. Thus, initially at least, no overt clinical evidence of endocrine disease may be discerned by the clinician.

HYPOTHALAMIC HYPOTHYROIDSM

The use of the hypothalamic hormone thyrotropin releasing hormone (TRH) now often permits the clinician to identify patients whose hypothyroidism appears to be due to a hypothalamic defect. Although the test is valid in determining the primary site of functional impairment in some cases, it must be emphasized that it may not be definitive in all instances. Hypothalamic hypothyroidism can be seen as an isolated defect, but more commonly, particularly in children, it is found in association with other manifestations of anterior pituitary hormone deficiency. Although additional stigmata of central nervous system dysfunction, such as dysplasia of the optic nerves, anatomic defects of midline structures, and absence of the corpus callosum, have been described in some of these patients, most of them have not manifested such defects. In light of the postulated pathogenesis of this syndrome such patients could theoretically be managed by repeated administration of exogenous TRH. Indeed, such a regimen has induced a reversal of the hypothyroidism in a few such patients, which further buttresses our concepts of the pathophysiology of this syndrome. However, given our present state of knowledge, patients with hypothalamic hypothyroidism are best handled by administration of thyroid hormone.

I treat such patients in the same manner as I manage patients with either conventional hypopituitarism or primary hypothyroidism. I generally prescribe 100–200 mcg per day of synthetic L-thyroxine administered as a single dose. I should emphasize that I titer the dose for each patient individually; a few may require lower or higher doses. For the experienced endocrinologist, clinical evaluation provides the best yardstick of adequacy of therapy. However, one of the advantages of this approach is that when L-thyroxine is given in this manner, measurements of plasma thyroxine and triiodothyronine are of considerable assistance, since they accurately reflect circulating thyroid hormone levels and values should fall within the normal range. To my mind the main advantage of L-thyroxine therapy is that it permits delivery of a stable level of thyroid hormone to the tissues. I also adhere to the same precautions in commencing thyroid replacement that I observe for patients with all forms of thyroid deficiency. To minimize potential risk to the coronary vessels and myocardium, I initiate thyroxine therapy in a stepwise fashion with 25-mcg increments at biweekly intervals, commencing with 25 mcg of L-thyroxine per day until optimal replacement is achieved. In selected patients and in those with known coronary artery disease an even more cautious gradual replacement program is often desirable. Except in patients with such problems as urgent impending (nonthyroidal) surgery or in instances of depressed consciousness and myxedema coma where more rapid replacement is clearly warranted, little is lost with this more gradual approach. It is usually well tolerated, and I believe it is probably safer than more rapid physiologic hormone replacement, although admittedly this has never been rigorously demonstrated.

DECREASED GROWTH HORMONE SECRETION SECONDARY TO HYPOTHALAMIC DISEASE

Therapy for so-called idiopathic growth hormone deficiency is discussed in Chapter 14. Individuals with this disorder manifest the clinical picture of growth hormone (GH) retardation in conjunction with impaired GH responses to standard stimuli in the absence of evidence of any systemic disease or pituitary tumor. Although categorized under anterior pituitary disease, this form of short stature is actually more likely to be a result of hypothalamic disease. The postulated etiologic agent would be deficient secretion of growth hormone releasing factor (GHRF) either on the basis of a specific dysfunction of the GHRF secreting neurons, or alternatively, secondary to deranged control of GHRF release by neurotransmitters (for example, excessive inhibitory beta-adrenergic tone). Of course, until GHRF is actually isolated and chemically characterized this evidence will remain inferential. Likewise the emotional deprivation GH deficiency syndrome may well have a hypothalamic basis. Moreover, organic hypothalamic lesions, discussed specifically in a later section of this chapter, can cause temporary or permanent impairment of growth hormone secretion, probably again as a result of dysfunction of the GHRF neurons. At present there is no practical implication of the distinction between a hypothalamic and an anterior pituitary origin. Specific therapy for all of these forms of growth hormone deficiency is limited to the prepubertal period and, as discussed in detail in Chapter 14, consists of human growth hormone. However, GHRF, or conceivably pharmacologic alteration in neurotransmitter tone, may provide alternative therapeutic approaches in the future.

DIMINISHED SECRETION OF ACTH SECONDARY TO HYPOTHALAMIC DISEASE

Some of the earliest stigmata of disordered neuroendocrine control in a variety of intracranial diseases are derangements in the diurnal rhythm of ACTH secretion and in the normal suppressibility of ACTH. Thus it is all the more surprising that diminished secretion of ACTH secondary to hypothalamic dysfunction is considerably less common than that for other pituitary hormones. Isolated impairment of ACTH secretion is quite rare. ACTH deficiency has been observed considerably more frequently in association with diminished secretion of other pituitary hormones, particularly in children, and there is inferential evidence that the ACTH impairment is secondary to hypothalamic disease. However, it must be emphasized that methods for pinpointing a hypothalamic or extrahypothalamic etiologic agent for these derangements of hypothalamic-pituitary function are even less precise than was the case with TSH or the gonadotropins. Investigators currently employ arginine vasopressin and hypoglycemia for this purpose because corticotropin releasing factor (CRF) is not yet available for clinical testing. A potent ovine CRF has recently been isolated and shown experimentally to induce ACTH release in normal persons. It is likely that use of this more direct stimulus will supplant these indirect approaches in the near future.

It is well established that adrenal insufficiency of any origin can be life-threatening, particularly in times of stress. Patients with this deficiency on a hypothalamic basis are currently best managed in the same manner as patients with ACTH deficiency on the basis of pituitary insufficiency. Most such patients should be well controlled on 25 mg of cortisone or its equivalent in 2 equally divided daily doses, although a few will require slightly higher or lower doses. The fact that ACTH deficiency does not lead to complete mineralocorticoid deficiency is the reason that additional mineralocorticoid in the form of fludrocortisone acetate or deoxycorticosterone acetate (DOCA) is rarely needed. Indeed, some authorities recommend the use of prednisone for patients with secondary hypoadrenalism. I prefer cortisone or hydrocortisone, since partial mineralocorticoid deficiency is often present and occasional patients have frank aldosterone deficiency. It is important to bear in mind that under conditions of stress (such as a febrile illness or significant trauma) these patients will require two or three times their normal dosage, which must be gradually tapered with recovery as their condition warrants. One sometimes troublesome complication is the development of euphoria and even frankly psychotic behavior when full replacement or greater doses are administered; therefore, the minimal effective dose of steroid should be utilized. Patients should wear an appropriate medical identification bracelet at all times. Moreover, a prudent precaution is to advise such patients to be accompanied by a companion and to carry a supply of injectable steroids when they venture into areas where modern medical care may not be readily available. A final problem worthy of mention is the fact that the initiation of glucocorticoid therapy may trigger the appearance of overt diabetes insipidus.

In conclusion, although I have mainly highlighted therapeutic problems in this section, the response to judicious glucocorticoid therapy in affected patients is usually rapid and gratifying.

GONADOTROPIN DEFICIENCY

Hypogonadotropic hypogonadism is a congenital deficiency in gonadotropin secretion which affects both sexes and is frequently familial. Hypothalamic hypogonadism is defined as diminished pituitary and gonadal function secondary to hypothalamic dysfunction with decreased, abnormal, or absent secretion of gonadotropin releasing hormone, or GnRH, and it is well known to occur in association with organic hypothalamic disease. Considerable circumstantial evidence also points to a hypothalamic origin for cases of hypogonadotropic hypogonadism in the absence of any observable pathologic changes. Therapy for these disorders, widely considered to be on a hypothalamic basis, will be described in this chapter, although admittedly, conclusive direct evidence for this hypothesis awaits development of radioimmunoassay methods sufficiently sensitive to determine GnRH concentrations in the peripheral blood.

Hypothalamic Hypogonadism in Males

In males the syndrome usually presents as delayed puberty with no evidence of sexual maturation and impaired testosterone secretion. Some patients with this syndrome have hyposmia or anosmia in addition to the hypogonadism, which is apparently due to developmental failure of the olfactory lobes. Also associated with the disorder to a variable extent are congenital deafness, harelip, cleft palate and other craniofacial asymmetries, color blindness, and mental retardation. Often, however, the clinician will observe patients with this disorder (referred to as Kallmann's syndrome) who have only anosmia or hyposmia. In the absence of any of the congenital stigmata of the syndrome, an absolute diagnosis is often possible only retrospectively, since puberty can be delayed in some boys until the age of 18 or 19. The anosmia

and or hyposmia is worth searching for very carefully with a meticulous history and specific testing, since it has considerable practical importance. Even in its absence, wherever a sufficiently strong suspicion exists I personally favor administering testosterone therapy to such patients by the age of 18 or 19 and certainly in the early twenties.

My rationale for advocating such a course is as follows: it is well documented that the longer the deficiency is allowed to remain untreated, the longer it takes to achieve an adequate response. Indeed, failure to treat early may preclude full restoration of normal male development irrespective of treatment duration. Moreover, stimulation of spermatogenesis with gonadotropins can be undertaken in the future when procreation is desired, since responsiveness to these agents is unimpaired by testosterone. Finally, in those individuals who might be mistakenly treated with testosterone, testicular growth will usually occur in the course of gonadal therapy, permitting the clinician to discontinue testosterone. I personally utilize a testosterone dosage equivalent to 12–15 mg per day intramuscularly in the form of testosterone enanthate or proprionate in a dose of 200–300 mg every 2 or 3 weeks. Parenteral preparations are safest and cheapest. Details of therapy are further discussed in Chapter 68, but basic criteria for adequate dosage include libido, potency, and beard growth. Patients should be cautioned that many months of therapy may be required for an adequate response. With toxic doses acne, nightmares, disturbing sexual urges, gynecomastia, and edema formation are often noted. A potential undesirable side effect that is actually a physiologic effect of testosterone and unavoidable in genetically susceptible individuals is the development, or more accurately, the expression, of genetically determined baldness.

If untreated these patients will remain in their prepubertal state indefinitely and many of these individuals may be undiagnosed for many years. Particularly in those cases in which adults in their thirties or even older are to be treated, the psychosexual aspects of therapy must be carefully borne in mind. The life styles, customs, vocations, avocations, and interactions with their marital partners may have been established and become firmly ingrained in the context of and in a manner appropriate to an ongoing long-term lack of sex drive. These psychologic factors may prove formidable barriers to therapy.

Infertility in hypopituitary men is more difficult to treat but can be overcome in some instances by chronic therapy with menotropins in the form of Pergonal, and FSH-rich preparation from urine of postmenopausal women, for 70 or more days followed by human chorionic gonadotropin for approximately 20 days. Such treatment is time-consuming and successful in inducing live sperm in only about 30 percent of cases. However, there are currently in progress several clinical trials with LHRH. Continuous therapy is not efficacious, since it causes down regulation of the receptors. Instead LHRH must be given by repeated intermittent injection for several months. Other investigators are attempting to achieve the same result with newer synthetic analogues of LHRH which are effective intranasally. Thus the chances are excellent for a new more physiologically efficacious and convenient therapy for this disorder in the near future.

Hypothalamic Hypogonadism in Females

As is the case for the male, newer insights into the mode of action and appropriate means of administration of LHRH and its analogues are likely to revolutionize our approach to therapy of hypothalamic hypogonadism in the female in the next few years. These developments will be discussed in their appropriate context at the conclusion of this section. However, in accordance with the purpose of this text, the major focus of this presentation will center upon optimal therapy with currently available modalities. A rational approach to such therapy requires a careful consideration of the age of onset, the nature of the underlying cause and its reversibility, the severity of the hypogonadism—or more specifically whether or not clinically significant hypoestrogenic symptoms are present—and finally whether or not fertility is desired.

Age of Onset and Nature of the Underlying Cause: In prepubertal girls, the presence of hypothalamic hypogonadism results in failure of normal sexual maturation and primary amenorrhea accompanied in some cases by other pituitary hormone deficiencies, also on a hypothalamic basis. Occasional cases of female Kallmann's syndrome have been described. Postpubertal hypogonadism (which occurs primarily in women) presents as secondary amenorrhea or oligomenorrhea or much less often is manifest as infertility associated with anovulatory cycles. Secondary amenorrhea of this type is commonly observed in women with so-

called functional or psychogenic amenorrhea. It may also be found in cases of hyperprolactinemia of any origin, in alterations in weight, including all instances of profound changes in either direction; and with exercise. Thus amenorrhea is virtually universal in anorexia nervosa and is quite common in ballerinas and female athletes. Less commonly hypogonadism is seen in conjunction with certain rare, poorly understood organic diseases of the central nervous system, such as Lawrence Moon, Bardet Biedl, and Prader Willi syndromes.

Rationale and Selection of Therapeutic Modalities: In prepubertal girls with amenorrhea, therapy at present consists of gonadal steroids for the development and maintenance of secondary sexual function and at an appropriate age gonadotropins for promoting fertility.

In the postpubertal female, therapy of the underlying disease process should be attempted wherever possible. Thus if associated hyperprolactinemia is present (as it may be with hypothalamic lesions), therapy should initially focus on restoring the prolactin to normal (See Chapter 10). Hypoestrogenic symptoms and signs can usually be treated with one of several estrogen preparations, but this should be undertaken only with specific precautions (see below). Supplementation with small doses of androgen is necessary to restore libido in panhypopituitary women. When desired, restoration of fertility is also achievable in many of these gonadotropin deficient women with clomiphene citrate, or alternatively, combined therapy with preparations possessing LH and FSH bioactivity.

Induction of ovulation is often an expensive procedure and can be dangerous. It should be reserved for patients who desire fertility and in whom no other specifically treatable causes of chronic anovulation or contraindications to pregnancy have been unearthed in a careful screening evaluation, which should include an evaluation of the adequacy of the husband's sperm. I would caution that in my view, induction of ovulation in this fashion should be attempted only in close consultation with an experienced gynecologist.

Gonadal Therapy and Induction of Ovulation: Estrogen therapy can be accomplished with a variety of estrogen preparations and birth control pills. I usually employ ethinyl estradiol for this purpose. Dosages from 5–20 μg per day are generally advised, but in my experience, a dosage in the range of 10 μg per day is probably adequate for the premenopausal adult female.

In light of recent still controversial evidence of an increase in cases of endometrial cancer, the prudent clinician will employ the smallest effective dose of estrogen. Also for this reason, I believe it is imperative that patients receive progesterone to induce menses because of the documented ability of progesterone to reverse endometrial hyperplasia. I accomplish this by limiting ethinyl estradiol administration to the first 25 days of each month and by inducing a menstrual period with medroxyprogesterone, 5–10 mg per day given on days 21 to 25 inclusive. I also specify that my patients have periodic breast and gynecologic evaluation by qualified specialists every six months, including cervical exfoliative cytology (Pap test).

Although current methods entail some risk (slight for the mother with appropriate precautions) and considerable time and trouble, it is possible to restore fertility to a substantial number of these patients. As I have indicated, only patients who have had a careful infertility work-up, including study of the husband's semen, are candidates for this mode of treatment. In many such patients clomiphene citrate therapy induces ovulation, and I try this approach in all my patients at the outset. I begin by administering the drug in a dosage of 50 mg per day for 5 days commencing on the fifth day of the menstrual period that I have previously induced with medroxyprogesterone acetate. If ovulation is successfully induced, it usually occurs between five and ten days after the course of clomiphene is completed. Therefore, patients are instructed to have intercourse every other day between the fifth and fifteenth day after cessation of clomiphene. If the 50-mg dose is unsuccessful in triggering ovulation during 2 successive months, I raise the dosage to 100 mg per day for 5 days and then to 150 mg per day for a similar interval. When ovulation is successfully induced as judged by basal body temperature and in some selected instances by plasma progesterone or urinary pregnanediol measurements, clomiphene is continued at the minimally effective dose until the patient conceives. I believe that clomiphene should be thoroughly tried before considering a course of gonadotropins because it is relatively simple and inexpensive, and most importantly, because it has fewer untoward effects than the gonadotropins. It should not be forgotten, however, that side effects do occur with clomiphene and can be quite troublesome. The most common is ovarian enlargement, which can occur with or without cyst formation. This possibility provides the principal reason for careful follow-up of patients on clomiphene and is also why the presence of ovarian cysts or tumors is a clear contraindication to its administration. The vasomotor symptoms of the hot flush are sometimes seen but are usually mild and limited to the period when clomiphene is actually taken. Abdominal discomfort and bloating can be a problem. Nausea, vomiting, headaches, blurring of vision with spots or flashes of light, and a variety of other side effects are found less frequently. The most feared complication, massive ovarian hyperstimulation, is increasingly rare. The incidence of multiple births is 10 percent with clomiphene. Therapy is successful in inducing ovulation in 70 percent of patients and pregnancy in 40 to 50 percent of treated subjects.

Hypoestrogenic patients often fail to respond, and these subjects, as well as all those who fail to ovulate after successive trials of clomiphene therapy at the 150-mg dose, are candidates for combined therapy with human gonadotropins. The FSH preparation available commercially in the United States, known as Pergonal, is a preparation of human menopausal gonadotropins supplied in vials standardized to contain 75 IU of FSH and 75 IU of LH. The preparation is given intramuscularly daily for 10 to 15 days. The goal is to produce the normal preovulatory growth of the follicle. Because of the variability of individual response, I begin with a single vial daily for this period and sequentially monitor follicular maturation by means of the estrogen response either by measuring total urinary estrogen or plasma estradiol levels. A competent gynecologic endocrinologist should be available to supervise this therapy. Estrogen measurements are also an indispensable adjunct and should be performed in every case. Excessively high preovulatory estrogens (certainly above 300 mg of urinary estrogen per 24 hours) indicate that ovarian hyperstimulation may have occurred, and the clinician should interrupt efforts to induce ovulation with human chorionic gonadotropins (HCG). Once estrogens have returned to baseline levels, therapy can resume at a lower daily dose of Pergonal. If an appropriate individualized dose of Pergonal has been administered, there is a rise of plasma estradiol to 500 to 1000 pg/ml or urinary estrogen to 50–150 μg per day. If this level of estrogen is not seen within a week of cessation of Pergonal, the daily dose of the drug should be increased. If the dose of Pergonal has achieved the desired estrogen level, ovulation can usually be induced by a single injection of 10,000

IU of HCG 24 hours after the last dose of Pergonal. To ensure the presence of sperm in the genital tract at the time of ovulation, patients are instructed to have intercourse the night preceding HCG administration and on the following two days.

The incidence of multiple gestation with this therapy is about 20 percent, but the pregnancy success rate is around 60 to 70 percent. Careful observation of excessive ovarian enlargement is critical. Simple measures of the patient's weight and abdominal girth must be supplemented with clinical estimates of ovarian size and estrogen assays to avoid the hyperstimulation syndrome. If severe, this is a potentially fatal complication and hospitalization is mandatory. Fortunately it has become much less common now that the precautions outlined have been followed in most clinics. Arterial thrombosis has rarely been described. It appears that the hypercoagulability is related to the hyperstimulation and not to the gonadotropin therapy itself. In addition to the hyperstimulation syndrome, multiple gestation must also be viewed as a complication, since multiple pregnancy increases the antenatal and perinatal loss and is generally undesirable. Finally, it should not be forgotten that this therapy carries with it a heavy emotional strain which in many instances is felt by both partners.

Future Therapeutic Directions: It has been recognized that luteinizing hormone releasing hormone (LHRH) offers unique advantages over other agents. It affords the potentia to (1) utilize endogenous gonadotropins and (2) incorporate physiologic feedback mechanisms to ensure release of the precise amounts of FSH and LH required to ripen and ovulate a single follicle and therapy avoid the ovarian hyperstimulation seen in some cases with exogenous gonadotropins. Pulsatile administration with a portable infusion pump of small physiologic doses of LHRH every 2 hours to LHRH deficient patients has been successful in initiating endogenous LH pulses. Intranasal forms of LHRH are also under development. These ingenious studies remain experimental at present but should revolutionize our therapy for this disorder in coming years.

ANTERIOR PITUITARY DISEASE

HYPOPITUITARISM

LAWRENCE A. FROHMAN, M.D.

Anterior pituitary hormone deficiency may exhibit markedly varying clinical manifestations depending on whether one hormone is involved or many and whether the deficiency is partial or complete. Treatment therefore requires a detailed assessment of the function of individual hormones and an appreciation that impaired secretory responses may be secondary to lack of other hormones and thus reversible with appropriate therapy. For example, growth hormone secretion is decreased in hypothyroidism but returns to normal with thyroxine therapy. In addition, impaired pituitary hormone secretion in patients with pituitary tumors may be corrected after tumor excision. Therefore the timing of pituitary hormone testing is important. It is also necessary, at least with respect to certain pituitary hormones, to distinguish between pituitary and hypothalamic etiologic factors, since therapies may be different.

Partial hypopituitarism, such as that seen with Sheehan's syndrome or with a slowly growing pituitary tumor, may exist for long periods of time without detection, and the patient may exhibit minimal symptoms if no severe medical, surgical, or psychologic stress occurs. In this type of patient the diagnosis requires a high index of suspicion and careful testing of the hypothalamic-pituitary (and, at times, target organ) axis. In contrast, complete hypopituitarism (panhypopituitarism) may occur acutely (as in a patient with pituitary apoplexy); the consequences may be life-threatening and immediate therapy is required. Treatment based on proper diagnostic testing will first be discussed for each anterior pituitary hormone and then consideration given to acute or urgent treatment.

TSH DEFICIENCY

The goal of therapy in patients with TSH deficiency is to restore normal thyroid function. The finding of a low thyroxine level unassociated with an elevated TSH level in a clinically hypothyroid patient indicates pituitary TSH deficiency. Distinction between hypothalamic and pituitary etiologic factors can generally be made by TRH testing; a TSH response is seen in the former but not in the latter. In some patients with recognized destructive lesions of the pituitary, thyroid function may be intact and only impaired or absent TSH responses are observed. There are also rare patients who secrete immunologically active but biologically inactive forms of TSH, and the diagnosis in these individuals is somewhat more complicated.

Therapy for all types of TSH deficiency, however, is the same. The drug of choice is L-thyroxine and the principles of management, with one exception, are identical to those for primary hypothyroidism (see Chapter 17). Restoration of the euthyroid state and of normal circulating thyroid hormone levels can be accomplished by an oral dose of 0.1–0.2 mg of L-thyroxine daily. This hormone is preferable to triiodothyronine, which has a shorter duration of action. In contrast to patients with primary hypothyroidism, in whom circulating TSH levels may be effectively used as a guide to replacement therapy, patients with TSH deficiency must be followed by measuring circulating T_4 levels in association with assessment of clinical symptoms.

In patients with partial TSH deficiency, less than full replacement may be required. Some physicians therefore, prefer to use smaller doses of L-thyroxine with periodic monitoring of serum T_4 levels on a long-term basis. I do not favor this approach because (1) more frequent monitoring is required and (2) progression from partial to complete TSH deficiency is unpredictable, particularly in patients with pituitary tumors who have received therapeutic irradition. If total hormone replacement is used, it is generally unnecessary to continue monitoring serum T_4 levels once a euthyroid state is achieved. Since endogenous T_4 production is decreased in the sixth and seventh decades, patients with TSH deficiency on L-thyroxine replacement will frequently require a reduction in dosage at this time to avoid signs and symptoms of hyperthyroidism.

Since patients with pituitary hypothyroidism rarely exhibit true myxedema, therapy can generally be initiated at the expected maintenance dosage. In patients with coronary heart disease, however, a smaller dose should be used initially and gradually increased to maintenance level. In patients with concomitant ACTH deficiency, treatment with glucocorticoids (see below) must be initiated prior to or simultaneously with thyroxine to avoid the possibility of cardiovascular collapse.

TSH and TRH are not of value in the treatment of TSH deficiency. TSH must be administered parenterally, bovine TSH is immunogenic, and human TSH exists only in very small quantities. Even if human TSH were to be readily available, it would provide no advantage over thyroxine. TRH also must be administered parenterally for maximal effectiveness. In large doses it is active after oral administration in normal persons and in patients with hypothalamic hypothyroidism, but it has no role in either long-term or short-term treatment.

ACTH DEFICIENCY

Deficiency of ACTH secretion results in partial or complete adrenocortical insufficiency. Patients may not have the typical signs and symptoms of primary adrenal insufficiency because of a significant preservation of mineralocorticoid secretion, which is under renin-angiotensin as well as ACTH control. As a result, patients may exhibit no evidence of volume depletion, even with virtually undetectable plasma cortisol levels. In patients with overt symptoms of adrenocortical insufficiency, immediate therapy is indicated. However, in those with minimal or no symptoms under nonstressful living conditions, careful assessment of stress-responsive ACTH or cortisol release is essential for therapeutic decision making. The most frequently used stimulus for evaluating ACTH secretory reserve is insulin hypogly-

cemia. This test should be used cautiously and never is a patient with overt clinical findings of adrenocortical insufficiency. It has been proposed that the cortisol response to synthetic ACTH injection can provide a rapid substitute for the insulin hypoglycemia challenge. There are, however, occasional patients in whom this test gives misleading information, and I do not recommend its use for this purpose. Within the next few years corticotropin releasing factor may provide a safer and easier assessment of coricotroph reserve.

The treatment of ACTH deficiency is based on the use of glucocorticoids (see Chapter 27). Although some mineralocorticoid deficiency is present, replacement therapy with synthetic mineralocorticoids is unnecessary. Originally, cortisone or hydrocortisone was used for treatment. However, comparable results can be obtained with synthetic glucocorticoids, such as prednisone, at considerably less expense. In contrast to patients with primary adrenal insufficiency, patients with ACTH deficiency often do not require full replacement therapy, and furthermore, if full substitution is used, signs and symptoms of glucocorticoid excess (obesity, hypertension, edema) may occur. In addition, children who are also growth hormone deficient may have impaired responses to human growth hormone therapy if given full glucocorticoid replacement (see Chapter 14 for details of dosages during childhood). The dosage regimen appropriate for most patients is prednisone, 2.5 mg p.o., b.i.d. Should this not be sufficient, the morning dose is raised to 5 mg. Other synthetic glucocorticoids can be used but they have no advantage over prednisone.

Patients with ACTH deficiency should be given the same advice given to those with primary adrenal insufficiency with respect to therapy during stress. When patients experience acute bacterial or viral infections with fevers greater than 101°F, the dose of prednisone should be doubled and then tapered as the clinical situation improves. Should the patient be unable to take medication orally, hydrocortisone hemisuccinate (Solu-Cortef), 25 mg i.m. every 6 to 8 hours, or cortisone acetate, 50 mg every 12 hours, should be given.

A question arises as to the treatment of patients with only relative ACTH deficiency, who manifest signs or symptoms of adrenocortical insufficiency only during stress. Most patients are best treated as described above, as though they had total ACTH deficiency. However, selected patients who possess a reasonable understanding of the nature of their disease can be managed without maintenance therapy, as long as they (1) understand the need to take oral or parenteral glucocorticoids during times of stress, and (2) have been properly instructed in the use of both.

Patients with partial or complete ACTH deficiency are advised to wear an identification tag (bracelet or pendant) indicating that they have hypopituitarism and require glucocorticoid therapy in the event of an emergency in which they are unable to communicate this information.

Acute and complete ACTH deficiency, as may be seen with pituitary apoplexy, is a life-threatening disorder and requires immediate treatment. The therapy of choice is hydrocortisone, 100 mg i.v. followed by 50 mg every 6 hours i.m. The route of administration can be switched to oral as tolerated and the dosage gradually tapered to maintenance.

GONADOTROPIN DEFICIENCY

Gonadotropin deficiency results in two problems: decreased gonadal steroid production leading to signs and symptoms of androgen or estrogen deficiency, and infertility. Each requires a different therapeutic approach. The manifestations and treatment also vary with age, (prepubertal, postpubertal, or postmenopausal/postclimacteric).

Females

The principles of therapy in hypogonadotropic females are similar to those in males. Ovarian steroids are used to allow development and/or maintenance of secondary sexual characteristics and to permit cyclic menstrual bleeding. Gonadotropins are used to promote fertility, and in women with hypothalamic hypogonadism, clomiphene or LHRH may also be effective.

Estrogenization of girls with prepubertal hypogonadotropic hypogonadism is usually started in the midteens, after considering the patient's height, psychosocial development, and the need for growth hormone therapy. The same considerations apply to girls as to boys receiving growth hormone in that initiation of estrogen therapy should be withheld as long as practical. Therapy should be started with conjugated estrogens, that is, Premarin, 5–10 mg p.o. daily for as long as is necessary to promote maximal breast development. The patient should then be switched to one of the low-dose estrogen oral contraceptives and maintained in a standard cyclic manner (see Chap-

ter 81). The continued use of estrogen through the reproductive years is indicated to maintain secondary sexual characteristics, libido, vaginal lubrication, and possibly to prevent osteopenia. In the postmenopausal period the same considerations apply to therapy with ovarian steroids as in women with normal pituitary function. In girls with hypopituitarism estrogen therapy will not produce growth of pubic or axillary hair, since this is normally caused by adrenal androgens. Full libido may also not be restored in some women with estrogen alone, and, if desired, a therapeutic trial of a small dose of androgen—fluoxymesterone, 2–5 mg p.o.—may be of value.

Fertility in women with pituitary gonadotropin deficiency is accomplished by inducing ovulation with gonadotropins. Follicular development is promoted by daily injections of a gonadotropin preparation with a high FSH-to-LH ratio, and serum estradiol or total serum estrogens are monitored daily. When the appropriate levels are reached, HCG is added to stimulate ovulation. This therapy is effective in inducing ovulation but can be associated with numerous problems, such as hyperstimulation and multiple pregnancies. It should therefore be carried out only by physicians experienced in its use.

In women with a hypothalamic origin for hypogonadotropism, clomiphene, 50 mg per day for 5 days beginning on the fifth day following a spontaneous or induced menstrual bleed, often causes a release of endogenous gonadotropins, stimulation of follicular growth, and ovulation. The ovulatory surge of gonadotropins usually occurs between five and ten days after the first dose of clomiphene. If cyclic bleeding does not occur, the dose is gradually increased to a maximum of 200 mg per day for 5 days. Three to four cycles of clomiphene are required before considering the therapy a failure.

Patients with prepubertal hypothalamic hypogonadotropism will not respond to clomiphene but may be successfully treated with intermittent (pulsatile) LHRH administration.

Males

Gonadotropin deficiency during childhood will prevent puberty and the testes will remain in an unstimulated prepubertal state. Androgen therapy must be coordinated with growth hormone therapy, if indicated, so that maximal linear growth is permitted to occur before closure of long bone epiphyseal cartilage plates (an effect of androgens). The decision to begin androgen administration must also take into consideration psychologic effects of delayed appearance of secondary sex characteristics during the teenage years.

Androgen therapy is best provided by one of the long-acting parenteral preparations of either testosterone cypionate or testosterone enanthate, 200 mg i.m. every 3 weeks. Full androgenization can be achieved in most patients, though in some the process remains incomplete. Patients can expect an increase in overall hair growth, increased penile development, improved musculature, voice deepening, prostatic growth, development of libido, and the ability to perform sexual intercourse. The ejaculate, however, will not contain sperm and testicular size will not be altered. Therapy can generally be monitored by clinical assessment, though if inadequate response is suspected, measurement of plasma testosterone prior to hormone injection can be helpful.

The treatment of hypogonadism occurring during adult life is generally more likely to result in full restoration of androgen function, in part because the period of androgen deprivation is usually of shorter duration. The details of therapy are identical to those listed above. Special consideration must be given to adult males discovered to be hypogonadal since the pubertal or prepubertal period. Lack of androgen during this time can profoundly affect psychosocial behavior and development relating to choice of marital partners and living patterns. The behavioral effects of androgen administered after these patterns have been established may create significant problems for the patient.

Gonadotropins can achieve the same effects but are not used because of the expense and the need for more frequent injections. Their use if reserved for treatment of infertility, as described below (see also Chapter 70). LHRH and LHRH analogues (the latter are still in an investigational state at present) can be used to increase endogenous gonadotropins and testosterone in patients with hypothalamic hypogonadism in whom pituitary gonadotropin secretory capability remains intact. Pulsatile administration of LHRH is required to prevent the development of pituitary insensitivity (due to "down regulation" of gonadotroph LHRH receptors). This can be accomplished either by giving several injections per day or by the use of an infusion pump programmed to give repeated bolus injections.

Spermatogenesis requires both FSH and high concentrations of intragonadal testosterone. This is accomplished in hypogonadotropic hypogonadal patients by treatment with exogenous gonadotropins. Prior treatment with testosterone does not impair responsiveness, but testosterone must be discontinued when gonadotropin therapy is intiated. Therapy is started with human chorionic gonadotropin (HCG), which exhibits LH-like actions and results in testicular growth and endogenous testosterone production. Dosage varies from 2000–4000 IU i.m. 3 times weekly. Testicular size and serum testosterone levels are monitored until they reach the normal range. This may require up to 12 to 18 months of therapy. At that time a sperm count is performed, since occasional patients will respond to HCG alone. If the patient is still azospermic, FSH is added (150 IU i.m. 3 times weekly), and combined therapy is continued for another 1 to 3 months. Those patients who respond will do so in this period. While sperm counts may not reach levels observed in normal males, fertility can be restored with considerably lower levels. Because of the expense and inconvenience, before initiating therapy both partners should be examined carefully to exclude other disorders that might prevent conception. It is also not practical to continue therapy for longer than necessary, and when it is discontinued, testosterone injections should be substituted. LHRH has also been reported to restore spermatogenesis in hypothalamic hypogonadal men. Its use at present, however, is still investigational.

GROWTH HORMONE DEFICIENCY

Treatment with growth hormone is at present almost always limited to the pediatric population. Many subjects are treated through the teenage years and for as long as the epiphyseal growth centers have not been closed by exposure to endogenous or exogenous sex steroid hormones. As long as these conditions persist, patients in their twenties and possibly even older can respond to growth hormone therapy. Ideally, treatment should be continued until the patient reaches an acceptable height, at least 5 feet 4 inches, taking into consideration his or her genetic potential. Full details of therapy are provided in Chapter 14.

NONFUNCTIONING PITUITARY TUMORS

PETER O. KOHLER, M.D.
and STEVENSON FLANIGAN, M.D.

Nonfunctioning pituitary tumors cause clinical symptoms by compromising nearby tissues, including the normal pituitary and the optic chiasm. Since small pituitary adenomas are frequent incidental findings at postmortem examination, it would appear that nonfunctioning adenomas are often not associated with morbidity. However, when a pituitary tumor reaches sufficient size that it begins to impair hormone secretion or visual function, treatment is indicated. The type of therapy depends to a large degree on the clinical status of the patient involved. Numerous individual considerations are necessary, including the age and general health of the patient (Table 1). The therapeutic goals generally include preservation of vision, control of tumor growth, and preservation of normal pituitary function to the degree possible. Assessment of pituitary function prior to treatment provides both information concerning the need for replacement hormone treatment and a baseline for documenting efficacy of treatment and/or the degree of tumor progression.

The types of therapy for patients with nonfunctioning tumors include those listed in Table 2. No therapy may be indicated other than hormone replacement in patients with other serious illnesses and a shortened life expectancy. However, if the patient is otherwise relatively well, but has endocrine deficits or radiographic evidence of tumor growth, such as bony erosion or visual disorders, treatment should be initiated. Several forms of medical therapy have been tried in the past. However, only bromocriptine seems to cause shrinkage of a few nonfunctioning tumors, in addition to prolactin- and growth-hormone-secreting adenomas. External radiation may be carried out with conventional supravoltage treatment or cobalt 60. There are several variations in administration of the irradiation, but an arc type or multiple port therapy seems desirable to avoid excessive doses to the brain. Heavy particle therapy has been used successfully with either protons or alpha particles, and this may be delivered by stereotactic techniques. Finally, surgery can be performed. Depending on the size of the tumor, either a transfrontal or transsphenoidal approach may be utilized. Techniques used at surgery may include hypophysectomy, thermal ablation, or implantation in the sella of a radioactive source, such as yttrium 90 or gold 198.

In the past, a frequent strategy for managing a patient with large pituitary tumors was to irradiate initially with conventional irradiation and then to operate only if there were evidence of progressive visual or endocrine loss. However, with improvement in surgical techniques and increased utilization of transsphenoidal hypophysectomy, most patients with large pituitary tumors now have an initial surgical approach to the tumor. If tumor removal is incomplete, as is frequently the case with very large tumors, irradiation can be utilized for control of subsequent tumor growth. Substantial experience has documented that incomplete tumor removal that is not followed by irradiation ultimately leads to continued tumor growth and visual or hormone function loss. The role of medical treatment other than for hormone replacement (see Chapter 5) is in the investigative stages at present. Each form of therapy is discussed below.

TABLE 1 General Considerations in Treatment of Large Nonfunctioning Pituitary Tumors

Age	Degree of visual loss
General health	Degree of hypopituitarism
Tumor size and extension	CSF rhinorrhea

TABLE 2 Therapies Used For Large Pituitary Tumors

None
Medical
External irradiation
    Conventional ^{60}Co or supravoltage
    Heavy particle
        Proton
        Alpha particles
Surgical
    Transfrontal or intracranial
    Transsphenoidal
Combinations

MEDICAL TREATMENT

In the past, medical treatment for nonfunctioning pituitary tumors has generally been considered ineffective. Recently, however, Wollesen and colleagues have indicated that treatment of patients with nonfunctioning tumors with high doses of bromocriptine (15–60 mgm per day) appears to show a reduction in tumor size, both in patients who had also received irradiation and those who had not. Reduction in tumor size by a median of 32 percent occurred in 9 of the 11 patients treated. These results suggest that high doses of bromocryptime may be useful in selected patients with nonfunctioning tumors. Additional experience is needed to document the efficacy of this form of treatment. The disadvantages of this treatment include the probable need to continue bromocriptine for extended periods of time, the cost of the medication, and the side effects. Since expansion of hormone secreting tumors when bromocriptine is discontinued has been described, this may also occur in the nonfunctioning tumors that respond to initial bromocriptine treatment. However, bromocriptine now provides a potentially useful treatment in patients who have contraindications to surgery or irradiation. This would include patients who have previously received maximally tolerable doses of irradiation.

IRRADIATION

Extensive experience with the use of conventional irradiation with supravoltage or cobalt 60 for pituitary tumor treatment has been documented. Conventional irradiation has been used for pituitary tumor control for several decades. Fager has reported improvement in 65 percent of 273 patients initially treated with irradiation alone. Initially, two bitemporal ports were frequently used for delivering the radiation dose. Subsequent refinements have included multiple ports or an arc type technique to avoid excessive irradiation to areas of the brain other than the pituitary tumor. Experience has shown that side effects of the irradiation can be decreased by frequent small treatments over a five- to six-week period. Attempts to shorten the overall treatment period or to increase the individual doses have been accompanied by increased side effects, such as visual loss. The complications of irradiation treatment include the potential risk of swelling or infarction of the tumors with loss of vision during the treatment. In actual practice this rarely occurs. However, several authorities recommend monitoring visual fields periodically during the irradiation treatment. A few rare tumors, such as sarcomas, have been reported several years following treatment. Also, small areas of brain necrosis have infrequently been reported as complications of irradiation therapy.

Cystic tumors, which appear to have a frequency of about 15 percent in nonfunctioning adenomas, seem not to respond as well to irradiation. Prior to the development of sophisticated CT scanning techniques this led to the recommendation that biopsy be performed prior to irradiation. However, the refinements in surgical techniques have made it seem more logical that if biopsy is to occur, an attempt to remove the tumor should also take place. At the present time, some cystic pituitary tumors can usually be demonstrated by CT scanning with contrast material. In these tumors a surgical approach seems more appropriate for the initial form of therapy. This also would appear to be the case with many solid tumors.

Heavy particle irradiation with proton beam and a stereotatic technique or with alpha particles is also extremely effective in nonfunctioning pituitary tumors. The response to irradiation of a nonfunctioning tumor is much more difficult to document than that of a functioning tumor that secretes measurable hormones. However, the results from the groups at Massachusetts General Hospital in Boston and in Berkeley, California, appear to indicate that proton beams with the delivery of a potentially larger dose than conventional irradiation provide an effective means to control nonfunctioning adenomas. The complications tend to be more frequent and may in fact be common in patients who have previously received maximally tolerable doses of conventional irradiation. These complications include visual field deficits and cranial nerve palsies.

SURGICAL THERAPY

In treating patients with nonfunctioning tumors surgical therapy is frequently combined with irradiation for optimal results in patients in whom complete surgical removal of the adenoma is not possible. Transfrontal craniotomy with removal from above is still used by many neurosurgeons for the largest pituitary tumors (grade IV) with significant suprasellar extension. However, the advances in transsphenoidal surgery have now made possible the approach to many tumors previously operated on only from above.

Considering first the transsphenoidal procedure, decompressive removal of an intrasellar pituitary adenoma is undertaken to protect residual gland function. With tumor escaping the confines of the sella turcica into the cranial vault, the procedure is designed to forestall compression of other functional structures in the vicintiy, most commonly the visual apparatus. This is still performed preferentially from below. Erosion through the floor of the pituitary fossa results in a mass in the sphenoid sinus which can present a problem in differential diagnosis. Angiography is occasionally necessary in differential diagnosis of a parasellar mass and for operative design. With the advent of CT scanning to the degree of resolution possible today, endocrinologic abnormalities are commonly localized to the pituitary gland long before the lesion extends beyond the confines of the fossa.

Preoperative review of risks must recognize the potential loss of residual gland function requiring replacement therapy. In many instances (except in dealing with microadenomas) there is a disturbance in water balance in the early postoperative period. Not infrequently the antidiuretic hormone response to the stress of anesthesia and operation reverses the day after the operation. The excessive urine output has raised concern that diabetes insipidus is occurring. With the more common transsphenoidal approach the potential for CSF leak is anticipated.

In the absence of a history of allergy, a sulfa drug for diffuse tissue penetration is started 24 hours prior to the procedure and resumed as soon as the patient can manage oral intake postoperatively; intravenous methicillin is also administered that day. The patient should be aware of the remote complications, such as infection, adverse reaction to anesthesia, and hemorrhage. Barring complications the patient can anticipate discharge on the fifth postoperative day. A transient numbness of the upper lip and the incisors should be anticipated.

Preparation for operation includes vigorous dental hygiene and an antiseptic wash of the abdominal wall. The patient should be in a stable state of health and the adequace of replacement therapy should be tested. Thyroid replacement in the face of chronic hypothyroidism is especially important. Because of the potential manipulation of the pituitary stalk, a major dose of supplemental steroids is administered the morning of the operation and in the immediate postoperative period. Tapering to maintenance dosage is planned if the patient has already required replacement therapy.

When diode goggles are used as a light source for visual cortical evoked responses (VER), they are draped out. A transverse incision at the mucosal reflection onto the inner surface of the upper lip permits a subperiosteal exposure of the septal spine and the floor of the nostril. Removal of bone is kept to a minimum (avoided if possible), but there is need for an aperture sufficient to accommodate the self-retaining speculum.

A submucosal detachment of the cartilaginous septum permits displacement to either side. The ventral edge of the bony vomer is separated from the cartilage and resected back to the floor of the sphenoid sinus as one piece to be used to reconstruct the floor of the pituitary fossa.

Opening the sphenoid sinus on one or both sides and avulsion of the sinus mucosa permits exposure of the promontory of the sella turcica. With the speculum in place x-ray confirmation of the direction of approach is obtained. A generous portion of the ventral bony wall of the fossa is removed and the dura is incised in a cruciate fashion, up to the circular sinus and laterally to the carotid groove. When the tumor has eroded into the sphenoid sinus the extrusion is encompassed and simply followed through bone and dura into the pituitary fossa.

With the intact gland exposed, a vertically oblique incision is made midway laterally on the side of the adenoma, visualized on 1.5 mm CT planes through the gland. Normal glandular tissue is moderately firm and tan. The capillary and sinusoidal vascularity will redden the cut surface. The adenoma is usually soft, gray, and will often "ooze" out through the cut. It is important at this point to collect all of the abnormal tissue for pathologic examinations. A 1-mm cube is put immediately in glutaraldehyde, anticipating electron microscopic examination for granules. The remainder is put in formaldehyde for light microscopic description of tumor architecture and peroxidase, antiperoxidase reactions. The walls are then curetted to normal gland and coagulated thoroughly with bipolar forceps.

An adenoma greater than a centimeter in diameter usually generates a capsule of compressed tumor tissue that can be "peeled" away. Again, cautery of the wall of the cavity is important. That is usually the cause of transient postoperative diabetes insipidus. The plane of pars intermedius and the soft and ghostly white nature of the pars nervosa are easily discernible. The larger tumor adheres to the dura and the undersurface of the arachnoid when it presents through the aperture of the diaphragma sellae. Dissecting the tumor capsule away often produces a rent in the ballooning arachnoid. With completion of the resection that rent should be plugged with Gelfoam and supported with the fat graft. The fat is supported in the fossa with the plate of vomer tailored just larger than the length of the opening in one plane or another. This is the point at which VER may show changes with compression form below with too much fat. Herniation of the optic apparatus into the pjituitary fossa and insufficient fat support can also be reflected in alterations in wave form. With adequate reconstruction of the floor of the pituitary fossa and with no escape of CSF on Valsalva stress, packing of the sphenoid sinus is not necessary.

The nasal passageways are re-established, reconstructing the septum in the midline. The lip is simply compressed into approximation of the edges of the incision with gauze pack outside the upper lip. With the gauze pack removed from the mouth, the hypopharynx is cleared before extubation. Postoperative diabetes insipidus is managed with aqueous Pitressin subcutaneously. If necessary, cerebrospinal fluid fistulization can be stopped with decompression by repeated lumbar punctures or a closed drainage with a lumbar subarachnoid catheter.

Adenomas less than 1 cm in diameter can be totally removed 90 percent of the time. Larger tumors still contained within the fossa can be eradicated surgically two-thirds of the time. For individuals with these tumors radiation therapy can be delayed for evidence of recurrent growth. Large tumors extending beyond the confines of the sella turcica are commonly so adherent to the walls of the cavernous sinus that expectations for surgical cure are less than one in three. If there is any question of incomplete resection, radiation therapy should be added within two or three months following the procedure.

The Cushing "subfrontal" craniotomy is selected for the tumor with mass laterally into the middle fossa. Another indication for the subfrontal approach is the "dumbbell" tumor with obvious constriction at the level of the diaphragma sellae. However, the appearance of calcification of the dorsal portion of the diaphragm extending in a gentle curve upward from the dorsum sellae can

be reassuring in the decision to approach resection from below.

With the subfrontal approach the potential for additional complications relates to transgression of the frontal sinus, venous congestion of the frontal pole, contusion of the frontal brain with retraction, loss of the olfactory tract on one side, and trauma to the optic apparatus and the hypothalamus. A large suprachiasmatic extension of tumor in the presence of short optic curves can be approached through the attenuated lamina terminalis. An extension principally laterally can be managed more easily from a ventrolateral approach.

SURGICAL MANAGEMENT OF CRANIOPHARYNGIOMAS

JOSEPH RANSOHOFF, M.D.

Craniopharyngiomas develop primarily during childhood and are among the most common intracranial tumors of nonglial origin in this age group. They also, however, present sporadically in young and middle-aged adults and are seen as well in the sixties and seventies. These neoplasms are thought to arise from embryonic squamous cell rests and incompletely involuted hypophyseal pharyngeal ducts. These cell rests, which are in the pituitary stalk and infundibulum, can develop into tumors of squamous epithelium, growing slowly and encroaching upon surrounding structures. Some of these may be solid and partially calcified; however, in the vast majority of cases, degenerative products cause some cystic changes in the center of the tumor mass as well.

The problems that develop as these tumors grow depend not only upon the relationship of the tumors to surrounding structures but also upon the age at which the tumor becomes symptomatic. Signs and symptoms that may develop as a result of craniopharyngioma include visual disturbances;

disturbances in hypothalamic function related to body growth, behavioral patterns, sexual development, electrolyte imbalance, and thermal regulatory mechanisms; and obstructive hydrocephalus with resultant papilledema, headache, nausea, and vomiting. Neuroendocrine symptoms are apt to be more pronounced in the younger age group, although sexual dysfunction can be seen in the adult male population as well. Visual symptoms may go unrecognized during the first several years of life and the tumors may grow to considerable size before symptoms become obvious. Visual impairment becomes obvious as the patient approaches school age. Thereafter, any combination of symptoms may present in all age groups.

DIAGNOSIS

The diagnosis of craniopharyngioma has been dramatically influenced by the development of computerized transaxial tomography (CT). The CT scan demonstrates these lesions with great accuracy, and the presence of a cyst or partly cystic tumor in this region with calcification is almost diagnostic. Plain skull films may or may not show calcification, but they generally demonstrate erosion or thinning of the region of the sella turcica. Hydrocephalus may be documented on CT scan, as may distortion of the anterior third ventricle. Examination of the optic fundi may demonstrate optic atrophy as a result of compression of the optic nerves and chiasm, with visual field and visual acuity changes or papilledema if the tumor has grown posteriorly with compression of the third ventricle and acute hydrocephalus. Digital intravenous angiography (DIVA) is useful for demonstrating the displacement of normal vessels and tumor vascularity, as well as for excluding giant aneurysms, which may closely mimic the CT picture of craniopharyngioma in adults. Endocrine defects may be recognized by appropriate tests of basal and stimulated pituitary function.

TREATMENT

There have been major advances in the therapeutic management of craniopharyngiomas, related not only to the improved diagnostic capacities as a result of the development of CT scanning, but also to the greatly improved ability to manage the neuroendocrine deficits that result from operative manipulation of this complicated region. The

development of the operating microscope has dramatically improved the neurosurgeon's capacity to achieve total or near total removals of craniopharyngiomas while sparing the important adjacent neurovascular structures.

The therapeutic goals of surgical intervention vary, of course, depending upon the age group of the patient and the related symptoms. In childhood and early adult life, every effort should be made to achieve a total or as close to a total removal as possible. In the author's experience, as well as from numerous reports in the literature, in patients with craniopharyngiomas in whom total excision has been presumed to be achieved, the recurrence rate with ten or more years of follow-up was less than 20 percent, clearly indicating that complete surgical excision is a distinct possibility. These recurrences may be seen as long as 15 years postoperatively. Such recurrences may be treated by reoperation and postoperative radiotherapy or with radiotherapy alone. Simple aspiration of the cystic component of the craniopharyngioma is rarely associated with any meaningful long-term relief of symptoms. However, cyst aspiration or ventricular shunting for the relief of acute hydrocephalus may enable the patient to be brought under better neuroendocrine control prior to attempting a more definitive surgical procedure.

There are two basic operative approaches to the tumor: frontal and frontotemporal. The frontal approach is the most commonly utilized and provides excellent access to the optic nerves and chiasm, as well as the adjacent carotid arteries. The tumor can generally be entered between the nerves and chiasm with aspiration of the cystic contents and, thereafter, careful microdissection of the tumor capsule from the adjacent regions of the hypothalamus, optic pathways, and the carotid artery. Whereas these tumors often extend posteriorly and displace the vertebral artery, they are almost never attached to the vertebral artery or its branches. A fair amount of dissection may be required to achieve a total removal of the posterior and inferior aspect of the capsule where it may be adherent to the base of the skull in the region of the posterior clinoids and clivus. The frontotemporal approach along the sphenoid wing is advantageous where the tumor presents posteriorly and superiorly, displacing the chiasm forward and presenting mainly into the region of the hypothalamus with obstruction of the third ventricle. The inferior surface of the chiasm and the anterior cerebral complex with its important perforating vessels into the region of the hypothalamus are best visualized via this approach. At times, of course, a combination of the frontal and temporal approaches becomes necessary to achieve the maximal therapeutic result.

The pre- and postoperative neuroendocrine management of these patients is important. Adequate preparation with corticosteroids (see Chapter 63) is essential, and careful control of diabetes insipidus (see Chapter 1) and related electrolyte disturbance is critical in the early postoperative care of the patient.

Long-term asymptomatic survivals of up to 20 years have followed radical subtotal removal when only a small fragment of capsule is allowed to remain adherent to vital structures, such as the undersurface of the chiasm or the medial wall of the carotid artery. However, review of the recent world literature reveals a recurrence rate of 75 percent following subtotal excision alone.

A major controversy in neurosurgery revolves around the issue of radiation therapy in the treatment of craniopharyngiomas. There seems to be little question, however, that radiation therapy does have a role in the management of these tumors, although it is not indicated as a primary therapeutic approach. The improvements in accuracy of delivery of radiation therapy, as well as improvement in radiation therapy equipment, have reduced the subsequent complication rate, especially with regard to long-term radiation necrosis. In terms of our current capacity to evaluate the recurrence rates of craniopharyngiomas that have been "totally" removed, it is probably best to withhold radiation therapy until evidence of recurrence can be demonstrated via the use of periodic postoperative CT scanning. In those patients in whom a large residual tumor mass clearly remains following surgical intervention, particularly in the younger and middle-aged groups, radiation therapy should certainly be considered after recovery from surgery. A total dose of between 5000 and 6000 rads, carefully focused based on the postoperative scan, over a period of 6 to 7 weeks probably represents the current regimen for optimal radiation therapy. There are numerous well-documented instances in which regrowth of tumor has been arrested following the use of radiation therapy, and hence this modality must always be included in the overall management regimen of these benign tumors. Review of the world literature reports a 30 percent recurrence rate when subtotal excision is combined with radiotherapy. Our own experience parallels this report. In 20 cases we have been able to follow undergoing combined therapy, 4 have shown recurrent symptoms, 1, however, being related to radiation damage rather than to tumor growth; 3 have been reoperated with further improvement in visual symptoms. Two small children have died months after surgery as a result of progressive hypothalamic neuroendocrine dysfunction. In the past decade we have had no operative deaths in either children or adults.

CONCLUSIONS

Craniopharyngioma is a benign tumor that produces neuroendocrine and visual symptoms in all age groups. With the recent advances in endocrine management, the advent of microneurosurgery, and the major developments in radiation therapy, these tumors can be managed with very low mortality and morbidity rates. In all age groups, unless the tumor is extremely large, calcified, and extending into the hypothalamus, an effort should be made to achieve a total surgical excision. Radiation therapy is effective in controlling regrowth if significant residual tumor can be seen on postoperative CT scans. *All* patients should be followed with periodic CT scans.

In the very young, in whom the long-term effects of radiation therapy on the developing brain may be deleterious, and in patients in the seventh and eighth decades of life, the decision to utilize radiation therapy following surgery may be delayed until definite evidence of tumor regrowth is demonstrated.

EMPTY SELLA

HAROLD E. LEBOVITZ, M.D.,
and FRANCIS A. NEELON, M.D.

An empty sella turcica is a sella whose volume is incompletely filled by the pituitary gland; cerebrospinal fluid and the suprasellar subarachnoid space extend below the diaphragma sellae to occupy the portion of the pituitary fossa that is not filled by the pituitary gland. As a result, when the subarachnoid space is drained of cerebrospinal fluid, as during pneumoencephalography or at craniotomy, the sella appears more or less "empty," the pituitary sometimes being reduced to a rim of tissue along the margin of the sella. Such an empty sella is anticipated following surgical or radiation therapy for a pituitary tumor and is known as a "secondary empty sella." It causes no symptoms unless an adhesive inflammatory reaction occurs and exerts traction on the optic chiasm, impairing vision.

Much more common is the "primary empty sella" for which no clear inciting cause is evident. In such cases an incompletely formed sellar diaphragm (found in 20 percent or more of adults) is thought to be a prerequisite. We believe that when even minimal or intermittent elevation of cerebrospinal fluid pressure occurs in such individuals (for example, with arterial hypertension, pulmonary disease, obesity, or benign intracranial hypertension), the sella is remodeled and enlarged and the pituitary gland is compressed against the sellar margin. In general this anomaly may be considered a benign anatomic variant, and it does not predispose to the development of any of the disorders (for example, pituitary tumor, hypofunction, and so on) to which the pituitary gland is susceptible.

DIAGNOSIS

The possibility of a diagnosis of a primary empty sella usually arises during a consideration of causes of an enlarged sella turcica. Such enlarged sellas are often found serendipitously (that is, in the absence of hormonal or visual symptoms of a pituitary lesion) on skull radiographs taken for some unrelated reason, such as headache, trauma, or sinusitis. In such a case, the demonstration that the sella is not filled by tumor is all that is needed. This is best accomplished at present with a high resolution (thin slice) computed tomogram (CT) of the skull in the coronal plan. Intravenous contrast enhancement may help identify the pituitary stalk and aid in CT resolution. When CT itself cannot demonstrate an empty sella, intrathecal injection of metrizamide may succeed by showing contrast material within the sella. Finally, one may resort to fractional pneumoencephalography (autotomographic) in the brow-up position; this is usually considered the most accurate method, but it should be used sparingly because of its discomfort and occasional danger.

CLINICAL CHARACTERISTICS

Table 1 outlines the salient clinical features of the empty sella. The vast majority of reported cases occur in females and are associated with obesity. Arterial hypertension is present in about a third of the patients. Pseudotumor cerebri seems to predispose to the development of an empty sella. A significant complication of the empty sella is the high incidence of CSF rhinorrhea.

HORMONAL ASPECTS

In general, we believe that no consistent hormonal abnormality can be associated with the empty sella; hence there is no "empty sella syndrome" as such. Defects in growth hormone secretion have been seen, but these are compatible with the obesity many patients have. Other hormonal deficits are rare and usually clinically obvious. Our practice has been to treat patients with proven empty sellas as we do those with normal sellas: We evaluate hormonal status only when there is some independent clinical indication. Of course, since any pituitary abnormality (including prolactin, corticotropin, and growth hormone secreting microadenomas) may be present in a patient with an empty sella, full pituitary evaluation should be carried out when indicated.

TREATMENT

Primary empty sella needs no specific therapy. Weight reduction or antihypertensive therapy may be indicated when the condition is present, but no change can be anticipated in the sella turcica. Nor is there any need for routine surveillance of hormonal or visual function in these patients, since we do not believe they develop problems in

TABLE 1 Clinical Characteristics of Primary Empty Sella*

Female	205/245	83.7%
Obesity	127/162	78.4%
Hypertension	50/164	30.5%
Pseudotumor cerebri	26/247	10.5%
CSF rhinorrhea	24/247	9.7%

*From Jordan, R. M., Kendall, J. W. and Kerber, C. W.: "The Primary Empty Sella Syndrome" Am J Med 62:569–580, 1977.

these areas any more frequently than the patient with a normal sella.

When benign intracranial hypertension (pseudotumor cerebri) accompanies the empty sella (pseudotumor hypophysei), careful ophthalmologic examination is indicated, as is treatment directed at the raised intracranial pressure: dietary sodium restriction (less than 2 gm salt per day), diuretic therapy (hydrochlorothiazide or furosemide), and therapeutic lumbar puncture at weekly intervals (removing enough cerebrospinal fluid to lower the CSF pressure to normal).

Spontaneous CSF rhinorrhea may complicate primary empty sella. This diagnosis may be established by detection of radioiodinated serum albumin in the nasal discharge following intrathecal installation of the appropriate tracer. Thin section polytomographic radiographs may identify a sellar defect. CSF rhinorrhea requires surgical correction and therefore referral to an experienced neurosurgeon or otolaryngologist. When the defect can be localized, repair can be attempted via the nasopharynx, packing the sellar defect with muscle and fascia. In resistant or recurrent cases, craniotomy may be required and the sella packed from above. In general, the outcome of such surgery is quite satisfactory and the hazard of meningeal infection is eliminated.

Secondary empty sella is generally a symptomless concomitant of prior radiation or surgical treatment. On rare occasions scar formation occurs, entrapping the optic chiasm in fibrous tissue. The resulting sellarward traction impairs vision, creating scotomas on visual field testing. Such patients may require open craniotomy with lysis of adhesions and careful visual field monitoring. The outcome after surgery is guarded, since no large series or long-term follow-up study is available.

SUMMARY

The primary empty sella is a common and benign anatomic variant that needs no specific treatment. The goals of therapy are to prevent unnecessary procedures and to correct associated abnormalities, as summarized in Table 2. Sophisticated computed tomography will usually suffice for definitive diagnosis of an empty sella, which, in the absence of hormonal or visual symptoms or signs, needs no further evaluation or long-term surveillance. An empty sella may occasionally be found in patients with any disorder of pituitary function; in these cases diagnostic and treatment

TABLE 2   Goals of Therapy for Primary Empty Sella

Prevent unnecessary radiation or surgical treatment
Prevent unnecessary endocrine testing
Treat benign intracranial hypertension if present
Surgical treatment of CSF rhinorrhea

plans should be formulated as for patients without empty sellas. Secondary empty sella syndrome consists of visual defects developing after radiation treatment (with or without surgery) of pituitary tumors. Progressive loss of visual fields is an indication for operation and lysis of adhesions.

PROLACTINOMA

MICHAEL O. THORNER, M.D.

The therapy for prolactin secreting pituitary tumors has changed considerably over the past five years. Initially it was thought that all pituitary tumors, including those secreting prolactin, should undergo active therapy directed primarily at the tumor itself, that is, surgery or radiotherapy or both. In this Chapter I will consider the various therapeutic options that are open to the clinician in treating a patient with a prolactinoma and then specify why I believe that the primary mode of therapy for the vast majority of these tumors should be medical.

BACKGROUND

Prolactin secreting pituitary tumors may present in a variety of ways. The female patient may complain to the gynecologist of menstrual disorders or infertility, and the male patient may go to the urologist because of impotence. Patients of either sex may consult a neurologist or ophthalmologist with complaints of headaches and visual field disturbances. In the past the mode of presentation has dictated the choice of therapy for the patient. For example, a patient presenting with visual field defects would automatically be immediately referred to a neurosurgeon for evaluation of a suprasellar mass compressing the optic chiasm, and almost certainly the patient would ultimately undergo surgery. Today, however, rather than approaching the management of pituitary tumors in a reflex manner, it may be beneficial to reconsider the objectives of the treatment of such tumors, especially in view of the advances in medical management. I consider the objectives to be (1) reduction or removal of the tumor mass, (2) preservation of anterior pituitary function, (3) correction of the hyperprolactinemic state, and (4) prevention of recurrence of the disease.

Prior to any treatment, it is imperative that the anterior pituitary function be properly assessed. I therefore always obtain, at the very least, measurements of basal (0800 hours) plasma cortisol, serum thyroxine and T_3 resin uptake, serum TSH, serum LH and FSH and, in addition, serum estradiol in women and serum testosterone in men. If all these are normal, and causes for the hyperprolactinemia, such as ingestion of drugs (which may elevate serum prolactin levels), have been excluded, no further endocrine studies need be performed. If there is any doubt about the interpretation of the basal hormone values we proceed to dynamic function tests; we perform a thyrotropin releasing hormone test (TRH) for measurement of TSH and prolactin reserve and an insulin tolerance test (ITT) for growth hormone and ACTH reserve measurements. Evaluation of the anatomy of the pituitary is essential, and methods of doing this have changed in the last few years. In the past plain skull x-rays, including a Caldwell (occipitomental) view and lateral view, were performed, and if these were equivocal tomography of the sella was also performed. These evaluations have now been virtually completely replaced in major centers in the United States by CT scanning with fourth or later generation scanners. Using these scanners it is possible to discern not only the bony contour of the pituitary fossa but also to (1) see the soft tissues of the pituitary; (2) diagnose empty sella, and (3) diagnose both microadenomas and macroadenomas in the pituitary. It is also essential to get a neuro-ophthalmologic examination, including measurement of the visual fields on the Goldman apparatus.

THERAPEUTIC APPROACHES

When the diagnosis of prolactinoma has been established, the options for therapy are (1) to ob-serve the patient and not treat; (2) to treat with external pituitary irradiation; (3) to treat with pituitary surgery (using a transsphenoidal approach); and (4) to treat with dopamine agonist drugs. One of the dilemmas in the evaluation of the optimal mode of therapy for this condition is that its natural history is not established and is clearly variable; however, the majority of microadenomas remain small and do not progress to macroadenomas. Unfortunately we cannot predict which will progress. Nevertheless, in my view any patient who is diagnosed as having significant hyperprolactinemia, particularly if he has gonadal dysfunction, deserves active intervention to restore gonadal function. An occasional patient will spontaneously develop return of gonadal function and lowering of prolactin levels, but this is highly unusual, and active treatment should be considered for the typical patient. Radiotherapy, either with conventional external pituitary irradiation, with proton beam therapy, or with implantation of radioactive yttrium, has been utilized to prevent further growth of the tumor and to reduce tumor size. Its effects on prolactin secretion are poorly described in the literature; however, the consensus is that serum prolactin levels fall in a similar way to serum growth hormone levels in acromegaly. Following external pituitary irradiation prolactin levels fall slowly; the nadir may not be achieved until up to ten years later and levels rarely reach the normal range. Therefore radiotherapy is not a satisfactory treatment for the prolactinoma. In the United States the most popular method for treatment of prolactinomas has been transsphenoidal surgery, an approach pioneered by Hardy and Guiot.

Results from several groups in the United States which have specialized in transsphenoidal surgery suggest that when prolactinomas are small, surgical therapy produces very good results; that is, if the prolactin level is less than 200 ng/ml, the chances of restoration of prolactin levels to normal and return of gonadal function are greater than 75 percent. However, these results are limited to centers that have the greatest experience. In centers where neurosurgeons do not operate on the pituitary every day, the results of surgery are less satisfactory and only a minority of patients are cured by surgery. Also, as the length of follow-up of patients after surgery increases, the number of patients with recurrence of their disease also increases and may be as high as 14 percent. Results of surgery are quite different when one is considering large prolactinomas with high prolactin levels (that is, those with prolactin levels greater than

250 ng/ml). In these cases, even in centers with the greatest experience, the chances of normalizing the prolactin levels and restoring gonadal function fall exponentially with the increase in the size of the prolactin secreting tumor and the pretreatment basal level of prolactin. As an example, in Hardy's experience women with pretreatment prolactin levels of >250 ng/ml have only a 29 percent chance of normal prolactin levels postoperatively. Furthermore, if there is any evidence of invasion of the dura by the prolactinoma the results of surgery are extremely poor (<20 percent with normal prolactin levels).

MEDICAL THERAPY FOR PROLACTINOMAS

In 1971 the first prototype dopamine agonist drug was introduced for clinical trials. The drug, bromocriptine, is a semisynthetic peptide ergot. It was developed specifically as an inhibitor of prolactin secretion before it was known that dopamine could inhibit prolactin secretion directly at the anterior pituitary or that dopamine was itself one, if not the only, prolactin inhibiting factor. Initial studies with bromocriptine showed that, regardless of whether a pituitary tumor was present, prolactin levels were suppressed by the administration of this compound and that when therapy was withdrawn prolactin levels rose once more. Not only were prolactin levels lowered (usually into the normal range) by bromocriptine therapy, gonadal function was also restored. This occurred in both men and women. Bromocriptine was in use in clinical research for the treatment of hyperprolactinemia for five years before it was realized that it also had profound effects on the volume of prolactin secreting tumors. Most investigators initially treated patients with large prolactin secreting tumors either with surgery or with irradiation, and when the patient was left with hyperprolactinemia bromocriptine therapy was started.

Studies in several centers, including our own, have clearly demonstrated that the majority of large, prolactin secreting tumors respond to bromocriptine therapy with lowering of prolactin levels by over 80 percent (often into the normal range), restoration of gonadal and anterior pituitary functions, and a reduction in pituitary tumor volume. The size reduction of the tumors may occur very rapidly, (within days of the initiation of therapy) and lead to decompression of the optic chiasm and to resolution of headaches and other symptoms and signs of raised intracranial pressure. These results may be expected in over 80 percent

of patients (based on our own 18 cases). However, there does appear to be a spectrum of sensitivity of the tumors in terms of size reduction. Some tumors appear to be exquisitely sensitive and will shrink over 80 percent within six weeks of initiation of therapy.

Mechanism of Size Reduction by Bromocriptine

Based on animal data, it was considered that size reduction of these tumors possibly resulted from an antimitotic effect of bromocriptine. It has been clearly shown that bromocriptine can reverse the estrogen-induced increased rate of mitosis of the in situ pituitary in the rat. However, the mitotic activity in human prolactinomas is, in general, rather low. We have recently had the opportunity of studying pituitary tissue from untreated patients with prolactinomas, patients treated with bromocriptine, and patients withdrawn from treatment. Bromocriptine causes marked changes in the volumes of the prolactin secreting cells. These marked reductions in cell volume are accounted for by reduction in both cytoplasmic and nuclear volumes. In the cytoplasm the amount of rough endoplasmic reticulum and size of the Golgi apparatus are markedly reduced, and the cell changes from appearing highly active to being quiescent. There is a similar reduction in both the nuclear and nucleolar areas. The changes are reversed after bromocriptine withdrawal.

An Approach to the Patient with Hyperprolactinemia

The correct approach to a patient with a prolactinoma depends on a variety of different factors. These include the sex of the patient (and, in women, whether pregnancy is desired); the expertise in a given medical center where the patient is being seen; and the "prejudice" of the physician who is looking after the patient. My own personal view is that this disease process, which presumably reflects a spectrum from hyperplasia to isolated adenoma, is best treated by medical means. However, there are a number of problems with medical management, including (1) the risk of swelling of the tumor during pregnancy, (2) the cost of long-term treatment, and (3) the unknown effects of lifelong medical therapy.

If a patient has a small microadenoma and a prolactin level of less than 200, there is a good chance that transsphenoidal surgery performed by a skilled surgeon will be successful; under such circumstances, the patient will have an 80 to 90 percent chance of being euprolactinemic postoperatively and of needing no other form of treatment. However, in the patient who does not have a clear microadenoma, that is, one who has a prolactin level of less than 100 and an absolutely normal CT scan of the pituitary, or in a patient who may have a microadenoma but has a prolactin level of over 200, the chance of surgery being successful is probably less than 50 percent, even in the best hands. Similarly, in patients with very large prolactinomas and very high prolactin levels, (above 250 ng/ml), the chances of restoring prolactin levels to normal by surgery are less than 30 percent. Thus surgery may be successful in decompressing the tumor but will usually not be successful in curing the disease. With these large tumors the chance of surgically inducing hypopituitarism is considerable. It is interesting that these patients rarely have ACTH or TSH deficiency preoperatively. In my view all patients with hyperprolactinemia who do not have a clear microadenoma, or who have a prolactin level of over 200 ng/ml, should be treated primarily with medical therapy. I would also treat such patients with microadenomas with medical therapy, provided they understand that the therapy probably has to continue throughout their lives; it is very unusual for a patient to remain euprolactinemic following the withdrawal of bromocriptine therapy, even after one or more years of such therapy.

At the present time only one drug has been approved by the FDA for the treatment of hyperprolactinemia in patients *without* tumors for up to six months only, and for treatment of infertility. Bromocriptine may be given starting with 1.25 mg taken with food on retiring. The dosage is gradually increased every 2 to 3 days to 1.25 mg b.i.d., then t.i.d., and then increased to 2.5 mg t.i.d. Sometimes when patients have very large tumors, and 7.5 mg/day is not sufficient either to reduce the size of the tumor or to lower the prolactin levels by greater than 80 percent, it may be necessary to increase the dosage up to 15 mg per day. At the present time the drug has not been approved for treatment of prolactinomas, only for patients without obvious pituitary tumors.

I believe that patients with large prolactinomas should undergo primary therapy with bromocriptine rather than undergoing surgery. If there is good documentation of reduction in tumor size the therapy should be continued indefinitely. If reduction in tumor size has not occurred within three months, it is unlikely that it will occur and medical therapy should be abandoned. However, if it does occur, size reduction may continue progressively up to one year or longer. We have seen no serious complications of this form of therapy other than return of the tumor to its pretreatment size following withdrawal of therapy as outlined above. One patient, after approximately 18 months of therapy, developed a hemorrhage into the pituitary which led to an increase in the volume of the pituitary. However, with conservative management this expansion spontaneously resolved, and the patient has remained on bromocriptine throughout. The rest of his anterior pituitary function was not compromised by this event. It is theoretically possible that bromocriptine may prevent the progress of prolactin secreting pituitary tumors, although this had not yet been proved.

Pregnancy and Bromocriptine

Many women with hyperprolactinemia are infertile and desire pregnancy. The administration of bromocriptine lowers the prolactin levels and restores gonadal function. Thus there is little problem about the ability of the patient to conceive. There are, however, several considerations that must be stressed and recognized both by the physician and by the patient. First, the question of exposure of the fetus to bromocriptine and possible teratogenic sequelae merits consideration. There is no evidence for teratogenicity in animal studies. Furthermore, in over 1400 pregnancies in women who were taking bromocriptine when they conceived (and documented by Sandoz) there is no evidence of increased incidence of abortion, multiple pregnancy, or fetal abnormalities. However, until these babies have lived their own complete life cycles, the possibility of unexpected late effects cannot be excluded. So that the fetus is not exposed to bromocriptine for any longer than necessary, it is suggested that when the mother is initially treated with bromocriptine she takes mechanical contraceptive precautions. Once she has had three regular menstrual cycles she may discontinue contraceptive precautions and in that way pregnancy can be suspected as soon as her period is 48 hours overdue. At that time a serum beta HCG assay should be performed to confirm pregnancy and the patient should discontinue bromocriptine. Thus the fetus is exposed theoretically to bromocriptine for a maximum of 16 days.

The second problem relates to the risk of expansion of the tumor during pregnancy. There is little doubt that patients with pituitary tumors run a small but significant risk of expansion of the tumor during pregnancy. It is very difficult to assess the absolute risk. With microadenomas the incidence appears to be less than 1 percent and probably less than 0.5 percent. In patients with macroadenomas the incidence is probably higher; it may be between 5 and 20 percent. This risk is unrelated to bromocriptine therapy prior to the pregnancy; rather, it may occur when pregnancy is induced with other drugs, including exogenous gonadotropins and clomiphene, and even when no drug therapy is employed in patients with pre-existing pituitary adenomas.

In practice the problem of pregnancy is not great, since the vast majority of women who present with hyperprolactinemia only have microadenomas. To avoid major problems, it is extremely important that the patient undergo careful endocrine, neuroradiologic, and neuro-ophthalmologic evaluation prior to treatment. If there is no suprasellar extension and the patient harbors only a microadenoma, then the risk of swelling of the pituitary is extremely small and it is suggested that the patient be clinically evaluated at two-month intervals throughout the pregnancy. If the patient has a macroadenoma and suprasellar extension, a strong case can be made for decompression of the tumor prior to pregnancy. However, it is possible for even these patients to go through pregnancy without developing visual disturbances. It is vital for patients to understand about their condition and to take part in the choice of therapy. Outside the United States trials are underway evaluating the effects of continuing bromocriptine therapy throughout pregnancy in patients with macroadenomas in the hope of preventing swelling. I believe it is better to treat those patients who develop problems, rather than treating all patients throughout pregnancy in the hope of avoiding this problem.

If visual field defects or headaches from tumor expansion occur during pregnancy, a number of options are open. It should be stressed that thus far no patient has become permanently blind following expansion of the tumor during pregnancy. Following termination of the pregnancy, either by abortion or delivery, the tumor has become smaller with resolution of visual symptoms and headaches in all cases. Thus the approach will depend on at what stage of pregnancy the symptoms occur. If they occur early in the pregnancy, abortion may be indicated. If they occur in the eighth month of pregnancy, premature delivery of the baby may be decided upon, although if the field defects and symptoms are minor, careful observation may be all that is required. The most difficult time is when the field defects and symptoms occur in the middle trimester of the pregnancy. At that time I would suggest starting the patient on bromocriptine again in the hope of reducing the tumor size and at least preventing further swelling. If this is unsuccessful, high-dose dexamethasone can be used to achieve the same ends. This also has the advantage that, if the baby needs to be prematurely delivered, the chances of fetal respiratory distress syndrome are reduced. As a last resort, transsphenoidal surgery during the pregnancy can and has been used to decompress the tumor. In all events this complication is fortunately extremely rare, and for this reason no one has accumulated any large experience in dealing with it.

HYPERPROLACTINEMIA OF UNDEFINED ETIOLOGY

ANDREW G. FRANTZ, M.D.

The development since 1971 of sensitive radioimmunoassays for human prolactin has led to the widespread use of this test in clinical practice. The chief reasons for measuring serum prolactin have been the discoveries that hyperprolactinemia frequently accompanies pituitary tumors, and is also a common cause of amenorrhea. When elevated levels are found, the first task facing the clinician is to rule in or out, if possible, a pituitary tumor. This is now best accomplished by high resolution CT scanning. If there is no clear evidence of tumor, the physician then turns to other causes of hyperprolactinemia, a list of which is given in Table 1. A detailed discussion of differential diagnosis is beyond the scope of this chapter, but it will be seen that most causes listed in Table 1 can be ruled out by history. Even if it appears that such causes have been ruled out, certain considerations must be borne in mind before it can be concluded that the hyperprolactinemia is truly unexplained.

TABLE 1   Factors That May Increase Serum Prolactin

CNS Disorders—Pathologic
    Pituitary tumors
    Hypothalamic disorders
    Interruption of hypothalamic—pituitary
       connections
    Empty sella syndrome
	Miscellaneous
	    Pregnancy
	    Post partum (first few weeks)
	    Hydatidiform mole
	    Nursing
	    Breast manipulation
	    Sexual intercourse—women only
	    Hypothyroidism
	    Hypoglycemia
	    Post seizure
	    Ectopic hormone production (very rare)
	    Renal failure
	    Hepatic failure

CNS Alterations—Physiologic
    Sleep, and first 2–3 hours after waking
    Stress	

Drug Related
    Estrogens, birth control pills
    Phenothiazines
    Butyrophenones
    Pimozide
    Reserpine
    Aldomet
    Tricyclic antidepressants
    Metoclopramide
    Opiates and opioids
    Cimetidine
    Isoniazid
    Arginine
    TRH	

WHAT IS UNDEFINED HYPERPROLACTINEMIA?

Among the factors that may explain otherwise undefined hyperprolactinemia, the following deserve brief mention.

Pituitary Tumor

Until the advent of CT scanning, hypocycloidal polytomography of the sella turcica was considered the best way of identifying small pituitary tumors, sometimes referred to as microadenomas. Recent studies have shown a surprisingly high frequency of both false negative and false positive interpretations of polytomograms. Early CT scans lacked the resolution necessary to identify small tumors. More recent high resolution, or "fourth generation," CT scans have improved to the point where they are now the best available radiologic tool. Nevertheless, it is beginning to be apparent that such scans occasionally fail to detect adenomas large enough to be theoretically well within their diagnostic range. Tumors below this range, for example, on the order of 1 to 2 mm in diameter, will of course be missed. One must therefore always remain alert to the possibility that "undefined" hyperprolactinemia may in fact represent a pituitary tumor, in spite of negative x-rays. The degree of elevation of the serum prolactin correlates well with the likelihood of tumor. Above a certain value, which may vary somewhat from laboratory to laboratory but is in the range of 200–300 ng/ml, an elevated serum prolactin level indicates a pituitary tumor with essentially 100 percent certainty, whatever the x-rays may show.

Time of Day When the Sample Is Drawn

It is well known that serum prolactin levels rise during sleep. If a patient is awakened from sleep to have a blood specimen drawn, the value may be above the normal range. Less well known, though clearly apparent from the first studies that were done, is the fact that serum prolactin does not decline to true baseline levels until at least 2 hours after waking. If there is doubt about a mildly elevated value, therefore, it may be worthwhile to find out when the sample was drawn, and to consider obtaining another sample at some time in the middle of the day.

Stress

Stress, including psychologic stress, is a well-documented cause of hyperprolactinemia in humans as well as in experimental animals. In my experience, however, the normal anxieties associated with illness and hospitalization cause little, if any, increase in serum prolactin. One should therefore be wary of attributing otherwise unexplained persistent elevations of the hormone to stress.

Transient Elevated Values

Prolactin, like other pituitary hormones, is secreted episodically. Occasionally a transiently elevated value may be encountered, perhaps as a result of a brief secretory peak, which is not confirmed on subsequent testing. Mild elevations—indeed, all elevations that are unexpected—should lead to repeat testing to rule out this factor as well as the ever present possibility of laboratory error.

Laboratory Variation

Different laboratories may have slightly different standards of what constitutes the normal range of serum prolactin. In addition, the prolactin radioimmunoassay is subject to somewhat greater disturbance and error than that for growth hormone. This is probably due to the greater likelihood of prolactin damage from both iodination and prolonged storage. The latter factor may cause the solutions used to calibrate the standard curve, if kept frozen for long periods of time, to lose immunoactivity. This will result in falsely high readings on serum specimens. Furthermore, because of alteration in the molecular form of either the standards or the circulating prolactin itself, serial dilution of the serum specimen may yield a curve that does not parallel that of the standard. Typically, assays carried out at higher dilutions may result in higher values than those done at lower dilutions. It is important to be sure that the laboratory is a reliable one with considerable experience in prolactin radioimmunoassays and a reasonably high weekly volume of determinations. Small hospital laboratories are unreliable and probably should not do these assays.

Abnormal Forms of Circulating Prolactin

Circulating prolactin is heterogeneous and includes some immunoactive material of high molecular weight which has reduced biologic activity as determined by receptor assay. On rare occasions one may encounter apparent hyperprolactinemia in an otherwise normal subject who has a greater than usual proportion of circulating high molecular

weight material but does not exhibit any clinical signs associated with excess prolactin. The frequency of such occurrences is probably not great, but it is not known with certainty because of the difficulty of doing serum fractionation and receptor assays.

In summary, "undefined" hyperprolactinemia implies a disturbance of hypothalamic or pituitary function even though no etiologic agent can be assigned; although by definition there is no evidence of pituitary tumor, the presence of the latter must always remain a possibility.

SHOULD HYPERPROLACTINEMIA BE TREATED? ARGUMENTS IN FAVOR OF TREATMENT

The availability of powerful prolactin-lowering drugs reinforces the natural impulse—present to some extent in all physicians—to correct an abnormality once it has been discovered. There are good arguments for as well as against treating hyperprolactinemia. In some cases the decision is clear-cut, in others doubtful. In doubtful cases my preference is generally not to treat. In the discussion that follows, however, the arguments in favor of treatment will be given first.

Restoration of Fertility

Without question the single most compelling reason to treat undefined hyperprolactinemia is to restore fertility, provided the latter is desired. The mechanisms by which hyperprolactinemia interferes with the normal functioning of the hypothalamic-pituitary-gonadal axis are still not completely understood. Nevertheless, there is a very high likelihood that reduction of serum prolactin to, or very close to, the normal range will result in restoration of menses in hyperprolactinemic, amenorrheic, premenopausal women. The menses so induced will be ovulatory in the great majority of cases, and the use of bromocriptine or similar drugs to achieve fertility represents a signal advance over the use of gonadotropins, since bromocriptine carries with it no increased risk of inducing multiple pregnancies or the ovarian hyperstimulation syndrome. There is also no evidence to date that bromocriptine causes any increased incidence of fetal abnormalities or of gestational difficulties. In men, hyperprolactinemia is a less frequent cause of infertility than it is in women, and its correction may be less likely to restore fertility. Nevertheless, there is no question that reduction of serum prolactin should be the first line of therapeutic approach in treating a hyperprolactinemic male who is suffering from impotence, oligospermia, or both.

Cessation of Galactorrhea

Galactorrhea of some degree is present in approximately two-thirds to three-quarters of women with hyperprolactinemia. In hyperprolactinemic men, by contrast, galactorrhea is much rarer, occurring in only 10 percent or so. Most women with galactorrhea are not seriously bothered by it, and in my experience the elimination of galactorrhea is seldom by itself a sufficient reason for instituting therapy. In some women, however, galactorrhea is sufficiently profuse to be a real nuisance. In such cases bromocriptine or a similar drug is the treatment of choice. Galactorrhea is not always totally eliminated, but it is almost invariably reduced to the point where it is no longer at all troublesome.

Restoration of Menses and Normalization of the Estrogenic Milieu—Prevention of Premature Osteoporosis in Women

Except when it seems indicated for psychologic reasons, there is no particular benefit in restoring menses per se in amenorrheic premenopausal women. Since the amenorrhea is usually associated with at least a mild state of hypoestrogenism, however, there may be some reason to correct the latter abnormality. Possible benefits include better maintenance of vaginal epithelium, and perhaps also better maintenance of skin texture and breast fullness, though abnormalities of the latter two are rarely evident. The strongest reason for wishing to restore a normal estrogenic milieu is the possible prevention of premature osteoporosis. A recent study has suggested that there is accelerated loss of calcium from the skeleton in hyperprolactinemic, amenorrheic, premenopausal women, and that restoration of menses by administration of bromocriptine may correct this abnormality. In my opinion, more study of this question is needed before confident recommendations can be made. Women differ considerably from one another in their susceptibility to postmenopausal osteoporosis, and the degree of hypoestrogenism in premenopausal amenorrhea is usually much less severe than that in the postmenopausal state. Evidence of pre-existing osteoporosis, documentation of excess calcium loss by appropriate means, perhaps a strong family history of postmenopausal osteoporosis, might all be reasons for favoring drug treatment of hyperprolactinemia in premenopausal women. It could be argued that a simpler and less expensive mode of treatment, in women who did not desire fertility, might be cyclic estrogen therapy. An objection to such a course could be the increased stimulus that might ensue to the growth of a hitherto undiscovered pituitary tumor. Also, the increased prolactin secretion that would probably result could conceivably synergize with the estrogens to produce an undesirable degree of breast hypertrophy. On the whole it seems preferable to avoid estrogen therapy in the face of unexplained hyperprolactinemia. The contraindication to estrogen use would be greater, naturally, if a pituitary tumor were actually demonstrable.

Restoration of Libido and Potency

An increase in libido and potency, occasionally greater than that obtainable with testosterone alone, is not infrequently seen in hyperprolactinemic men with pituitary tumors who are treated with ergot derivatives. Sometimes there is also a sense of increased general well-being, not clearly related to improved libido or potency. Although unexplained hyperprolactinemia, particularly of a degree likely to affect gonadal function, is less common in men than in women, it would be entirely appropriate to try ergot drug therapy in such a situation if diminished libido or potency were present. Passing mention should be made of the fact, not often discussed in the literature, that women with hyperprolactinemia may also suffer from diminished libido. Increased libido may accompany return of menses, and this may constitute a rationale for drug therapy, at least on a trial basis, independent of the aim of restoring fertility.

Possible Prevention of the Development or Growth of a Pituitary Tumor

Small, unrecognized pituitary adenomas may be present in some patients with unexplained hyperprolactinemia, or may emerge during a period of observation. Since ergot drugs are known to shrink some prolactinomas and probably inhibit the growth of most, a rationale might be made for the use of these drugs as preventive therapy. I believe the risks of developing a tumor in patients with undefined hyperprolactinemia, as well as the character of such tumors themselves once developed, are not sufficiently threatening to warrant long-term use of ergot derivatives on an essentially preventive basis in cases in which no tumor can be demonstrated.

ARGUMENTS AGAINST TREATMENT OF UNDEFINED HYPERPROLACTINEMIA

The chief argument against treating undefined hyperprolactinemia is the lack of evidence that it is in any way harmful, aside from the possible disturbances of gonadal function already referred to. Specifically, there is no indication as yet that long-term hyperprolactinemia is associated with any increase in the incidence of breast cancer or other neoplasms, or with any significant metabolic abnormalities. Normalization of serum prolactin per se is therefore not a therapeutic goal to be striven for.

A second argument against treatment is that undefined hyperprolactinemia may disappear spontaneously. I am aware of several such cases, including one of a girl in her late teens with primary amenorrhea whose prolactin went gradually from 130 to 17 ng/ml over a 2-year period with the spontaneous onset of normal menses toward the end of that time. It should also be mentioned that even when there is evidence of an accompanying pituitary tumor, hyperprolactinemia may sometimes spontaneously resolve in a gradual fashion not suggestive of pituitary apoplexy, and that this may be accompanied either by lack of evidence of progression of the tumor, or in a few cases by actual regression in size of the tumor. The mechanisms by which this occurs are not known. There is evidence that a few cases of sella turcica enlargement interpreted as tumor actually represent hyperplasia. The latter may be dependent on a hypothalamic disturbance, either lack of normal inhibition or excess of stimulation, which in some cases may be a transitory phenomenon.

There are three additional reasons against treatment, aside from the known side effects of the drugs. First, there is the possibility of new, currently unrecognized side effects of ergot derivatives emerging after prolonged treatment, in a manner somewhat similar to the late appearance of tardive dyskinesia after chronic treatment with neuroleptic drugs. To date there is no evidence to suggest such a phenomenon, even after periods of treatment with bromocriptine of up to ten years. Second is the fact that to be effective, treatment, must be chronic; whatever the etiology of the hyperprolactinemia, it tends to return as soon as drug therapy is withdrawn. Third is the matter of expense. Bromocriptine, the only currently approved effective drug, is relatively expensive, and at high dosage levels may become prohibitively so.

For the majority of patients with undefined hyperprolactinemia, I believe that no treatment is indicated except for the special situations previously discussed. The physician should measure the serum prolactin levels at intervals of a few months to a year or so, depending on the elevation of the hormone and the apparent stability of the pattern. He or she should also check the skull x-rays, preferably by CT scan, at somewhat less frequent intervals, particularly if a rising prolactin level suggests a change in pattern or the possible growth of a hitherto inapparent tumor.

TREATMENT OF HYPERPROLACTINEMIA: THE USE OF ERGOT DERIVATIVES

The only drugs of proven clinical effectiveness in the treatment of hyperprolactinemia are the ergot derivatives, and the only one currently available on prescription in the United States is bromocriptine (Parlodel, Sandoz). Several similar drugs are currently under investigation, and at least one of these (pergolide mesylate) may have certain advantages in terms of longer duration of action and possibly, if marketed, lower cost.

Treatment with bromocriptine is usually initiated by giving one 2.5-mg tablet accompanied by a snack at bedtime. Under these circumstances nausea is usually not a severe problem. Beginning the next morning, the patient may start on a dosage schedule of 2.5 mg twice a day. Nausea, if present, usually disappears soon after treatment is begun, and may be minimized by taking the medication with food. If nausea is unusually severe, the starting dose may be lowered to 1.25 mg, given only once a day for a few days before building up to a dose of 2.5 mg b.i.d. Mild postural hypotension occurs not infrequently, and about 1 percent of patients may experience an unusually severe form of postural hypotension after the first dose only, which does not occur to the same degree after subsequent doses. Like nausea, postural hypotension tends to disappear with continued treatment. Other side effects encountered in a minority (less than 20 percent) of patients are, in order of decreasing frequency: headache, dizziness, fatigue, abdominal cramps, lightheadedness, vomiting, nasal stuffiness, constipation, and diarrhea.

About 5 percent of patients find they cannot tolerate the drug because of one or more side effects, chiefly nausea. Treatment with bromocriptine is contraindicated in patients with schizophrenia and it should be used with care when given together with other blood pressure lowering medications.

After a week or two of therapy the serum prolactin level should be measured again; if lowering of prolactin is insufficient, the dose of bromocriptine may be raised to 2.5 mg 3 times a day, or even higher. A total dosage of 7.5 mg/day, however, can be expected to be effective in the great majority of patients with undefined hyperprolactinemia.

ACROMEGALY

PHILLIP GORDEN, M.D.
ELI GLATSTEIN, M.D.
and JESSE ROTH, M.D.

Acromegaly results from persistent hypersecretion of human growth hormone (HGH). When the disorder occurs prior to epiphyseal fusion it is referred to as gigantism. In both cases the disease results from hypersecretion of HGH from the pituitary gland; no cases of ectopically produced HGH have been clearly documented. Various pituitary disorders associated with acromegaly are listed in Table 1. Since macroadenoma is the pre-

TABLE 1 Pituitary Disorders Associated with Acromegaly*

Macroadenoma: ~85–90% of cases
Microadenoma:~10–15% of cases
Pituitary hyperplasia: rare†

*Acromegaly may occur as a part of multiple endocrine adenomatosis (type I), associated with carcinoid tumors and ectopic ACTH secretion or in association with other syndromes of multiple endocrine neoplasia associated with testicular tumors.

†This occurs in association with islet cell and other extrasellar tumors and presumably results from the release of a growth hormone releasing factor from the tumor. The distinction between hyperplasia and adenoma may be difficult or impossible.

dominant lesion, the sella is enlarged in acromegaly in 85 to 90 percent of patients.

Growth hormone action on cartilage and the skeletal system is mediated by an insulinlike growth factor known as IGF-I or somatomedin C. While some patients with large non-islet cell tumors and hypoglycemia may have "acromegaloid features," this is not usually a problem in the differential diagnosis of acromegaly. Thus for the purpose of this discussion, we will consider only therapeutic modalities directed against hypersecretion of HGH from the pituitary gland.

CLINICAL AND LABORATORY DIAGNOSIS

The acral and soft tissue features of the disease are well known; these include the typical facies, large hands and feet, a history of excessive or inappropriate sweating, lack of stamina, and pain and parethesias in the distal extremity. In women amenorrhea is common, and in both men and women hypopituitarism may be a prominent manifestation of the disease. Other features that should be sought are hyperglycemia, hypertension, hypercalciuria, arthritis, and cardiac dysfunction. Since the mean duration of the disease, as determined historically, is on the order of ten years before diagnosis, the clinical features are usually well established and the diagnosis can be made without elaborate testing.

The most important laboratory test is the measurement of human growth hormone by radioimmunoassay. The HGH concentration should be persistently above 5 ng/ml and not suppressible below this level by oral glucose (that is > 5 ng/ml 2 hours after the oral administration of 100 gm of glucose). Elevated concentrations of somatomedin-C/IGF-I may also be used to confirm the diagnosis. This test is expensive, however, and offers no important advantage over the growth hormone measurements with respect to follow-up examination. Studies that should be carried out prior to therapy are listed in Table 2.

THERAPEUTIC MODALITIES

Therapy is directed against two features of acromegaly: the pituitary tumor, its capacity to extend out of the sella, producing visual impairment or other mass effects; and the elevated concentration of HGH.

TABLE 2 Laboratory Studies that Should Be Performed Prior to Therapy

Hematology

Immunoassay of HGH in basal resting state (preferably upon arising in a.m.)
Immunoassay of HGH 2 hours after 100 g or oral glucose
Somatomedin-C/IGF-I (optional)
Serum calcium, phosphate, and creatinine
Blood glucose
Prolactin
LH, FSH, estradiol, and testosterone
TSH, T_4, T_3, and free T_4
Serum cortisol

Radiology

Skull films
CT* scan of pituitary
Chest x-ray for heart size
Films of large joints

Urinalysis

24-hour calcium and creatinine concentration

*Computed tomography

Three different therapeutic modalities are in general use, including irradiation of several types, transsphenoidal microsurgery, and pharmacologic agents (Table 3). Irradiation and transphenoidal surgery are the most widely used primary forms of therapy. If we define an ideal therapy as one that eliminates the pituitary tumor and the attendant hypersecretion of HGH in a uniformly effective, totally safe fashion and without risk of hypopituitarism, then none of the currently available modes of therapy is ideal. Since at the NIH most

TABLE 3 Therapeutic Modalities in Acromegaly

Irradiation

Conventional supervoltage, generally available
Heavy particle, available only in Berkeley, California
Proton beam, available only in Boston, Massachusetts

Surgical

Transphenoidal microsurgery, available in most large medical centers

Pharmocologic

2-bromo-α-ergocryptine (Parlodel), generally available but not specifically approved for use in acromegaly
Estrogen, generally available but high degree of side effects

of our experience relates to the evaluation of conventional supervoltage irradiation, we will describe in detail how this is carried out and discuss the results of this form of therapy against the other methods of treating acromegaly.

Conventional Supervoltage Irradiation as Administered at the Clinical Center of the National Institutes of Health

Because acromegaly tends to be associated with relatively modest-sized pituitary neoplasms, tumor volumes of 5 to 6 cm are typically adequate to encompass the area. However, in those patients who have computerized axial tomography (CT) evidence of significant suprasellar extension, or who have tomographic evidence of extension into the sphenoid sinus, more generous fields may be required. Confidence in tumor localization will permit the construction of relatively small tumor volumes, since histologically benign tumors, such as eosinophilic or chromophobic adenomas, do not require the same generous margins to account for infiltration that are generally necessary in the radiation treatment of most malignant tumors.

Technically, the equipment required for modern treatment of the pituitary region includes a simulator and a megavoltage radiotherapy unit with rotational isocentric capability. The simulator is essential to set up the radiotherapy portals in such a way that the tumor volume is consistently within all treatment portals but the eyes are carefully excluded from the radiation beams. Since radiation is both attenuating and diverging as it transverses tissue, special care with respect to the eyes must be taken before radiation is actually delivered.

An essential element in the arrangement of the radiation portals is absolute immobilization of the patient's head during treatment. This will usually require a head board when the patient is recumbent, or a bite block that has been customized the fit the patient's teeth, or both.

Beam direction and field size are established by simulation. This process refers to a mock-up procedure that will duplicate everything to be done in the treatment room, except that a diagnostic x-ray beam is used rather than a megavoltage beam. Because of the preferential absorption according to atomic number, with a diagnostic, low-energy x-ray beam, radiologic detail can be seen in arranging the portals with a simulator film. Inasmuch as a megavoltage beam does not absorb according to atomic number, anatomic detail cannot be identified well by looking at megavoltage films. A headboard is used to elevate the neck and head at an angle of approximately 30° with respect to the top of the treatment couch. This elevation effectively moves the eyes out of the plane of axis of the rotating gantry, and thus allows the orbits to be excluded from the tumor volume of interest, not only for the entering photon beam, but also for the exiting photon beam. Fluoroscopy and image intensifiers help to visualize the field during simulation. When the patient is comfortably positioned on the headboard, we prefer to mark three separate points on the skin to serve as the definition of the critical plane for rotational arcing of the gantry. These three points are obtained by laser light markings that correspond to the isocenter from three separate directions, based on simulator imaging. This type of laser light system is available both in the simulation room and in the treatment room. Our general approach is to utilize 220° arcing or rotational field treatment. For very large lesions, we may resort to a three-field isocentric arrangement, utilizing two large wedged lateral fields and one anterior field.

Although any megavoltage beam is adequate to treat pituitary tumors, higher energies have more skin sparing and result in a more homogeneous radiation dosage across the central tumor volume than does ^{60}Co equipment. Accordingly, 6 to 15 MeV x-ray beams from a linear accelerator are probably optimal conventional energies for the treatment of pituitary lesions.

Because the pituitary region is central within the skull, and because the skull is curving in several different planes, a wedge of approximately 45° is commonly employed in the treatment of pituitary tumors to compensate for the sloping contours of the skull. We prefer a 220° arcing rotational field in the coronal plane, above the level of the orbits, as advocated by Kramer and colleagues. We utilize a 45° wedge starting counterclockwise at the lowest edge of the treatment field (from an approximately 200° angle), with the thick edge of the wedge pointed upward toward the top of the skull; as the gantry rotates to the vertex (90°), the treatment is stopped and the wedge is rotated 180° so that the thick edge of the wedge will ultimately point downward as the arc resumes. The treatment is then continued to complete a 220 arc (to −20°). If a three-field isocentric treatment plan is used, wedges are used on the two lateral fields to optimize their integration with the anterior field by eliminating any hot spot. Opposing lateral fields as the sole means of treatment of the pituitary are not recommended, inasmuch as they imply that higher doses will be delivered to the temporal lobes of the brain than will be received by the pituitary region itself, and thus potentially predispose to neurologic injury.

The dose that is recommended is 4500–5000 rads over 5 to 6 weeks. Treatment delivery is 5 days a week at the rate of 180 rads a day. The total tumor dose to the volume in question does not exceed 5000 rads over 6 weeks, thereby eliminating most of the major complications of radiation therapy resulting from the pituitary treatment. It is important to realize that most of the radiation injury reported from the treatment of pituitary tumors is seen either following doses in excess of 5000 rads or when similar doses of radiation have been delivered in very short periods of time, rather than at the rate of 180 rads per day. If the treatment has been properly planned and well administered, the major complications should be negligible, since the major areas of risk (other than the pituitary region itself) should be outside the high-dose tumor volume.

Results of Conventional Supervoltage Irradiation

The mean concentration of HGH in our patients prior to therapy is 60 ng/ml (range 5–280 ng/ml). The mean percentage fall in HGH is 52 percent up to two years after irradiation and 77 percent by five to ten years after treatment. While the major fall in HGH concentration occurs between two and five years, there is a more gradual decline in hormone concentration up to ten years after treatment. In terms of absolute concentration of HGH, values of ≤ 5 ng/ml are achieved in 42 percent of patients at 5 years and in 69 percent of patients 10 years after therapy. Values of ≤ 10 ng/ml are achieved in 73 percent at 5 years and 81 percent at 10 years after therapy. Similar results are obtained in patients who have undergone unsuccessful surgical therapy prior to irradiation.

Changes in skeletal features are difficult to document objectively, but as best we can determine, they remain stable or moderately improved. It must be remembered that if the disease has been present for a significant period prior to therapy, many of the features of the disease are not reversible.

None of the patients developed clinical signs or symptoms of extrasellar extension after irradiation. In approximately 75 percent of patients with headaches prior to therapy there was improvement in symptoms, but in about 10 percent of patients without headaches prior to treatment, headaches ensued. There is a significant decrease in serum phosphorus and in both basal glucose values and glucose tolerance.

With regard to untoward effects, one patient developed a transient visual field cut 3 months after irradiation; a second patient, however, 18 months after therapy developed severe bitemporal field defects and dementia. Though the patient had CNS sarcoidosis in addition to acromegaly, we attribute this defect to radiation necrosis. There are no predictors of this type of complication, which fortunately is exceedingly rare.

With respect to other pituitary dysfunction, there is a progressively increased incidence of hypopituitarism, so that by ten years after therapy approximately 19 percent of patients are hypothyroid, 38 percent hypoadrenal, and up to 50 percent hypogonadal. These figures take into account those patients who had hypopituitarism prior to treatment as well as the cumulative risk of hypopituitarism as a function of time. These figures include both the natural history of the pituitary tumor as well as the possible additive effect of irradiation on the induction of pituitary insufficiency.

An additional endocrinologic feature of acromegaly is that about one-third of patients have elevations of serum prolactin concentration. Since HGH has a biologic potency equivalent to prolactin, the sum of prolactin + HGH = total prolactin activity. Under these circumstances the total prolactinlike activity of plasma is elevated in the majority of acromegalic patients. Thus apparent hypogonadotropic hypogonadism can result from destruction of gonadotropin-producing cells or from inhibition of gonadotropin secretion secondary to total prolactin elevation. After pituitary irradiation, serum prolactin concentration tends to fall in those patients in whom it was initially elevated and to rise modestly over the first two years following therapy in those patients in whom it was normal or low.

Transsphenoidal Pituitary Microsurgery

With the rediscovery of transsphenoidal surgery and more recent advances in microsurgical techniques, there is considerable enthusiasm for the use of this mode of therapy in the treatment of acromegaly. Our own experience has been limited in this form of treatment, but several generalizations can be made from the 7 to 8 papers that have reported on approximately 400 patients.

When therapy is successful the fall in HGH is immediate. Thus the cumulative results from all reports suggest that about 75 percent of patients will achieve normal HGH concentrations (that is < 5 ng/ml) following surgery. There are features of special note:

1. The results of treatment are stratified; patients with microadenoma do best and patients with infiltrating, erosive, and extrasellar tumors do worse.

2. Most surgical results are reported within days to weeks after treatment. It is now clear that some of these patients have recurrences over a longer period.

3. If hypopituitarism occurs, it is immediate.

4. The complications of surgery include a mortality rate that is now probably less than 1 percent overall, and morbidity that can include CSF rhinorrhea, meningitis, diabetes insipidus, and so on. These complications are relatively uncommon but are directly proportional to the size and erosive properties of the tumor and inversely proportional to the experience of the surgeon.

Proton Beam and Heavy Particle Irradiation

Proton beams and heavy particles offer two additional forms of irradiation therapy. The results of these forms of therapy are similar to those with conventional supervoltage irradiation; in addition, the complications and side effects of these therapeutic modalities are similar to those from supervoltage irradiation. For most patients, proton beam and heavy particle irradiation are roughly equivalent to conventional supervoltage therapy. The major advantage of the two former methods is that they can be completed in a few days, whereas supervoltage therapy requires several weeks. This must be balanced against the availability of supervoltage therapy in many centers around the world and the availability of heavy particle and proton beam therapy in only two centers in the United States.

Pharmacologic Therapy

An effective "pill" for the treatment of acromegaly is highly desirable. Many agents have been tried and most abandoned. For instance, high-dose estrogen (1 mg ethsinyl estradiol per day) may be useful for the treatment of selected features of acromegaly. These include hypercalciuria and hyperglycemia. The side effects of these high doses of estrogen, however, usually prohibit their use except in a few highly selective circumstances.

The most recently employed drug, 2-bromo-α-ergocryptine (Parlodel), has received a mixed review. While it is clear that this drug dramatically decreases prolactin in prolactinoma and in acromegaly, and in some instances actually decreases tumor size, its efficacy in decreasing HGH in acromegaly is controversial. While in a number of uncontrolled studies bromocriptine was found to decrease HGH concentration and produce symptomatic benefit, more recent controlled clinical trials have failed to demonstrate either reduction in HGH or symptomatic improvement.

It is our own tentative conclusion that bromocriptine in doses 2 to 3 times greater (that is 20–40 mg per day) than those used to treat prolactin excess decreases plasma HGH in as subpopulation of patients, approximately 30 percent of acromegalic patients. These patients cannot be prospectively identified, and if one elects a trial with this agent, patients must be carefully followed with frequent HGH determinations. If the physician feels that reduction of HGH has been achieved, the drug should be stopped so that the reduction can be further verified. The major problem in using this agent is that symptomatic improvement is hard to quantitate and relate to the specific drug without a placebo control, and the natural fluctuation of plasma HGH makes it difficult in some patients to demonstrate a sustained change in HGH concentration. The principal acute side effects of bromocriptine are gastrointestinal intolerance and postural hypotension.

Treatment of Special Features of Acromegaly

Hypopituitarism is a prominent feature of acromegaly either as a result of the pituitary tumor directly or indirectly or as a consequence of therapy. Replacement of thyroid hormone, adrenal steroids, testosterone in men, or estrogen in women should be given as described in other chapters.

Fasting hyperglycemia occurs in 10 to 15 percent of patients. If HGH is decreased by therapy the hyperglycemia is usually promptly decreased.

The microangiopathic features of diabetes rarely occur in acromegalic patients, but ketoacidosis can develop in some cases. If symptomatic hyperglycemia is present, insulin therapy should be instituted. These patients are typically insulin-resistant and require relatively large doses of insulin. If they are not resistant, hypopituitarism should be suspected.

Hypertension occurs in 20 to 30 percent of patients with acromegaly and should always be treated. Usually the hypertension can be effectively treated with typical antihypertensive drugs, such as diuretics and β-blockers.

THERAPEUTIC CHOICES

Situations in Which the Pituitary Tumor Is Dominant

In patients with major visual impairment or other manifestations of extrasellar extension of the tumor, the therapeutic decision must be made in collaboration with a neurosurgeon. Each case must be individualized. Usually surgery, and in some instances surgery plus irradiation, is required. Careful attention should be paid to associated hypopituitarism; hypothyroidism should be treated, as this may aggravate the situation. More recently it has been noted that bromocriptine therapy can, in some instances, actually reduce tumor size. This is especially true in prolactinoma. Reduction in tumor size is less clear in acromegaly, and it is possible for the drug to decrease HGH concentration while the tumor mass actually increases. If the physician elects to use bromocriptine to control the mass effect of the tumor, this should be done only under very close supervision of the patient and after more standard forms of therapy have failed.

Situations in Which the Elevated Concentration of HGH Is Dominant

This can be divided into at least two parts. First, are individual patients in whom it is deemed necessary to reduce the HGH concentration rapidly. This includes patients with congestive heart failure. While the relationship of acromegaly to the pathogenesis of a specific cardiomyopathy is unclear, it is clear that patients with acromegaly and coexistent heart disease, regardless of cause, do poorly. Thus management of coexistent heart disease and possibly severe hypertension is facilitated by successful treatment of acromegaly. Other situations include arthritis and joint fixation. This is relatively uncommon in acromegaly, and it is not clear whether, once the arthritic process is established, treatment of the acromegaly ameliorates the arthritis. Nevertheless, severe arthritis represents an indication for rapidly decreasing the HGH concentration. In some patients there may be a sense of urgency because of the severity of symptoms, for example, sweating, loss of stamina, renal stones and hypercalciuria, etc. In instances in which it is deemed necessary to decrease HGH concentration rapidly, transsphenoidal microsurgery is the treatment of choice. If it is unsuccessful, irradiation should be given.

Second, the typical acromegalic patient is one who is middle-aged, has had the disease for ten years or longer at the time of diagnosis, and is only moderately symptomatic. At present, therapeutic choices for this type of patient are made by regional preference and expertise. There is no available information that tells us whether one therapy or another is beneficial with respect to longevity; we cannot even be certain whether rapid reduction in HGH is beneficial with respect to morbidity. The therapeutic dilemma for the majority of patients is as follows: Conventional supervoltage irradiation produces a consistent but slow reduction in HGH; this is independent of the size of the pituitary tumor or its erosive properties. In most instances the pituitary tumor is stabilized, and over a period of five to ten years the growth hormone concentrations return to normal in about 75 percent of patients. Those who do exceptionally well cannot be identified in advance. If a patient has a very large pituitary tumor and HGH concentration > 100 ng/ml, it is less likely that this patient will achieve a normal growth hormone concentration. There is less morbidity with irradiation than with surgery.

Transsphenoidal microsurgery will reduce HGH rapidly in about 75 percent of patients, at least in the hands of the most experienced surgeons. The results are stratified, that is, microadenomas do best and erosive and expansive tumors worst. The mortality rate is probably < 1 percent, and morbidity is clearly greater than that from irradiation and includes acute hypopituitarism. Thus once the patient and his physician understand the risks of surgery, they must also understand there is a one in four chance that results will not be satisfactory and that some fraction of those with an immediate satisfactory result will suffer recurrences.

In summary, there are two clear options open for therapy. Decisions must be made on an individual basis. If one elects surgery, then irradiation can be used if surgery is not successful. The decision can also be made the other way around, irradiation first and surgical intervention at a later date, if necessary. At present, bromocriptine therapy should be used only for those patients in whom irradiation, surgery or both has been unsuccessful. In selected cases it may be used as an adjunct to irradiation to achieve a more rapid reduction in HGH. It should be monitored closely, however, and discontinued if efficacy cannot be shown by reduction in plasma HGH concentration.

INAPPROPRIATE TSH SECRETION

IONE A. KOURIDES, M.D.

Inappropriate thyrotropin (TSH) secretion can be defined as TSH hypersecretion in the presence of high circulating levels of thyroid hormones (T_4 and/or T_3). Not only must the total concentration of thyroid hormones (bound to thyroid binding proteins) be elevated, but also the free or unbound thyroid hormone levels must be increased. This definition eliminates disorders caused by increased thyroid binding proteins from further consideration. Moreover, patients with elevated thyroid hormone levels and detectable levels of immunoactive TSH can be considered to have inappropriate TSH secretion even if the concentration falls within the "normal" range (0.5–3.5 µU/ml). This is true because all other forms of hyperthyroidism except pituitary hypersecretion of TSH are characterized by a suppressed serum concentration of TSH (< 0.5 µU/ml) in a highly sensitive and specific TSH radioimmunoassay.

Patients with inappropriate TSH secretion can be separated into two major groups: patients with TSH secreting pituitary tumors and those with a non-neoplastic disorder. The patients with the non-neoplastic disorder all have pituitary thyrotroph resistance, and some also have variable degrees of peripheral resistance to the action of thyroid hormone. Isolated pituitary resistance is associated with clinical hyperthyroidism, but generalized resistance to thyroid hormones may be associated with no apparent problem except a goiter. However, when these latter patients are found to have elevated thyroid hormone levels and a goiter, their inappropriate treatment with antithyroid drugs can cause hypothyroidism. A brief summary of the laboratory and clinical findings in these syndromes is presented in Table 1.

THERAPY

Since the therapies for TSH secreting pituitary tumors and for non-neoplastic TSH hypersecretion are completely different, these disorders will be dealt with separately.

TSH Secreting Pituitary Tumors

Once this diagnosis has been made, based on radiography and the criteria shown in Table 1, treatment should be directed at the tumor itself. Patients with TSH secreting pituitary tumors have to date been identified only when they have large tumors, probably because they have often been previously misdiagnosed as having conventional hyperthyroidism (Graves' disease or a toxic nodular goiter). Thus surgery or radiotherapy directed at the pituitary tumor is appropriate therapy, either because of compression of the residual normal pi-

tuitary and subsequent destruction of its hormonal function, or because of impairment of vision due to compression of the optic nerve tracts. Moreover, pituitary tumor TSH hypersecretion tends to respond poorly to most medications that normally decrease TSH secretion. For example, almost no patient with a TSH secreting pituitary tumor has demonstrated decreased TSH secretion after treatment with exogenous thyroid hormone. In addition, these patients are already thyrotoxic and thus can potentially develop worsening signs and symptoms of hyperthyroidism after such treatment. Patients with TSH secreting pituitary tumors are usually more than 50 years of age and consequently less likely to be able to tolerate prolonged hyperthyroidism.

Pituitary tumor TSH secretion also most often appears to be autonomous when other agents capable of decreasing TSH secretion have been tested. Somatostatin and dopamine agonists, such as bromergocriptine, rarely decrease TSH secretion or improve the hyperthyroidism in patients with TSH secreting pituitary tumors. Although somatostatin can decrease non-neoplastic TSH secretion, it has minimal effects on neoplastic TSH secretion. Moreover, it can be administered only by continuous intravenous infusion, making it a highly impractical therapeutic modality even if it were effective. Bromergocriptine can decrease non-neoplastic TSH hypersecretion, but it has rarely been effective when tested in patients with TSH secreting pituitary tumors. We have used bromergocriptine in an attempt to treat only one

TABLE 1 Laboratory and Clinical Findings in Patients with Inappropriate TSH Secretion

	Thyroid Hormone Levels	Serum TSH (µU/ml)	TSH Response to TRH	Alpha Subunit (ng/ml)	Metabolic Status
TSH secreting pituitary tumors	↑	> 0.5	0	> 2.5 (> 9 postmenopausal women)	Hyperthyroid
Isolated pituitary resistance to thyroid hormones	↑	> 0.5	↑	< 2.5 (< 9 postmenopausal women)	Hyperthyroid
Generalized resistance to thyroid hormones	↑	> 0.5	↑	< 2.5 (< 9 postmenopausal women)	Euthyroid or hypothyroid
Conventional hyperthyroidism (Graves' disease or nodular goiter)	↑	< 0.5	0	< 2.5 (< 9 postmenopausal women)	Hyperthyroid
Normal	normal	0.5–3.5	↑	< 2.5 (< 9 postmenopausal women)	Euthyroid

patient with a TSH secreting pituitary tumor, and it was completely ineffective in decreasing either TSH or alpha subunit (of TSH) secretion. On the other hand, TSH secretion from a pituitary tumor will decrease after the administration of high doses of glucocorticoids. We have previously shown that TSH hypersecretion will decrease after dexamethasone administration (2–4 mg orally every 6 hours), whether the TSH hypersecretion is caused by primary thyroid gland failure, a TSH secreting pituitary tumor, or non-neoplastic inappropriate TSH secretion. Not only will TSH secretion decrease, but the increased alpha subunit secretion also will decrease. In fact, in one patient with an extensive TSH secreting pituitary tumor who was not cured by surgery or radiotherapy, glucocorticoids were used both to control tumor compression of normal tissue and the TSH hypersecretion by the tumor.

Therapy directed at the thyroid gland, such as radioactive iodine or thionamide antithyroid drugs, may control the hyperthyroidism, but it will do nothing to stop the progression of the TSH secreting pituitary tumor. Patients have inadvertently been treated with ^{131}I because of a mistaken diagnosis of primary thyroid disease or purposefully treated with thionamide antithyroid drugs (in the United States methimazole or propylthiouracil) to control the signs or symptoms of hyperthyroidism prior to pituitary surgery.

The only definitive therapy for TSH secreting pituitary tumors is either surgery, selective adenomectomy, and/or radiotherapy directed at the pituitary tumor. Surgery has usually been performed via a transsphenoidal approach; however, for large tumors a transfrontal approach has occasionally been used (Table 2). Although an attempt to remove only the pituitary tumor is made, partial or complete hypopituitarism is a possible result of the therapy. Complete anterior pituitary hormone function should therefore be tested several weeks postoperatively. Patients with TSH secreting pituitary tumors may be given large doses of glucocorticoids in the perioperative period; such patients may also have received thionamide antithyroid drugs prior to surgery to control the hyperthyroidism. Both medications should be tapered and then stopped prior to testing anterior pituitary gland function postoperatively. Diabetes insipidus may well occur immediately after surgery, but it is unlikely to be a persistent problem. If patients cannot meet their urinary output by oral intake of fluids, vasopressin injections may be used temporarily until endogenous vasopressin secretion has recovered. The most relevant parameters to follow to determine the success of surgery are of course regression of hyperthyroidism and normalization of the serum TSH level.

Sometimes pituitary surgery alone is inadequate to control the TSH induced hyperthyroidism or remove the pituitary tumor, in which case conventional radiotherapy is often added, usually in a dose of approximately 4500 rads. Radiotherapy alone could be used in patients who are a poor surgical risk although few patients have been treated only with radiotherapy so the radiosensitivity of these tumors has not been definitively established. It is important to point out that these tumors may recur after both pituitary surgery and irradiation, sometimes with hyperthyroidism and sometimes with no evidence of increased TSH secretion or hyperthyroidism. However, in the latter instances, serum alpha subunit (of TSH) is usually elevated; serum alpha may be the most sensitive indicator of either recurrence or residual pituitary tumor.

Resistance to Thyroid Hormone

Since the mechanism for both the pituitary and the peripheral resistance to thyroid hormones has not yet been elucidated, patients with the non-neoplastic disorder present a greater therapeutic dilemma. Binding of thyroid hormones to nuclear receptors in accessible tissues, such as circulating mononuclear cells and skin fibroblasts, has been studied in a number of these patients with generalized resistance. Nuclear binding of thyroid hormones has usually been normal. If mononuclear cells and fibroblasts are representative of resistant tissues, then the thyroid hormone resistance appears to be a postreceptor defect. Moreover, in the few patients studied with TSH hypersecretion, there does not appear to be a defect in the monodeiodination of T_4 to T_3. If exogenous T_4 or T_3 is given to patients with non-neoplastic TSH hypersecretion, both thyroid hormones will cause decreased TSH secretion, although the TSH secretion is not completely suppressed, as it would be in a normal individual with high circulating thyroid hormone levels.

Patients with generalized resistance to thyroid hormones should not be treated with thionamide antithyroid drugs, since such therapy may make the patient hypothyroid, further increase TSH secretion, and increase goiter size. Because there is at least a theoretic risk that prolonged TSH hypersecretion can lead to thyrotroph hyperplasia and

TABLE 2   Therapy for Inappropriate TSH Secretion

	Treatment	Effects
TSH secreting pituitary tumors	Pituitary adenomectomy and/or radiotherapy	Hypopituitarism and/or diabetes insipidus
	Antithyroid drugs prior to surgery	Control hyperthyroidism
	Glucocorticoids if inoperable	Decrease TSH and tumor compression
Isolated pituitary resistance to thyroid hormones	Therapy directed at the thyroid gland (antithyroid drugs, radioactive iodine, subtotal thyroidectomy)	Increase TSH secretion, increase goiter size, possible recurrent hyperthyroidism
	Propranolol	Block thyroid hormone action peripherally
	Exogenous T_3	Decrease TSH secretion, shrink goiter, may make hyperthyroidism worse
	Bromergocryptine	Decrease TSH secretion, decrease goiter size, alleviate hyperthyroidism
Generalized resistance to thyroid hormones	Exogenous T_4 or T_3	Decrease TSH hypersecretion, reduce goiter size

eventually to the development of a TSH secreting pituitary adenoma, these patients should rather be treated with agents that decrease TSH secretion. The exogenous administration of either T_4 or T_3 may be useful in these patients because they have peripheral resistance (Table 2). As long as the peripheral resistance exceeds the pituitary resistance, the patient will not become hyperthyroid, but TSH secretion will decrease, as will the thyroid gland enlargement. A judicious trial of increasing doses of either T_4 (starting with 0.1 mg p.o. daily) or T_3 (starting with 25 μg p.o. daily) may be beneficial. Success can be evaluated by "normalization" of the serum TSH level and goiter size. Although the TSH concentration will decrease into the normal range (0.5–3.5 μU/ml), it is important to remember that it is still inappropriately elevated in relationship to the high circulating thyroid hormone levels.

The patient with selective pituitary resistance but peripheral sensitivity to thyroid hormone is the most difficult to treat (Table 2). Since such patients do have evidence of hyperthyroidism, it is not unreasonable to direct therapy at the thyroid gland. Thionamide antithyroid drugs (propylthiouracil or methimazole) or radioactive iodine will decrease thyroid hormone levels. However, pituitary TSH hypersecretion will then increase, with the potential risk of the development of a pituitary tumor; moreover, goiter size may increase. A subtotal thyroidectomy will also cause increased TSH secretion and possibly recurrent hyperthyroidism in the residual thyroid tissue. Propranolol may be useful in blocking the peripheral effects of thyroid hormone excess in patients with peripheral sensi-

tivity to thyroid hormone; propranolol can be used in a dose of 10 to 40 mg p.o. every 6 hours. The side effects of propranolol are the same as those observed when propranolol is used to treat other conditions: slow pulse, hypotension, feeling faint, and so forth.

What is needed in the treatment of selective pituitary resistance to thyroid hormone is an agent that will decrease both the TSH hypersecretion and the high thyroid hormone levels. As has been mentioned, somatostatin will decrease the TSH secretion, but it cannot currently be used therapeutically because it has to be given by continuous intravenous infusion. Glucocorticoids will also decrease the TSH secretion, but the potential side effects of pharmacologic doses of glucocorticoids outweigh their benefit in reducing TSH secretion. One group of investigators has suggested that 25 or 50 μg of T_3 p.o. daily in a single dose can be used to decrease TSH secretion and thus to cause subsequent decreases in circulating T_4 and T_3, resulting in amelioration of the hyperthyroidism. Therapy with T_3 would probably work only in those patients who have relatively greater peripheral than pituitary resistance to thyroid hormone. Otherwise, the increase in circulating T_3 levels would acutely exacerbate the hyperthyroidism.

The dopamine agonist bromergocryptine appears to have the greatest potential to decrease both TSH secretion and, subsequently, thyroid hormone levels. Several groups of investigators are currently testing bromergocryptine in doses of 2.5 to 7.5 mg p.o. daily (usually given in divided doses twice a day) as therapy for patients with pituitary resistance to thyroid hormone. In one patient whom we have been treating with 2.5 mg of brom-ergocryptine p.o. twice daily, the serum TSH has "normalized" and thyroid gland size has dramatically decreased; however, thyroid hormone levels have not yet changed significantly. An evaluation of the utility of bromergocryptine in these patients should be available within a year or so. The side effects of bromergocryptine therapy include nausea, constipation, and postural hypotension. The drug should be therefore taken with food or at bedtime or both.

Increased awareness of the possibility of inappropriate TSH secretion has led to an increase in the number of patients recognized as having these syndromes. Any patient with elevated circulating thyroid hormone levels should have a serum TSH concentration measured to avoid inappropriate or unnecessary therapy.

FSH-SECRETING PITUITARY ADENOMAS

PETER J. SNYDER, M.D.

Pituitary adenomas that hypersecrete FSH are presumably adenomas of gonadotroph cells. Although normal gonadotroph cells secrete both FSH and LH, adenomas of gonadotroph cells that secrete only FSH are more common than those that secrete both FSH and LH or only LH. FSH-secreting adenomas have been recognized more commonly in men than in women; in men they constitute about 10 percent of all pituitary adenomas.

Because excessive secretion of FSH does not produce any signs or symptoms, FSH-secreting adenomas are generally not recognized clinically until they are very large. The spectrum of their clinical presentations is usually similar to that of other mass lesions originating within the sella turcica: neurologic manifestations, such as deterioration of vision and headache; and manifestations of hormonal deficiencies, including those of TSH, ACTH, and LH. The consequences of LH deficiency, via testosterone deficiency, are decreased libido, potency, and fertility, which seem ironic

in a patient who has a gonadotroph cell adenoma. If the adenoma secretes only FSH, however, and if it compresses the normal gonadotroph cells, LH secretion will diminish and, as a result, so will testosterone secretion. In fact, men who have FSH-secreting adenomas often have mild to moderate secondary hypogonadism.

The frequent occurrence of hypogonadism in these patients presents the only difficulty in differential diagnosis, because men who have primary hypogonadism of many years' duration may develop a large sella turcica, although generally not to the extent of suprasellar extension. In contrast to men who have an enlarged sella turcica as the result of longstanding primary hypogonadism, men who have an FSH-secreting pituitary adenoma will generally have a history of normal sexual development and fertility, normal virilization and testicular size, a basal serum LH concentration that is usually not elevated, even when the serum testosterone level is subnormal, and a marked increase in serum testosterone level after administration of human chorionic gonadotropin. Also in contrast to men who have primary hypogonadism, men who have FSH-secreting adenomas may have FSH responses to TRH, exaggerated LH responses to TRH, and higher FSH beta-subunit concentrations (Table 1).

Once the diagnosis of an FSH-secreting pituitary adenoma is made, therapeutic considerations are generally similar to those for other, large, pituitary adenomas.

SURGERY

Because FSH-secreting pituitary adenomas are usually not detected until they are very large and extend well above the sella and impair vision, as well as extend into the sphenoid sinus, surgical excision of as much of the adenoma mass as possible is often desirable to relieve compression of the optic chiasm rapidly. A comparison of treatments for these adenomas is found in Table 2.

Transsphenoidal Surgery

The preferred initial surgical procedure is transsphenoidal microsurgery, even though the adenoma usually extends above the sella turcica, because this procedure is less hazardous than approaching the pituitary via a transfrontal craniotomy, because the greater volume of the adenoma usually is within the sella, and because as

TABLE 1. Comparison of Characteristics of FSH-Secreting Pituitary Adenomas and Primary Hypogonadism

	FSH-Secreting Pituitary Adenoma	*Primary Hypogonadism*
Puberty	Normal	Often incomplete
Fertility history	Normal	Subnormal
Testicular size	Normal	Small
Serum testosterone	Low to normal	Low to normal
Testosterone response to HCG	Marked, to within normal range	Subnormal
Serum FSH	High	High
Serum LH	Usually normal	High if testosterone is low
FSH response to TRH	Present in 50% of patients	Absent
LH response to TRH	Exaggerated	Absent
FSH beta-subunit	Very high	High

soon as the intrasellar portion of the adenoma is excised, the suprasellar portion may drop into the sella so that it can also be excised during the transsphenoidal procedure.

The outcome of transsphenoidal pituitary surgery can be considered both neurologically and endocrinologically. Neurologically, the outcome in patients who have FSH-secreting adenomas is similar to that in patients who have transsphenoidal surgery for other large pituitary adenomas. The reduction in adenoma mass, while often not complete, is usually dramatically large, as judged by computerized tomographic (CT) scanning. Marked reduction in adenoma mass was seen by CT scanning in 10 of 11 patients who had transsphenoidal surgery for FSH-secreting pituitary adenomas at the Hospital of the University of Pennsylvania. Ten of these 11 patients had impaired vision before surgery, and 8 of the 10 had improvement in vision, both in fields of vision and visual acuity, after surgery. Improvement in vision, however, while occasionally dramatic, was usually of a lesser magnitude than the reduction in adenoma size by CT scanning. The more modest improvement in vision presumably reflects the irreversibility of some of the damage produced by optic chiasmal compression of many years' duration. Of the two patients who did not experience an improvement in vision following surgery, one had no change either in adenoma size by CT scan or in vision, but the other had a worsening of vision in spite of a decrease in adenoma mass. This worsening was likely the result of surgical damage to the optic chiasm and illustrates one of the neurologic complications of transsphenoidal surgery. Other neurologic complications include oculomotor nerve damage, hematoma formation, and CSF rhinorrhea, which predisposes to meningitis.

Endocrinologically, the outcome of transsphenoidal surgery is generally an improvement on many of the abnormalities present before surgery, but occasionally impairment of hormonal

TABLE 2 Comparison of Treatments for FSH-Secreting Pituitary Adenomas

Treatment	*Indications*	*Complications*
Transsphenoidal surgery	Intrasellar mass with suprasellar extension and severe impairment of vision	Worsening of vision, oculomotor palsy, diabetes insipidus, hypopituitarism, CSF rhinorrhea
Transfrontal surgery	Large, residual, symptomatic, suprasellar mass following transsphenoidal surgery	Worsening of vision, oculomotor palsy, hypothalamic and frontal lobe syndromes, diabetes insipidus, hypopituitarism
Radiotherapy	Intrasellar mass with only mild suprasellar extension and mild impairment of vision	Hypopituitarism, worsening of vision
Testosterone	Pituitary enlargement antedated by long-standing primary hypogonadism	Gynecomastia
Observation only	Adenoma confined to sella, patient elderly or infirm	

functions that had been normal before surgery. Ten of the 11 patients described above had a decrease in their initially elevated serum FSH concentrations to within the normal range following surgery; the only exception was the man who had no reduction in adenoma mass as seen by CT scan. FSH responses to TRH and exaggerated LH responses to TRH are also generally reduced following surgery, and also generally in proportion to the amount of pituitary tissue removed. The serum testosterone concentration is usually unchanged or somewhat lower following surgery, but occasionally it may be increased from subnormal to well within the normal range, indicating that removal of the gonadotroph cell adenoma may relieve pressure on the normal gonadotroph cells and allow recovery of their function.

Pituitary hormonal function that is normal before surgery usually remains normal afterward as well, but excision of normal pituitary tissue should be recognized as an occasional complication of transsphenoidal surgery. Hypothyroidism, hypocortisolism, and even hypogonadism may occur after surgery. Diabetes insipidus may also occur and, although ususally transient, may be permanent.

Local complications of transsphenoidal surgery include obstruction to the nasal passages requiring surgical correction, and persistent sinusitis.

Transfrontal Craniotomy

If transsphenoidal surgery is not successful in removing a sufficient amount of pituitary tissue to relieve compression of the optic chiasm or to relieve other neurologic symptoms caused by suprasellar extension of the adenoma, excision via a transfrontal craniotomy should be considered. The frequency and severity of significant neurologic complications, however, including oculomotor palsies and hypothalamic and frontal lobe syndromes, are greater with this type of procedure than with transsphenoidal surgery. The most common endocrinologic complication of this approach is diabetes insipidus, and deficiencies of any of the anterior pituitary hormones can be produced as well.

Postoperative Management

Management of the patient following surgery is similar whether the surgery has been transsphenoidal or transfrontal. In the immediate postoper-

ative period diabetes insipidus should be looked for and treated, if present, with aqueous vasopressin. If diabetes insipidus persists until the time of discharge from the hospital, desmopressin acetate should be prescribed for outpatient management (see Chapter 1). The pharmacologic doses of glucocorticoids used during the perioperative period should be decreased by the time of discharge to a maintenance dosage of hydrocortisone for outpatient use. No other hormonal medications need be given at this time. Prior to discharge, CT scan and determinations of fields of vision and visual acuity should be repeated.

Approximately six weeks after surgery, pituitary function, including serum concentrations of FSH, LH, testosterone, and thyroxine, and ACTH reserve should be tested. On the basis of these tests and the postoperative CT scan and vision, the needs for further surgery or radiation (described below) and for hormonal replacement are determined. Subsequent tests of adenoma size and pituitary function should be made in six months and then yearly.

RADIATION

Radiation therapy for FSH-secreting pituitary adenomas should be considered in several situations, because these adenomas are generally radiosensitive. A total dose of 4500–5000 rads of supravoltage radiation from a linear accelerator or ^{57}Co source is administered over 4 to 5 weeks. Radiation can be considered as the primary treatment if the adenoma is large enough to require treatment but is not causing neurologic symptoms that require immediate surgery. An example of such a situation is a man who on CT scan has a contrast-enhancing mass within the sella but extension only slightly above the sella and who has no more than a small defect in vision.

Radiation can also be used as secondary treatment following surgery. When the CT scan and the serum FSH concentration indicate that some adenoma tissue remains after surgery, radiation therapy will generally not only prevent continued growth of the remaining tissue, but also cause a further decrease in adenoma mass.

The outcome of radiation therapy, like surgery, can be considered both neurologically and endocrinologically and has many similarities to the results of radiation for other, large pituitary adenomas. Although experience with radiation as primary therapy for known FSH-secreting adenomas is limited, improvement of vision may occur in weeks to months. Neurologic complications of supravoltage radiation are expected only rarely; they include a transient worsening of vision during radiation, a complication that should be detected by testing vision during the course of radiation. Endocrinologically, the response to radiation takes at least many months, and possibly several years. The elevated serum FSH level generally will fall, but any of the pituitary hormones that had been secreted normally before radiation could also decrease, become subnormal, and need to be replaced. Transient side effects of radiation include nausea and lethargy; temporal hair loss may be transient or permanent.

The response to radiation should be assessed once a year and should include determination of the size and function of the adenoma by serum FSH concentration, visual fields and acuity, and CT scan, and determination of the function of the nonadenomatous pituitary.

TESTOSTERONE

Although FSH secretion in normal men and in men who have primary hypogonadism can be decreased by increasing the serum testosterone concentration, attempts to decrease FSH secretion from FSH-secreting adenomas and to decrease their size by long-term administration of testosterone have not yet been reported. If such a treatment were to be attempted, it would best be done in a patient who has little or no neurologic impairment, given the uncertainty of the results.

On the other hand, if a patient has sellar enlargement as a consequence of documented primary hypogonadism of long duration, administration of testosterone to a man, or estrogen and progestin to a woman, would be expected to decrease the size of the pituitary, although not for several months.

NO TREATMENT

Because FSH-secreting adenomas generally grow slowly, observation—but no treatment—of the adenoma could be considered for a patient whose adenoma is detected before neurologic impairment occurs, especially if the patient is elderly or chronically ill. Cortisol and thyroxine deficiencies, if present, should be corrected.

SUMMARY

Pituitary gonadotroph cell adenomas that secrete FSH generally grow slowly and, because excessive FSH secretion produces no symptoms, are often not detected until they are large enough to impair vision. When vision is severely impaired, transsphenoidal surgery is required to relieve pressure on the optic chiasm rapidly. Radiation therapy is also acceptable as primary treatment if vision is no more than mildly impaired, and it should be employed as a secondary treatment to prevent further growth of residual adenoma tissue following surgery. If vision is not impaired and if the patient is elderly or chronically ill, treatment of the adenoma may not be necessary. The results of treatment, as well as possible recurrence, should be monitored by measurement of the serum FSH concentration, CT scan, and assessment of vision. Hormonal deficiencies should be corrected whenever they are found.

SHORT STATURE

MARGARET H. MACGILLIVRAY, M.D.

NORMAL VARIANTS OF SHORT STATURE

Genetic or Familial Short Stature

At present, reassurance and psychologic counseling are the only means of helping children who are genetically short. Androgen therapy is contraindicated because use of these agents may further compromise adult height. Pharmacologic doses of growth hormone (GH) will undoubtedly be offered as treatment when supplies of the hormone become abundant through recombinant DNA technology. The risks of glucose intolerance, diabetes mellitus, and antibody formation will have to be weighed against the potential gains in statural growth. Health must take precedence over height in any research project that involves the use of pharmacologic agents to alter height of genetically short children.

Constitutional Growth Delay

In most situations, children with constitutional growth delay should not be given androgens, because the acceleration of bone maturation may not be offset by sufficient gains in height. Patients need to be educated about the nature of their delayed growth pattern and about their excellent prognosis for adult height. Boys are more frequently affected than girls. If early signs of puberty are detected (testicular enlargement, gonad >2.5 cm in length), it is sufficient to give reassurance that more rapid growth and spontaneous sexual maturation will soon occur. For prepubertal boys with pronounced growth delay (-3 to -4 S.D. in height and prepubertal), a 6 month course of androgen therapy is justified. Oxandrolone, 0.05 to 0.1 mg/kg body weight per os per day, will stimulate the rate of linear growth as much as 50 to 100 percent. Assessment of bone maturation (x-ray of left wrist and hand) should be done prior to and at the completion of the six months of treatment. Height and weight should be evaluated at zero, three, and six months during treatment and at three- to six-month intervals thereafter. These boys frequently continue to grow at improved growth rates, and older patients (ages 13 to 15) may even experience onset of puberty after androgen treatment is discontinued. Alternative androgen treatment regimens may be used if there is a need to stimulate genital as well as statural growth (fluoxymesterone, 2 mg/M^2 per day per os *or* testosterone enanthate, 50–100 mg i.m. every month). The criteria previously given for oxandrolone are used to monitor the growth response.

Preliminary studies indicate that some patients with pronounced growth delay respond dramatically to growth hormone therapy; however, the potential benefits and risks of such treatment cannot be critically assessed until the supplies of growth hormone have increased.

PATHOLOGIC SHORT STATURE

Growth Hormone Deficiency

Dose, Frequency, Sites

Treatment consists of growth hormone (GH) extracted from human pituitaries obtained at autopsy. The standard dose used is 0.1 U/kg body weight given intramuscularly 3 times weekly (Monday, Wednesday, and Friday). In obese ad-olescents, the dose of GH can be reduced to 0.08 U/kg to conserve hormone. It is important to use a 3-ml syringe with a 1-inch, 22-gauge needle to guarantee delivery into the muscle site. Tuberculin syringes with 5/8-inch, 25-gauge needles should be avoided. Also, the injection sites must be rotated to maximize absorption. Use of the muscle mass in the anterior thighs and buttocks areas will yield ample sites for drug administration.

Treatment Period and Response

In the prepubertal years, most GH-deficient children are treated for nine to ten months each year and are given a rest period during the summer months. Once sexual maturation has begun, it is imperative to treat continuously with GH in order to maximize final height.

Treatment should continue until heights of 5'4" to 5'6" are attained or until there is no further response to growth hormone administration. As the availability of GH increases, the goal of treatment will be to help patients attain adult heights compatible with their genetic endowment.

These patients must be carefully monitored throughout the treatment course. *Precise height* (preferably with a stadiometer) and weight measurements are obtained prior to and every three to four months during therapy. Initial and final body measurements must coincide with the onset and cessation of GH administration, respectively. Growth rates, extrapolated to centimeters per year, are calculated for each treatment interval in order to compare current progress with previous responses. *Bone maturation* is usually determined from an x-ray film of the left hand and wrist at the start and completion of each treatment period or at 6- to 12-month intervals. *Serum thyroxine* concentrations are measured prior to and every 6 to 12 months during treatment to detect the onset of secondary hypothyroidism which may follow GH treatment.

In the first year or two of therapy, most GH-deficient children grow at rates in excess of 9 cm per year. Therafter, the usual growth response falls to 6–8 cm per year and a small number of children fail to respond. Patients who cease to benefit from GH therapy may be noncompliant or using poor technique; alternatively, they may be developing antibodies, acquiring hypothyroidism, or experiencing closure of their epiphyses during sexual maturation. If noncompliance persists after counseling and re-education, it is essential to transfer the responsibility for GH administration from the parents to a visiting nurse, school nurse, or family physician. Hypothyroidism that develops during GH treatment must be treated with L-thyroxine, 2–3 µg/kg per day per os. Growth hormone therapy should be discontinued if failure to respond results from advanced bone maturation during puberty (bone age > 15 years).

Concomitant Therapy

Androgens. During the prepubertal years, small doses of anabolic/androgenic agents given simultaneously with GH will provide faster rates of linear growth than will GH given by itself. Oxandrolone, 0.05–0.1 mg/kg per day per os, will augment the response to GH without causing phallic enlargement. When micropenis is present, GH combined with fluoxymesterone, 2 mg/M^2 per day per os, or testosterone enanthate, 50 mg i.m. once monthly, will stimulate penis growth as well as augment growth velocity. Androgen therapy must never be used without concurrent GH administration in hypopituitary children because the rate of bone maturation will increase without compensatory gains in height. Consequently, ultimate stature may be compromised.

The following precautions must be taken if androgens are given simultaneously with GH: (1) Obtain bone age at start and completion of the treatment period with combined therapy (usually this amounts to six-month intervals); and (2) withhold androgens if baseline bone age is significantly ahead of height age *or* if bone age moves ahead of height age during any treatment period. In either situation, the preferred treatment is GH used by itself.

In gonadotropin-deficient males, the main goals of treatment include attainment of (1) satisfactory adult height (at least 5'4" to 5'6"); (2) full virilization; and (3) fertility (optional). Once sufficient statural growth has been achieved, testosterone enanthate, 200 mg i.m., may be administered every 2 to 3 weeks. We have observed that many of these patients fail to grow beards and fully virilize despite years of testosterone treatment. Gonadotropin administration, described in Chapter 70, will stimulate the growth of facial and body hair, testicular volume and sperm production.

Thyroid Hormone. L-thyroxine, 2–3 µg/kg per day per os, is prescribed for individuals with seconday/tertiary hypothyroidism.

Glucocorticoids. ACTH deficient individuals with symptomatic glucocorticoid insufficiency are treated with 10 mg hydrocortisone/M^2 per day given in 2 divided doses. Hypopituitary patients are unusually sensitive to small doses of glucocorticoid and may need even lower doses of hydrocortisone to obtain optimal responses to concomitant GH administration. During high fever, serious illness, or surgery, these patients require stress doses of cortisone (hydrocortisone, 60 mg/M^2 per os per day given in 3 or 4 divided doses or cortisone acetate, 60 mg/m^2 given i.m. each day).

Growth hormone resistance (Laron Dwarf) is a serious growth disorder for which there is no successful treatment.

Hypothyroidism

The treatment of primary hypothroidism is L-thyroxine, 6–10 µg/kg in the first 12 months of life and 3–4 µg/kg per day per os after the first year. The maximum is 150–200 µg/per day. For each patient, the actual dose is that which will maintain serum thyroxine concentrations in the normal range. Children with longstanding primary hypothyroidism will experience a temporary period of personality upheaval and disinterest in school after thyroid replacement is started. For this reason one-half of the calculated replacement dose is given for the first two weeks, followed by the full amount thereafter. Measurements of height, weight, serum thyroxine, and thyroid-stimulating hormone are obtained every 3 to 6 months during the first year and subsequently every 6 to 12 months.

The treatment of children with secondary/tertiary hypothyroidism is L-thyroxine, 2–3 µg/kg per day per os.

Glucocorticoid Excess

Growth failure due to glucocorticoid excess is most frequently seen in children receiving pharmacologic doses of cortisone or related compounds for asthma, various cancers, collagen vascular disease, immune suppression, postrenal transplantation, or aplastic anemia. The only means of helping these children is to institute an alternate-day glucocorticoid treatment regimen if it will not aggravate the primary disease. In a significant number of these children, growth is of secondary importance because survival requires daily high doses of cortisone.

Children with Cushing's syndrome due to unilateral adrenal adenoma or carcinoma require unilateral adrenalectomy. Concomitant glucocorticoid replacement is necessary until the contralateral adrenal resumes function. Micronodular adrenal disease (Black adrenal) is treated with bilateral adrenalectomy. Bilateral adrenal hyperplasia due to pituitary adenoma responds well to transsphenoidal removal of the tumor by an experienced neurosurgeon. The care of children with bilateral adrenal hyperplasia who have no detectable lesion in the pituitary-hypothalamic region is controversial. Because of the limited experience with pituitary radiation in children who have this type of Cushing's syndrome and the urgency to correct the growth problem, we have continued to use bilateral adrenalectomy followed by cortisol replacement (Hydrocortisone, 15–20 mg/M^2 per day per os) and 9 α-fluorhydrocortisone (Florinef), 0.1 mg/day. During stressful illnesses, the dose of hydrocortisone is increased to 60–75 mg/M^2 per day per os or i.m. as outlined previously.

Gonadal Dysgenesis

There is no uniform opinion on the treatment of these girls. Androgen therapy with oxandrolone, 0.05 to 0.1 mg/kg per day, has been used intermittently (6 months on, 6 months off) or continuously. Fluoxymesterone, 2–3 mg/M^2 per day, has also been prescribed. Both hormones yield temporary improvements in growth velocity followed by declining responsiveness. It is preferable to restrict the use of anabolic drugs to girls whose bone age is retarded by 2 or more years and whose chronologic age is 10 or more years. Bone age measurements every six months should be closely followed to enable one to assess the impact of the treatment and decide on further therapy. The decision to start sex hormone therapy depends upon the level of emotional maturity and the opinion of the patient concerning the importance of height versus sexual maturation. Most girls wish to start estrogen therapy by age 14 or 15 and express a willingness to forfeit some adult height in order to feel comfortable with their age mates. Conjugated estrogens (Premarin), 0.625–1.25 mg per day for 4 to 6 months, will initiate breast growth in the majority of girls. Thereafter, Premarin on calendar days 1 through 20 and medroxyprogesterone (Provera), 10 mg on calendar days 15 through 20 inclusive, will provide cyclic vaginal bleeding and additional breast growth. Periodic gynecologic examination, including vaginal and endometrial cytology, are essential.

In a recent study, the growth response to combined treatment with GH (0.08 U/kg i.m. per day) and oxandrolone gave better results than either drug used alone. The National Pituitary Agency has an ongoing collaborative program to evaluate the benefits of GH, 0.2 kg 3 times weekly, in girls with Turner's syndrome who have normal glucose tolerance. The potential benefits and risks of GH used singly or in combination with androgen administration are being actively investigated.

Environmental Deprivation Syndrome (Psychosocial Dwarfism, Emotional Deprivation Syndrome)

The management of these children consists of optimal nutrition in a happy environment. Dramatic improvements in growth and behavior confirm the diagnosis. It is usually difficult to help these children in their family setting. Foster care or hospitalization are alternative means of providing an atmosphere filled with affection, psychologic support, and good nutrition (140 cal/kg per day are advisable). Prolonged foster care is preferable to returning these children to disturbed home situations. However, legal restraints frequently mandate that these patients rejoin their parents with a less than satisfactory outcome.

Skeletal Disorders (Chondrodystrophies, Vitamin D-Resistant Rickets, etc.)

There is no safe or effective treatment for disproportionate short stature due to the chondrodystrophies and other biochemical abnormalities of bone growth. Androgen treatment is contraindicated because it will further compromise adult height.

Vitamin D-resistant rickets (hypophosphatemic rickets) is effectively treated with 1,25 (OH)$_2$ D$_3$ (20–80 ng/kg per day per os) and phosphorus supplementation (1.5–2 gm per day per os). The aims of treatment include maintenance of serum calcium in the normal range and serum phosphorus above 4 mg/dl. Clinical and biochemical evaluations should be done at one-month intervals in the first year and every three months thereafter. Increased growth rates, bone strength, and loss of genu valgum have been observed in children treated during early childhood.

Intrauterine Growth Failure

Persistence of pathologic short stature beyond the age of 2 years in a child who was small at birth for gestational age indicates the presence of a permanent insult to the growth process. Growth hormone treatment with or without concomitant androgen therapy has proved beneficial in selected cases. Alternatively, anabolic/androgenic agents have been administered alone with variable results. In a small percentage of these patients there is no effective treatment, and psychologic support becomes the most important means of helping them to gain self-confidence and independence as adults.

Growth Failure Associated with Chronic Disease

Correction of short stature due to chronic disease depends almost entirely upon successful treatment of the primary disorder. Growth failure due to hypoxemia from a hemoglobinopathy or bone marrow aplasia can be successfully managed by chronic transfusion therapy. The major risk is iron overload. Poor growth due to malabsorption requires an accurate diagnosis and precise diet. Celiac syndrome is successfully treated with a high-caloric diet free of gluten, sucrose, and lactose, to which supplements of calcium, iron, folic acid, zinc, and other vitamins are added. The growth response to this treatment is usually dramatic. Chronic inflammatory bowel disease is a frustrating cause of growth failure. The anorexia and chronic diarrhea cause severe malnutrition. High-caloric diets have resulted in significant improvements in growth once the underlying disease has been controlled. In severely ill children parenteral nutrition has been used with variable success. Congenital heart disease interferes with growth in young children if there is accompanying hypoxemia or heart failure. Successful medical and surgical correction is soon followed by improved rates of linear growth and weight gain. There is no effective therapy for the growth failure of children who have severe central nervous system disease. Patients with end-stage renal disease may exhibit catch-up growth following successful renal transplantation, provided glucocorticoids can be used on an alternate-day schedule.

THYROID DISEASE

HYPERTHYROIDISM

MARTIN I. SURKS, M.D.

The treatment of hyperthyroidism requires a number of therapeutic decisions by the physician. To utilize appropriately the variety of treatment modalities available, one must have a knowledge of the etiologic factors and natural history of the various thyroid disorders responsible for hyperthyroidism as well as the current and potential impact of the disease on the hyperthyroid patient. Since there is no specific therapy for Graves' disease or hyperfunctioning thyroid adenomata, the current goals of therapy are to reduce elevated thyroid hormone concentrations to the normal range, to relieve hypermetabolism, to relieve symptoms, and to limit as much as possible the iatrogenic disorders associated with different treatment modalities. Although closely related, each of these objectives should be considered independently during the patient's management. For example, the clinician may alleviate severe symptoms by means of beta-adrenergic blockade even before treating the elevated serum hormone concentrations. In addition to these considerations, the physician should also define the short- and long-term goals of the management plan. These are frequently the same, but in some instances sharp distinctions may be drawn between them. Thus, in hyperthyroid patients of advanced age, the long-term goal may be to destroy the thyroid tissue with radioiodine but the short-term objective may be to return the patient to the euthyroid state by means of thioamide drug treatment. Another issue affecting the choice of therapeutic modality is the permanence of the destructive effects of radioactive iodine [^{131}I] iodide or surgery, and the lack of known long-term consequences of antithyroid drug therapy. Lastly, the patient's wishes and responsibilities in his own management are important factors in therapeutic decisions. Some individuals have strong feelings concerning surgery, ingestion of drugs, or radioactive iodine. Involvement of the patient in the therapeutic decisions generally improves reliability in ingestion of medications and follow-up evaluation. Although a number of etiologies of hyperthyroidism have been described, this chapter discusses only treatment of the common thyroidal disorders that are associated with thyrotoxicosis; namely, the hyperthyroidism that occurs with thyroiditis, hyperfunctioning adenoma, and Graves' disease.

THYROIDITIS

Both subacute (de Quervain's) thyroiditis and spontaneously resolving hyperthyroidism may be associated with thyrotoxicosis. Although these disorders may have a different origin, they are both self-limited; the hyperthyroidism persists for several weeks to several months. Patients with these disorders do not respond to drugs of the thioamide group, and treatment with radioactive iodine is neither indicated nor possible, since the activity of the iodine trap is markedly depressed. Because of these considerations, the physician's principal role is to diagnose these disorders accurately to prevent institution of inappropriate treatment, such as administration of antithyroid drugs. The patient should also be reassured that the disorder is indeed self-limited. The uncomfortable palpitations, inappropriate and excessive perspiration, and tremors that occur in some patients may be alleviated by treatment with beta-adrenergic antagonists such as propranolol. Doses of 10–20 mg 4 times each day are generally adequate for symptomatic relief. In my experience, the large doses of glucocorticoids that are occasionally administered to relieve severe anterior neck pain in subacute thyroiditis do not ameliorate the accompanying hyperthyroidism.

There is general agreement that thyroid function returns to normal after recovery from subacute thyroiditis and that this disorder is not associated with an appreciable incidence of hypothyroidism in later years. Thus these patients do not appear to require lifelong follow-up evaluation as do patients with Graves' disease. At the present time, a similar recommendation cannot be made for patients suffering from spontaneously resolving hyperthyroidism. Although the long-term consequences of this disorder may be similar to those in de Quervain's (subacute) thyroiditis, this has not yet been documented by adequate follow-up studies. The thyroid function of patients with this disorder should be assessed annually.

THYROID ADENOMA

From the therapeutic viewpoint, hyperthyroidism resulting from a single autonomous adenoma or from hyperfunctioning multiple adenomas (Plummer's disease) can be considered together. Since the hypersecretion of thyroid hormones occurs in thyroid tissue that is functioning autonomously, these disorders are not associated with natural remissions. Their natural history appears to be characterized by progressive growth of the lesion and thyrotoxicosis. The use of thioamide drugs in anticipation of an eventual remission is therefore inappropriate. When hyperthyroidism is present, there is little question that the patient should receive definitive treatment. However, the decision to treat patients with functioning adenoma who are clinically euthyroid is complicated by the fact that these lesions may progress very slowly. Thus some patients with functioning adenomas may never develop thyrotoxicosis. In my view, those patients who have autonomous adenomas that are greater than 2 cm in diameter and that result in suppression of the remaining normal thyroid tissue should be treated definitively, even if clinically significant thyrotoxicosis is not present. The erratic and frequently excessive iodine supply that prevails in this country places these patients at risk for the sudden development of hyperthyroidism. Thus a euthyroid patient with an autonomous adenoma who receives a medication that has a high iodine content or requires a radiographic procedure employing an iodinated contrast medium may become thyrotoxic several weeks later. Patients with lesions that are not yet suppressing the remaining thyroid tissue should be observed without specific therapy, since they may never develop hyperthyroidism. Re-evaluation at annual intervals is generally sufficient for these individuals.

The definitive treatment of hyperfunctioning adenoma is destruction of the abnormal tissue, either by surgical removal or by means of radioactive iodine. Although each of these modalities has been used effectively in different centers, my approach is to treat these disorders with radioactive iodine. Radioiodine has the advantage of destroy-

ing only the hyperfunctioning tissue, because the normal thyroid tissue that surrounds the adenoma is suppressed and thus exposed only to scatter radiation. The patient treated with radioactive iodine is also spared the discomfort of hospitalization and surgery as well as the risk of complications of thyroid surgery. The potential risk of radiation exposure in younger patients (see below) is not usually an important consideration, since toxic adenoma and Plummer's disease most frequently occur in middle-aged or older patients. Lastly, these patients do not have the high incidence of hypothyroidism that occurs after treatment of Graves' disease with radioactive iodine, because uninvolved thyroid tissue is suppressed and receives only a small dose of radiation.

Since radioactive iodine treatment generally results in exaggerated release of thyroid hormone stores during the first week after administration, patients of advanced age or patients with underlying cardiovascular disease should first be treated with thioamides in order to deplete the thyroid of its organic iodine stores and effect return to the euthyroid state. Either propylthiouracil, 100–200 mg 3 times each day, or methimazole, 10–20 mg 3 times each day may be used. These dosages, if taken reliably, adequately block thyroidal iodothyronine formation. Thyrotoxicosis should be improved within one to two weeks, and patients generally become euthyroid after three to six weeks of treatment. Patients should be advised of the allergic reactions that can occur with these drugs, predominantly skin rash, which occurs in about 5 percent of individuals. They should also be alerted to the signs of agranulocytosis: fever, sore throat, and rash. This complication occurs rarely, in less than 0.5 percent of patients.

Patients can be evaluated clinically every two to three weeks after starting thioamide treatment, and a measurement of serum T_4 concentration is carried out. When patients are euthyroid clinically and serum T_4 is also normal, antithyroid drugs are discontinued and the 24-hour radioiodine uptake is determined 4 to 7 days later. The radioiodine treatment dose is calculated from an estimate of thyroid size and the fractional 24-hour uptake of radioactive iodine. Since adenomatous tissue is relatively radio-resistant compared with thyroid tissue in Graves' disease, the dose is generally calculated to deliver about 150 µCi/g tissue. Patients are re-evaluated every three to four weeks after the radioactive iodine dose. Thioamide treatment at about one-half of the previous dose may be reinstituted for the first month after radioiodine administration in those patients who had significant hyperthyroidism that required thioamide treatment before radioactive iodine treatment. This prevents a clinical relapse during the three- to six-week interval that appears to be required for clinical improvement after radioactive iodine administration. In these individuals the thioamide should not be readministered until about four days after the radioiodine dose is given in order to ensure maximal uptake and organification of the radioiodine. The drug is discontinued after one month. Subsequent monthly visits for clinical evaluation and serum T_4, T_3, and TSH measurements, if necessary, should demonstrate the effectiveness of the radioactive iodine dose. Patients who remain hyperthyroid three to six months after radioactive iodine treatment probably require a second treatment dose. For patients who are euthyroid at this time, the follow-up evaluations can be made at three-month intervals for the first year, six-month intervals during the second year, and then, in some patients, at annual intervals. Although it is unnecessary to follow these radioiodine treated patients for the development of hypothyroidism, some patients should be evaluated for the late recurrence of hyperthyroidism. In these individuals radioiodine treatment may have reduced the size of the adenoma and ameliorated thyrotoxicosis. However, the adenoma may still have the propensity to grow slowly and produce hyperthyroidism again after many years.

GRAVES' DISEASE

There is general agreement that the hyperthyroidism of Graves' disease results from the binding of an autoantibody to the TSH receptor with subsequent stimulation of the thyroid. Since the thyroid tissue does not function autonomously in Graves' disease, a decrease in the concentration of the immunoglobulin that stimulates the thyroid results in amelioration of hyperthyroidism. In some patients complete—and possibly longstanding—remission of the disease occurs. Optimal treatment for these patients would be to control the hyperthyroidism with drugs of the thioamide group until remission occurs and then discontinue drug therapy. Unfortunately, only a minority of patients with Graves' disease, 25 to 30 percent in the United States, may enter a spontaneous remission. Therefore, one of the important therapeutic decisions to be made when considering management of new patients with Graves' disease is whether to employ

antithyroid drugs for long-term management or to proceed directly to radioactive iodine or surgery. Drug therapy should be reserved for patients who have a reasonable chance of entering spontaneous remission. Clinical factors favoring remission include sudden onset of hyperthyroidism, which may be associated with an emotional crisis and a small goiter, less than 60 grams in size. At the present time there are no generally available laboratory tests that can help determine whether or not patients are in remission or have a good chance for entering remission. In the future, measurements of the concentration of the thyroid stimulating immunoglobulin and determination of the HLA type may help the clinician in these therapeutic decisions.

Antithyroid Drugs

Because radiation in children is associated with an increased incidence of leukemia, thyroid nodules, and cancer, children with hyperthyroidism should not be treated with radioactive iodine; they should be given antithyroid drugs. Although similar adverse effects have not been documented after radioactive iodine treatment in adolescents, I still employ thioamide drugs in this age group, since the very long-term follow-up of radioiodine treated adolescents has not been well documented. Thioamide drug therapy is also recommended for most adults with hyperthyroidism who have a reasonable chance of entering remission based on above criteria. In the absence of these criteria, radioactive iodine treatment becomes the treatment of choice in adults, except in women who wish to bear children. Although an increase in congenital abnormalities has not been documented in the children of women who have been treated with radioiodine, the increased incidence of congenital abnormalities that occurs with other types of radiation is a cause for continuing concern and evaluation when considering radioactive iodine therapy. A balanced view of the therapeutic options and risks should therefore be presented to these patients and the patients' opinions strongly considered in the therapeutic decision. Patients treated with thiomide drugs will become euthyroid and can be maintained for many years on drug therapy. Moreover, in the absence of a natural remission, the antithyroid drugs can always be discontinued for definitive radioiodine treatment if the patient becomes frustrated by the persistent need for medication.

Propylthiouracil or methimazole is administered in initial doses of 300–600 mg per day or 30–60 mg per day, respectively. The larger doses are employed for patients with large goiters. Although both drugs affect the thyroid glands similarly, propylthiouracil has the added advantage of inhibiting T_3 production from T_4 in the peripheral tissues. These agents are most effective in divided doses, but hyperthyroidism can also be controlled when the daily dosage or a somewhat greater dosage of medication is administered once each day. Patients should be advised of the allergic reactions that occur in about 5 percent and the agranulocytosis that occurs in less than 0.5 percent of patients. Since the latter is frequently heralded by fever, sore throat, and rash, this syndrome should alert the patient to discontinue medication immediately and call the physician. Routine measurement of the white blood cell count does not have any predictive value for agranulocytosis.

Clinical improvement generally occurs within several weeks in most patients but may be delayed for one to two months in patients with large goiters. Clinical re-evaluation at intervals of two to four weeks with measurement of serum T_4 is thus necessary for good management. A significant decrease in serum T_4 generally indicates that clinical improvement will occur rapidly. In the average patient, clinical improvement and a decrease in serum T_4 generally occur within one month, and this necessitates a decrease in dosage of thiomides to about one-half to two-thirds of the starting dosage. Close monitoring of the clinical course and serum T_4 concentration dictates further reductions in the thioamide dosage until a maintenance dosage is reached. This dosage, 50–150 mg per day for propylthiouracil or 5–15 mg per day for methimazole for most patients, maintains the euthyroid state for a prolonged period of time. Further enlargement of the thyroid in conjunction with serum T_4 decreased to below the normal range and increased serum TSH concentration indicates that the patient has been overtreated with the thioamide and requires a reduction in dosage. An alternative method to that described above is maintenance of the starting dosage of thioamide for an extended period of time together with the introduction of a full replacement dosage of L-thyroxine to maintain the euthyroid state. I prefer to employ a small maintenance dosage of thioamide, since this requires only one medication for the patient and a smaller medication dosage.

Thiamide treatment is continued at the maintenance dosage until remission occurs. Since at the present time there are few objective findings to document remission in individual patients, the duration of treatment can be quite variable. Some clinicians discontinue treatment soon after return to the euthyroid state, while others continue thioamide treatment for years. In the future, measurement of human thyroid-stimulating immunoglobulin concentration should provide a good guide for the discontinuation of drug therapy. However, as of now, only a significant decrease in thyroid gland size suggests remission. In children and adolescents, I prefer to maintain thioamide treatment for one to two years before discontinuing in order to determine whether the patient is in remission. If relapse occurs, a second treatment course of one to two years is recommended. Subsequent relapse is an indication for subtotal thyroidectomy in these age groups, although some adolescents prefer to continue treatment with maintenance dosages of thioamide for a number of years, and then, as young adults, decide to have radioiodine treatment. Clearly, with regard to reliable ingestion of medication, these decisions must take into account the motivation of the patient.

A single course of treatment for one to two years is also carried out in adult patients. If relapse occurs radioiodine treatment is recommended. For patients who do enter remission, follow-up evaluations are made every two to three months for the first year after terminating thioamide treatment and annually thereafter. These evaluations should include serum T_4 and serum T_3 measurements, since an elevation in serum T_3 level may occur sooner than that of T_4 during a relapse. Serum TSH should also be measured during follow-up of patients who were treated with thioamide many years earlier, because hypothyroidism appears to be a very late consequence of Graves' disease in some patients even without treatment with radioactive iodine or surgery.

Radioactive Iodine

Radioactive iodine, $[^{131}I]$ iodide, is a safe, effective, and convenient treatment of hyperthyroidism for most patients. Although it is not recommended for children or adolescents because of the considerations listed above, it is the treatment of choice for adult patients who are not good candidates for a natural remission. This approach is modified for women of childbearing age who may prefer a trial of thioamides, even though their anticipated incidence of remission may be small. For women who plan to bear children within several years, however, the decision to treat the disorder with antithyroid drugs or with radioiodine may be a difficult one. With the former treatment, the patient may not go into remission and thus will still require thioamide drugs during pregnancy. The management of Graves' disease with antithyroid drugs during pregnancy is discussed below. With radioactive iodine treatment, thyrotoxicosis can be relieved permanently before conception. Radiation risks to mother or child are only hypothetic and have not been documented in available studies. Radioiodine treatment is also recommended for those patients who have been treated with thioamides but who did not enter a natural remission.

Radioactive iodine treatment is generally attended by an increase in the serum concentration of thyroid hormones due to radiation thyroiditis, which is generally painless. The increased hypermetabolism is rarely significant clinically in young individuals, but patients of advanced age or patients who have significant underlying cardiovascular disease may experience further decompensation of the cardiovascular disease. These patients should therefore receive thioamide drug treatment as described in the section above on the treatment of autonomous adenomas to restore the euthyroid state and to deplete the thyroid of stored hormones before radioiodine treatment. Radioactive iodine can be administered about four days after discontinuing the thioamide drugs. Calculation of the radioiodine dose involves determination of thyroid gland size, generally by palpation, and the fractional uptake of radioiodine, determined by the 24-hour radioiodine uptake. The delivered dose should be between 70–100 μCi/gm of thyroid tissue. The lower dose is attended by a lower incidence of early hypothyroidism but a higher incidence of treatment failure and need for a second treatment dose. The higher dose is more effective but also produces a greater incidence of early hypothyroidism. These considerations should be explained in detail to the patient to avoid unreasonable expectations from the treatment.

Clinical improvement is generally detectable within several weeks after the radioiodine treatment, but the maximal effect of radioiodine may not occur until two to four months later. During the interval between administration of the isotope and clinical improvement, patients with severe symptoms can be made more comfortable by the administration of a beta-adrenergic blocking drug, such as propranolol. Doses of 40–80 mg per day are generally sufficient to relieve tachycardia, in-

appropriate and excessive perspiration, and tremor. Patients should be re-evaluated at monthly intervals with clinical examination and measurement of serum T_4 and, if indicated, TSH levels. Failure to improve clinically and the absence of a significant decrease in serum T_4 after three months indicates that a second treatment dose of radioactive iodine is required. With the doses recommended above, approximately 20 percent of patients require a second treatment dose, and in less than 5 percent a third treatment dose is necessary. Some return to a euthyroid state after two to four months; this is documented by a normal serum T_4, T_3, and TSH concentration. These patients are then followed at two to three-month intervals until the end of the first year after radioiodine treatment, every six months for the second year, and at annual intervals thereafter. A few patients become hypothyroid clinically after two to four months. This is documented by decreased serum T_4 and increased serum TSH levels. Since some of these individuals may regain normal thyroid function, thyroxine treatment may be withheld for several months if the hypothyroidism is not severe. If clinically warranted, however, thyroxine treatment, 0.1–0.2 mg per day, may be instituted. In these patients thyroxine treatment should be interrupted one year after radioiodine treatment to determine whether thyroid hypofunction was transient or is permanent. If permanent, T_4 treatment is reinstituted and the patient followed at annual intervals indefinitely. Hypothyroidism that persists for six to nine months after radioiodine treatment is generally permanent and should be treated appropriately with L-thyroxine. In my experience, 10 to 15 percent of patients become hypothyroid during the first year after radioiodine treatment. The subsequent development of hypothyroidism occurs at a rate of 2 to 4 percent per year for the population at risk.

As indicated above, there is a delicate balance between the effective dose of radioactive iodine and the incidence of hypothyroidism in patients with Graves' disease. In younger individuals, lower doses may be used in the hope of reducing the incidence of hypothyroidism. However, the necessity for administration of a second dose is greater. In older individuals who have underlying cardiovascular disease, a larger dose of radioiodine may be selected to prevent an extended course of hypermetabolism. The resulting higher incidence of hypothyroidism may be considered acceptable because it is accurately and easily managed by L-thyroxine replacement therapy.

Surgery

Subtotal thyroidectomy is an effective treatment for Graves' disease and the treatment of choice in children and adolescents if thioamide therapy does not result in a remission of thyrotoxicosis. Surgery should also be considered in other settings in which radioactive iodine treatment is either contraindicated or not feasible. These include treatment of hyperthyroidism in pregnancy (see below) and in patients who refuse radioactive drugs. The major role of surgery as the principal treatment of Graves' disease in adults has changed dramatically since the introduction of radioactive iodine. Surgery was still a common treatment of adult hyperthyroidism for some years after radioactive iodine became widely available. This resulted from the belief that the incidence of hypothyroidism following subtotal thyroidectomy was only about 10 percent. Since it is now generally accepted that the late incidence of hypothyroidism after subtotal thyroidectomy is appreciable, albeit not as high as after radioactive iodine administration, the principal justification for surgical management as opposed to radioactive iodine treatment has been removed. In addition, with fewer thyroidectomies being performed, surgical experience with this once common procedure has diminished and the potential for postoperative complications, such as hypoparathyroidism and vocal chord injury, has increased.

Since surgery may precipitate thyroid storm in some hyperthyroid patients, hyperthyroidism should be relieved by drug therapy before elective subtotal thyroidectomy is performed. This is generally accomplished by thioamide drug therapy according to the principles outlined below. Many surgeons also prefer that iodides such as Lugol's solution or saturated solution of potassium iodide, 5 drops 2 or 3 times each day, also be administered during the last 2 to 3 weeks before surgery. Alternatively, preoperative preparation may be carried out in many patients with high doses of propranolol, 120–360 mg per day in divided doses. Some patients on this regimen for only several days undergo surgery without incident.

Pregnancy

Radioiodine is contraindicated during pregnancy because it crosses freely through the placenta to the fetal circulation and may cause injury to fetal tissues. Although subtotal thyroidectomy can be successfully employed to treat pregnant women with thyrotoxic Graves' disease, most patients can be successfully managed by the judicious use of thioamide drugs. Initial dosages of propylthiouracil or methimazole in the range of 300 or 30 mg per day, respectively, are decreased after the first month to one-half or less of that dosage. This generally results in reasonable, although sometimes not optimal, control of the mother's hyperthyroidism without significant fetal goiter or hypothyroidism. The smallest dosage of thiomide that satisfies these guidelines should be used. Iodides should never be employed in pregnant women because their use is associated with large fetal goiters.

THYROID STORM

LEWIS E. BRAVERMAN, M.D.

DIAGNOSIS

Thyroid storm is difficult to diagnose because there is such a fine line between severe thyrotosicosis and what has been termed thyroid storm. The diagnosis of thyroid storm in a severely ill patient is usually made on clinical grounds. These patients have a modest fever ($>100°F$); are frequently agitated, manic, restless, and occasionally psychotic, with hot, flushed skin that may be moist or dry depending upon the state of hydration; have tachycardia with various tachyarrhythmias, especially auricular fibrillation in the elderly; and display the other usual physical findings of thyrotoxic Graves' disease or toxic nodular goiter. In the elderly patient, apathy, severe myopathy, congestive heart failure, and profound weight loss are not uncommon, and thyroid enlargement may be minimal. As storm progresses, stupor leading to coma, hypotension and vascular collapse, and death may ensue within 48 hours unless active therapy is instituted.

Thyroid function tests do not often differentiate between severe thyrotoxicosis and thyroid storm. Serum thyroxine (T_4) concentrations are usually similar, although recent reports have suggested that the serum free T_4 concentration is significantly higher in the patients with storm, which might partially explain their more severe symptoms. The serum triiodothyronine (T_3) concentration is not higher in thyroid storm, and it may in fact be less elevated or even normal in these patients when the precipitating cause is an intercurrent illness or surgery. This is not surprising since a major source of the circulating T_3 results from the peripheral outer ring monodeiodination ($5'$-deiodination) of T_4, an enzymatic process that is markedly impaired in a wide variety of acute and chronic systemic illnesses. Liver function tests are frequently abnormal, especially in elderly patients in whom congestive failure is not uncommon. The mild elevation in total and free serum calcium which may accompany hyperthyroidism can be exaggerated. Occasionally these very ill patients do not have the expected leukocytosis and neutrophilia because the white blood count tends to be lower in hyperthyroid patients and a relative lymphocytosis occurs.

Prior to the use of iodides and then the antithyroid drugs, propylthiouracil (PTU) and methimazole (Tapazole, MMI), in the preparation of hyperthyroid patients for thyroid surgery, thyroid storm was most frequently seen during and after subtotal thyroidectomy. It is now rarely seen in this context, owing to the restoration of euthyroidism prior to surgery with PTU or MMI and iodides. Propranolol has also been used in a few large centers as sole therapy before surgery, but it must be remembered that the circulating thyroid hormones remain elevated because the synthesis and release of the hormones are not affected by the beta-blockers. More recently it has been reported that the use of propranolol for six weeks and the addition of iodides two weeks prior to surgery results in normal serum T_4 and T_3 concentrations at the time of surgery.

In view of the proper preparation of hyperthyroid patients for thyroid surgery, thyroid storm now occurs most commonly in patients with rather severe underlying thyrotoxicosis, frequently undiagnosed, who become ill for other reasons, such as infections and pulmonary and cardiovascular disorders, the latter often aggravated by the thyrotoxicosis. Thyroid storm may also be precipitated during and after nonthyroid surgery, including orthopedic surgery for fractures. The widespread use of radioactive iodine (I^{131}, RAI) as the primary treatment for hyperthyroidism, especially in older patients, may also precipitate thyroid storm because of the release of large quantities of T_4 and T_3 during radiation destruction of thyroid. This most often occurs approximately 10 to 14 or more days after the administration of large doses of I^{131} to patients with very large goiters who have not been recently treated with PTU or MMI. Although propranolol will usually suffice to reduce the symptoms of this transient worsening of the thyrotoxicosis, propranolol alone will not necessarily prevent thyroid storm. To avoid this rare but worrisome complication of I^{131} therapy, it is advisable to use PTU or MMI to deplete thyroid stores of T_4 and T_3 in older patients with severe thyrotoxicosis prior to I^{131} therapy. The antithyroid drugs should be discontinued for approximately four days and, if deemed necessary, restarted four days after I^{131} treatment. Propranolol should also be employed unless contraindicated by bronchospastic lung disease.

Iodide-induced hyperthyroidism, or Jod-Basedow's disease, is not uncommon in areas of endemic iodine-deficient goiter or in areas such as Western Europe where iodine intake is marginal. It is now a problem in Europe, where Jod-Basedow's disease not infrequently occurs following the administration of iodine-containing x-ray contrast dyes and drugs such as Amiodarone. As noted below, iodides also block release of T_4 and T_3 from the thyroid so that these patients are at least partially protected while pharmacologic quantities of iodine remain in the circulation. However, worsening of the thyrotoxicosis and thyroid storm can ensue when the blocking effect of iodide on hormone release has dissipated and large quantities of excess stored hormones are released into the circulation. Although not common in the United States, where iodine intake is sufficient, this syndrome must be considered. Recently, cardiac deaths, probably due to ventricular arrhythmias, have been reported following the acute ingestion of massive doses of thyroid hormones, certainly a form of thyroid storm.

THERAPY

Underlying Illness

As noted earlier, nonthyroidal illness and surgery in previously undiagnosed or only partially treated patients with hyperthyroidism are the most common causes of thyroid storm. Vigorous therapy of the precipitating disease should be undertaken, especially since death in patients treated for thyroid storm is now primarily due to the underlying illness (Table 1). It should be emphasized that cardiac arrhythmias and congestive failure re-

TABLE 1 Treatment of Thyroid Storm

Vigorous therapy of underlying intercurrent illness with digoxin, diuretics, antibotics, intravenous fluids supplemented with the B vitamins, and insulin for diabetic ketoacidosis

Cooling blanket and/or antipyretics (perhaps not aspirin) for hyperpyrexia

Beta-adrenergic blocking drugs or, far less commonly, drugs that deplete catecholamines:

    Propranolol (beta$_1$ and beta$_2$ blocker)
        1 mg i.v. per minute for a total dose of 2–10 mg
        40–80 mg p.o. every 4–6 hours

    Metoprolol (beta$_1$ blocker)
        100–400 mg p.o. every 12 hours

    Atenolol (beta$_1$ blocker)
        50–100 mg p.o. daily

    Reserpine
        Test dose with 0.25 mg i.m., then initial dose of 1–5 mg
        1–2.5 mg i.m. every 4–6 hours

    Guanethidine
        1–2 mg/kg p.o. every 4–6 hours

Inhibit synthesis of the thyroid hormones

    Propylthiouracil
        Approximately 800 mg p.o. stat and 200–300 mg every 8 hours

    Methimazole
        Approximately 80 mg p.o. stat and 40 mg every 12 hours

Block release of thyroid hormones from the thyroid

    Iodides
        Saturated solution of potassium iodide (SSKI), 5 drops p.o. every 8 hours
        Lugol's solution, 10 drops p.o. every 8 hours
        Sodium iodide, 1 gm i.v. infusion over 12 hours every 12 hours

    Telepaque or Oragrafin (1 gm p.o. daily)

    Lithium—requires careful monitoring
        800–1200 mg p.o. daily
        Serum lithium concentrations range from 0.5–1.5 mEq/l

Inhibit peripheral 5′-monodeiodination of thyroxine (T$_4$) to triiodothyronine (T$_3$)

    Corticosteroids, equivalent to 300–400 mg hydrocortisone daily, especially dexamethasone, 2 mg every 6 hours

    Propranolol

    Propylthiouracil

    X-ray iodine containing contrast agents
        Telepaque, 1 gm daily
        Oragrafin, 1 gm daily

    Amiodarone—efficacy in thyroid storm not yet tested
        Approximately 80 mg p.o. and 40 mg every 12 hours

Remove thyroid hormone from the circulation

    Plasmapheresis
    Peritoneal dialysis

quire approximately twice the dose of digoxin needed in euthyroid patients, and refractory arrhythmias should alert the physician to the presence of thyrotoxicosis. Similarly, more insulin may be required to treat diabetic ketoacidosis. Since diabetes mellitus and Graves' disease occur more frequently in the same patient, owing to the autoimmune etiology of both diseases, deterioration in the control of diabetes should suggest the onset of thyrotoxicosis. It is evident that adequate antibiotic therapy, careful fluid and electrolyte balance, vigorous pulmonary therapy, and careful pre- and postoperative care must be given to these patients. If emergency surgery is required in a thyrotoxic patient, propranolol, iodides, and perhaps corticosteroids should probably be given prior to, during, and after surgery.

Specific Therapy

A cooling blanket should probably be used if the temperature rises above 101°F. Antipyretics may also be given, although large doses of aspirin displace the thyroid hormones from the serum binding proteins, and therefore slightly increase the free hormone concentrations. More recently, aspirin has been reported to decrease the peripheral conversion of T$_4$ to the far more biologically active hormone T$_3$, and this might negate the possible adverse effects of aspirin noted above. Until this question is resolved, it is advisable to use other antipyretic drugs.

Many of the clinical manifestations of hyperthyroidism can be alleviated by the administration of drugs that deplete or block the peripheral action of the catecholamines. Prior to the availability of beta-adrenergic blockers, drugs that deplete catecholamine stores—reserpine and guanethidine (blocks release also)—were used with some success. However, parenteral reserpine has troublesome side effects, the most severe being resistant hypotension. If this drug must be used, a test dose of 0.25 mg i.m. should be administered and blood pressure carefully monitored. Somnolence, diarrhea, and flushing can also occur following the large doses of reserpine required to deplete peripheral catecholamines. Thus reserpine should be used only in patients in whom the beta-adrenergic blocking agents are contraindicated. Oral guanethidine has also been employed in the treatment of storm, but its effect is not evident for approximately 12 hours, and, like reserpine, it can cause diarrhea and postural hypotension.

Propranolol and its derivatives are potent beta-adrenergic blocking agents and are now the drugs of choice in alleviating the catecholamine dependent signs and symptoms of thyrotoxicosis and thyroid storm. The greatest experience has been achieved with propranolol, and the cardiac and psychomotor manifestations of thyrotoxicosis are improved within minutes following its intravenous administration. Propranolol can also be administered orally; the route of administration depends upon the severity of the cardiac symptoms and the speed required to correct the tachycardia or tachyarrhythmias. Since propranolol may be contraindicated in patients with congestive heart failure, it is frequently debated whether to use the beta-blockers in patients with severe thyrotoxicosis or thyroid storm and congestive failure. Tachycardia and tachyarrhythmias are major contributing factors to the congestive failure in many of these patients, and it is, therefore, recommended that propranolol be used along with digoxin and other cardiotropic drugs and diuretics. Propranolol has the added advantage of partially blocking the peripheral conversion of T_4 to T_3, which the specific beta$_1$-adrenergic blocking agents, metoprolol and atenolol, do not have. Since propranolol is contraindicated in patients with asthma, these beta$_1$-blocking drugs may be used with less risk.

PTU and MMI are potent inhibitors of the synthesis of both T_4 and T_3. Although they partially block synthesis rapidly, it takes many weeks to deplete the thyroid of stored hormones, and the clinical effects of these drugs are therefore not observed for weeks. Since they are not available in a parenteral form, oral administration is required, often necessitating the use of a gastric tube in severely ill patients. As noted below, PTU but not MMI has the added advantage of partially blocking the peripheral conversion of T_4 to T_3. Thus PTU may be the drug of choice. Either drug should be administered at least 1 hour before iodides are given in order to prevent the excess thyroid hormone synthesis that occurs in the hyperfunctioning gland treated with iodides. PTU or MMI is continued long after iodides have been discontinued to maintain the euthyroid state so that definitive ablative therapy can be carried out. It should be emphasized in this regard that I^{131} therapy cannot be given to patients receiving iodides or for weeks after iodides have been withdrawn, since the thyroid RAI uptake is suppressed.

Iodide administration plays a major role in the treatment of thyroid storm owing to its rapid inhibition of thyroid hormone release from the gland. This effect occurs almost immediately after the oral or intravenous administration of iodide. Some inhibition of hormone synthesis may also occur in the thyrotoxic gland. Either Lugol's solution or saturated solution of potassium iodide (SSKI) is given orally, or a slow intravenous infusion of sodium iodide is administered to patients unable to take oral medication. Iodide therapy will result in dramatic improvement and should be maintained until the serum T_4 and T_3 concentrations are normal or near normal. Some escape from the iodide effect occurs, especially when PTU or MMI is not employed. Lithium, a relatively weak inhibitor of thyroid hormone release, also partially inhibits thyroid hormone synthesis and may relieve the manic behavior occasionally seen in thyroid storm. However, its margin of safety in severely ill patients is limited, and other more efficacious drugs are available, as already noted.

It is generally believed that the major thyroactive hormone is T_3, that the major source of circulating T_3 is derived from T_4, and that most, if not all, of the metabolic effects of T_4 result from the intracellular generation of T_3 from T_4. A variety of drugs are now available which impair the outer ring monodeiodination of T_4 to T_3 and offer a new dimension to the treatment of thyroid storm by decreasing the peripheral generation of T_3. As noted above, propranolol and PTU impair the conversion of T_4 to T_3, although the former is a relatively weak inhibitor. The corticosteroids, especially dexamethasone, are potent inhibitors when given in high doses. The survival rate in thyroid storm was improved when corticosteroids were administered. Until studies appeared demonstrating that dexamethasone inhibited 5'-deiodination of T_4, resulting in decreased T_3 generation, it was suggested that the improved survival rate was due to the relative adrenal insufficiency believed to be present in thyroid storm. Although there is some evidence of impaired conversion of cortisone to the more active corticosteroid hydrocortisone, and plasma cortisol concentrations may not be as elevated as expected, suggesting a degree of decreased adrenal reserve, the major effect of the glucocorticoids, especially dexamethasone, is most likely due to decreased peripheral generation of T_3. The gallbladder dyes, Telepaque and Oragrafin, are extremely potent inhibitors of 5'-deiodinase and also partially block the entrance of T_4 into the liver. They also have the advantage of containing large quantities of iodine, which can be released from the dyes and block release of T_4 and T_3 from the thyroid. Preliminary studies have suggested that these agents may be extremely efficacious in the treatment of thyroid storm. Although not as yet approved for use in the United States, the antiarrhythmic and antianginal drug Amiodarone inhibits 5'-deiodinase activity, is rich in iodine, and may also block entrance of T_4 into the cell. Although the drug has been implicated as a cause of iodine-induced hyperthyroidism in Europe, where iodine intake is marginally low, it might prove to be extremely useful in the treatment of thyroid storm, especially in the United States where iodine intake is high and the risk of Jod-Basedow's disease is therefore low.

In view of the multifaceted approach to the therapy of thyroid storm and the subsequent marked improvement in the survival rate to as high as 93 percent in some series, it is unlikely that plasmapheresis or peritoneal dialysis will be required in the treatment of this life-threatening disorder.

It is evident that each patient must be treated individually and that a set protocol cannot be advised for all patients. Specific therapy should be directed toward inhibiting the synthesis and release of T_4 and T_3 from the thyroid, blocking the peripheral conversion of T_4 to T_3, relieving the catecholamine mediated effects by beta-adrenergic blockade, and treating the possibility of decreased adrenal reserve with corticosteroids. Associated and precipitating diseases should of course be vigorously treated.

PRIMARY HYPOTHYROIDISM

DAVID H. SARNE, M.D.
and SAMUEL REFETOFF, M.D.

In primary hypothyroidism, the thyroid gland fails to achieve tissue levels of thyroid hormone adequate to maintain euthyroidism. Patients with hypothyroidism form a clinical and biochemical spectrum. Myxedema is characterized by gross cardiorespiratory, neuromuscular, and gastrointestinal dysfunction. In subclinical hypothyroidism, a lack of symptoms is accompanied by normal serum thyroid hormone levels. All patients will have an elevated basal level of serum TSH (thyroid stimulating hormone, thyrotropin) and an exaggerated TSH response to TRH (thyrotropin releasing hormone). The goal of therapy is to restore thyroid hormone in tissues to a level sufficient to relieve all symptoms and reverse all the biochemical abnormalities of hypothyroidism.

Primary glandular dysfunction is the most common cause of hypothyroidism. In the United States, chronic (autoimmune) thyroiditis and iatrogenic hypothyroidism are the most common etiologies in adults, while in infants, congenital athyreosis and inborn errors of hormonogenesis are more common. Irrespective of the cause, the treatment remains the same: exogenous hormone replacement. Exceptions are rare and include the administration of iodine to patients with an iodide trapping defect or deiodinase deficiency and the withdrawal of iodine from patients with iodine induced myxedema.

The normal thyroid gland synthesizes L-tetraiodothyronine (L-T_4) and L-triiodothyronine (L-T_3) within a large protein molecule, thyroglobulin. In this form, they are stored in the colloid of the thyroid follicles. As needed, the colloid is resorbed and hydrolyzed, and the hormones are released into the circulation. The normal intrathyroidal T_4 to T_3 molar ratio is 10 to 1. Whereas T_4 is synthesized only in the thyroid gland, 80 percent of the extrathyroidal T_3 is derived from peripheral monodeiodination of T_4.

PREPARATIONS AVAILABLE FOR CLINICAL USE

Thyroid hormone is available as synthetic hormone or as a crude extract from animal thyroid glands (Table 1). Natural preparations include hydrolyzed extracts and intact thyroglobulin. Synthetic hormone is available as L-T_4, L-T_3, or a mixture of both.

The sodium salt of L-T_4 (sodium levothyroxine) is the most commonly used synthetic preparation. The use of a pure chemical assures uniform potency. Absorption after an oral dose varies from 30 to 90 percent. The half-life of the absorbed T_4 is six to nine days. Most is reversibly bound to plasma proteins and only the free fraction is immediately available to tissues. These properties are usually advantageous. Therapy may be taken once daily and, although less desirable, can if necessary be administered on a once weekly basis (1.5–2 mg per week). Once a steady state is achieved, ingestion of the daily dose and even an occasional missed dose do not alter the serum concentrations of T_4, T_3, or TSH.

Available strengths for oral administration range from 25 to 300 µg. The colors of the various

TABLE 1 Thyroid Hormone Preparations Available for Oral Administration

Preparation	Generic Name	Common Brand Name*	Available Strengths
Synthetic			
Sodium L-Tetraiodothyronine (L-T$_4$)	Levothyroxine	Levothroid	0.025, 0.05, 0.1, 0.125, 0.15, 0.175, 0.2, and 0.3 mg
		Synthroid	0.025, 0.05, 0.1, 0.15, 0.2, and 0.3 mg
Sodium L-Triiodothyronine (L-T$_3$)	Liothyronine	Cytomel	5, 25, and 50 μg
Mixture of L-T$_4$ and L-T$_3$	Liotrix	Euthroid	½, 1, 2 and 3 grain equivalents (1 gr eq = 60 μg T$_4$ plus 15 μg T$_3$)
		Thyrolar	¼, ½, 1, 2 and 3 grain equivalents (1 gr eq = 50 μg T$_4$ plus 12.5 μg T$_3$)
Crude Hormone			
Powered thyroid glands	Desiccated thyroid	Desiccated thyroid	½, ½, 1, 1½, 2, 3, 4, and 5 gr
		Thyroid Strong Tablets†	½, 1, 2, and 3 gr
		S-P-T‡	1, 2, 3, and 5 gr
	Thyroglobulin	Proloid	½, 1, 1½, 2, and 3 gr

*Listed in the 36th edition, *Physician's Desk Reference* (Oradell, NJ: Medical Economics, 1982).
†1 gr is equivalent to 1½ gr of other desiccated thyroid products.
‡An encapsulated suspension in soybean oil

dosages have been standardized by the manufacturers.* Tartrazine (yellow dye #5), used in the 100 μg (yellow) and 300 μg (green) tablets may produce adverse reactions in patients sensitive to the dye. Sodium levothyroxine is also available in solution (100 μg/cc) for intravenous or intramuscular administration or lyophilized in mannitol (500 μg to be reconstituted in 5 cc NaCl) for intramuscular use.

A sodium salt of L-T$_3$ (sodium liothyronine) is also available. As with levothyroxine, the use of a pure chemical assures uniform potency. After an oral dose, about 90 percent of the drug is absorbed. The half-life of the absorbed T$_3$ is one day. The drug is best administered in two or three daily doses. Even after a steady state is achieved, each dose produces a detectable postabsorptive rise in the serum hormone level. This variation in the hormone level should not produce symptoms. T$_3$ has a more rapid onset of action following the institution of therapy and its effects disappear more rapidly after its discontinuation. T$_4$ and T$_3$ have distinct advantages. T$_3$ is the drug of choice when a rapid onset of action is needed, as in the treatment of myxedema, or when rapid dissipation of the hormonal effect is useful, as in the temporary withdrawal of therapy from thyroid cancer patients prior to scanning.

*25 μg, orange; 50 μg, white; 100 μg, yellow; 125 μg, purple; 150 μg, blue; 175 μg, turquoise; 200 μg, pink; and 300 μg, green

Liothyronine for oral administration is available in strengths from 5 to 50 μg. There is no commercially available preparation for parenteral administration unless obtained by special arrangement from Smith, Kline and French. It can, however, be prepared by dissolving crystalline L-T$_3$ in a slightly alkaline solution that is sterilized by passage through a Millipore filture.

A synthetic mixture of L-T$_4$ and L-T$_3$ (liotrix) in a molar ratio of 4 to 1 is available for oral use only. The product was developed to supply T$_4$ as well as T$_3$ in order to provide a more normal hormonal milieu. Only later was it recognized that most extrathyroidal T$_3$ is generated from T$_4$ in peripheral tissues. The absorption and half-life of each component remain the same as when they are administered separately. These preparations should be administered on a once daily basis. Their hormonal potency is identified by approximate equivalence to desiccated thyroid. Despite the similar ratio of T$_4$ to T$_3$, the two available synthetic mixtures differ in their hormone content. One grain equivalent of Euthroid contains 60 μg L-T$_4$ and 15 μg L-T$_3$, while 1 grain equivalent of Thyrolar contains 50 μg L-T$_4$ and 12.5 μg L-T$_3$.

Dose equivalents in terms of approximate biologic activity of the synthetic products are 100 μg L-T$_4$, 40 μg L-T$_3$, and 1 grain equivalent of the L-T$_4$/L-T$_3$ mixtures. The usual adult replacement dose is 100–200 μg L-T$_4$ per day (25 μg L-T$_3$ b.i.d.–t.i.d. or 1 to 2 grain equivalents L-T$_4$/L-T$_3$ per day).

Crude hormone preparations have been successfully used to treat hypothyroidism for over 75 years. Thyroid hormone extracts are prepared from the glands of slaughterhouse animals, usually cattle and pigs. The molar ratio of T_4 to T_3 in these products is usually 3 or 4 to 1, but pure pork products have even more T_3, with a ratio of 2.5 to 1. The U.S. Pharmacopeia sets a standard based only on the organic iodine content (0.17 to 0.23 percent). Determination of the actual content in T_4 and T_3 is not required, and thus inactive preparations primarily containing other iodinated compounds have been marketed in the past. There is no legal safeguard to prevent a variability in potency. However, reputable manufacturers currently standardize their own products by bioassay or chemical analysis, and any serious variation in potency is unlikely. Nevertheless, with the increasing use of generic prescriptions, the use of preparations from different manufacturers may lead to an inadvertent change in dosage. There are no side effects specifically associated with the crude hormone preparations.

These preparations can only be used orally. Available strengths range from 0.25 to 5 gr. Tablets of more than 3 gr desiccated thyroid contain hormone in excess of normal replacement therapy, and they should be avoided. Among the various preparations, the biologic potency per grain is roughly equivalent except for Marion Thyroid Strong Tablet, which is 1.5 times more potent than most desiccated thyroid products. The approximate equivalent of 100 μg L-T_4 is 1 gr of desiccated thyroid. Thus the usual adult replacement dosage is 1–2 gr daily.

Crude hormone in the form of pork thyroglobulin is also available. This compound is especially high in T_3 content. It offers no advantages over other biologically active extracts and is more expensive.

As the price difference between the synthetic products and crude extracts has decreased, the former have become the drugs of choice. Except for special circumstances requiring rapid alterations in hormone effect, L-T_4 is preferable to L-T_3 because its longer half-life allows replacement with a single daily dose and provides a more stable hormonal blood level. As most tissue T_3 is normally derived from T_4, we do not ordinarily use the combination products.

INSTITUTION OF THERAPY

The rapidity with which normal thyroid hormone levels should be restored depends on a number of factors, including age, duration and severity of hypothyroidism, and the presence of other disorders (Table 2). In a young, otherwise healthy

TABLE 2   Administration of L-T_4

Patient	Initial Dose	Next Increase	Added Doses	Maintenance
Adult				
Under 45 years old, mild hypothyroidism	100 μg T_4 daily	50 μg T_4 at 4–8 weeks	50 μg T_4 at 4–8 weeks	100–200 μg T_4
Under 45 years old, marked hypothyroidism *or* Over 45 years old, mild hypothyroidism, and without known cardiac disease	50 μg T_4 daily	50 μg T_4 at 4 weeks	50 μg T_4 at 4–8 weeks	100–200 μg T_4
Over 45 years old, marked hypothyroidism *or* Known cardiac disease*	25–50 μg T_4 daily	12.5–25 μg T_4 at 4 weeks	12.5–25 μg T_4 at 4–8 weeks	100–200 μg T_4
Myxedema coma	500 μg T_4 i.v.	25 μg T_3 q 6 h‡		100–200 μg T_4
Child				
Infants, neonates	25 μg T_4 daily	12.5 μg T_4 at age 6 months	12.5 μg T_4 at age 1 year	
2–10 years†	50 μg T_4 daily	12.5–25 μg T_4 at 4–8 weeks	12.5–25 μg T_4 at 4–8 weeks	150–200 μg T_4

*Recommended dosages may produce unacceptable exacerbation of angina.
†Maintenance dosage is usually about 3.5 μg/kg body weight.
‡Until condition is improved, T_3 should then be discontinued and the patient should be treated with 100 μg T_4 daily.

individual with a recent onset of hypothyroidism, therapy may be instituted with 100 μg L-T$_4$ daily. Further adjustment, usually an increase, is made at monthly or bimonthly intervals until the patient is euthyroid. In patients with recent onset of hypothyroidism after radioiodide treatment, hormone replacement should not be instituted until serum TSH levels have been elevated for seven to ten days without a documented increase in serum T$_4$ levels. In younger patients with longstanding hypothyroidism and in patients over the age of 45 but without known heart disease, we begin therapy with 50 μg L-T$_4$ daily and after 4 weeks increase the dosage to 100 μg per day. The dosage is further adjusted as above. In adults, the usual replacement dosage is 100–200 μg L-T$_4$ daily, with only 20 percent of adults requiring the higher dose and very few requiring more than 200 μg daily.

In older patients with severe hypothyroidism and in patients with known ischemic heart disease, the initial dose should be only 25 μg L-T$_4$ daily. An EKG should be obtained before beginning therapy. The patient must be closely followed as the daily dose is increased by 25 μg increments at monthly intervals. Some patients may tolerate increments of only 12.5 μg L-T$_4$. In a few patients angina may actually improve, but in most the frequency and severity of the attacks could increase with higher doses of thyroid hormone. Even with the addition of beta-blockers and nitrates, some patients cannot achieve euthyroidism without an unacceptable exacerbation of angina. Such patients should be evaluated for coronary artery bypass, and if they are otherwise appropriate candidates, they can undergo surgery despite having only partial hormone replacement.

In hypothyroid neonates and infants, full maintenance therapy should be instituted rapidly to prevent or minimize the deleterious effects of thyroid hormone deprivation on the still developing nervous system. We recommend beginning therapy with 25 μg L-T$_4$ daily, which should be increased to 37.5 μg by age 6 months and to 50 μg daily by age 1 year. It should be noted that the usual maintenance dosage in children is, on average, 3.5 μg/kg body weight per day* rather than 2.1 μg/kg body weight per day as in adults.

Myxedema coma is the end stage of severe, long-neglected, or undiagnosed hypothyroidism. The treatment of this condition is described in detail in Chapter 18. It is a medical emergency with a high mortality rate even with proper treatment. If the diagnosis is apparent on clinical grounds,

*Or 100 μg T$_4$/m^2 body surface area

treatment should be instituted without awaiting laboratory confirmation. However, a blood sample for serum thyroid hormone determination should be obtained prior to the initiation of therapy. The proper method for hormone replacement in this condition remains controversial. Our goal is to restore serum levels of free T$_4$ and T$_3$ rapidly, this requires a loading dose to saturate the hormone-binding serum proteins. We recommend an intravenous bolus of 500 μg L-T$_4$ followed by 25 μg L-T$_3$ every 6 hours via nasogastric tube until improvement is noted. The dosage is then reduced to normal maintenance level. Adjunctive therapy, including cautious administration of intravenous fluids, ventilatory assistance, and treatment of hypothermia, infection, and other complications, should be administered in an intensive care unit setting.

Patients with subclinical hypothyroidism have no signs or symptoms of hypothyroidism. Serum levels of T$_4$ and T$_3$ may be within the normal range. The condition is detected by an elevated basal serum TSH level and an exaggerated TSH response to TRH. The question of need for treatment in this entity remains controversial. We supplement these patients with thyroid hormone when such treatment does not pose any significant risk, since therapy may reverse subtle abnormalities and some of these patients ultimately develop clinical hypothyroidism.

In patients with suspected adrenal dysfunction, evaluation of the hypothalamic-pituitary-adrenal axis should be performed and full replacement glucocorticoid therapy instituted prior to initiating thyroid hormone therapy. In patients with inadequate adrenal reserve, thyroid hormone may precipitate adrenal crisis. If rapid treatment is required, cortisol levels before and 1 hour after the administration of cosyntropin should be obtained and hydrocortisone administered before giving thyroid hormone. Any patient with secondary (pituitary) or tertiary (hypothalamic) hypothyroidism must also be evaluated for adrenal insufficiency (see Chapter 27). If a patient requiring elective surgery is found to be hypothyroid, the operation should be postponed until the patient is made euthyroid. If the operative procedure is urgent, it may be carried out with relative safety unless the hypothyroidism is quite severe.

MAINTENANCE THERAPY

Once euthyroidism is achieved, patients can be maintained on the same single daily dose of L-T$_4$. Adjustments are rarely needed unless other disorders intervene. No dosage change is usually required during pregnancy because, although total T_4 levels are increased secondary to increased levels of thyroid binding globulin (TBG), the absolute amount of thyroid hormone degraded each day remains unchanged.

With concomitant severe illness, the peripheral conversion of T_4 to T_3 is reduced. As appropriate serum levels of T_3 in·this setting are not known, we do not alter thyroid hormone therapy in these patients.

MONITORING THERAPY

No available test can clearly document the achievement of physiologic tissue levels of thyroid hormone. Basal metabolic rate, cholesterol, CPK, and other parameters that indirectly quantitate the effect of thyroid hormone on peripheral tissues vary for other reasons and are not reliable indicators of euthyroidism. In the past, measurement of protein bound iodine (PBI) and later total T_4 and T_3 in serum were used to monitor therapy. Interpretation of results requires particular attention to the hormone preparations used, and in some instances, the timing of blood sampling in relation to the treatment schedule. The ability to measure serum TSH levels has greatly improved the accuracy with which thyroid hormone replacement can be monitored. The response of TSH to TRH is the most sensitive indicator of the adequacy of thyroid hormone replacement. Once a normal TSH response is achieved, an increment of only 5 µg of T_3 is sufficient to abolish it. In most cases, though, the basal serum TSH level is an adequate index of the proper replacement dosage. We increase the dosage of thyroid hormone in the manner described above until the basal TSH level is within the normal range.

Although an elevated TSH level indicates inadequate replacement, the inability of most current routine assays to discriminate between low and normal TSH values limits its use to detect overdosage. The failure of TSH to respond to TRH does suggest overdosage in patients with primary hypothyroidism. The daily dosage of T_4 should be decreased by 25 µg, with further monthly decrements according to the resulting TSH level. The appropriate dosage is then the lowest that maintains the TSH within the normal range. Alternatively, a TRH test can be performed with each decrement, with the appropriate replacement dosage being that which no longer suppresses the response to TSH.

In patients with secondary hypothyroidism (pituitary dysfunction), serum free hormone levels interpreted in light of the hormone preparation and an understanding of usual maintenance dosage must be used to judge the adequacy of therapy. In patients with tertiary hypothyroidism (hypothalamic dysfunction), although the basal TSH will not be a reliable indicator, the TSH response to TRH can be used for monitoring therapy.

While on L-T_4 therapy, at a dosage sufficient to restore the TSH level to normal, most patients with primary hypothyroidism will have normal values for total T_4 (TT$_4$), free thyroxine index (FTI), and total T_3 by radioimmunoassay (TT$_3$). TT$_4$ and FTI values tend to be high normal and TT$_3$ values low normal. In 10 to 15 percent of patients, TT$_4$ and FTI values will be above the upper limit of normal. However, since the TSH will remain elevated with a lower dosage, we presume this reflects the somewhat lower levels of TT$_3$.

Patients treated solely with L-T_3 will characteristically have low TT$_4$ and FTI values and elevated levels of T_3. Pituitary conversion of T_4 to T_3 appears to play a major role in the normal regulation of thyroid hormone; thus in the face of a low serum T_4, the serum T_3 level necessary to achieve TSH suppression is higher.

If clinical or biochemical evidence of hypothyroidism persists despite suppression of TSH to normal, the response to TRH should be evaluated. If it remains exaggerated, the dosage of thyroid hormone should be increased. If the response to TRH is normal or suppressed, either the abnormalities are not related to thyroid hormone lack or the patient may have peripheral but not pituitary resistance to the action of thyroid hormone.

Some patients who became hypothyroid after the definitive treatment of Graves' disease require very small doses to achieve euthyroidism. Their glands most likely retain autonomous function but lack sufficient capacity to maintain euthyroidism.

TREATMENT FAILURES

Most adults achieve euthyroidism with a daily dosage of 200 µg L-T_4 or less. If after a 2- to 6-month trial on 200 µg L-T_4 daily the patient has still not become euthyroid, the following should be considered (Table 3). The most common reason is failure to take the medication as prescribed. This can be documented by administration of the hormones under supervision. Other explanations include incorrect diagnosis, malabsorption, rapid

TABLE 3 Evaluation of Patients Requiring Unusual Doses of L-T₄ for Subjective Improvement

			Etiologies	Recommendation
Subphysiologic dose (< 100 μg/day)	Basal TSH normal	FTI low	1. T_3 toxicosis 2. Recent decrease in replacement dosage 3. Taking preparation rich in T_3 4. 2° or 3° hypothyroidism 5. Taking drugs that alter T_4 binding and metabolism (e.g., Dilantin) or suppress TSH (e.g., bromocriptine)	Check T_3 Repeat TSH, FTI in 2 weeks Check T_3 TRH test Check drug history, increase T_4 if TSH is affected
		FTI normal	1. Proper replacement	Verify with TRH test, continue with same dosage
		FTI high	1. Nonsuppressible endogenous T_4 2. Patient taking more than prescribed dosage	Reduce dosage Check history, reduce dosage
	Basal TSH high	FTI low or normal	1. Inadequate replacement	Increase dosage
		FTI high	1. Inappropriate TSH secretion (pituitary adenoma or resistance to thyroid hormone)	Evaluation for adenoma vs. resistance
Supraphysiologic dose (> 200 μg/day)	Basal TSH normal	FTI low or normal	1. Poor absorption 2. Rapid metabolism 3. Inactive preparation 4. Patient taking less than prescribed dose	Check absorption Check metabolism Change preparation, recheck Check history
		FTI high	1. Overtreatment 2. Peripheral resistance to thyroid hormone	Reduce dosage 25 μg, repeat TSH, FTI in 4 weeks Evaluate for resistance
	Basal TSH high	FTI low or normal	1. Poor absorption 2. Rapid metabolism 3. Patient taking less than prescribed dose 4. Inactive preparation 5. Unusually high requirement	Increase dosage 25 μg, repeat TSH, FTI in 4 weeks Check metabolism Check history Change preparation Increase dosage 25 μg, recheck TSH, FTI in 4 weeks
		FTI high	1. Pituitary and peripheral resistance to thyroid hormone	Evaluate for resistance

degradation or excretion of the hormone, use of an inactive preparation, and resistance to thyroid hormone. The last two circumstances are rare, while incorrect diagnosis is much more common. Re-evaluation of the clinical and laboratory data should ensure the accuracy of diagnosis. Proper re-evaluation may require withdrawal of replacement hormone.

As thyroid hormone is recycled via the enterohepatic circulation, the failure of biliary reabsorption as well as intestinal absorption may lead to increased fecal loss. Steatorrhea, the use of binding resins, such as cholestyramine, and,

rarely, a high soy bean diet may lead to excessive fecal loss of the ingested hormone. We have also observed a patient with inadequate absorption secondary to severe achalasia. Malabsorption may be documented by the measurement of protein bound radioactive iodine following the simultaneous administration of oral and intravenous thyroid hormone, each labeled with a different iodine isotope. Rapid metabolism can be demonstrated by kinetic studies using radiolabeled hormone. An estimate of metabolic clearance can be made using the levels of bound and free hormone on the usual replacement dosage, provided regular ingestion can be documented. Other than treatment of the underlying cause, increasing the daily dosage of hormone should provide adequate replacement in the above conditions.

Direct chemical analysis or bioassay can confirm the presence of an inactive preparation, but in practice, simply changing the preparation is sufficient. Resistance of the pituitary and peripheral tissues to thyroid hormone is a rare condition. With current techniques, the proof is time consuming and requires a sophisticated investigation. It should be suspected when the other causes of treatment failure have been excluded.

SIDE EFFECTS

Although a very rare patient may have a reaction to the dyes or other additives, true allergic or idiosyncratic reactions to the hormone are unheard of. Most common toxic effects relate to overdosage and are those of thyrotoxicosis. Headaches, palpitations, and anxiety are the most common complaints. Treatment consists of temporary cessation of therapy and resumption at a lower dosage. Deleterious effects in the setting of adrenal insufficiency or cardiac disease have already been discussed. Nonspecific complaints that appear to be psychologic in origin and gastrointestinal symptoms can sometimes be relieved by changing the time of drug ingestion or by administering the hormone with meals or in divided doses.

DRUG INTERACTIONS

Since alterations in metabolic status can affect the handling of a variety of drugs, patients should be carefully observed during the institution of therapy; the dosages of other drugs may need adjustment. Requirements for insulin or oral hypoglycemic agents often increase with thyroid hormone therapy. The effects of anticoagulants are increased, while those of digitalis and propranolol may be substantially decreased. Particular attention should also be paid to the dosages of diuretics, sedatives, and opiates. As mentioned previously, cholestyramine and other binding resins may decrease the absorption of thyroid hormone.

WITHDRAWAL OF THERAPY

Re-evaluation of the diagnosis of hypothyroidism and the treatment of thyroid carcinoma with ^{131}I require the cessation of thyroid hormone therapy. Even with replacement dosages of L-T$_4$, suppression of TSH may persist for four to six weeks after this hormone is discontinued. During this period there is a progressive fall in the level of thyroid hormone, and transient signs and symptoms of hypothyroidism may develop even in patients who ultimately prove not to be hypothyroid. Only if serum T$_4$ levels fail to increase over a period of seven to ten days during which TSH has been elevated is the presence of primary hypothyroidism confirmed.

To shorten the period during which patients are subjected to the symptoms of hypothyroidism, we switch patients from L-T$_4$ to an equivalent dosage of T$_3$ administered b.i.d. or t.i.d. four weeks before hormone therapy is discontinued altogether. With this regimen, serum TSH should start rising within 10 to 14 days; however, on occasion at least 21 days must elapse. Patients with thyroid carcinoma resume therapy immediately after the scan is completed, unless they will be receiving a treatment dose of radioactive iodine, in which case the replacement is delayed until 24 hours after ^{131}I therapy.

This chapter was supported in part by U.S. Public Health Grants AM 15,070, AM 07011, and RR 55.

MYXEDEMA COMA

BASIL RAPOPORT, M.B.

Myxedema coma is a medical emergency with a reported fatality rate as high as 80 percent. As its name suggests, this condition involves a diminished level of consciousness in association with severe hypothyroidism. Fortunately, myxedema coma is encountered relatively rarely in clinical practice, and only approximately 100 cases have been reported in the literature. This figure must be considered in the light of hypothyroidism being a common clinical condition. That is, very few patients with hypothyroidism develop myxedema coma. In recent years, however, with increasing attention being focused on the problem, the diagnosis of myxedema coma is being made more frequently. One possible reason for its apparent rarity is that cases of myxedema coma may remain unrecognized. Thus seriously ill persons dying with a multitude of medical problems, such as respiratory failure and infection, may have unrecognized hypothyroidism that contributes to their demise.

Myxedema coma may present as the end manifestation of chronic, severe primary thyroid failure. In this situation, patients with untreated hypothyroidism, with all the classic signs and symptoms of this condition, slowly lapse into stupor, coma, and then death. A more common presentation, however, is that of myxedema coma precipitated in patients with moderate or unrecognized hypothyroidism by a superimposed acute medical illness, particularly an infection, or following the administration of sedatives or narcotics. Myxedema coma should therefore be considered in all stuporous or comatose patients, particularly when hypothermia is also present and when a reason for the diminished level of consciousness is not clearly evident.

WHEN TO TREAT

Recent evidence suggests that the early and aggressive therapy of myxedema coma significantly reduces its mortality rate (Table 1). Indeed, in the absence of irreversible or untreated associated illness, recognized myxedema coma should now rarely be a direct cause of death. Important factors determining the mortality rate in myxedema coma are the duration of coma and the speed with which therapy is instituted. For this

TABLE 1   Summary of the Treatment of the Acute Phase of Myxedema Coma

1. Treat on suspicion
2. Maintain adequate ventilation:
    tracheal intubation or tracheostomy
    mechanical ventilation
    monitor blood gases
3. Treat shock with plasma expanders rather than adrenergic agents
4. T_4, 300–500 µg i.v., then 75–100 µg i.v. daily
5. Hydrocortisone, 50–100 mg i.v. every 8 hours
6. Treat hypothermia by passive warming
7. Intravenous fluids:
    provide free water sparingly
    provide intravenous glucose if hypoglycemic
8. Treat precipitating illness
9. Provide all medications intravenously

reason, and because laboratory confirmation of myxedema may be delayed for hours or even days, therapy should begin when the diagnosis is seriously suspected, even before it has been established with certainty. The rationale for this approach is that the regimen to be described below is of little risk if the patient ultimately proves to be euthyroid. Euthyroid individuals tolerate the short-term administration of a large dose of thyroxine very well. In contrast, as mentioned above, the delay of therapy can make the difference between survival and death.

MAINTENANCE OF VITAL BODY FUNCTIONS

Respiratory failure is a major cause of death in myxedema coma and may occur for many reasons. Severe myxedema decreases the sensitivity of the brain-stem respiratory centers to hypoxia and hypercarbia. In addition, as discussed below, a frequent precipitating event in myxedema coma is pneumonia or an exacerbation of chronic obstruction pulmonary disease.

While the development of respiratory failure may be insidious, it may also occur very rapidly and need immediate treatment. The airway should first be inspected and, if necessary, cleared. In particular, enlargement of the tongue that may be associated with longstanding hypothyroidism may contribute to upper airway obstruction. If the respiratory failure is acute, artificial ventilation should be initiated immediately, either mouth to mouth or with an Ambu bag and an airway. Forward pressure on the mandible is important because of the possibility of tongue enlargement. At the earliest opportunity the patient should undergo tracheal intubation and mechanical ventilation should be instituted. Arterial blood should be obtained and sent to the laboratory for the analysis of blood gases to ensure that adequate ventilation is being achieved. A tracheostomy should be performed if mechanical ventilation is prolonged.

In cardiopulmonary arrest from any cause, the patient's electrocardiogram should be monitored during the acute phase and an intravenous line inserted for the administration of medications. Hypotension is particularly ominous and difficult to treat, because hypothyroid patients are relatively insensitive to adrenergic agents. Alpha-adrenergic agents should be avoided because patients with profound myxedema already have severe peripheral vasoconstriction. In addition, the combination of adrenergic agents together with large doses of thyroid hormones (see below), particularly triiodothyronine (T_3), has been associated with serious tachyarrhythmias. Because myxedematous patients usually have a diminished plasma volume, it is more important to provide volume in the form of plasma expanders while central venous pressure is being monitored.

The patient should be transferred as soon as possible to an intensive care unit where vital signs are more easily monitored and specialized nursing care is available. With the patient now being adequately ventilated and perfused, venous blood should be drawn and sent to the laboratory for the determination of serum T_4, T_4 index, TSH, cortisol, hemoglobin, hematocrit, white blood count and differential, serum electrolytes, BUN, creatinine, glucose, creatine phosphokinase (CPK), SGOT, and LDH. Some of these tests will be important for later management, while others, such as the white blood cell count and serum sodium, are for more immediate management. Patients with longstanding myxedema may be anemic for a variety of reasons and whole blood may be administered if the hematocrit is below 25–30.

The above description is for management of myxedema stupor or coma with acute respiratory failure. In other patients, the onset of anoxia and hypercarbia with progressive mental impairment may be slow and insidious, and it may be revised by other measures (see below) without the need for emergency cardiopulmonary resuscitation.

Assisted ventilation may be necessary for a prolonged period of time, as long as one or two weeks after the institution of thyroxine therapy. The author has observed this phenomenon in a patient with unrecognized hypothyroidism who underwent elective surgery and in whom the diagnosis of myxedema coma was made postoperatively when the patient failed to regain consciousness or to resume spontaneous ventilation. The reasons for the prolonged acute respiratory failure are not clear but may include intercostal and diaphragmatic muscle weakness, obesity, atelectasis and pneumonia.

THYROID HORMONE ADMINISTRATION

Thyroid hormone should be administered as soon as adequate respiration and perfusion have been established. It should be appreciated that there is considerable controversy as to the correct form of thyroid hormone therapy in myxedema coma. Because of the rarity, gravity, and complicated nature of the condition, it is unlikely that controlled clinical trials with different hormone regimens will ever be performed. It is the author's view, however, that available evidence supports the likelihood that the improvement in the mortality rate in myxedema coma, as reported in more recent series, follows the early use of a large dose of intravenous thyroxine (T_4).

There is obviously a paradox in this form of therapy, in that severe myxedema in the absence of coma is traditionally treated very cautiously by administering small doses of thyroid hormone and waiting for the effects to be fully developed before increasing the dose. In the case of myxedema coma, however, the immediate threat to life from the myxedema itself takes precedence over the potential deleterious effects of too-rapid thyroid hormone administration. In other words, the risk of a serious cardiac arrhythmia is the price that must be paid for the more immediate and far greater risk of death from myxedema coma itself.

L-thyroxine should be administered as an intravenous bolus of 300–500 μg, depending on the size of the patient (approximately 7 μg/k with a maximum of 500 μg). The rationale for this dose is that the T_4 pool size is approximately 700 μg in the average euthyroid 70 k adult. The use of intravenous T_4 rather than T_3 is preferable for a number of reasons. First, an intravenous preparation of T_4, unlike T_3, is commercially available. Second, the disposal rate of T_4 is considerably slower than that of T_3. It is therefore possible to administer T_4 as a single daily dose rather than as multiple doses throughout the day. Third, in humans extrathyroidal thyroxine is the major source of T_3 production in that T_4 undergoes monodeiodination to T_3 in the peripheral tissues. The relatively stable T_4 pool functions as a depot, so that the peripheral T_3 concentration remains relatively stable. In contrast, when T_3 is administered, serum T_3 levels fluctuate widely and may be associated with a higher incidence of cardiac arrhythmias. Fourth, it is easier to monitor levels of T_4 than T_3 in serum because of the simpler and more widely available assays for T_4.

As mentioned above, not all endocrinologists would use T_4. An alternative is to administer T_3 (20–40 μg) intravenously at 6 hourly intervals during the acute phase of myxedema coma. The rationale for this is that the metabolic effects of T_3 occur more rapidly than do those of T_4. In addition, it is argued, the acute illness that generally coexists with myxedema coma decreases the peripheral conversion of T_4 to T_3, and T_3 therefore bypasses this metabolic block. Despite these theoretic advantages of T_3, however, the most recent reports on therapy of myxedema coma, in which T_4 was used, have indicated survival rates superior to those previously reported when T_3 was administered. Although the author prefers the use of T_4, it must be admitted that the most important factor influencing survival is probably the early recognition and treatment of myxedema coma with thyroid hormone in any form, as well as management of the usually very serious underlying precipitating condition.

If intravenous thyroxine is not available, or if one chooses to administer intravenous T_3, the preparation may be made by dissolving T_4 or T_3 powder in a few drops of 0.1 N NaOH. The solution is then diluted with sterile normal saline containing 1 percent albumin (to prevent nonspecific binding of the thyroid hormone to the container) and passed through a sterile Millipore filter (0.22 μ). Alternatively, crushed tablets may be administered through a nasogastric tube. In this case the dose should be doubled, that is, 1000 μg of T_4, because absorption of T_4 from the gastrointestinal tract is approximately 50 percent in euthyroid individuals. However, intragastric administration is less reliable that the intravenous route in severe hypothyroidism because of decreased intestinal motility and absorption.

Further T_4 administration is dictated by the clinical response. If the patient remains stuporous or comatose and is unable to take oral medications, 75–100 μg of T_4 should be administered intravenously in a single daily dose. It should be recognized that in severe hypothyroidism the metabolic clearance of T_4 is diminished, and that these doses of intravenous T_4 may temporarily elevate the serum T_4 levels above the normal range. These values will normalize as euthyroidism is attained and the metabolic clearance of T_4 returns to normal. However, this aspect of therapy does not present much difficulty, as serum T_4 levels may be monitored and T_4 administration adjusted accordingly.

When the patient is able to take medications by mouth, a physiologic replacement dose of T_4 (150–200 μg per day) should be instituted. As discussed above, the requirement for a greater oral than intravenous dose reflects the fact that only about half of ingested thyroxine is absorbed.

It is not recommended that serum T_3 levels be monitored, because values may not attain the normal range during the acute phase, especially if the patient has a severe coexisting illness or is also receiving glucocorticoids. Serious nonthyroidal illness as well as glucocorticoids decrease the peripheral conversion of T_4 to T_3. As mentioned above, however, the results with T_4 therapy have been satisfactory, even in patients receiving glucocorticoids in whom the T_3 level remains suppressed. Elevated TSH levels associated with primary hypothyroidism usually begin to decrease within 24 hours of initiation of T_4 treatment, and subsequently normalize over a period of a few days to a week. It should be recognized, however, that glucocorticoids also suppress TSH secretion and make interpretation of the serum TSH level difficult.

On the second day of treatment, if the serum T_4 level is less than 5 μg percent, and the patient is still stuporous or comatose, a second intravenous dose of 300–500 μg of T_4 should be administered. This is particularly important if there is coexistent bacterial infection, such as pneumonia. The rationale for this approach is that bacterial infection may seriously diminish the response to T_4 because polymorphonuclear leukocytes metabolize thyroxine and render the T_4 metabolically inactive.

GLUCOCORTICOID ADMINISTRATION

Hydrocortisone should be administered intravenously at stress doses (50–100 mg 3 times a day). While there has been no clinical study to support this therapy, and neither is it likely that such a study will ever be undertaken, this approach is justified because of the increased risk of associated adrenal insufficiency. Thus coexisting primary adrenal insufficiency may occur together with autoimmune primary hypothyroidism (Schmidt's syndrome). In addition, hypothyroidism may be secondary to pituitary insufficiency, in which case ACTH reserve may also be impaired, leading to secondary adrenal insufficiency.

Steroid hormone metabolism is decreased during hypothyroidism. That is, during hypothyroidism, limited adrenal steroid production may be sufficient for a normal response to stress. With the restoration of euthyroidism, however, adrenal steroid utilization is greatly increased. This, together with the frequently coexisting severe illness, will increase the need for adrenal glucocorticoid production, which may be beyond the capacity of the adrenals if their functional reserve is diminished. This situation increases the risk of acute adrenal insufficiency and shock. As mentioned above, it is important to draw a blood sample for analysis of serum cortisol concentration prior to beginning hydrocortisone therapy. If this level is elevated, consistent with the stress of the coexistent acute medical illness, and if there is rapid clinical improvement within a few days (before significant pituitary-adrenal axis suppression is induced), the dose of hydrocortisone may be tapered rapidly and the hormone discontinued. Obviously, if the endogenous serum cortisol level is subnormal during the period of stress, cortisol therapy must be continued and may be tapered to physiologic replacement doses as the illness resolves.

HYPOTHERMIA

Temperatures as low as 75°F have been recorded in myxedema coma. Severe hypothermia (less than 90°F) is of serious prognostic significance. Despite the hypothermia, shivering does not occur in this condition. It is important to recognize that monitoring body temperature in patients with myxedema coma is only possible with a low-reading thermometer. If a routine clinical thermometer is used, the hypothermia may not be appreciated. Despite the hypothermia, active warming with a heating blanket is not recommended. Instead the patient should be passively warmed with an ordinary blanket. Thyroid hormone administration is the most effective way to restore body temperature to normal. A rise in body temperature from subnormal levels should be evident within 24 hours of thyroid hormone therapy. Active warming with a heating blanket is potentially dangerous because patients with myxedema coma typically have a decreased plasma volume and intense peripheral vasoconstriction. Peripheral vasodilatation under these circumstances may produce shock.

TREATMENT OF THE PRECIPITATING ILLNESS

Although myxedema coma my occasionally occur because of profound hypothyroidism per se, the condition is more frequently caused by a coexistent acute medical illness. The most common cause is infection, either pneumonia or of the urinary tract. The diagnosis of acute infection may be obscured in myxedema coma because fever and leukocytosis may appear only at a later stage, following the administration of thyroid hormone. It is therefore important to obtain blood cultures as well as a portable chest x-ray at an early stage during the management of myxedema coma. Careful examination of the urine is also mandatory. Although recommended by some, the author would not suggest the use of empiric broad-spectrum antibiotic therapy unless a source of infection is clearly demonstrated. Other common precipitating causes of myxedema coma include drugs (particularly sedatives and narcotics), gastrointestinal bleeding, myocardial infarction, and chronic obstructive pulmonary disease. If present, these should be treated by the usual means. If the patient does not regain consciousness within 24 hours, the possibility of cerebrovascular accident should be considered, even if localizing neurologic signs were not present at the outset.

Intravenous fluids should be administered carefully. Hyponatremia is frequently present in myxedema coma because of diminished free water clearance in severe hypothyroidism. This may occur because of increased vasopressin activity as well as because of decreased glomerular filtration. It is therefore very important to avoid excess intravenous free-water administration. Despite the hyponatremia, total body sodium and water content is increased. The hyponatremia is best treated by correction of the hypothyroidism with thyroxine. Hypertonic saline should only be given if the hyponatremia is profound. Adequate thyroid hormone therapy is associated with a gratifying diuresis and return of the serum sodium to normal. Hypoglycemia is rarely present but should be considered, especially when hypothermia is present. The treatment is intravenous glucose.

During the acute phase of myxedema coma all drugs, such as digoxin for coexisting congestive heart failure, should be administered intravenously. This is because peripheral vasoconstriction may decrease absorption of medication given by other routes. It must also be appreciated that the clearance of administered drugs is usually impaired during the hypothyroid phase.

The rationale for measuring serum CPK, SGOT, and LDH values at the outset of therapy is that serum levels of these enzymes are commonly elevated in severe hypothyroidism because of their decreased metabolic clearance rate. With thyroid hormone therapy, these enzyme concentrations will gradually return to the normal range. Their use for the diagnosis of myocardial infarction may therefore be unreliable, unless serum values are known prior to the institution of thyroid hormone therapy. Thus elevated serum enzymes do not in themselves support a diagnosis of myocardial infarction. On the other hand, a failure of these enzyme concentrations to decrease as euthyroidism is restored, or an increase above already elevated levels, should raise the suspicion of tissue damage.

As for any comatose patient, careful and specialized nursing is essential. The patient requires frequent turning, and urinary retention and fecal impaction should be recognized and treated appropriately.

PROPHYLAXIS OF MYXEDEMA COMA

One last important, and frequently overlooked, feature of myxedema coma is its prevention. With the advent of the use of radioactive iodine for the treatment of hyperthyroidism, there is an increasingly large population of intrinsically hypothyroid patients requiring exogenous thyroxine treatment. It is important to reinforce continually in these patients the need for lifelong thyroxine ingestion and the potential consequences of the discontinuation of this therapy. All too frequently patients discontinue their medications because they ''feel so well'' on the medication that they don't appreciate the need for this agent.

ENDEMIC GOITER AND CRETINISM

JOHN B. STANBURY, M.D.
and GEORGE RICCABONA, M.D.

Endemic goiter is an exceedingly common disease in many regions of the developing world. In countries where it is severe, its treatment imposes a major drain on the resources of the medical care system. Treatment of sporadic cretinism (1 in 4000 live births) and of endemic cretinism is unsatisfactory unless begun within the early months of life, and even then the results may not be satisfactory. Both endemic goiter and endemic cretinism should never occur, since their appearance indicates failure to institute simple and inexpensive preventive measures.

ENDEMIC GOITER

Indications

There are four indications for treatment of an endemic goiter: (1) pressure symptoms on the trachea or esophagus or recurrent laryngeal nerve, or obstruction at the superior thoracic strait; (2) a mass in the neck that is unacceptable for cosmetic reasons or is unduly burdensome because of its mass; (3) unrelieved suspicion of malignant degeneration; and (4) supervening thyrotoxicosis. The vast majority of persons in an endemic goiter region are without goiter or have only modest enlargement of the thyroid which requires no treatment. The goiters of many adolescent males disappear in a few years. Many goiters slowly enlarge with the passage of time. At times, with or without recognized trauma, an acute painful focal swelling of the thyroid may signal a hemorrhage into a cyst, and may rarely require emergency decompression either by thyroidectomy or by needle aspiration.

Medical Treatment

Iodine

Occasionally a diffusely hyperplastic thyroid in an endemic region will melt away within a few days to two weeks or so of administration of three to five drops of Lugol's solution or saturated solution of potassium iodide, but usually nothing happens unless the goiter is small and recent. Occasionally the added iodide enables hyperplastic and autonomous elements of the gland to produce more hormone than is needed, and thyrotoxicosis occurs (Jod Basedow). The same events may occur after injection of iodized oil, but in this instance the iodine cannot be withdrawn. Iodide (or iodized oil) may have its only therapeutic role in the treatment of the child or adolescent who has a small goiter of recent origin. Disappearance of these small goiters occurs frequently in the course of prophylactic programs with both iodide and iodized oil.

Thyroid Hormone

If the patient is available for continuing follow-up, thyroxine (0.1–0.2 mgm per day) or triiodothyronine (75–100 μg per day in divided doses) may be tried or, if they are unavailable, desiccated thyroid may be used. Dramatic partial or complete resolution of the goiter may occasionally be achieved, but this program carries the same risk of inciting thyrotoxicosis as does iodide administration. The advantage of thyroid hormone administration over iodide is that the therapeutic result may be achieved more quickly, but the full therapeutic result may not be achieved for 12 to 18 months. During this time the patient should be watched for evidence of thyrotoxicosis. An increase in size of the goiter in spite of medication would suggest malignant degeneration.

Radioiodine

Success has been reported in reducing the size of endemic goiters with ^{131}I. Generally the dose has been large—25 MC and more—and at times has been given respectively. Radioiodine has been used when treatment was required but surgery was contraindicated. The risk of radiation-induced swelling of the thyroid must be kept in view, and transient thyrotoxicosis has been described. Since goiter is a response to reduced hormone synthesis, radiation damage to the goiter reduces thyroid function still further and necessitates that all hormone requirements be permanently satisfied with thyroxine or equivalent medication.

Surgical Treatment

The surgical approach to endemic goiter and its complications is quite different from that in nonendemic areas: Whereas in the latter, hyperthyroidism and suspicion of malignancy are the major indications for thyroid surgery, in endemic goiter districts many persons will have nontoxic goiter, some with severe signs of airway obstruction and esophageal narrowing; some will have toxic nodular goiters; and there will be a few cases of advanced and highly aggressive thyroid cancer. Without adequate prophylaxis these goiters will recur in 10 to 20 percent of operated patients, and they will sometimes be associated with recurrent nerve paralysis or latent tetany arising from the previous intervention.

Preoperative Care

Initial evaluation may disclose dyspnea from tracheal stenosis, congestion of the jugular veins from pressure on the thoracic aperture, hoarseness from recurrent nerve compression, Horner's syndrome due to compression of the cervical sympathetic nerves, and stridor. The examination may include indirect laryngoscopy for recurrent nerve function, and a search for evidence of cardiac or pulmonary limitation. Particular attention should be paid to the possibility of underlying thyrotoxicosis. The evaluation should include, if possible, radiographic study for tracheal or esophageal obstruction and possible extension of the goiter into the mediastinum; definition of thyroid function by measurements of FT_4I, FT_4, T_3, TSH, and possibly the TRH test; thyroid scan for size and configuration, and regional function of the thyroid; possibly fine needle biopsy of cold nodules; and, in previously operated patients, measurements of plasma phosphorus and calcium concentrations.

If surgery is considered necessary, one may proceed as follows.

Nontoxic Nodular Goiter. With compression of the trachea of more than one-third of the diameter adequate decompression can be obtained in most cases when the adventitia is spared and no calcified tracheal cartilage prevents postoperative dilatation of the trachea. Generally a *bilateral resection* is done under general anesthesia with orotracheal intubation. Thyroid remnants of 15–25 grams (gm) are left in place and the wound drained for 24 to 48 hours postoperatively. In *recurrent goiters* with scarring and difficulty in anatomic orientation and with unilateral large nodular lesions a unilateral resection should be employed for benign thyroid diseases.

Thyroid Cancer. For thyroid cancer (proven if possible at intervention by frozen section) the goal of the procedure is a "near total" thyroidectomy (for example, total lobectomy on the side of the primary lesion, subtotal resection of the contralateral lobe) with lymph node exploration and modified neck dissection if necessary. This ideal therapy will often be impossible, especially in endemic goiter areas, because of the advanced stages of the disease. Under such circumstances the surgeon should try to remove as much as of the tumor as possible without doing much harm to the patient.

Hyperthyroid Goiters. A distinction should be made between isolated "toxic adenomas" (hot nodules) and disease involving the whole thyroid gland. While in single "toxic adenomas" enucleation or unilateral resection will yield an adequate result, other forms of hyperthyroid goiters should be treated by bilateral, subtotal resections leaving 5–15 grs. of thyroid tissue. Clinically definitely "toxic" patients should be made euthyroid

TABLE 1 Postoperative Complications After Thyroid Surgery in Endemic Goiter Areas

Years	Unilateral Vocal Chord Paralysis (%)	Bilateral Vocal Cord Paralysis (%)	Tetany (%)	Fistulas (%)	Other (%)	Total (%)
1958–1969	6.8	1.5	0.77	1.53	0.12	10.72
1970–1980	4.2	0.3	0.35	0.7	0.01	5.56

Courtesy of Universitats Klinik, Innsbruck, Austria. Iodized salt was introduced just before 1970.

by antithyroid drug medication (carbimazole, methimazole) for three to four weeks prior to surgery. Adrenergic β-blocking agents, such as propranolol, can be added, as can mild sedatives. In less severe cases β-blockers, sedation, and Lugol's solution are usually preparation for surgery. With thyroid storm and large goiters, plasmapheresis together with an antithyroid medication and iodine can make surgery possible 7 to 14 days later.

Results

Results of thyroid surgery in endemic goiter areas are listed in Tables 1 and 2. Therapy of thyroid cancer in an endemic goiter is usually not only surgical but will include ^{131}I treatment, percutaneous irradiation with megavolt sources, and sometimes cytostatic drugs such as cis-platinum, vincristine, and adriamycin. While these thyroid cancer patients frequently have unfavorable prognoses, a combined therapeutic approach can provide actual cures in a significant number of cases.

Postoperative Care

Since the pathogenetic factor responsible for thyroid enlargement in an endemic goiter area is not eliminated by surgery, patients should be started at discharge on thyroid hormone medication (usually one-half the daily requirement) to establish adequate prophylaxis against recurrence of goiter. Since hypothyroidism after surgery can occur years after the intervention, a long-term follow-up of patients is necessary. The thyroid medication should be adjusted to the given situation, and calcium metabolism should also be monitored.

Thyroid surgery is a valuable therapeutic approach in any endemic goiter area if adequate diagnostic resources permit a reasonable surgical strategy, and adequate technical and sanitary conditions prevail. Postoperative follow-up will be an important factor for satisfactory long-term results.

Complications

In an endemic region there may be many "thyroid cripples," as a result of spontaneous, or surgically or ^{131}I-induced hypothyroidism resulting from the overzealous attention of physicians. Recurrent nerve damage and tetany are also seen fairly often in regions where the presence of endemic goiter has provoked frequent surgical attention.

Jod Basedow. This uncommon complication of the treatment of endemic goiter with iodide, thyroid hormone, or iodized oil is generally mild in nature and easily treated. If possible, the inciting medication is withdrawn and the patient treated with rest, an antithyroid drug, such as methimazole (10 mgm every 8 hours), and possibly with propranolol (20–40 mg every 8 hours). When the patient is euthyroid, iodide or thyroid hormone can be reinstituted cautiously, or if indicated the thyroid can be removed surgically.

Pregnancy. There is little information regarding the course and outcome of pregnancy in women with endemic goiter. Fetal wastage and deformities of the neonate are said to occur more often than in normal persons. The physiologic rise in thyroxine, binding globulin, and plasma thyroxine concentration may fail to occur. Many newborns in areas of unusually severe endemic goiter are hypothyroid. One may presume that it would be advantageous to both mother and fetus to meet hormone needs with L-thyroxine, 100–200 μg

TABLE 2 Late Results of Thyroid Surgery for Benign Goiters in Endemic Goiter Areas

Years	Clinically Hypo (%)	"Latent" Hypo (%)	Persistent Hyper (%)
1956–1969	11.4	?	4
1970–1980	20.5	25.5	2

Courtesy of Universitats Klinik, Innsbruck, Austria

daily, or equivalent medication throughout pregnancy and during lactation. Since the only sources of iodine for the infant are the mother's milk and such food supplements as are given, and the latter may be low in iodine, the nursing mother should be given at least 200 μg iodine per day or replacement doses of thyroid hormone.

Intercurrent Disease. In general the euthyroid state should be sought in the endemic goiter patient with intercurrent disease. This can be achieved with T_3, 75 μg daily in 3 divided doses, or less quickly by 1–200 μg thyroxine daily. Thyroxine may be given intravenously in moderately alkaline solution in extreme cases. Caution must be exercised in restoring the euthyroid state too rapidly in patients with congestive heart failure, angina pectoris, myocardial infarction, severely limited respiratory exchange, as in emphysema, or if pituitary or adrenal failure is present. In the last instance adrenal cortical support is required.

CRETINISM

Sporadic Cretinism (Congenital Hypothyroidism)

This disorder arises because of congenital absence of the thyroid or when only a remnant of functioning thyroid remains, or because an inborn metabolic error prevents or impairs thyroid function. The essence of successful treatment is early diagnosis, and this is now possible as a result of screening programs in most states, Canada, and Europe. While early treatment vastly improves physical development, it is not yet established whether neural functioning develops normally in all.

Our opinion is that a *presumptive* diagnosis of congenital hypothyroidism in the neonate is sufficient to warrant immediate replacement medication. We would prefer to see a cautious program of treatment started on the basis of a positive initial screen as soon as blood has been drawn for confirming tests. This inevitably will mean that some infants will be treated who do not need it, but this will do no harm and can be stopped if the confirming tests are normal. We do not advise metabolic studies on the infant with an inborn error of the thyroid; these can await the passage of a few years, when withdrawal of thyroid medication while the diagnostic tests are performed will do no harm.

If a diagnosis of congenital hypothyroidism is made beyond the neonatal period, treatment can

TABLE 3   Approximate Hormone Dosage

Age Range	Desiccated Thyroid, mg/day	Thyroxine, μg/day	Triiodothyronine, μg/day
0–12 months	40–60	50–75	25–50
12–24 months	60–90	75–125	25–75
2–4 years	90–120	100–150	50–75
4–12 years	90–180	100–300	50–100

be instituted according to Table 3). As the age of beginning treatment advances, less long-term benefit can be expected. If medication does not begin before 1 year of age, permanent retardation is certain; it is probable if treatment is not begun before 3 months. An important variable controlling the outcome is the quantity of functioning thyroid, if any, present during fetal life and before medication is begun in the neonatal period. Treatment of the older subject with congenital hypothyroidism may be accompanied by unacceptable behavior problems. A dose level must be sought which avoids overt hypothyroidism but allows socially tolerable activity.

Hypothyroid infants and children have poor control of salt and water metabolism. If parenteral fluids are necessary for intercurrent illness, care must be taken to avoid fluid and electrolyte overload.

Endemic Cretinism

Virtually no information exists regarding the results of early treatment of the endemic cretin. The disease generally occurs far from medical resources among medically unsophisticated populations. The condition is rarely recognized until developmental retardation is well advanced. Hopefully, as screening programs are begun in endemic goiter regions, the thyroprivic neonate will be identified and treated, and the question of reversibility of retardation will be answered. Cretins with hypothyroidism and unclosed epiphyses may grow rapidly with replacement medication. Whether there is any catch-up in the nervous system is unestablished. One should give the younger endemic cretin the benefit of any doubt, and provide a trial of hormone replacement for at least several months to take advantage of any potential for growth and development, paying careful attention to possible undesirable emotional or behavioral deterioration.

SPORADIC NONTOXIC GOITER

MONTE A. GREER, M.D.

Nontoxic goiter is a very common affliction. Although thyroid enlargement occurring in nonendemic goiter areas is usually classified as "sporadic," this term is somewhat misleading. Sporadic is defined as occurring in isolated, single instances. This is not precisely the case in sporadic goiter, since there is a strong family pattern of thyroid enlargement, regardless of the geographic region within which the patients reside. Fifty percent of patients with goiter in nonedemic areas have one or more close relatives with thyroid enlargement.

The etiologic agent of nontoxic goiter in an individual patient is rarely definitely determined. Some cases may represent thyroid neoplasia, chronic thyroiditis, or early Graves' disease without thyrotoxicosis. Treatment of these various categories is discussed elsewhere in this book. This chapter covers treatment primarily in relation to patients in whom a specific pathologic diagnosis has not been made.

TREATMENT

Thyroid Hormone

The primary weapon in treating nontoxic goiter is exogenous thyroid hormone. The rationale for the use of thyroid hormone is based on the negative feedback control of TSH secretion by circulating thyroid hormone. For each patient, there is an individual "set-point" for plasma thyroid hormone concentration. The sensor is located in the pituitary thyrotroph, which functions like a thermostat, and the thyroid like a furnace. When the efficiency of a furnace is impaired, as by a blocked fuel line or a malfunctioning burner, the thermostat sends signals more frequently and the furnace must work harder to provide an adequate amount of heat. The analogy holds for the pituitary-thyroid relationship. Impaired production of thyroid hormone, caused by a subtle biosynthetic defect that is not diagnosable by current techniques or caused by inhibitory drugs, allows an adequate production of thyroid hormone only if TSH secretion is increased. This higher concentration of TSH, in addition to increasing the output of thyroid hormone, also causes hypertrophy and hyperplasia of the gland. As soon as the thyroid is stimulated sufficiently to produce enough hormone to reach the set-point concentration in the thyrotroph, TSH secretion shuts off. A lower concentration of TSH is necessary to maintain normal production of thyroid hormone if a goiter is present, since thyroid secretion is proportional to the mass of functional thyroid tissue. This explains why plasma TSH concentration is rarely above normal in euthyroid patients with nontoxic goiter.

The objective of treatment is to reduce the size of the goiter or alleviate the complaints of the patient by the most innocuous, simple, and inexpensive technique available. Providing thyroid hormone exogenously meets this goal in the majority of patients.

Although the underlying etiologic factor in nontoxic goiter is rarely ascertained, this makes little practical difference in management. Whether the goiter is caused by impaired production of thyroid hormone due to deficient enzymatic machinery in the cell, destruction of tissue by chronic thyroiditis, or inadequate iodine substrate, treatment is basically identical. Exogenous thyroid hormone will reduce TSH secretion and allow regression of the hypertrophied gland to the same degree as would be attained by surgical hypophysectomy.

Although any form of physiologically active thyroid hormone will depress TSH secretion, levothyroxine (T_4) has generally supplanted all other substances. Being a synthetic product, T_4 is readily standardized and of uniform potency among reputable manufacturers. Since T_4 is the major secretory product of the thyroid and undergoes extensive extrathyroidal degradation to triiodothyronine (T_3), essentially normal plasma levels of both T_4 and T_3 can be maintained by the administration of T_4 alone. T_4 has a relatively long half-life in plasma of seven days, and the conversion of T_4 to T_3 (primarily in liver and kidney) goes on at a steady rate. Therefore the administration of the required daily quantity of T_4 in a single daily dose maintains a stable plasma concentration of both T_4 and T_3, similar to the situation that would exist if all thyroid hormone were being secreted directly from the thyroid.

T_3, on the other hand, has a short half-life in plasma (approximately one day), and supplying this hormone in a single daily dose causes marked fluctuations in plasma T_3 concentration. Although it has not been shown that these swings in plasma T_3 concentration are deleterious, there is a potential risk that marked elevations of thyroid hormone concentration above the normal physiologic limits, even for relatively short durations, might increase the damage to an impaired myocardium. T_3 is also considerably more expensive than T_4. Since in physiologically equivalent doses it is not more efficacious in suppressing TSH secretion, it is illogical to use this hormone instead of T_4.

Preparations from animal thyroid glands, such as desiccated thyroid or purified thyroglobulin, have proven their effectiveness in almost a century of use. However, since they come from a pool of animals with an uncertain history, their concentration of thyroid hormone and their ratio of T_4 to T_3 can vary from batch to batch and from manufacturer to manufacturer. Since the cost of desiccated thyroid is only slightly less than that of T_4, T_4 is generally preferred.

A combination of T_4 and T_3 in approximately the ratio found in the human thyroid gland is also commercially available. However, the cost of this material is considerably more than that of T_4 alone, and since oral ingestion of this combination also causes spikes in plasma T_3 concentration, its employment is not generally favored.

The quantity of thyroxine necessary to suppress plasma TSH secretion completely varies among different individuals, but the average daily requirement is 0.2 mg. I have seen nontoxic goiter develop in patients who were receiving 0.1 mg daily of T_4 for inappropriate reasons (for example, the treatment of obesity) in whom the goiter shrank dramatically when the dosage of T_4 was increased to 0.2 or 0.3 mg daily.

Theoretically, the minimum quantity of T_4 required to reduce plasma TSH concentration to subnormal levels should be employed. Unfortunately, current commercial assays are inadequate to distinguish between a subnormal and low normal plasma TSH concentration. Therefore, I usually begin treatment with an average daily maintenance dosage of 0.2 mg T_4 in an otherwise healthy individual. If the goiter regresses promptly, the dosage is continued until a minimum size has been maintained for several months, at which time the dosage can be reduced to 0.1 mg daily and the patient observed further. If no in-

crease in the size of the gland occurs, a dosage of 0.1 mg can be maintained indefinitely. If some re-enlargement of the gland occurs when the dose of T_4 is reduced, treatment with the previously effective larger dose can be reinstituted.

If no reduction in the size of the goiter is produced by 0.2 mg daily, the dosage is increased to 0.3 mg daily. If no reduction occurs after treatment for three months with this dosage, a radioiodine uptake is performed to ascertain that there has been adequate suppression of TSH secretion and of thyroid function. A TRH test is performed if the radioiodine uptake is still in the normal range to ascertain that 0.3 mg of T_4 daily is adequate to abolish the normal TRH-induced increase in TSH secretion. A very small minority of patients require more than 0.3 mg of T_4 daily to suppress TSH secretion adequately.

Suppressive therapy with T_4 does not change the underlying problems that caused the goiter in the first place. Therefore, if T_4 is discontinued after the goiter regresses, it will recur in the overwhelming majority of patients. For this reason, I recommend that T_4 therapy be continued for the patient's lifetime.

The longer the goiter has been present, the more likely that it will develop "nodular" areas rather than presenting as a diffuse, relatively symmetric mass. These nodules are often histologically different from the paranodular tissue and from each other. They presumably represent geographic areas withing the thyroid which have developed from aberrant clones. One or more of the nodules may develop autonomy from TSH and undergo little regression with treatment with T_4, in comparison to the paranodular tissue or to the TSH-sensitive nodules. This allows the nodules to be more readily delineated as the paranodular tissue shrinks under therapy and may suggest actual growth of the autonomous nodules, giving rise to alarm that the nodules may be malignant.

In some patients thyroid enlargement represents a nonthyrotoxic stage of Graves' disease or of multinodular toxic goiter. The differentiation from Graves' disease may be particularly difficult before hyperthyroidism develops or if the patient is in remission from thyrotoxicosis after treatment with antithyroid drugs. A significant goiter may exist, radioiodine uptake may be normally suppressed, and the TSH response to TRH may be normal. Treatment with thyroid hormone will not decrease the size of the goiter and is contraindicated, since it will probably give rise to a supranormal concentration of thyroid hormone through the combination of both exogenous and endogenous contributions if the patient's thyroid function is independent of TSH. Eventually, manifest thyrotoxicosis appears in many of these patient.

Special Considerations

In elderly patients, or those with known coronary insufficiency, it is best to start with a lower dose of T_4 to minimize the risk of myocardial infarction. I usually begin with 0.1 mg of T_4 daily and increase this to 0.2 mg daily if there are no adverse effects and the goiter has not decreased in size. Elderly patients have almost always had their goiter for many years and are unconcerned about the cosmetic problem. Since the probability that thyroid enlargement will decrease significantly with T_4 therapy is inversely proportional to the length of time it has been present, observation rather than therapy may be the wisest course in the aged, unless subliminal hypothyroidism is a concern. As long as a normal pituitary-thyroid feedback relation exists and the amount of administered T_4 does not exceed the physiologic equivalent of thyroid secretion, no increased metabolic effect will be produced by thyroid hormone therapy.

In a few patients the goiter is caused by ingestion of drugs (for example, high doses of iodide or lithium) that inhibit formation of thyroid hormone in susceptible individuals and thus reduce negative feedback on TSH secretion. Removal of the offending agent from the patient's regimen will suffice to produce regression of the enlarged gland. When this is not possible, thyroid hormone can be added, as above.

Surgery

Surgery should be reserved for patients who do not respond adequately to medical management and for whom the cosmetic problem is important. If the goiter is due to an underlying biosynthetic defect in hormone formation, extirpation of a major portion of the gland will only compound the problem by removing the compensatorily increased mass of tissue that allows the patient to produce sufficient thyroid hormone. Although the patient is euthyroid before thyroidectomy, there is a high probability that hypothyroidism will ensue after thyroidectomy. The risk of the surgery is gen-

erally justified only if a serious cosmetic problem exists or, in rare instances, if the gland is large enough to cause physical disability by tracheal or esophageal compression. It is important to choose an experienced thyroid surgeon to minimize the risks of hypoparathyroidism and recurrent laryngeal nerve paralysis.

SINGLE THYROID NODULE

MARVIN C. GERSHENGORN, M.D.

Management of the single (or solitary) thyroid nodule is based upon deciding whether a particular nodule is likely to be a carcinoma so as to increase the proportion of malignant lesions operated upon and decrease the number of excisional biopsies performed for benign disease. A small number of thyroidologists recommend that all lesions should be excised, while others, also a small group, advise excision only if malignancy is highly suspected. I assume that all single nodules may harbor a carcinoma and utilize a series of diagnostic maneuvers yielding information that would suggest an increased or decreased likelihood of a nodule being malignant. The observation that the detection rates of thyroid carcinoma in surgical series range from 20 to 60 percent, a far greater prevalence than in the general population, attests to the validity of this type of approach.

CLINICAL CONSIDERATIONS

The clinical history of the patient with a single thyroid nodule offers the first insight into the likelihood that a nodule might harbor a carcinoma. A reliable observation that indicates that the nodule is of recent development and/or is growing perceptibly increases the chance of malignant disease. The risk is increased further if either of the aforementioned has occurred while the patient is taking thyroid hormone replacement or suppression medication. The age of the patient is important, since most thyroid nodules are found in patients over 40, but most cases of papillary carcinoma, the most common form of malignancy, occur in patients under 40. Thus the younger the patient, the more likely that a nodule is a carcinoma. The patient's sex is important because nodular thyroid disease occurs in females approximately four times more frequently than in males, but the female to male ratio for carcinoma is only about two to one. Thus a nodule in a male is more likely to be malignant than in a female. A history of radiation exposure to the head, neck, or anterior chest, especially if the dose received was greater than 100 rads and longer ago than 5 years, increases the likelihood of malignancy, since exposure to ionizing radiation has been found to be associated with an increased incidence of nodular thyroid disease in general and an increased proportion of nodules that harbor a carcinoma. (Although it had been feared that carcinomas found in patients who have been exposed to ionizing radiation may behave very aggressively, up to the present time, most tumors in these patients have been papillary carcinomas whose biologic behavior appears to be identical to similar tumors in nonirradiated patients.) A history that includes voice change, stridor, or dyspnea suggesting vocal cord paresis or paralysis, a Horner's syndrome suggesting cervical sympathetic nerve damage, dysphagia suggesting impingement on the esophagus, or a superior vena cava syndrome increases the likelihood of malignancy significantly. Lastly, a family history of thyroid carcinoma suggests that a nodule may be a medullary carcinoma.

The finding on physical examination of a single thyroid nodule is very important, since although apparently uninodular glands are commonly shown to contain multiple nodules at surgery, the likelihood of a clinically solitary nodule being a carcinoma is significantly greater than that of a nodule in a multinodular gland. In contrast to some thyroidologists, I believe that a single, dominant nodule in a multinodular gland must also be viewed with increased suspicion of harboring a carcinoma. Several characteristics of the nodule are important. Its consistency has limited value, since a firm or hard nodule may be caused by calcification following hemorrhage into a benign lesion, and soft nodules can be malignant. In the absence of calcification, however, a firm, sharply demarcated nodule is more likely to be malignant. Evidence of extension beyond the thyroid capsule or fixation to surrounding tissues is highly suggestive of malignancy. Rapid growth,

especially when the nodule is also tender, usually is due to hemorrhage into a benign lesion; cystic lesions are also usually benign. However, because malignant lesions may have cystic components and since hemorrhage may occur in any nodule, especially those greater than 2.5 cm in diameter, these findings do not exclude malignancy. Enlargement of the cervical lymph nodes and laryngeal and cervical sympathetic nerve impairment strongly favor malignancy.

LABORATORY EVALUATION

Laboratory evaluation of patients with nodular thyroid disease, especially the radioisotopic "thyroid scan," plays a major role in determining the likelihood of malignancy. Measurements of thyroidal iodine metabolism (radioiodine uptake), serum thyroid hormone and thyroid-stimulating hormone (thyrotropin, TSH) levels, and antimicrosomal and antithyroglobulin titers are employed to exclude known causes of nodular thyroid disease and to determine the patient's thyroid status. Serum thryoglobulin determination is not of diagnostic value, although it is useful in following patients after initial therapy for thyroid carcinoma.

Scintillation scanning with radioactive iodine or ^{99m}Tc-pertechnetate is an extremely important test in the evaluation of the thyroid nodule. Its value is based on the fact that most malignant neoplasms accumulate little or no radioiodine and appear as nonfunctioning ("cold") or hypofunctioning areas on the scintiscan. This is so because thyroid cancers almost invariably are less efficient in their capacity to take up radioiodine than normal thyroid tissue. The finding of a "cold" nodule on the scintiscan, however, indicates only that there is an increased likelihood of malignancy; most "cold" nodules are benign. Conversely, a clinically palpable nodule that appears to function as well as the surrounding tissue and is not delineated on the scan may, in fact, be hypofunctioning; it is important to note that to be detectable a hypofunctioning nodule must measure at least 0.8 cm, and even then it may be undetectable if situated at the margin of the gland, if surrounded by sufficient normally functioning thyroid tissue, or if radioiodine uptake by the thyroid is low. Such errors are less common when the location of the nodule on physical examination is carefully noted at the time of scintiscanning, and when imaging is performed with ^{123}I-iodide or ^{99m}Tc-pertechnetate—which allows for very high count rates—employing the gamma camera with pinhole collimator and taking both frontal and oblique views. Then a nodule may be classified as hypofunctioning when there is unequivocal demonstration of radioiodine within it, but less than in the surrounding tissue. The function of other nondelineated but clinically palpable nodules should be classified as indeterminate. The finding of a hyperfunctioning ("hot") nodule (toxic adenoma) that suppresses function in the remainder of the gland weighs most heavily against the likelihood of malignancy, since this type of nodule is very rarely, if ever, malignant. Most cases in the literature which purport to document the finding of a malignant hyperfunctioning nodule are clearly instances of incidental "occult" carcinoma in patients with toxic adenoma. In most instances ^{99m}Tc-pertechnetate may be substituted for radioactive iodine for scintiscanning in the evaluation of a thyroid nodule. There have been several reports, however, of nodules that appeared functional on technetium scintiscan but were nonfunctional ("cold") on radioiodine scan, presumably owing to their ability to trap iodide but not bind it to proteins.

Ultrasound examination of the thyroid is useful in differentiating cystic from solid lesions. This is important because a solid lesion is much more likely to be malignant. The finding of a simple cyst on ultrasonogram which corresponds exactly to a palpable nodule strongly suggests that the lesion is benign. In contrast, many benign and malignant neoplasms, especially those larger than 2.5 cm, will have cystic areas within them, but these are distinct from simple cysts.

I employ two other tests that generally offer less helpful information, but when positive, they strongly suggest that a nodule is malignant. The first is soft tissue roentgenograms of the neck. These may disclose punctate calcifications within the nodule which appear to correlate with psammoma bodies. This finding significantly increases the likelihood of papillary carcinoma. In contrast, dense calcifications, which are sometimes found in association with medullary carcinoma, have little predictive value, since they usually are found in areas of hemorrhage in benign or malignant lesions. The second of these tests is measurement of the calcitonin concentration in blood. When plasma calcitonin is found to be elevated, a diagnosis of medullary carcinoma or its premalignant state, C cell (or parafollicular cell) hyperplasia, may be made with virtual certainty.

Fine-needle aspiration and large-bore needle biopsy have measurably improved the preoperative diagnosis of thyroid nodules. In my personal experience, the fine-needle aspiration technique, which employs a 22-gauge or smaller needle, is easy to perform, allowing for sampling of multiple sites within a suspicious lesion, and is without serious complications. The theoretical complication of spread of tumor along the needle track has not occurred in several large series. I do not attempt routinely to make a specific diagnosis of the thyroid lesion but try more generally to differentiate malignant from benign conditions. In my experience, as well as that of others, satisfactory specimens are obtained in over 95 percent of cases and are correctly categorized in approximately 90 percent. A false negative diagnosis is made in approximately 6 percent of aspiration specimens, while the incidence of false positive diagnoses is less than 5 percent. For best results it is very important to have the aspiration sample analyzed by a cytopathologist who has gained experience with this type of specimen. If the aspiration specimen demonstrates a malignancy, surgery is recommended. If a malignancy is not found, a trial of suppression therapy is initiated. The fine-needle technique is of value also in the management of simple cysts, because their total evacuation without reaccumulation of fluid can obviate the need for surgical excision. In contrast to preference for aspiration biopsy, several groups have advocated using large-bore needle biopsy and have reported a high rate of correct diagnoses. False negative and false positive diagnoses occur about as often as with the fine-needle technique. However, even in experienced hands, the large-bore needle biopsy procedure can be complicated by hematomas, tracheal puncture, and transient laryngeal nerve palsy. In my opinion, since the fine-needle aspiration biopsy technique appears to be at least as accurate as large-bore needle biopsy and is virtually free of complications, it is the procedure of choice for preoperative diagnosis of solitary thyroid nodules and should be employed routinely.

THERAPEUTIC PLAN

The use of a trial of suppression therapy with thyroid hormone in patients in whom there is no contraindication, such as coronary artery disease or in the elderly, has been advocated. Even in the latter group of patients careful adjustment of the hormone dosage can permit a cautious trial of suppression therapy. The utility of this procedure is based on the observation that thyroid tissue, including adenomas, grows in response to TSH stimulation and involutes when pituitary TSH secretion is inhibited by thyroid hormones and circulating TSH levels decline. Adequate suppression usually cannot be estimated by measuring serum TSH alone but is documented by demonstrating radioiodine uptake of less than 2 percent or lack of response of serum TSH to administration of thyrotropin releasing hormone (TRH). A nodule that fails to regress or continues to grow with adequate suppression therapy is more likely to be malignant. Some nodules will become impalpable with thyroid hormone therapy and almost certainly repre- sent benign lesions. Many nodules, however, tend to diminish somewhat in size but remain clinically palpable, a finding that is not helpful in judging whether it is benign or malignant, since even some thyroid carcinomas can have a growth response to TSH.

The following is my approach to the management of a single thyroid nodule (Fig. 1). After the initial history and physical examination, all patients have their thyroid status assessed by determining serum concentrations of thyroid hormones and TSH, an index of the thyroxine binding proteins and measurement of antithyroid antibodies,

Figure 1 Management of Single Thyroid Nodule[1]

Hyperfunctioning Nodule[2]
  Hyperthyroid (''hot'' nodule)—administer bovine TSH to verify function of extranodular tissue:
    Over 40 years of age ⟶ RADIOIODINE
    Under 40 years of age ⟶ SURGERY OR RADIOIODINE
  Euthyroid—administer T_3 (25 mcg q.i.d. for 7 to 10 days) and repeat scintiscan
    Suppresses ⟶ SUPPRESS[3]
    Does not suppress
      Over 40 years of age ⟶ RADIOIODINE
      Under 40 years of age
        Smaller than 2.5 cm ⟶ OBSERVE
        Larger than 2.5 cm ⟶ SURGERY OR RADIOIODINE

Nonfunctioning (''cold'') or hypofunctioning[2, 4] nodule or a nodule of indeterminate function:
  Ultrasound
    Simple cyst ⟶ ASPIRATE AND SUPPRESS
    Solid or solid with cystic areas
      Clinically suspicious[5]
      Calcitonin elevated
      Soft-tissue x-ray positive ⟶ SURGERY
      Fine-needle aspiration biopsy malignant

    None of the above:
      Trial of suppression therapy
        ''Cold'' or indeterminate nodule of larger than 1 cm in a male or female
          under 40 years—for 3 months
            Unchanged or enlarges ⟶ SURGERY
            Regresses to smaller than 1 cm
              or less than 20% of original size ⟶ SUPPRESS
        Hypofunctioning nodule or indeterminate nodule larger than 1 cm in a female
          over 40 years of age—for 6 to 12 months
            Enlarges ⟶ SURGERY
            Unchanged ⟶ SUPPRESS OR SURGERY
            Regresses to smaller than 1 cm or
              less than 20% of original size ⟶ SUPPRESS
        Nodule of smaller than 1 cm—long-term
            Enlarges ⟶ SURGERY
            Unchanged or regresses ⟶ SUPPRESS

[1]History is obtained and physical examination is performed. If a nodule is found, serum levels of T_4, T_3, an index of T_4 binding, TSH and antithyroid antibodies are measured and then thyroid scintiscan is obtained.

[2]Uptake demonstrated with ^{99m}Tc-pertechnetate should be confirmed with ^{123}I-iodide except when the surrounding tissue is suppressed.

[3]Suppression therapy may be contraindicated in the elderly, in patients with cardiovascular disease, and so on.

[4]Definitely functioning but less than surrounding tissue.

[5]Clinically suspicious nodule is one in a patient who is under 18 years of age or who has ''high-risk'' radiation exposure or a nodule associated with cervical lymphadenopathy, fixation to surrounding tissues, or pressure symptoms.

and have a thyroid scintiscan. The scintiscan is best performed with ^{123}I-iodide or ^{99m}Tc-pertechnetate and the gamma camera with pinhole collimator. A nodule that appears to function with ^{99m}Tc-pertechnetate should be retested with ^{123}I-iodide, except when the surrounding tissue is suppressed. Oblique views are taken if the nodule is not well delineated by frontal scan. Patients with a "hot" (or hyperfunctioning) nodule that is suppressing the remainder of the thyroid have very little chance of harboring a malignancy. A nodule which on the scintiscan shows substantially more radioactivity within it than in the surrounding normal thyroid is also generally benign. In the patient with an apparent solitary "hot" nodule who is hyperthyroid, prior to radioiodine therapy or surgical thyroidectomy, I evaluate the functional capacity of the extranodular thyroid tissue by measuring its radioiodine uptake after administration of bovine TSH. In hyperthyroid patients over 40 years of age I recommend treatment with radioactive iodine. I administer a dose of 300 uCi ^{131}I retained per gram of nodular tissue after 24 hours to destroy its function and reduce its size. Repeat ^{131}I treatment is given at six-month intervals as required. In hyperthyroid patients under 40 years of age I recommend surgical excision of the nodule. Preoperative treatment with antithyroid drugs and/or propranolol may be given. In some patients between the ages of 20 to 40 years, ^{131}I treatment may be used; however, the theoretical possibility of the development of radiation-associated cancer in the perinodular tissue and of the development of hematopoietic malignancies must be considered.

In euthyroid patients with an apparently hyperfunctioning nodule, I perform a T_3 (triiodothyronine) suppression test by administering 25 mcg of T_3 4 times a day for 7 to 10 days so as to determine whether the nodule is functioning autonomously or whether it is simply hypertrophic thyroid tissue and can be suppressed with thyroid hormone. If the nodule is hypertrophic, I administer suppression therapy indefinitely. If the nodule is functioning autonomously and the patient is over 40 years of age, I recommend treatment with radioactive iodine to prevent the development of hyperthyroidism. If the patient is under 40 years of age my recommendation is influenced by the size of the nodule. If the nodule is larger than 2.5 cm I recommend surgical excision or radioactive iodine treatment while the patient is taking thyroid hormone for suppression of the extranodular tissue, since, with time, nodules of this size tend to enlarge and then produce hyperthyroidism. If the

nodule is smaller than 2.5 cm, I observe for the possible development of hyperthyroidism and for tumor growth. The patient may be treated with thyroid suppression therapy, but extra care is taken to avoid hyperthyroidism. The patient is observed for possible progression to a "hot" nodule.

Further work-up for the possibility of malignancy is performed in glands that contain "cold" or hypofunctioning nodules, or in which a palpable nodule is so situated that the presence or absence of function cannot be confidently decided by scintiscan. An ultrasound examination is obtained to differentiate cystic and solid lesions. Simple cysts, which appear as globular structures with smooth, thin walls and without internal echoes, are evacuated with fine-needle aspiration technique, and the straw-colored cyst fluid is sent for cytologic analysis. Cysts that arise in thyroglossal duct remnants are treated in a similar fashion. The patient is usually then given thyroid suppression medication and followed for reaccumulation of fluid. Reaspiration can be performed as often as necessary. Cysts that repeatedly accumulate fluid, especially if the nodule cannot be obliterated by aspiration, are sometimes cancerous, even though cytology shows them to be benign, and may ultimately merit excision. In patients with solid or mixed cystic-solid lesions, I perform fine-needle aspiration biopsy at multiple sites within the nodule(s). I may obtain soft-tissue roentgenograms of the neck, and measure plasma calcitonin levels. Patients with a family history of medullary carcinoma or of other components of the multiple endocrine neoplasia syndrome are evaluated with stimulated as well as basal plasma calcitonin measurements. The soft tissue roentgenograms are obtained to look for punctate calcifications of psammoma bodies. Surgical excision is recommended when the plasma calcitonin level is elevated, when punctate calcifications are present, or when there is a cytologic diagnosis of malignancy. It is important to note that, at present, I do not consider the cytologic diagnosis of benign disease definitive. I will recommend surgery also in the absence of the above-mentioned criteria if the patient is a child (less than 18 years old), there is cervical lymph node enlargement, fixation to surrounding tissues or pressure symptoms, and when there is a history of "high-risk" radiation exposure, especially more than 5 years previously.

The remaining patients are given a trial of suppression therapy. This will only last 3 months in patients whose risk of harboring a malignancy is high, that is if there is a definite solid, "cold" nodule, greater than 1 cm in diameter, in a male, or in a female under 40 years of age. If such a nodule does not substantially decrease in size, surgical excision is recommended. If the size is decreasing progressively, suppression therapy is maintained. If the size later stabilizes at 1 cm or larger (or greater than 20 percent of its original dimension in the case of a very large nodule), surgical excision is recommended. In my experience approximately 10 to 20 percent of these nodules will regress sufficiently to obviate the need for surgery. I assume that some tumors that respond to suppression therapy may be differentiated carcinomas; however, it appears safe to continue suppression if the nodule does not increase again in size and there are no findings strongly suggesting malignant behavior.

Patients with a 1 cm or larger nodule that is hypofunctioning on scintiscan, that is, radioactivity is definitely present within the nodule but is less than in the surrounding normal thyroid, may have a lesser risk of malignancy. In this group of patients and in females over 40 years of age who have a "cold" or indeterminate nodule of larger than 1 cm, I administer suppression therapy for 6 to 12 months. If the nodule regresses, suppression therapy is continued indefinitely. If the nodule enlarges during suppression, surgical excision is recommended. If the nodule neither regresses nor enlarges during suppression, a rather common finding, I recommend continued suppression therapy or surgical excision. Two factors influence the decision for surgery. First is the patient's age; in older patients, particularly women, most seemingly "single" nodules are actually dominant nodules in small multinodular glands, and the cancer yield is small. A second factor is size; the prognosis of thyroid cancer is much worse when the presenting nodule is more than 4 or 5 cm in diameter, and the hazards of postponing surgery are presumably greater. Therapy is individualized on the basis of these factors. Older women who have small "cold" or hypofunctioning lesions are maintained on suppression therapy; the younger the patient, especially a male, and the larger the lesion, the more likely surgical referral becomes. Lastly, patients who have a nodule that is less than 1 cm in diameter are placed on long-term suppression therapy. If the nodule enlarges, surgical excision is recommended. If the nodule remains unchanged or regresses, suppression is continued indefinitely.

I believe that it is now well documented that employing an approach to the management of the single thyroid nodule such as that outlined herein, which includes both ultrasonography and fine-needle aspiration biopsy, substantially increases the accuracy of preoperative diagnosis. This results in a decrease in the number of excisional biopsies performed for benign disease and in a reduction in the number of carcinomas left in situ.

GOITROUS AUTOIMMUNE THYROIDITIS (HASHIMOTO'S DISEASE)

ROBERT D. UTIGER, M.D.

The goitrous form of chronic autoimmune thyroiditis is the most common cause of diffuse goiter. It is an autoimmune disorder, characterized by the presence in serum of antithyroglobulin, antithyroid microsomal, thyroid cytotoxic and other antithyroid antibodies, sensitization of B lymphocytes to thyroid antigens, and deficient suppressor T lymphocyte activity. The major clinical manifestation is thyroid enlargement, with or without hypothyroidism. Patients with goitrous autoimmune thyroiditis typically have a small or moderate-sized firm diffuse or slightly irregular goiter. Most patients are clinically euthyroid. Their serum thyroxine (T_4) concentrations are in the lower range of normal or unequivocally low, and serum TSH concentrations are often elevated. About 25 percent have symptomatic hypothyroidism with low serum T_4 and elevated serum TSH concentrations. (Hyperthyroidism due to autoimmune thyroiditis is discussed in Chapter 15.) The diagnosis is most readily confirmed by the finding of positive serum tests for antithyroglobulin or antithyroid microsomal antibodies, since they are present in high titer in nearly all patients. The major diagnostic alternative is nontoxic multinodular goiter.

The two disorders usually can be differentiated by (1) the findings on thyroid palpation, (2) the tendency to higher serum T_4 and normal serum TSH concentrations in patients with nontoxic multinodular goiter and lower serum T_4 and elevated serum TSH concentrations in those with goitrous autoimmune thyroiditis, and (3) the finding of positive antibody tests in patients with goitrous autoimmune thyroiditis. The natural history of goitrous autoimmune thyroiditis is quite variable. In some patients there is no change in thyroid size or function over a period of years. In others thyroid enlargement increases, hypothyroidism develops, or both. Rarely, goitrous autoimmune thyroiditis spontaneously remits or has an intermittent course, or hypothyroidism develops coincident with reduction in thyroid size.

TREATMENT

The indications for treatment are thyroid enlargement and hypothyroidism. Patients who have a small goiter and no clinical or biochemical manifestations of hypothyroidism need no treatment. When thyroid enlargement is greater, unsightly, or causes neck discomfort or other local symptoms, T_4 therapy in doses of 0.1 to 0.2 mg daily should be given. T_4 therapy is obviously indicated in those patients with clinical hypothyroidism, whatever their degree of thyroid enlargement. The benefit of treating those patients who have a small goiter and are clinically euthyroid but who have low serum T_4, elevated serum TSH concentrations, or both is uncertain. In general, because of the difficulty of recognizing clinical hypothyroidism when it is mild, the possibility of the development of further thyroid enlargement or hypothyroidism, and the safety and low cost of T_4 therapy, treatment is recommended for these patients as well.

T_4 therapy results in some reduction in thyroid enlargement in most but not all patients. The decrease in goiter size may occur within a few weeks, but more often the response occurs over a period of several months. With continued therapy the thyroid gland becomes normal in size in about 20 percent of patients, and substantial reduction in goiter size occurs in 50 to 60 percent of patients. A larger initial T_4 dose probably results in more rapid reduction in thyroid size. Moreover, greater responses might be expected in those patients with high serum TSH concentrations. However, neither of these suppositions has been documented. In those patients whose goiter does not decrease in size during T_4 therapy, the thyroid enlargement is probably due mostly to cellular infiltration and fibrosis. There is little evidence that T_4 therapy directly alters the serum levels of antithyroid antibodies, and measurements of them cannot be used to predict responses to therapy.

The goals of therapy are complete amelioration of the clinical and biochemical manifestations of hypothyroidism and persistent reduction in goiter size. Monitoring of the adequacy of T_4 treatment of hypothyroidism is discussed in Chapter 17. If thyroid enlargement persists after full amelioration of hypothyroidism, a small increment in T_4 dosage, such as 0.05 mg daily, may be tried for several months. This may result in further reduction in goiter size and is unlikely to cause iatrogenic hyperthyroidism. The same empiric program may be used in those who were not previously hypothyroid.

Most patients should receive lifelong T_4 therapy, since withdrawal is usually followed by recurrence of goiter and development of hypothyroidism, even when it was not present originally. There are exceptions, however, particularly in younger patients. Therefore, there is no reason not to discontinue T_4 therapy after several years in a patient who is willing to be re-evaluated periodically thereafter.

WELL-DIFFERENTIATED THYROID CANCER

EUGENE W. FRIEDMAN, M.D.
and ARTHUR E. SCHWARTZ, M.D.

Well-differentiated thyroid cancer comprises papillary, mixed papillary-follicular, and follicular carcinomas. These are slow-growing, low-grade tumors with a generally good prognosis. Even the presence of widespread metastatic disease in lymph nodes, lungs, or bones is compatible with long-term survival. Although patients succumb to systemic disease, the most common threat to life is uncontrolled recurrent midline tumor involving the airway or major blood vessels.

FEATURES OF THYROID CANCER AND THEIR INFLUENCE ON PROGNOSIS

Histology

Most thyroid malignancies present as mixtures of papillary and follicular elements, particularly if multiple sections are taken. In 72 percent of our patients with well-differentiated thyroid cancer, the tumors were classified as papillary or mixed papillary-follicular. The remaining 28 percent of tumors were reported to be follicular carcinomas. Histologic features have a bearing on prognosis. Whereas papillary and mixed papillary-follicular carcinomas have a similar and benign course, follicular carcinoma, as reported by most but not all observers, behaves more aggressively. In our experience it is associated with increased recurrence and lower overall survival rates. Of our patients with follicular cancer, 16.6 percent have died over a 15-year period, as compared with 4.6 percent of those with papillary and mixed papillary-follicular carcinoma of the thyroid (Fig. 1).

Age and Sex

The age of the patient at the time of onset of the cancer is a major prognostic factor and may well have more influence on survival than the surgical approach or postoperative management. All

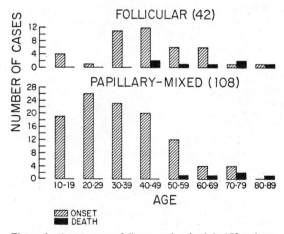

Figure 1   Age at onset of disease and at death in 150 patients with well-differentiated thyroid cancer followed for more than 15 years.

observers report a greatly improved prognosis in younger patients; we have not seen a death from disease in a patient whose carcinoma appeared before the age of 40, even though the condition is common in this age group. Figure 1 illustrates the relationship of age of onset to prognosis in our series.

We observed a female to male ratio of 3:1 in well-differentiated thyroid cancer in a group of patients followed more than 15 years. In 42 patients with follicular carcinoma, the age range was 10 to 87 with a median of 45 years. In 108 patients with papillary and mixed papillary-follicular carcinoma, the age of patients ranged from 17 to 79 with a median of 35 years. The decreased survival rate for those patients with follicular carcinoma and the fact that their ages at the onset of the cancer averaged ten years more than those with papillary and papillary-follicular carcinoma may be significant. There was no difference in prognosis between men and women.

Size and Extent of Primary Tumor

The size and extent of the thyroid cancer have been proven to have an impact on prognosis. Those malignancies that had grown beyond the capsule of the thyroid or had invaded adjacent structures were associated with a decreased survival rate. All patients in our series who died of disease had large (over 2.5 cm) primary tumors, most of which resulted in uncontrolled local recurrence.

Pregnancy

Pregnancy has had no apparent effect on tumor growth or prognosis. Five patients with papillary-follicular carcinoma who became pregnant within two years of surgery have remained well. Another patient with papillary-follicular carcinoma who had surgery during her pregnancy went on to deliver a normal baby and has remained well since that time. Two patients who developed follicular carcinoma within six months of delivery also remain well. Three patients had miscarriages within a two-year period following surgery for papillary-follicular carcinoma.

RESULTS OF THERAPY

Seven of our 42 patients with follicular thyroid cancer died over a 15-year period. Six of these had extensive local recurrent neck disease; 2 of these patients died from hemorrhage into the trachea. One patient died of pulmonary metastases. The length of survival ranged from 6 months to 12 years with an average of 4.5 years.

Five of our 108 patients with papillary and mixed papillary-follicular carcinoma died over a 15-year period. Three succumbed to extensive local recurrence in the neck, and two died with pulmonary and systemic metastases. The length of survival ranged from 6 to 17 years with an average of 9.2 years.

All patients who died of disease and were examined post mortem were found to have extensive systemic metastases; lungs, brain, and bone were the most common sites.

PROBLEMS IN EVALUATING THERAPY FOR WELL-DIFFERENTIATED THYROID CANCER

Many of the surgical and some of the medical aspects of management of well-differentiated thyroid carcinoma remain controversial. The rarity, protracted course, and low mortality rate of this condition, regardless of the method of therapy, make it difficult to evaluate alternative methods in the treatment of this disease. These factors also make prospective randomized studies frustrating to pursue. The frequent presence of foci of microscopic carcinoma in the thyroid gland and lymph nodes, which sometimes remain quiescent for the lifetime of the patient, makes it impossible to predict accurately the behavior of the disease from microscopic findings. However, although much remains unresolved, observation of the results of selective plans of management over a period of many years has validated some guidelines.

How Much Thyroid Should Be Removed?

Should the entire thyroid gland be removed for a carcinoma confined to one lobe? There are many studies demonstrating a high frequency of microscopic foci of cancer in the opposite lobe; these rates range from 10 to 40 percent on routine histologic examinations, the incidence depending mainly on how many sections are taken. On serial sections, it has been reported to be 58 percent. It is impossible to determine whether these represent intraglandular dissemination of disease or multiple primary foci. Despite the frequent incidence of occult disease in the opposite lobe, the practice of removing only the involved lobe and isthmus has resulted in a high rate of cure. Most institutions

employing lobectomy and isthmusectomy report a recurrence rate in the opposite lobe of approximately 5 percent, with one-half of these patients being salvaged by later resection of the opposite lobe. Those who succumb often do so from systemic manifestations of disease rather than from local recurrence. This has been true of patients with both follicular and mixed papillary-follicular cancers.

It is certainly well established that the presence of microscopic foci of occult carcinoma in the uninvolved thyroid lobe far exceeds the clinical incidence of recurrent disease, by a factor in the range of 8 to 1.

In a series of 31 lobectomies for follicular cancer and 70 for papillary and mixed papillary-follicular carcinoma clinically confined to one lobe and followed for 15 years, we have observed four patients who developed disease in the opposite lobe. Three of these patients had mixed papillary-follicular carcinoma, one had follicular carcinoma. Two patients had disease involving the trachea which could not be completely resected at the original procedure. These patients died of local recurrent disease. Another patient who had follicular carcinoma required removal of the opposite lobe 7 years after the original lobectomy and now remains well 25 years after the original operation. A fourth patient with papillary-follicular carcinoma died of local extension 11 years after the original lobectomy. Thus our rate of recurrence in the opposite lobe following lobectomy and isthmusectomy for well-differentiated thyroid cancer confined to one lobe was 3.9 percent (Fig. 2). Since two of these patients had unresectable tracheal disease and a third was salvaged by subsequent removal of the opposite lobe, only one death can possibly be attributed to a failure to perform an initial total thyroidectomy. This patient, how-

	Patients	Recurrence Opposite Lobe
Mixed P-F	70	3
Follicular	32	1
TOTAL	102	4 (3.9%)

Figure 2 Incidence of recurrent clinical disease in the opposite lobe of 102 patients with well-differentiated thyroid cancer confined to one lobe, treated by thyroid lobectomy and excision of the isthmus and followed more than 15 years.

ever, had massive retropharyngeal disease at the first procedure, and this may have accounted for his subsequent recurrence.

If a few additional patients could be saved, should a routine total thyroidectomy be performed? The main concern in total thyroidectomy is not the risk of injury to the recurrent laryngeal nerve. In the hands of experienced surgeons throughout the country, this is a rare complication with an incidence of 1 percent or less. Were it not for the specter of permanent hypoparathyroidism, total thyroidectomy would be universally accepted as the treatment of choice for well-differentiated thyroid carcinoma. The incidence of this complication, which may be more debilitating than the original cancer, has ranged from 10 to 30 percent in major institutions with extensive experience in managing thyroid carcinoma. Although there have been occasional reports of series of total thyroidectomies with only a 2 percent incidence of hypoparathyroidism, these results have not been reproduced by other thyroid surgeons. The risk of hypoparathyroidism reflects the inherent hazard of removal or devascularization of the glands during the total thyroidectomy and paratracheal and upper mediastinal node dissection. Our incidence of this complication in total thyroidectomy has been 5 percent.

We therefore continue to rely on hemithyroidectomy and resection of the isthmus for papillary and papillary-follicular carcinomas of the thyroid which are clearly localized to one lobe, have not extended beyond the thyroid capsule, and where no nodules are palpable in the opposite lobe. These constitute the great majority of cases of well-differentiated thyroid cancer. The presence of nodularity or extension of disease in the isthmus or the opposite lobe mandates total thyroidectomy.

Although past results have been favorable, indications in recent years for total thyroidectomy have been extended to include those patients in whom certain factors suggest a more guarded outlook. These include those patients in whom a diagnosis of follicular carcinoma is made on frozen section, those in whom foci of anaplastic tumor can be identified within well-differentiated tumors, and those patients with carcinoma who have had an exposure of the head and neck to ionizing radiation in childhood. Because most deaths have occurred in patients with large primary tumors, those papillary and mixed papillary-follicular carcinomas confined to one lobe but more than 2.5 cm in size, or occupying most of one lobe and penetrating its capsule, are managed by lobectomy and resection of the isthmus with a subtotal lobec-

tomy performed on the opposite lobe (to protect the parathyroids). If the opposite subtotal lobectomy specimen shows evidence of cancer on frozen section, the procedure is converted to a total thyroidectomy. Papillary and papillary-follicular carcinomas in the isthmus which are small and limited can be managed by resection of the isthmus and portions of both lobes, leaving a remnant of tissue at the posterior margin of both lobes to protect the parathyroids. If frozen section reveals carcinoma on either side, the involved lobe is completely removed.

TECHNIQUE OF THYROIDECTOMY

The recurrent laryngeal nerve is routinely identified and traced throughout its course when either lobectomy or total thyroidectomy is undertaken. During the performance of every thyroidectomy, diligent efforts are made to identify all parathyroid glands and preserve them with their blood supply. More instances of hypoparathyroidism are probably the result of devascularization of the parathyroid glands than of their actual removal; therefore, when a parathyroid gland appears devascularized or is located on the surface of the thyroid and cannot be preserved with its blood supply, it is resected, minced into small fragments, and transplanted into the sternomastoid muscle. Recent reported success rates of over 70 percent with parathyroid transplants hold out the hope of improved protection against hypoparathyroidism with this method.

LATERAL JUGULAR NODE DISEASE

Should a routine neck dissection be performed in the absence of clinically positive lymph nodes? The incidence of metastatic disease in jugular lymph nodes is high, even in the absence of clinical enlargement. Before 1970, it was our standard practice to perform routine radical neck dissections for well-differentiated thyroid cancers. In 87 neck dissections performed for papillary and mixed papillary-follicular carcinoma, the overall incidence of microscopic metastases to neck nodes was 80 percent; 58 percent of those necks that were clinically free of disease showed metastases. In cases of follicular carcinoma, in which some observers report a low incidence of lateral node metastases, routine neck dissections in 29 patients disclosed an overall incidence of 83 percent metastases; in those patients in whom the necks were clinically negative, the incidence of node involvement was 70 percent. On the basis of these findings, most patients were formerly advised to undergo, and usually accepted, prophylactic neck dissections. Those who refused prophylactic neck dissections were followed with great interest; only 20 percent later developed jugular node disease, and in all patients the disease was controlled by neck dissection. Since these observations were made, the use of prophylactic neck dissection has been discontinued; a neck dissection is now performed only when there are clinically involved lymph nodes.

We have not found the presence of metastases in jugular, paratracheal, or upper mediastinal lymph nodes to affect the prognosis of well-differentiated thyroid cancer adversely. The survival rate for those patients who had metastatic neck node involvement was not different from that for patients whose neck nodes were not involved, regardless of the extent of metastases. This was the case in both follicular and papillary-follicular carcinoma and has been the experience of most observers.

It has also become evident that modifying the standard neck dissection to spare the sternomastoid muscle and spinal accessory nerve has produced a satisfactory operation; we have not had to re-explore any patient for recurrence following such a neck dissection. A complete dissection is performed, removing the jugular vein and associated lymph nodes. This can usually be accomplished through a transverse extension of the original thyroid incision up toward the mastoid tip, so that an adequate flap can be raised. Since the cosmetic and functional results of such a neck dissection are excellent, and local recurrence following such procedures is extremely rare, we do not see any reason for repeated local excisions of lateral neck nodes as they develop. We have no enthusiasm for this "berry-picking" method of handling lymph node metastases in thyroid carcinoma, preferring instead a single modified neck dissection if positive nodes develop. We have never had a patient die because of our inability to control lateral neck dissection.

PARATRACHEAL AND UPPER MEDIASTINAL NODE DISSECTION

Most deaths in our series have been the result of uncontrolled midline disease, and therefore paratracheal and upper mediastinal node dissections have become routine parts of our surgical procedure for thyroid carcinomas. The nodal and fatty tissue in the tracheoesophageal groove and in the upper mediastinum is thoroughly removed leaving a bare trachea and a skeletonized recurrent laryngeal nerve. Although the microscopic incidence of metastatic nodes is high, the frequency of local recurrence when gross disease does not involve the tracheal structures has been minimal.

APPROACH TO THYROID NODULE SUSPECTED TO BE MALIGNANT

Considerably fewer than 20 percent of all explored thyroid nodules prove to be malignant. Although a thyroid mass may be suspected to be a cancer, the conclusive diagnosis must be established by surgical neck exploration.

The preferred procedure for diagnosis should be the excision of the entire involved lobe and isthmus, rather than an excision of the nodule itself. If the nodule appears in the isthmus, the entire isthmus and adjacent portions of the right and left lobes should be removed. At times, the pathologist may have difficulty in diagnosing well-differentiated thyroid cancer on frozen section. It is not unusual for a benign report at frozen section to be revised to a diagnosis of carcinoma when permanent sections are reviewed. Follicular tumors present particular problems, often requiring capsular or vascular invasion for the diagnosis of cancer. This evidence is often not apparent on frozen section examination, and the physician is confronted with a diagnosis of carcinoma several days later. It is satisfying at that time to know that the entire lobe and isthmus have been removed. If the isthmus is clear of tumor and the carcinoma is limited to one lobe, we do not re-explore the patient, foregoing the usual paratracheal and upper mediastinal node dissection performed for papillary, papillary-follicular, and follicular carcinomas. Small papillary and papillary-follicular cancers of the isthmus are also not re-explored. We have not seen locally recurrent disease as a result of this method of management.

Although past results have been good, the finding of pure follicular cancer in one lobe, the presence of poorly differentiated elements within well-differentiated cancer, a history of radiotherapy to the head and neck, or the presence of follicular cancer in the isthmus would now be factors in advising re-exploration, total thyroidectomy, and paratracheal and upper mediastinal node dissection.

TABLE 1 Summary of Management of Well-Differentiated Thyroid Cancer

I. Thyroid Procedure

A. Papillary or papillary-follicular cancer
   1. Confined to one lobe
      If larger than 2.5 cm and penetrating capsule

      Lobectomy and excision of isthmus
         Additional near-lobectomy of opposite lobe, without entering the area of the recurrent nerve. If malignant on frozen section, convert to total thyroidectomy
   2. Limited to isthmus
      Near-total thyroidectomy preserving the posterior shell of each lobe
   3. Involvement of one lobe with extension of nodularity in isthmus or opposite lobe
      Total thyroidectomy

B. Follicular carcinoma—lobe or isthmus
   Total thyroidectomy
C. Mixture of undifferentiated elements in well-differentiated thyroid cancer
   Total thyroidectomy
D. Well-differentiated thyroid cancer with history of radiotherapy to head and neck.
   Total thyroidectomy

II. Midline compartment node dissection (paratracheal and upper mediastinal)

A. With lobectomy
   Routine ipsilateral paratracheal and upper mediastinal dissection
      If an ipsilateral dissection is done and positive nodes are present on the opposite side, then a total thyroidectomy and bilateral paratracheal and upper mediastinal dissection are performed, even if no nodules are felt in the opposite lobe
B. With total thyroidectomy
   Bilateral paratracheal and upper mediastinal dissection

III. Lateral (jugular) node dissection
   For clinical node disease only

IV. Thyroid suppression
   Lifetime maintenance on .15 to .2 mg levothyroxine in all patients

V. Postoperative ^{131}I scanning and ablation of residual thyroid tissue
   All patients with total or near-total thyroidectomy

VI. Thyroglobulin assays and routine interval follow-up with ^{131}I scanning
   All patients who have had a total or near-total thyroidectomy with ablation of residual thyroid tissue

POSTOPERATIVE THYROID SUPPRESSION

Almost all observers report improved survival and decreased recurrence rates with the use of TSH suppression for well-differentiated thyroid cancers. All of our patients with this diagnosis are maintained on .15 to .2 mg of levothyroxine per day. This is usually sufficient to suppress TSH levels below 2μU/ml.

POSTOPERATIVE RADIOTHERAPY

We are unable to evaluate the effect of postoperative radiotherapy on well-differentiated thyroid cancer. It has been employed only occasionally in those patients in whom extensive local disease in the area of the larynx and trachea could not be resected, and in these patients it was difficult to perceive any beneficial effect. Physicians have hesitated to use it for a disease with a very protracted course, since ionizing radiation itself may be carcinogenic. Certainly radiotherapy should not be used prophylactically after neck dissections for metastatic nodal disease in the neck; this is well controlled by surgery.

RADIOACTIVE IODINE THERAPY AND THE USE OF THYROGLOBULIN ASSAYS

Much of the impetus for total thyroidectomy has been the result of the increased interest in employing radioactive iodine routinely after total or near-total thyroidectomy for well-differentiated thyroid cancer to detect any remaining functional thyroid tissue and destroy it with an appropriate dose of ^{131}I. Elimination of all functioning thyroid tissue provides two methods of detecting recurrent thyroid cancer: the appearance of areas of concentration of radioactive iodine on subsequent total body scan, and the detection of increased levels of serum thyroglobulin by radioimmunoassay. Should either method detect recurrent or metastatic thyroid cancer, ablative therapy with radioactive iodine can be instituted. Approximately 75 percent of well-differentiated thyroid malignancies are reported to concentrate radioactive iodine. A number of our patients with pulmonary metastases have survived 15 to 20 years in spite of extensive disease. Radioactive iodine was concentrated by many of these tumors and an associated decrease in size was noted following therapy. In all instances, however, the lesions recurred.

Thus the value of radioactive iodine in the management of metastatic or recurrent thyroid cancer remains controversial. While some observers report improved survival rates, others find no difference. Most observers concede that should recurrence ensue, iodine is almost never curative.

At this time, all patients at our institution who have had total or near total thyroidectomies are scanned six weeks following surgery, and any remaining thyroid tissue is ablated with [131]I. They are then followed by total body scans and thyroglobulin assay for possible recurrence.

The sensitivity of thyroglobulin as a marker for recurrent thyroid cancer is an innovative development and is proving to be reliable; it is hoped that improvements in the diagnosis of metastases may be matched by better methods of treatment. Conventional chemotherapy has not been useful.

MEDULLARY THYROID CARCINOMA

CHARLES L. BERGER, M.D.,
SAMUEL A. WELLS, JR., M.D.,
GEOFFREY MENDELSOHN, M.D.,
and STEPHEN B. BAYLIN, M.D.

Medullary thyroid carcinoma (MTC), which represents 5 to 10 percent of all thyroid neoplasms, arises from the small numbers of calcitonin secreting parafollicular or C cells of the thyroid. In 80 percent of patients, MTC occurs in a sporadic form and is diagnosed retrospectively during surgery for a thyroid mass. The remaining 20 percent of patients with MTC have genetic disorders in which MTC is often accompanied by pheochromocytomas of the adrenals, parathyroid hyperfunction, and more rarely, multiple neuromas and gastrointestinal ganglioneuromatosis.

The proper treatment of MTC is intimately connected with the mode of diagnosis in a given patient, the stage of the disease at the time of initial therapeutic intervention, the type of MTC present (sporadic versus genetic), the presence of any associated conditions (such as pheochromocytoma or hyperparathyroidism), and a working knowledge of the natural history of the disease. Before discussing treatment, this chapter must include discussions of diagnostic maneuvers currently employed to screen for this tumor and the behavior of MTC as a function of stage and type of disease. With this background information in mind, the current surgical and nonsurgical aspects of the treatment of MTC can be placed in proper perspective.

DIAGNOSIS OF MTC

Sporadic versus Genetic Disease

Patients with the sporadic form of MTC present with palpable thyroid nodules that cannot be distinguished clinically from other types of thyroid enlargement. We know of no practical way to diagnose these individuals prospectively. Although all of these patients with clinical disease will have increased basal levels of circulating calcitonin, the low incidence of MTC makes it impractical to screen all patients with thyroid nodules for elevations of calcitonin. Consequently, the diagnosis of sporadic MTC remains serendipitous and is made during histologic examination (frozen or permanent sections) of a thyroid mass removed at the time of surgery.

The diagnosis of inherited MTC is a critically different matter. The goal in this form of the disease is to establish a positive family history and to make the earliest possible diagnosis of MTC. Indeed, only those patients operated upon for subclinical disease have the highest percentage chance for "cure."

The central question is when should the inherited form of the disease be suspected? It is safe to say that all patients with MTC must be suspected of having the genetic form of the disorder until a careful work-up has ruled it out. The index case for any given kindred will, of course, present with clinically overt disease. In the main, such individuals cannot prospectively be differentiated by physical examination from patients with sporadic MTC. There is, however, one important exception to this rule which involves those patients with the rarest form of MTC, so-called multiple endocrine neoplasia type IIb or III (Table 1). These individuals have a classic set of clinical features, including variable numbers of neuromas over the lips, eyelids, tongue, and oral mucosa, plus a Marfanoid habitus. In addition, 50 percent of this group of patients have functioning pheochromocytomas and all have gastrointestinal ganglioneuromatosis characterized by a proliferation of ganglionic plexuses throughout the gastrointestinal tract. As will be discussed below, the virulence of MTC in this syndrome is extraordinary, and it is essential that children with these clinical features be identified immediately and offered early therapy. Although this disease is genetically determined, a family history is usually not present. Kindreds, however, with MEN-III are well described and involvement of multiple family members must be carefully ruled out.

TABLE 1 Characteristics of Medullary Thyroid Carcinoma

	Sporadic	MEN-II (IIa)	MEN III (IIb)
Mean age at diagnosis (years)			
With clinical disease	53*	34†	13‡
By provocative testing	Not applicable	20.5†	No statistics available
Location in thyroid gland	Usually unilateral	Bilateral	Bilateral
Earliest recognized lesion	Carcinoma	C-cell hyperplasia (CCH)	Not identified but probably CCH
Characteristics of metastasis	Local and distant Variable in aggressiveness	Local and distant Variable in aggressiveness and dissemination	Local and distant Very aggressive
Physical findings	Thyroid mass	Thyroid mass in late disease Normal physical examination in early stages	Thyroid mass in late disease Marfanoid habitus (100%) Neuromas of lips, tongue, eyelids (100%)
Associated conditions	None recognized	Pheochromocytomas (50%) Hyperparathyroidism (10–25%)	Pheochromocytomas (50%) Mucosal neuromas (100%) Gastrointestinal ganglioneuromatosis (100%)
Treatment	Total thyroidectomy if disease initially recognized as MTC; modified radical neck if disease obvious in cervical nodes Rule out pheochromocytoma Rule out hyperparathyroidism Screen immediate family members to rule out familial disease	Rule out pheochromocytoma Total thyroidectomy; modified radical neck if disease obvious in cervical nodes Treat hyperparathyroidism if present Intense screening of family members to identify earliest stages of disease	Rule out pheochromocytoma Total thyroidectomy; modified radical neck if disease obvious in cervical nodes Intense screening of family members to identify earliest stages of disease

*Khairi MR, et al: Medicine 54:89, 1975
†Wells SA, et al: Ann Surg 188:377, 1978
‡Norton JA, et al: Surg Clin North Am 59:109, 1979

Patients with the more common type of genetic MTC, multiple endocrine neoplasia type II or type IIa, do not have the physical stigmata of the patients described above. Therefore genetic disease must be ruled out by finding (1) a family history of multiple thyroid problems, (2) a history of hyperparathyroidism and consequences of hypercalcemia, or (3) a history of adrenal tumors and/or complications resulting from pheochromocytomas.

The findings at the time of initial surgery can also be helpful in the search for familial disease. MTC in both lobes of the thyroid is the exception in patients with sporadic disease but is the rule in patients with the genetic type. Likewise, the histologic finding of associated areas of so-called C-cell hyperplasia in patients with MTC is felt by some investigators to be characteristic only of inherited MTC.

The Use of Calcitonin (CT) Assays in Diagnosis of MTC

Once a history of genetic or familial MTC is documented, optimal treatment aims at screening family members (especially children) at risk for the presence of subclinical disease. This task depends entirely on determining the concentration of circulating calcitonin (CT).

Patients with inherited, subclinical MTC most often do not have abnormal basal levels of circulating CT. It is thus mandatory that provocative testing for CT secretion be performed. A number of such tests have been devised and changes in format have occurred with time and trial and error. We now prefer a combination test devised in our laboratories which employs a 1-minute infusion of calcium gluconate (2 mg of elemental calcium/kg) followed by a 5- to 10-second bolus of Pentagastrin (Peptavlon, Ayerst Laboratories, 0.5 μg/kg). Heparinized blood samples are taken at 0, 2, 3.5, 5, and 7 minutes of the test for determination of plasma calcitonin concentrations.

The precise levels of provoked calcitonin secretion which differentiate normal from an abnormal response remain controversial. Different radioimmunoassays have different sensitivities. Some reliably detect levels of calcitonin in normal individuals and some do not. It is safe to say, however, that studies from most investigators suggest that blood calcitonin concentrations in normal individuals do not rise above 200 pg/ml either in basal samples or during provocative testing. In our

hands, any individual at direct genetic risk whose blood calcitonin concentration rises above 200 pg/ml during provocative testing is a candidate for thyroidectomy. It is critical, however, that the physician screening patients for MTC know the calcitonin assay being used and its track record in diagnostic use for designating individuals with MTC.

Some important caveats with regard to the use of calcitonin assays must be mentioned. Occasional individuals have been recognized whose basal concentrations of calcitonin are over 200 pg/ml (generally 200–400 pg/ml) but whose values fail to rise further during provocative testing. In these cases one must seriously consider that the plasma or serum samples contain substances interfering with the radioimmunoassay. Indeed, several investigative groups have stated that the delta for calcitonin during the provocative test is as important as the actual peak value reached. Again, in our experience, a rise upwards of 200 pg/ml over basal is diagnostic for patients at risk. To help document this fact, we have catheterized (simultaneously placed catheters in the inferior thyroid veins and in a peripheral vein) individuals at risk for MTC whose peak levels during initial provocative tests ranged from 200 pg/ml to 1000 pg/ml. All individuals who had peripheral levels of 200 pg/ml or higher on one or more previous provocative tests had thyroid venous blood levels of greater than 400 pg/ml (even if the peripheral blood levels were simultaneously less than 200 pg/ml during the venous catheterization study). All of these patients have had C-cell hyperplasia or microscopic MTC at the time of surgery. We feel that such catheter tests are not clinically necessary for patients at direct risk whose peak CT levels are 250 pg/ml or greater. This procedure may occasionally be useful, however, for those few patients with more borderline tests and/or in those whom one suspects that interfering substances in plasma or serum are causing artifacts in the calcitonin immunoassay.

The Use of Immunohistochemistry in Diagnosis of MTC

It is our bias, after several years of experience, that performance of immunohistochemical staining for CT plays a vital role in MTC diagnosis. This is especially so for documenting the early stages of disease encountered in patients with the genetic forms of this disorder. Early C-cell hyperplasia and small microscopic tumors can sometimes be missed by examination of routine hematoxylin and eosin stained histologic tissue sections. Systematic examination of the entire thyroid gland combined with immunoperoxidase or immunofluorescent CT immunostaining can alleviate this problem. Virtually all cells in very early lesions of the neoplastic C-cell proliferative spectrum will stain intensely for CT and can thus be readily identified. We thus feel that close coordination between clinician and pathologist must be an integral part of managing patients with MTC.

APPROACH TO TREATMENT OF MTC

Sporadic Disease

At present, the only efficacious therapy for all forms of MTC is the surgical removal of as much tumor as possible. It is imperative to note that, in our hands, 80 percent or more of patients who present with clinically palpable disease will have continued abnormalities of CT secretion after thyroidectomy. This is probably owing to the propensity of MTC to metastasize (especially to cervical nodes) at a very early stage. By definition, then, patients with the sporadic form of MTC fall into this category. Thus the major therapeutic decisions really involve postoperative management.

The individual surgical approach to patients with sporadic MTC is essentially that for any patient who presents with a nonfunctioning thyroid nodule. If frozen sections during surgery are consistent with the diagnosis of MTC, we recommend total thyroidectomy. Even though a majority of these individuals will turn out, upon careful examination of the thyroid, to have unilateral disease, in the absence of a detailed family history and without having checked CT levels in immediate relatives, it is impossible to rule out the genetic form of the tumor. It is therefore safest to assume that the genetic form of MTC could be present.

Cervical node involvement is usually found at the time of initial surgery for palpable MTC. All visible lymph nodes should therefore be removed from the angle of the jaw down to the major vessels in the supraclavicular areas. If lymph nodes are obviously involved with tumor, modified radical neck procedures with preservation of the sternocleidomastoid muscles can be considered. There are absolutely no data to indicate that more radical and cosmetically deforming surgery offers any benefit to patients with clinically manifest MTC.

The postoperative care of patients with sporadic MTC presents several management decision problems. After surgical recovery and the replacement of thyroid hormone, patients should be tested for CT secretion as previously outlined. Since most patients will have residual abnormalities in such tests, decisions must be made about the need to localize the areas of remaining disease.

With regard to localizing residual disease, it is essential to note that 70 percent or more of patients with sporadic MTC have long-term survival expectations (five years or more) *whether or not* they have residual abnormalities in CT secretion. Some patients, even with documented metastases to distant sites such as lung and liver, can do remarkably well for long periods of time. Similarly, the majority of individuals with no objective signs of residual tumor but with presumed micrometastases do very well without any further surgical or medical intervention. Thus, while we are appropriately aggressive in trying to localize residual disease and to characterize fully the postoperative status of our patients with MTC, we usually follow the majority without additional therapy.

There are certain patients in whom further therapy must be particularly considered, once the patient has been staged postoperatively. One vexing problem involves patients in whom only a partial thyroidectomy was performed. In the absence of any family history of MTC, and given the relatively favorable prognosis for many patients with MTC, it does not seem to constitute poor management to defer further surgery in those individuals whose postoperative CT secretion studies are normal. A positive family history, as discussed earlier, markedly augments the possibility that the residual thyroid gland could harbor further tumor deposits. In such patients it is tempting to consider removal of the remaining gland whether or not the postoperative CT secretion is abnormal. Residual thyroid often is the site for recurrent or residual disease or both. Thus, in the absence of defined distant metastases in an otherwise healthy patient, it is reasonable to consider removing remaining thyroid tissue in an effort to normalize CT secretion. Also, removal of remaining intrathyroid tumor may prevent the local regrowth of MTC which can, in a few patients, cause extraordinary morbidity because of impingement on major cervical structures (vessels, pharynx, trachea).

Brief comment must be made about reports citing the efficacy of giving ^{131}I to ablate residual MTC. The mechanism proposed is that remnants of thyroid tissue will concentrate the ^{131}I, leading to a cytotoxic effect on MTC deposits that are nearby. In our analysis of these data, and from brief personal experience, this type of approach remains an unproven one, and more research will be required to place this approach in perspective. We believe that the administration of ^{131}I should not be considered a front-line approach to dealing with residual cervical MTC in the postoperative setting.

A second postoperative management problem involves decisions regarding radiation and/or chemotherapy. It is extraordinarily tempting for the concerned physician to feel that some form of treatment must be offered to a patient who retains evidence of residual MTC after initial surgery, even if the only evidence for this is an abnormality in CT secretion. This is especially understandable since the patient, by definition, has a malignancy–and since a small subset of patients with sporadic MTC may develop a virulent clinical course and die from disseminated tumor. However, we feel there are several reasons why most of these patients with the sporadic form of MTC should be simply monitored and not offered aggressive therapy.

First, no effective chemotherapeutic regimens have been identified for patients with MTC to date. Drugs such as Cytoxan, vincristine, adriamycin, and Streptozotocin have all been tried but no convincing responses have been documented. Combination protocols with the above types of therapies have also proven ineffective.

Second, we have seen several patients with minimal residual tumor (one with only a positive provoked CT response) in whom the morbidity of local radiation (to the cervical area) proved devastating. Patients with MTC appear to be particularly prone to a desmoplastic reaction to radiation which can lead to intense cervical scarring and fixation of vital structures in the neck and mediastinum. One unfortunate young individual in our patient population has recently undergone a laryngectomy for radiation induced tracheitis. There were no clinical signs of residual tumor at the time of repeat surgery and all that is retained is a distinctly abnormal postoperative provocative test for CT secretion. Although each patient must be the focus for individual therapeutic approaches, we are particularly conservative with the use of local radiation—and certainly would not recommend its use in an adjuvant setting. Local clinical recurrences that may pose a threat to the trachea, esophagus, or both are best surgically managed if feasible; they should be radiated only if surgical debulking is contraindicated.

Finally, one group of patients must receive serious consideration for postoperative therapy. As we have mentioned, the use of immunohistochemistry for tumor CT content plays an important role in precise diagnosis of MTC. Recently we have found that patients whose primary MTC lesions have a heterogeneous staining pattern for CT appear to have a poor prognosis. This heterogeneity is characterized by large areas of tumor cells—and occasionally the majority of the tumor—which stain poorly, if at all, for CT. Such a heterogeneous pattern is characteristic of distant metastases in patients who have died of disseminated MTC. Our retrospective studies have revealed that six of seven patients who have had such a staining pattern in their primary tumor have died of metastases within five years, and the seventh has required repeat surgery for a rapidly enlarging cervical mass within one year of initial thyroidectomy. Prospective studies need to be done to document the universality of our findings. Serious consideration might be given to administering adjuvant therapy to patients with heterogeneous CT staining patterns in their primary tumors. The rationale would be that such therapy might prove effective at a time when tumor burden is *low* and before extensive disease has developed.

Genetic Disease

Multiple Endocrine Neoplasia Type II (MEN-IIa—Sipple's Syndrome). The index case patient with this form of MTC will of course present with palpable thyroid disease. Save for the presence in some patients of symptoms that might suggest the presence of pheochromocytoma (which should be surgically managed before thyroidectomy is performed), hyperparathyroidism, or both, these patients may be approached essentially as outlined above for those with sporadic MTC. The same statistics given for patients with sporadic MTC regarding incidence of postoperative residual tumor and abnormalities in CT secretion apply to patients with MEN-II and clinically detectable MTC. Also, as for patients with sporadic MTC, most of these individuals have long survival times despite clinical and/or biochemical evidence of residual tumor. It is imperative that, once the familial form of MTC is documented, emphasis be placed on the performance of a total thyroidectomy. In individuals who may have received a partial thyroidectomy before the presence of genetic MTC was established, we favor performing additional surgery to approach the almost certain presence of additional tumor in the opposite lobe of the thyroid.

Once a family with MEN-II has been identified, careful screening of individuals at risk by provocative testing of CT secretion provides an opportunity for surgical intervention to cure MTC. Because individuals carrying the MEN-II gene(s) often manifest their C-cell proliferative disorder at a very early age, we now routinely test and identify children between 5 and 12 years of age. All of these young individuals have had no clinical disease and are identified only by low-level abnormalities of CT secretion during provocative testing with Pentagastrin and calcium. Pathologic evaluation has revealed that most such patients have had only bilateral C-cell hyperplasia or microscopic carcinoma localized to the thyroid. All have remained free of abnormal CT secretion patterns three years or more since their total thyroidectomies and bilateral cervical lymph node dissections.

One of the difficult problems in screening patients at direct risk for MEN-II is to establish an age above which continued testing may not be necessary. We have identified several individuals over 40 years of age in multiple kindreds who have had low-level abnormalities of CT secretion when first tested and who had microscopic evidence of abnormal C-cell proliferation at the time of thyroidectomy. We do not know, of course, that these individuals might not have had abnormal calcitonin secretion tests and early stages of disease as young children. We currently recommend 6- to 12-month testing of direct risk patients under 20 years age and, if tests are negative to this age, biannual testing from this point on.

Mention must be made of the treatment of the associated endocrine lesions in patients with MEN-II. In children with biochemical signs of early MTC and absence of palpable thyroid tumor, we have not yet identified one with pheochromocytoma. Many new urine and blood tests for catecholamine secretion are under study by several investigators to detect very early pheochromocytomas. At present, however, we have had no patients who experienced difficulties that could be attributed to excess catecholamine secretion at time of thyroidectomy if they have had repeatedly normal urinary VMA and metanephrine levels and normal computed tomographic scans of the adrenal glands.

We have not encountered abnormalities of the parathyroid glands in patients with only C-cell hyperplasia or microscopic MTC. Enlarged parathyroid glands have occasionally been found in patients with very small (1–4 mm) but grossly visible MTC lesions. We have approached the parathyroid disease in MTC by removing any enlarged glands seen. If all parathyroid tissue must be removed because of hyperplasia of all four glands, transplantation of small pieces of parathyroid tissue into the patient's forearm can prove quite effective. This procedure prevents postoperative hypoparathyroidism. At this site, easy removal of the tissue can be accomplished should hypercalcemia recur. In patients with large deposits of cervical MTC whose normal parathyroids may need to be removed during extensive surgery, the normal tissue may be reimplanted in the fascia of the sternocleidomastoid muscles.

Multiple Endocrine Neoplasia Type III (MEN-IIb). The behavior of MTC in patients with MEN-III is strikingly different from that in the patient categories discussed above. The tumor in these patients appears to arise at a younger age and to behave much more aggressively. Thus, as shown in Table 1, the mean age for presentation of MEN-III patients with palpable tumor in the neck is *lower* than that for biochemical detection of subclinical disease in patients with MEN-II. We have seen, among MEN-III patients, children less than 10 years of age with widely disseminated MTC, and individuals as young as 2 years have been diagnosed as having this form of the tumor.

It is thus imperative that babies and young children with the physical stigmata of MEN-III be recognized and offered total thyroidectomies. As in cases of MEN-II, the MTC is always bilaterally located in these patients. Although provocative testing for CT secretion may be used to screen for MEN-III, patients (especially young children) with good documentation of the physical stigmata for this syndrome should probably undergo total thyroidectomy regardless of the CT results. Of course, tests for pheochromocytoma should be carefully evaluated prior to performing surgery for MTC.

Despite the case made against the use of chemotherapy for most patients with sporadic MTC and MEN-II, the MEN-III syndrome may need to be considered differently in this regard. As in the other forms of MTC, patients with MEN-III who present with palpable cervical disease will almost always have residual tumor after thyroidectomy. Likewise, some of these patients will evidence this

residual disease only by abnormalities of CT secretion. Yet, unlike the majority of patients with
the other types of MTC, every patient with MEN-
III is at a very high risk for developing widespread
metastases and for dying at a young age from
MTC. Thus a more adjuvant approach might be
considered in these patients in order to administer
therapy at a time when tumor burden is low. It
must be emphasized that such an approach has not
yet been tried. Yet, as we have previously pointed
out in discussing patients who have heterogeneous
staining patterns in primary MTC lesions, the
known failure of chemotherapy to act efficaciously
in patients with MTC and large tumor burdens suggests that, with available modalities, early treatment in patients at high risk may be the only alternative approach.

GRAVES'
OPHTHALMOPATHY

JOSEPH P. KRISS, M.D.,
I. ROSS MCDOUGALL, M.D.,
and SARAH S. DONALDSON, M.D.

The ophthalmopathy accompanying thyroid
disease is most often associated with thyroid hyperfunction accompanying diffuse goiter (Graves'
disease). However, it occasionally may occur in
euthyroid patients with Hashimoto's thyroiditis, in
patients with myxedema who have never been thyrotoxic, and even in patients without any known
thyroid disease.

The severity of the eye disease often does not
parallel the degree of clinical toxicity or laboratory
parameters of thyroid function. Some patients with
severe thyrotoxicosis have no eye involvement
clinically, whereas in others ophthalmopathy develops or worsens while they are in a euthyroid
state. The eye condition may precede, accompany,
or follow the thyrotoxic state. In a significant proportion of patients the condition appears to be precipitated or aggravated by ablative therapy of the
thyroid. There is no satisfactory method of predicting the outcome or severity of the disease in

an individual patient. More severe ophthalmopathy
causing distressing symptoms or serious disability
occurs predominantly in persons over age 40. Eye
manifestations in younger individuals are likely to
be limited to mild symptoms, stare and proptosis.

The clinical manifestations of ophthalmopathy offer puzzling variations. They may be unilateral, bilateral, symmetric, or asymmetric. Occasionally a unilateral ophthalmopathy precedes
bilateral involvement. Clinical manifestations vary
greatly in degree and number from patient to patient, and even in the same patient over time; they
include proptosis, periorbital swelling, chemosis,
extraocular motor paresis, corneal abrasions, and
optic nerve damage. Accompanying ophthalmic
symptoms may include excessive lacrimation and
photophobia; burning, gritty, or pulling sensations;
diplopia; pain because of corneal abrasion, and
loss of visual acuity.

The recorded frequency of eye involvement
has depended on the criteria used to determine involvement. Severe involvement probably occurs
in no more than 2 percent to 10 percent of patients
with Graves' disease, but the incidence is higher
in older individuals. Clinical eye involvement of
any degree may vary from 50 percent to 90 percent. The female/male incidence of moderately severe ophthalmopathy is about 2:1; this represents
a relative increase of ophthalmopathy in males,
because the expected ratio for Graves' disease per
se is about 6:1.

A review of the pathologic features in Graves'
ophthalomopathy shows that the extraocular muscles bear the brunt of the disease; they become
greatly enlarged, firm, rubbery, and resistant to
passive stretching. The muscle volume may be increased to eight to ten times normal. This increased muscle volume causes anterior displacement of the globe. In vivo demonstration of muscle
swelling can be accomplished by orbital ultrasonography or computerized transverse axial tomography (CT scan). Using the latter technique, the
medial and inferior recti are seen to be the muscles
most often affected.

When there is loss of visual acuity, the CT
scan often shows marked enlargement of the muscles at the orbital cone near the optic foramen, an
observation that suggests the possibility that the
muscle swelling could damage the optic nerve by
compression.

Microscopically, the most dramatic changes
seen are edema and a marked inflammatory cellular infiltrate that consists predominantly of lymphocytes. The inflammatory collections are peri-

vascular and occasionally resemble lymph follicles with germinal centers. The inflammatory cells are sometimes distributed throughout the extraocular muscle. With time, fibrosis and shortening of the muscles may occur. In the inferior rectus, such a change may cause downward rotation of the eyeball, inability to look upward, and vertical diplopia.

CLINICAL ASSESSMENT

It is important in assessing any patient for the first time to address the following questions:

What is the severity of ophthalmopathy?

What is the extent of functional disability?

Is the ophthalmopathy progressive?

Is there coexisting thyrotoxicosis?

Did thyrotoxicosis exist previously?

If there is a negative history of thyrotoxicosis, is there any evidence of other autoimmune thyroid disease?

Have corticosteroids been given and with what results?

We recommend the use of a numerical rating scale (ophthalmopathy index) to assess the severity of ophthalmopathy. The index is calculated by first rating the severity of involvement of five categories (soft tissues, proptosis, extraocular muscle, cornea, sight loss) on a scale from 0–3, and then determining their sum (Table 1). This is helpful in comparing the extent of disease in different individuals or evaluating the results of treatment in a given person.

Progression is usually discernible over a time scale of weeks to months, rarely years. It is not difficult to evaluate if photographs, exophthalmometric readings, or repeated ophthalmologic examinations have been made, if the onset has been recent, or the involvement severe. Proptosis and/ or extraocular muscle dysfunction that has not changed over a six-month period may signify the existence of a stable ophthalmopathy, which is treated differently from progressive disease.

TREATMENT

The majority of the patients we have treated for ophthalmopathy have had thyrotoxicosis previously, which was treated successfully by radioiodine or thyroidectomy, and many have been maintained in a euthyroid state on oral replacement therapy. The clinical problem in such patients is relatively uncomplicated, and attention can be focused on the eyes. If the patient has coexisting thyrotoxicosis or is euthyroid only by virtue of continuing antithyroid drug therapy, then the therapeutic problem is more difficult and requires decisions regarding both the eyes and the thyroid and the timing of these treatments.

In our series of patients, the failure to respond to therapy (see below) has been associated mostly with the absence of previous thyrotoxicosis, that is, spontaneously developing euthyroid or hypothyroid Graves' ophthalmopathy. We recommend that an orbital CT scan be done in any patient with ophthalmopathy without a history of thyroid disease or laboratory evidence of thyroid dysfunction or thyroid autoimmunity. Such patients may have orbital pseudotumor rather than Graves' ophthalmopathy, and the CT findings are sufficiently distinctive to distinguish these clinical entities. (Orbital pseudotumor of the lymphocytic infiltrative type also responds very satisfactorily to the orbital radiotherapy program outlined here; the type characterized by fibrosis on orbital tissue biopsy responds poorly to all known modalities of treatment.)

TABLE 1 Categories of Eye Involvement

Soft Tissue	Proptosis	Eye Muscles	Cornea	Acuity	Severity Score
Slight redness, chemosis, periorbital edema, minimal symptoms	>20–23 mm	Infrequent diplopia, not in 1° gaze	Slight stippling	20/25–20/40	1
Moderately severe redness, chemosis, periorbital swelling and symptoms	>23–27 mm	Frequent diplopia, moderate limitation of movement	Marked stippling and symptoms	20/45–20/100	2
Conjunctival redundancy, marked edema, and severe symptoms	>27 mm	Severe constant muscle dysfunction	Ulceration	$\frac{20}{>100}$	3

Ophthalmic index = sum of scores for all 5 categories

Mild Ophthalmopathy

It is often unnecessary to prescribe any treatment for patients with mild ophthalmopathy (index score 1–3). Not infrequently the condition will subside spontaneously over a period of several months. Photophobia is generally reduced by wearing tinted glasses. When there are symptoms of burning or grittiness of the eyes, demulcent eye drops containing methylcellulose are most beneficial. However, before any local therapy is prescribed, it is important to ensure that there are no corneal abrasions, since the symptomatic relief afforded by the local treatment may allow corneal ulceration to progress unnoticed. Treatment with antibiotic eye drops or decongestant drops containing corticosteroids is not recommended; the former may promote the growth of resistant bacteria, the latter may produce cataracts. We do not use diuretics in an attempt to control periorbital edema.

More Severe Progressive Ophthalmopathy

Progression of ophthalmic disease to a more severe state (index score >3) generally is an indication to initiate oral corticosteroid treatment or supervoltage orbital radiotherapy. We favor the latter (many of our patients have failed to respond to corticosteroids), but the former is especially effective in controlling soft tissue symptoms and signs; it may also be effective in reversing optic neuritis. Prednisone in doses of 20 mg twice daily is almost always effective; it is usually necessary to continue the drug for many months to control the symptoms completely, tapering the dosage downward, if possible, to minimum effective dosage approximately every 3 weeks. Not infrequently it proves difficult to wean the patient from corticosteroid therapy without the recurrence of signs and symptoms. When relapse occurs, the dosage immediately should be raised to its former level and repeated attempts to taper therapy should be delayed for 2 weeks or more, and then done in decrements of only 2.5–5 mg. The usual precautions are taken to avoid the more serious side effects of long-term corticosteroid therapy, but they can almost never be avoided entirely. Physical features of Cushing's syndrome develop in most patients. Since most of the patients with more severe ophthalmopathy are in the age group of 40 to 70 years, osteoporosis is a major hazard of corticosteroid therapy. Occasionally the ophthalmopathy is so severe that one may be tempted to employ larger doses of prednisone, up to 100 mg per day. Such cases often have optic neuritis, severe eye muscle dysfunction, or both, in addition to soft tissue symptoms and signs. In such instances we prefer to start orbital radiotherapy immediately, with the expectation of a favorable response without the necessity of using adjunctive corticosteroid therapy. There is evidence that combined oral corticosteroid-orbital radiotherapy is more effective than corticosteroid treatment alone, but a comparable comparison of combined therapy with orbital radiotherapy alone (see below) has not yet been reported.

Since 1968 we have been treating patients suffering from progressive ophthalmopathy with index scores of 4 or greater with supervoltage orbital radiotherapy using a 6 Mev linear accelerator, delivering a well-collimated, high-energy x-ray beam to the extraocular muscles. Patients receive a total orbital dose of 2000 rads in 10 fractions given over a 2-week period. Alternating left and right lateral fields are used. An earlier technique employed posterior angulation of the beam to protect the cornea and lens. Modifications have since been made in our radiotherapy technique: A beam-splitting technique is used so that the central axis of the beam corresponds to the anterior border of the treatment field. This maneuver results in an improved and satisfactory distribution of the radiation dose to the orbital muscles, while shielding the cornea and lens. To be sure that the beam is correctly aligned, a double exposure film is obtained in which the first exposure is limited to the field to be treated, the collimators are opened, and the second exposure is made, thus superimposing the first exposure on the entire lateral skull. If during treatment a marked reduction in proptosis occurs, it is necessary to readjust the alignment of the treatment field. A small tattoo is placed on the skin just lateral to each eye to mark the anterior limit of the field. The retina is obviously incuded in the treatment field. The dosage employed was selected with the knowledge that the retinas of young patients treated for retinoblastoma can tolerate such levels (or higher) of radiation without significant ill effect. The pituitary gland is not included in the treatment field.

It is important to have a thorough ophthalmologic evaluation prior to starting radiotherapy. Sine most of these patients are over age 40, and many are over age 60, it is especially important to determine if a senile cataract is already present, so that its influence in causing impairment of vision may be known beforehand. Cataract is not a contraindication to radiotherapy treatment, but one would not want any loss of acuity occurring late in the follow-up period to be falsely ascribed to radiation therapy.

We recommend that orbital CT scans be obtained in patients whose clinical indications for radiotherapy may be borderline, such as long duration of symptoms with little clinical evidence of progression, or a relatively low ophthalmopathy index score. We particularly favor those machines that enable one to reconstruct a series of coronal or sagittal views of the orbit, thus identifying the degree of swelling of the four rectus muscles. We tend not to accept for treatment those patients who have little or no evidence of ocular muscle enlargment. Orbital CT scans may also provide information useful in planning the treatment ports for orbital radiotherapy.

The radiation treatment program is well tolerated by all patients. A transient moderate increase in periorbital and conjunctival edema may be observed during the first week in some patients. In some instances, objective and subjective improvement occurs during the two-week treatment period, usually continuing for weeks or months afterward; in others, improvement occurs more slowly and becomes manifest only weeks or months after treatment is completed.

The evaluation of response to treatment is made at approximately monthly intervals after treatment for the first year, employing the criteria in Table 2.

To date, follow-up data of 1 year or more after treatment have been recorded for 121 patients. Of these, 41 had surgery performed on the eye muscles or lids, with 81 percent having an excellent/good response to treatment. Of the 80 patients treated by radiotherapy alone, 67 percent had an excellent/good response, 10 percent had no response, but only 2 percent showed progression of disease despite treatment.

Improvement has been observed in all five categories of involvement. In this series the pretreatment frequencies of involvement by category were about 90, 80, 95, 35, and 60 percent for soft tissue, proptosis, extraocular muscle, cornea, and sight loss, respectively. Excluding the benefits of any subsequent eye surgery, the percentages of those involved who improved with radiotherapy alone, by category of involvement, were about 95, 60, 60, 50, and 85 percent, respectively.

The factors of age, sex, interval between onset of disease and treatment, presence of serum antithyroid antibodies, presence of eye muscle dysfunction, and orbital CT findings are not useful in distinguishing patients with an excellent/good response from those with no response.

The only factor correlating clearly with lack of response to therapy was absence of previous hyperthyroidism (8 of 12 patients).

Supervoltage radiotherapy, or the combination of radiotherapy and corrective eye surgery, is thus effective in reversing or arresting the progress of Graves' ophthalmopathy. The treatment has been especially effective in those with soft tissue signs and visual acuity loss. It tends to result in reduced intraocular tension, avoids the side effects of corticosteroid therapy, and relapses after initial improvement have been rare. The treatment may permit corrective eye surgery to be done sooner than would be the case without control of the disease process.

SPECIAL CONSIDERATIONS

Coexisting Hyperthyroidism and Ophthalmopathy

The patient who presents with coexisting ophthalmopathy and thyrotoxicosis poses an especially vexing dilemma, especially in patients

TABLE 2 Overall Evaluation of Response to Orbital Irradiation

Score	Response	Description
3	Excellent	Marked improvement or disappearance of signs/symptoms; marked improvement in functional capacity; off prednisone
2	Good	Moderate to marked improvement in most signs/symptoms, but some residual signs; improved functional capacity
1	Fair	Moderate to marked improvement in some, signs/symptoms (e.g., soft tissue), but little or no improvement in major problems (e.g., diplopia)
0	No response	No change in signs/symptoms
1	Worse	Progression of signs/symptoms after completion of therapy

over 40 years of age. Younger patients usually present with proptosis as the ophthalmopathic manifestation, and this usually does not worsen with ablative therapy or with prolonged antithyroid drug therapy. In older patients, however, ^{131}I therapy has a greater potential for aggravating the ophthalmopathy, while satisfactory control of the hyperthyroidism with antithyroid drugs is sometimes accompanied by progression of the ophthalmopathy, the symptoms of which come to dominate the clinical symptom complex. We recommend combined therapy in such patients, that is, ^{131}I therapy to treat the hyperthroidism definitively plus simultaneous prednisone therapy, 20–40 mg per day for about 3 months to forestall any worsening of the eye condition, or alternatively, simultaneous orbital irradiation if the eye condition is already severe. This recommendation is controversial; some clinicians prefer to treat with antithyroid drugs and prednisone and/or radiotherapy.

Relapses

A very few patients have experienced an initial favorable response to orbital irradiation but a few months after treatment experienced a relapse, usually less severe than before treatment and usually characterized by soft tissue symptoms and signs. Such patients are managed with prednisone, 5–30 mg per day, tapering the dosage judiciously but usually maintaining treatment for several more months before stopping therapy.

Orbital Decompression

Although surgical decompression can be beneficial, especially in severely affected patients whose sight is threatened, the procedure is unduly invasive and unnecessary for most patients with moderate or severe progressive disease. In the last 20 years we have recommended orbital decompression only twice in an attempt to control progressive loss of visual acuity in patients with severe ophthalmopathy. In one of these patients ophthalmopathy progressed despite surgery. The other improved, but she also received a second course of orbital radiotherapy.

However, we believe that orbital decompression does have a place in the management of some patients with *stable* ophthalmopathy associated with disfiguring proptosis, with or without marked lid-lag, and usually minimal or no eye muscle dysfunction or visual acuity loss. The candidates are almost invariably relatively young women, preoc-

cupied with their unsatisfactory appearance either because they have a strong sense of their former pulchritude or because their jobs require social intercourse. They cannot accept themselves despite frequent physician reassurances that their condition is mild, stable, and nonthreatening to vision. Their self-image also remains poor despite comforting statements from their spouses, family, or friends. They tend to resist suggestions to start psychiatric therapy—they don't want to *adjust* to their condition, they want to change it. We do not view such a situation as a cosmetic problem. Here we are dealing with a serious disruption of the individual's life, something she broods over frequently and which deeply affects her activities and emotions. Such patients may respond dramatically to decompressive corrective eye surgery.

Eyelid or Eye Muscle Surgery

In our experience about one-third of the patients with more severe degrees of ophthalmopathy will need some type of eye muscle or eyelid surgery to optimize ocular function, even if orbital radiotherapy, prednisone therapy, or both were employed. These procedures are best undertaken at a time when the inflammatory signs of ophthalmopathy have abated and other signs have stabilized. For those undergoing orbital radiotherapy, the appropriate time is usually six months to two years afterward. Many patients with mild, fixed diplopia benefit from being fitted with prisms. Retraction of the upper eyelid is usually treated by levator recession or by lateral tarsorrhaphy; we prefer the former because of the better cosmetic result. Correcting lower lid retraction generally requires a plastic procedure. Periorbital fat infiltration may be helped by blepharoplasty. In general, in contemplating surgical approaches to the treatment of stable Graves' ophthalmopathy, first consideration should be given to reduction of proptosis, then to repair of eye muscle dysfunction, and finally attention should be directed to the function and appearance of the lids. These considerations are probably best dealt with as a series of planned stages in reconstruction.

Alternatives

Since 1980 we have been employing an orbital radiotherapy treatment protocol of 3000 rads, delivered over a period of 3 weeks to determine if we could significantly reduce the percentages of patients whose benefit from orbital radiotherapy has been slight or nil—15 and 10 percent, respectively. An assessment of the patients treated under this revised protocol has not yet been made. We continue to recommend the standard 2000 rad dosage protocol for the present. We currently use combined supervoltage orbital radiotherapy and oral prednisone therapy only in special circumstances: (1) after ^{131}I therapy for coexisting thyrotoxicosis and (2) if the patient is already taking a maintenance dosage of prednisone to prevent relapse and orbital radiotherapy is to be added; in such cases, prednisone therapy is continued throughout the period of radiotherapy and for two to four weeks afterward, after which tapering of corticosteroid therapy is started. Treatment of ophthalmopathy with more aggressive schemes of immunosuppressive chemotherapy or with plasmapheresis should be regarded as experimental and awaits clear demonstration of benefit.

One group of investigators has strongly advocated and employed total thyroid ablation (surgical and/or radioiodine) as a prophylactic and therapeutic measure for ophthalmopathy. This recommendation has been highly controversial, and adverse effects of such treatment have been reported by several other groups. We cannot recommend this approach.

The question has been raised of the possible substitution of cobalt teletherapy for treatment by linear accelerator. It is more difficult to collimate the radiation using the former technique. Appreciable posterior angulation of the beam is required to avoid undue exposure of the cornea and lens, and consequently the dose distribution to the eye muscles is nonhomogeneous, there being a lower than desirable dose delivered to the anterior portions of the muscles. For these reasons cobalt teletherapy is not recommended.

ADRENAL DISEASE

PHEOCHROMOCYTOMA

STANLEY E. GITLOW, M.D.,
DEMETRIUS PERTSEMLIDIS, M.D.
and STANLEY W. DZIEDZIC, M.D.

Although considered to represent a medical curiosity, this tumor of the neural crest receives disproportionate attention because of the difficulty in differentiating it from one of our most common maladies, primary hypertension. The authors have had the opportunity to study 175 patients with proven pheochromocytomas who were originally referred for diagnostic evaluation and one of us (D.P.) performed the required surgical procedures for patients in this group on 63 occasions.

The treatment of these subjects can be divided conveniently into four categories: (1) the therapeutic approach to a patient suspected of harboring this tumor but whose biochemical diagnosis has not been attained; (2) the preoperative management of a patient whose diagnosis has been ascertained; (3) management during and after surgery; and (4) care of patients whose tumors cannot be fully resected.

THERAPEUTIC APPROACH WHILE ACHIEVING DIAGNOSIS

Since a clinical presentation of hypertension in its accelerated phase increases the likelihood of the diagnosis of pheochromocytoma, one should always evaluate such a patient initially for an alpha-adrenergic crisis. The appropriate treatment of a patient who presents with severe hypertension with or without substantive compromise of cerebral, cardiac, or renal function consists of the intravenous administration of 2 to 4 vials (10–20 mg) of phentolamine in 250 ml of fluid by microdrip. Within 3 or 4 minutes the patient's response to alpha blockade is known: a marked lowering and optimal control of the arterial pressure

while appropriate biochemical diagnostic studies proceed, or a more modest or negligible hypotensive response leading to an immediate change to alternate antihypertensive agents. It should be emphasized that not every alpha-adrenergic crisis stems from a neural crest lesion. Central nervous system (CNS) lesions (neoplastic or vascular) as well as essential hypertension associated with myocardial damage and β-blockade therapy may be responsive to alpha-adrenergic inhibition in the absence of a pheochromocytoma. The use of phentolamine in this manner is not for diagnostic purposes, but rather assists the clinician to avoid errors in the progressive management of the acutely ill hypertensive patient. The technique results in negligible delay. At no time should any patient be given phentolamine according to the manufacturer's prescription in the package insert. Intravenous administration of a few milligrams of phentolamine by direct "push" may result in irreversible shock in occasional patients with neural crest lesions and therefore should be avoided even in those patients with proven lesions and paroxysmal symptomatology. It is not unusual for a patient to require relatively large doses (10–100 mg per hour) of phentolamine for adequate control of the adrenergic state, but this is always administered by titration rather than as a bolus.

The relatively brittle clinical state of these patients must be emphasized. We know of subjects with these tumors who were treated with every antihypertensive agent currently available (even to the point of tumor resection during administration of the short-acting ganglioplegic, trimethaphan). In some instances, modest control of the hypertension and symptomatology was achieved; in others, the same drugs appeared to elicit no response, an exacerbation, or even precipitate a demise. Sudden death of cardiac or cerebrovascular origin is still unfortunately common in the presence of this tumor. One should never induce a paroxysm, whether for diagnostic purposes or otherwise. If the patient indicates that a crisis may be induced by drinking beer or by a certain body posture, he should be advised to avoid such actions until a reliable biochemical study has ruled out the presence of a pheochromocytoma. Similar caution extends to the physical examination of a patient suspected of suffering from this tumor: Avoid deep abdominal palpation.

Occasionally, patients with a severe alpha adrenergia will oscillate between enormous hypertension (diastolic pressures of 140–200) and shock. These swings in pressure follow one another within minutes and represent either fluctuations in the peripheral release of alpha agonist or, more commonly, variations in cardiac competency in the face of continued severe peripheral vasoconstriction. Again, not all of these patients have neural crest lesions. The treatment of choice, however, is the intravenous administration of (dilute) phentolamine, even though parenteral nitroprusside might be equally effective in lowering the blood pressure of such a patient. Indeed, in rare instances of alpha-adrenergic crisis stemming from CNS pathology, nitroprusside may be the best means of attaining blood pressure control for short periods of time.

Most patients suspected of having a pheochromocytoma do not present initially in the emergency room but rather in the company of and resembling subjects with essential hypertension, thyrotoxicosis, diabetes, cardiomyopathy, and recurrent paroxysmal symptomatology often attributed to "nerves." Although their troubles may seem to be of modest proportions, consider the advisability of administering an oral alpha-blocking drug while performing the required biochemical assays. Neither phentolamine nor phenoxybenzamine will modify catecholamine metabolism enough to elicit diagnostic difficulties with assays of total metanephrines or vanillylmandelic acid (VMA) excretion. Should you choose to avoid alpha blockade, under no circumstances administer a β-blocking drug until a pheochromocytoma has been ruled out. The commonly used diuretics, as well as alpha-methyl-dopa, hydralazine, clonidine, or guanethidine, may or may not effectively control an alpha-hyperadrenergic state, but more importantly they will rarely result in direct injury to the patient. Not so with the β-blocking drugs. Unfortunately, the introduction of propranolol resulted in a number of deaths in patients with neural crest lesions before it became evident that the β-blockade so induced resulted in substantively increased alpha sensitivity. Even in the presence of the less common epinephrine-secreting pheochromocytoma, the toxicity of increased alpha sensitivity markedly outweighs any benefit to be derived from β-blockade. Those very patients with

catecholamine myocardiopathy who might logically be expected to benefit the most from β-blockade may suffer calamitous results from the administration of these drugs. Even the most sanguine among us warn against their use before adequate alpha blockade has been achieved. We feel more strongly there is no excuse for using a β-blocking drug for a patient with or suspected of having a pheochromocytoma. Any need for an antiarrhythmic drug can be met through the use of agents that do not exhibit the counterproductive effects associated with the β-blockers. Patients with pheochromocytomas who, during surgery or otherwise, suddenly develop premature contractions or other dysrhythmias, are most commonly experiencing acute alpha adrenergia, the cardiac manifestations apparently resulting from an acute rise in systemic blood pressure. Increasing the rate of phentolamine infusion commonly controls such phenomena.

Phentolamine is available not only as a parenteral preparation but in 50-mg tablets as well. This drug is less effective when given orally than the alternate alpha-blocker, phenoxybenzamine. The latter, supplied as 10-mg capsules, demonstrates a relatively slower turnover but should be administered no less frequently than every 8 hours. The dosage should be titrated against the hypertension or other symptomatology, starting with 30–40 mg per day in divided doses. Do not hesitate to prescribe this drug for a patient with normal blood pressure suspected of having a pheochromocytoma. A stuffy nose and slight orthostatic phenomena are small prices to pay for protection against the sudden and capricious behavior of these tumors. It is not uncommon for a patient to require as much as 160–200 mg of phenoxybenzamine daily to block adequately the catecholamine release of some pheochromocytomas. The unpleasant side effects of this drug may become difficult to bear with such high dosages. Occasionally the addition of prazosin assists such a patient, but in no case should one rely on the alpha blockade achievable with this drug as the sole protection against a pheochromocytoma. Alpha-methyl-para-tyrosine was introduced as an inhibitor of catecholamine synthesis shortly after the role of tyrosine hydroxylase became appreciated. Unfortunately, the dosage required to modify substantively the biochemical behavior of these tumors is such as to result commonly in symptomatology of extrapyramidal neural dysfunction (cogwheel rigidity, masked facies, weakness). We have rarely found this drug to be clinically useful. Disulfiram was considered a likely prospect to modify catecholamine synthesis by inhibition of dopamine-β-hydroxylase. Our clinical studies failed to substantiate its usefulness, since significant enzyme inhibition required a dose far in excess of that tolerated by human subjects. The role of those drugs capable of eliciting combined alpha and beta blockade (labetalol) has not yet been elucidated.

Sensitive and specific assays of total metanephrines and VMA excretion eventually lead to biochemical diagnosis. It is sad that we continue to witness recommendations favoring pharmacologic manipulation of these brittle and precarious patients for the sole purpose of relieving the clinical laboratories of the responsibility of performing reliable testing. Once a reliable laboratory assay has established the presence of a neural crest lesion (and this can be accomplished in a noncomatose patient with over 99 percent certainty), no unnecessary manipulation of that patient should be tolerated. We have witnessed paroxysms precipitated by as little as a crudely performed sonography (from abdominal pressure with the probe). Mass demonstration may be helpful to the surgeon but is rarely essential for the patient about to have the initial laparotomy. The most reliable noninvasive techniques, sonography and CT scan, will occasionally ''detect'' lesions absent at surgery and fail to delineate some of the smaller tumors. Such studies do not relieve the surgeon of the necessity of performing a careful exploration to exclude the presence of unexpected multiple lesions. About 15 to 20 percent of adults, 50 percent of children, and more than 75 percent of familial cases and those with MEN II or neurocutaneous syndromes will have more than one pheochromocytoma.

Efforts aimed at tumor localization become essential in those patients who present with clinical and biochemical evidence of recurrent pheochromocytoma. Such cases often demand uncommon perseverance to delineate a lesion suitable for resection. Angiography and other invasive studies may be helpful, but none should be performed without the patient receiving intravenous phentolamine nor in the absence of a clinician experienced in the management of this illness.

A few studies are essential even for the patient presenting with a pheochromocytoma for the first time. Careful x-rays of the chest (PA, lateral, and both anterior oblique views) rarely miss the 1 to 2 percent of pheochromocytomas above the diaphragm. When these are negative, the surgeon may more securely prepare to enter and explore the abdomen as the source of excessive catecholamine synthesis. Finally, an IVP (or renogram in the dye-sensitive patient) should be done to confirm the presence of two functioning kidneys prior to attempting the resection of a tumor often desmoplastic and occasionally intimately related to the vasculature of one kidney.

Only routine preoperative testing should be permitted beyond those studies noted above. It is unnecessary to evaluate blood volumes or perform special studies to rule out a concomitant medullary carcinoma of the thyroid (MEN II) prior to surgery, since information so derived will not change the management of the case until after the removal of the pheochromocytoma. Only then should one proceed with a pentagastrin study or other endocrinologic investigations. Similarly, no effort should be made to discover or remove the cholelithiasis so common in these patients. Temptations to complicate the preoperative work-up, surgical preparation, or surgery itself should be assiduously avoided. Similarly, there should be no unnecessary delay in proceeding from diagnosis to resection. Our early hesitancy to operate upon subjects with biochemically proven neural crest lesions because of serious cardiac disease (previous myocardial infarction, congestive failure, dysrhythmia with pacemaker, and so on) resulted in attempts to carry them through their illness with alpha blockade rather than tumor removal. Unfortunately, the illness progressed and eventually escape from effective alpha blockade and excessive side effects from high phenoxybenzamine doses were seen. A careful surgeon can rectify this error. At present, delay in tumor removal is tolerated only if the lesion is unresectable (malignant or anatomically obscure). We believe that this principle should be applied to the patient whose disease is complicated by pregnancy as well: prompt resection of the tumor with as little unnecessary manipulation of the patient as possible.

PREOPERATIVE MANAGEMENT

Two decades ago, one of us (S.E.G.) viewed with concern the occasional use of phenoxybenzamine during and immediately prior to surgery for resection of pheochromocytomas. It seemed that one should have preferred an alpha blocker with a shorter half-life during an episode accentuated by physiologic change. For that reason, we utilized parenteral phentolamine as the drug of choice for preoperative stabilization and intraoperative control of vascular function. Removal of the tumor from the circulation, almost invariably resulting in acute fall in pressure, was the moment when the short action of this drug was most appreciated. From information available, however, it apparently mattered little which agent was used. On the other hand, one currently reads of the preference by some physicians to avoid alpha blockade in order to ease the difficulty experienced by the surgeon in anatomically locating all of the neural crest tumors. In our opinion, nothing could be more hazardous to the patient. Permitting the patient to experience paroxysms, whether preoperatively or during surgery, is literally equivalent to playing Russian roulette. Moreover, reasonable preoperative management demands that the patient's cardiovascular adjustment be returned to as close to normal status as possible. Circulating blood volumes, afterload levels, and cardiac function all improve during the few days in which parenteral phentolamine achieves alpha blockade. Although one might prefer a prolonged period of salutary physiologic control, the hazards of living with a pheochromocytoma demand its prompt resection. In practice, oral alpha blockade is used during the required brief work-up (3 to 4 days) and the parenteral agent is initiated 24 to 48 hours prior to surgery. The sole drawback to the use of parenteral phentolamine stems from its need for close monitoring. Thus the patient is usually transferred to a critical care unit for titration of the drug versus hypertension, sweating, dysrhythmias, tremulousness, abdominal pain, or other paroxysmal symptoms. The infusion rate is rarely changed more than 5 mg per hour every 10 to 15 minutes until resection. Large variations in dosage should be avoided. Whatever dosage is needed to control or prevent a paroxysm should be maintained between them. It is rare that excessive blockade elicits any injury. Modest hypotension (systolic pressure of about 90 mm Hg) is usually well tolerated with good cardiac and renal function.

MANAGEMENT DURING AND AFTER SURGERY

Although the presence of an informed internist and anesthesiologist at the operation might be desirable, nothing takes the place of a surgeon experienced with neural crest lesions, their clinical behavior, pathophysiology, and anatomic distribution. On the day of the surgery, 2 phentolamine solutions in dextrose/water are prepared: (1) 1 mg/ml (50 ampules in 250 ml), and (2) 5 mg/ml (100 ampules in 100 ml). The weak solution suffices for anesthetic induction and intubation, whereas the stronger is needed during dissection around the tumor. One hundred extra ampules of phentolamine should be available in prolonged operations for giant or multiple tumors. Atropine-like drugs should be avoided. Although the avoidance of general anesthetics known to sensitize the myocardium to catecholamines has elicited much comment over the years, surgery can probably be accomplished with any anesthetic agent currently in use. It is more critical that portals be available for the immediate parenteral administration of antiarrhythmic, pressor and alpha-blocking drugs. Volume replacement requires its own portal, since a disproportion between the vascular capacity and circulating volume might legitimately be expected to occur upon tumor removal. About 4–5 liters of crystalloid or colloid are usually needed to correct for this, with the bulk of volume repletion implemented after removal of the tumor. The precise fluid load can be more easily estimated by the routine use of a central venous line. A Swan-Ganz catheter is needed in all instances in which the patient's cardiac function is compromised. Cardiac monitoring (EKG) and a direct arterial line complete the preoperative arrangements. It should be emphasized that the intravenous portal for drugs should be arranged so that parenteral fluids might be switched without undue delay. A dilute solution of norepinephrine should be prepared but should rarely be required. Its requirement usually signifies inadequate intraoperative volume replacement.

A sudden appearance of dysrhythmia (usually PVCs) usually results from an acute elevation of blood pressure. This can be handled by increasing the rate of phentolamine infusion, deepening the anesthesia, or administering a bolus of 50–100 mg of lidocaine. Although parenteral propranolol may be used at such times, one of us (S.E.G.) has never witnessed an instance when it was needed.

In abdominal tumors, a transperitoneal approach is mandatory. An upper midline incision from the xiphoid process to below the umbilicus permits good access to both suprarenal areas, where 90 percent of pheochromocytomas are found.

In large adrenal or extra-adrenal tumors, the type of incision is dictated primarily by the size and anatomic location. Large adrenal tumors, usually single, are best approached by a subcostal incision.

Thoracic pheochromocytomas are resected via a posterolateral thoracotomy, and neck tumors are excised by incision along the sternocleidomastoid.

Thorough visual and manual exploration from the diaphragm to the pelvis is mandatory, with special focusing on the adrenals and para-aortic regions. Complete exploration must be accomplished, irrespective of the preoperative imaging results; there is no substitute for the surgeon's exploratory skills, particularly in view of the limited resolution of current imaging techniques.

Upon discovery of one adrenal tumor, resection is delayed until the other adrenal can be evaluated. This will assist one in making a decision regarding preservation of adrenocortical tissue. If the patient has a neurocutaneous syndrome or MEN II, bilaterality of the lesions reaches almost 100 percent (synchronous or metachronous) and a preoperative decision might have been made to perform a bilateral adrenalectomy with autotransplantation of normal cortical tissue into a peripheral muscle compartment.

The main technical difficulties are posed by the retropancreatic location of the left gland and the retrocaval position of the right adrenal. Such proximities to large vessels and the pancreas may create problems during dissection. Adrenal or extra-adrenal tumors may grow near or around the renal vessels and may be difficult to remove without disrupting the renal blood supply. The right adrenal vein is short (about 5 mm long), retrocaval, and enters the cava high, about 6 to 7 cm from the level of the renal veins. Pheochromocytomas, like carcinoid tumors, occasionally display pericapsular desmoplasia; this fibrotic reaction may be severe enough to mimic malignancy and render dissection more difficult.

Removal of each tumor from the vascular circuit usually results in a temporary fall in blood pressure. This is rarely great enough to compromise renal function (and can be monitored by urinary flow). Continued hypertension at that point signifies incomplete removal of the neural crest lesions. About 10 to 20 percent of patients have minimal residual hypertension, but this rarely becomes evident until after discharge from the hospital.

A continued requirement for postoperative pressor drugs is most likely related to retroperitoneal bleeding and represents an urgent indication for re-exploration. The swings in vascular pressure make such bleeding more common. Deep retroperitoneal fluid collections, occasionally septic (often staphylococcal) during surgery should be suspected when the patient moves one diaphragmatic leaflet poorly and becomes febrile. Bilateral adrenal resection obviously requires adrenocortical replacement. ACTH may be used periodically to stimulate cortical engraftment.

Total metanephrines excretion falls rapidly postoperatively but may remain above normal during a stressful postoperative course. VMA excretion, on the other hand, almost always approaches normal about two to four days after complete tumor resection.

MANAGEMENT OF NON-RESECTABLE TUMORS

Malignant pheochromocytomas fortunately occur in no more than 5 to 10 percent of the cases. Their bad and good news is represented by the relative infrequency with which they are responsive to therapy and their relatively slow growth, respectively. Even these circumstances are not universal. In rare instances radiotherapy appears to offer a temporary alleviation of the tumor's progress, especially in instances of bone metastases. On the other hand, the tumor occasionally "explodes" with rapid growth, metastatic nodules appearing within days in bones, lungs, liver, and local nodes. The more common slow-growing pattern favors debulking surgical procedures and management with phenoxybenzamine (often for years). We have not been impressed with any great improvement stemming from the use of alpha-methyl-p-tyrosine. The literature reflects that chemotherapy with various cytotoxic agents, including streptozotocin, has failed to elicit a reliable or consistent response. On the other hand, one of us (S.E.G.) now has experience with three such patients who have responded to streptozotocin. Two have experienced a long-term decrease in objective evidence of tumor size, catecholamine catabolite excretion, and need for alpha blockade therapy.

In the final analysis pheochromocytoma represents the needle in the hypertensive haystack. It is worthy of our attention because its near 100 percent mortality rate may be almost completely reversed by biochemically precise evaluation, gentle and efficient preoperative preparation, and experienced surgical care.

ADRENOCORTICAL INSUFFICIENCY

TERENCE D. WINGERT, M.D.
and PATRICK J. MULROW, M.D.

Primary adrenocortical insufficiency, or Addison's disease, is due to lesions of the adrenal glands resulting in reduced cortisol, aldosterone, and adrenal androgen production. The causes of primary adrenal insufficiency include idiopathic atrophy; granulomatous infections, such as tuberculosis or histoplasmosis; destruction by hemorrhage, tumor, or iron; and adrenalectomy. Lesions of the hypothalamus or anterior pituitary with decreased adrenocorticotropin (ACTH) production will result in secondary adrenal insufficiency. Cortisol and adrenal androgen secretion are reduced but aldosterone secretion is normal. Diseases of the anterior pituitary that cause secondary adrenal insufficiency include neoplasms, infarction, granuloma, hypophysectomy, and, rarely, infection. Suppression of the hypothalamic-pituitary-adrenal axis by administration of supraphysiologic doses of glucocorticoids can also result in secondary adrenal insufficiency.

The clinical presentation depends upon whether the process is primary or secondary. In primary adrenal insufficiency there is a deficiency in glucocorticoids and mineralocorticoids, as well as adrenal androgens. In secondary adrenal insufficiency the basic deficit is in glucocorticoid production, since ACTH is not the main determinant of mineralocorticoid secretion. In both primary and secondary adrenal insufficiency the presenting signs and symptoms may be subtle in the unstressed patient, and a high index of suspicion is required to make the diagnosis.

Very specific and effective steroid therapy is available for adrenocortical insufficiency. The more common steroid hormones and their relative potencies are listed in Table 1.

ADRENAL CRISIS

The diagnosis of adrenal crisis is based on the clinical presentation and is a medical emergency. It appears as a syndrome of weakness, fever, and hypotension. A precipitating event, such as infection or trauma, is often present. Most of the causes are caused by primary adrenal insufficiency.

Laboratory findings are nonspecific, but a low serum sodium level, increased serum potassium level, and an elevated BUN suggest the diagnosis. Treatment should be initiated after a blood specimen for cortisol measurement is drawn, but without awaiting the result, and consists of glucocorticoid replacement and volume expansion with 5 percent dextrose in normal saline intravenously. Mineralocorticoid therapy is not necessary initially. A careful search for precipitating causes should be made.

Hydrocortisone should be given parenterally and is available as a water soluble hemisuccinate or phosphate ester preparation. Maximal glucocorticoid secretion approximates 300 mg per day, so this is the dose we recommend. One hundred milligrams should be given as an intravenous bolus, followed by 100 mg every 8 hours as a continuous intravenous infusion. We do not use intramuscular cortisone acetate because of concerns about variable absorption in these gravely ill patients who may be in shock. Three hundred milligrams of hydrocortisone provide sufficient mineralocorticoid activity so that mineralocorticoid replacement is not needed. After the patient's condition is stable, the dosage can be reduced daily by approximately one-third until a maintenance dosage is achieved, usually within five days. More than twice replacement doses for prolonged periods should be avoided to prevent side effects from excess glucocorticoid. When the dosage is

TABLE 1 Relative Potencies of Some Common Steroid Compounds

Steroid	Glucocorticoid Activity	Sodium Retaining Potency
Short Acting		
Cortisol (hydrocortisone)	1	1
Cortisone	0.8	0.8
Intermediate Acting		
Prednisolone	4	0.8
Prednisone	3.5	0.8
Triamcinolone	3–5	0
Long Acting		
Dexamethasone	25–30	0
Fludrocortisone, Florinef	10	400
11-Deoxycorticosterone	0	20
Aldosterone	0.1	400

less than 100 mg daily, mineralocorticoid replacement is usually needed and fludrocortisone acetate therapy should be initiated.

During the crisis, replacement of fluids and electrolytes is equally important as hormonal replacement. These patients are volume depleted with severe sodium and water deficits. Initial therapy should be intravenous normal saline and dextrose at a rate determined by the degree of dehydration. Dextrose is necessary to treat the hypoglycemia that may occur in adrenal crisis. The first liter should be given over a period of ½ to 1 hour. Careful monitoring of central venous pressure or blood pressure will guide fluid treatment. Hypertonic saline is rarely indicated unless the serum sodium level is critically low. Its administration will exaggerate the dehydration of the intracellular space. Hyperkalemia usually responds to volume expansion and hormonal replacement and needs no specific therapy. Daily monitoring of body weight and electrolytes are necessary to assess treatment. Vasopressors for vascular collapse or bicarbonate for acidosis are rarely needed. The treatment of precipitating factors is crucial. We do not give antibiotic therapy routinely, but rather make this determination in each individual case based on clinical and laboratory evidence indicating the possibility of infection. The patient should generally improve within a few hours if the diagnosis of adrenal crisis is correct.

Treatment should not be withheld to establish the diagnosis if adrenal crisis is suspected. The plasma cortisol measurement will be of some help, but usually the result is available well after the crisis is over. If, in a critically ill patient, the plasma cortisol level is less than 10 μg/dl, one can strongly suspect adrenal insufficiency. To confirm the diagnosis, ACTH testing can be done at a later date while the patient is on maintenance therapy, usually with dexamethasone, since it does not interfere in the steroid measurement.

In secondary adrenal insufficiency, vascular collapse and hyponatremia are not usually present and skin pigmentation is not increased. The BUN and serum potassium level are normal. Hypoglycemia may be prominent if other pituitary hormones are diminished.

PRIMARY ADRENAL INSUFFICIENCY

Glucocorticoid Replacement

Replacement dosages are quite constant over a wide range of body weights. The dosage may need to be increased for the tall or very active person, while a slightly lower dosage might be appropriate for the elderly or for patients with hypertension. Certain drugs increase the metabolism of glucocorticoids, such as phenobarbital, diphenylhydantoin and rifampin, and higher dosages may be needed. Liver disease slows metabolism and the dosage may have to be reduced in patients with significant liver impairment.

The normal adult adrenal cortex secretes about 15–25 mg of cortisol daily in a diurnal secretory cycle. Replacement glucocorticoids are usually cortisone, hydrocortisone, or prednisone. These are usually administered in two doses to mimic the diurnal variation in cortisol secretion. Daily oral replacement in adults consists of hydrocortisone, 20–30 mg, with two-thirds in the morning and one-third in the early afternoon, or prednisone, 7.5 mg, split 2:1 on a twice a day schedule. In an occasional patient the dose may have to be given every eight hours for optimal results.

The adequacy of the replacement dosage is followed clinically. Reduction in the abnormal pigmentation may be used to judge the adequacy of the replacement dosage in primary adrenal insufficiency. We do not feel that measuring ACTH levels is necessary or useful.

Mineralocorticoid Replacement

Patients with primary adrenal insufficiency require mineralocorticoid replacement in addition to glucocorticoids. As oral aldosterone is ineffective, a synthetic mineralocorticoid for oral administration is used. The choice is fludrocortisone acetate (Florinef), which is prescribed in a dosage of 0.05–0.2 mg in a once daily dose. The replacement dosage is quite variable from patient to patient; we recommend starting at 0.1 mg once daily. A liberal sodium intake is also recommended.

The clinical guidelines to assess adequacy of replacement therapy include blood pressure, particularly the standing pressure; body weight, presence of edema; and plasma electrolytes, particularly the potassium level. Measurement of plasma renin levels is not generally necessary, but they may be elevated if too little fludrocortisone acetate is given or suppressed if too much is administered. After initially prescribing 0.1 mg once daily, we reduce the dose by 0.05 mg if hypertension, edema, or hypokalemia occurs. If orthostatic hypotension and/or hyperkalemia is present, we increase the dose in 0.05-mg increments. Once a dosage is established it remains remarkably stable, but periodic assessment should be carried out.

Adjusting Glucocorticoid Therapy for Stress

Patients need to be educated about their need for additional glucocorticoids during times of stress. They must know that they need to increase their dosage for minor stress; recognize symptoms of worsening adrenal insufficiency and report this to their physician; inform all medical professionals that they are steroid-dependent; and carry on their person a card or a "Medic Alert" bracelet stating that they are steroid-dependent. A kit containing dexamethasone phosphate for intramuscular use is a good idea for patients who do extensive traveling where medical care might not be readily available.

For treatment of minor stress, such as upper respiratory tract infections, fever above 100°F, or dental extractions, the dosage of glucocorticoid should be doubled until the stress or illness has resolved. Rarely should this increase be necessary for more than four to five days. If the illness is suspected to be serious or vomiting prevents administration of oral medication, the patient should be hospitalized.

Major stress, such as surgical procedures, myocardial infarctions, serious injuries, and sepsis, requires 300 mg of parenteral hydrocortisone daily. If the major stress is a planned event, such as surgery, we recommend beginning the hydrocortisone administration the day before, or at least a few hours before the stress. This is because there is a slight delay in the effect of glucocorticoids after administration. For example, we give 100 mg i.v. continuously on the night before surgery and every 8 hours until the patient is stable postoperatively. The glucocorticoid should be tapered to the replacement dosage as rapidly as recovery will allow, but this must be individualized to each patient.

There is no need to increase mineralocorticoid therapy for stress, as the high levels of glucocorticoids provide adequate mineralocorticoid activity. At times of severe stress when high doses of glucocorticoids are being administered, it may be best to omit the mineralocorticoid therapy temporarily.

The effect of pregnancy on the requirement for replacement steroids in humans has not been systematically studied. The usual recommendation is to continue the pregestational replacement dosage throughout pregnancy unless the clinical situation indicates a need for a dosage adjustment. If vomiting, hypotension, or hyperkalemia occurs, the glucocorticoid dose should be increased. The presence of hypertension, excessive peripheral edema, and hypokalemia would indicate that a reduction in the mineralocorticoid dose is warranted. Labor and delivery should be managed the same as severe stress.

The patient and physician should avoid increasing the replacement of glucocorticoids without objective indication of stress or indication of inadequate replacement. The patient may report subjective improvement in well-being on higher doses of glucocorticoid, but supraphysiologic doses can be hazardous. Acutely (within hours to days), excess glucocorticoids cause increased catabolism of muscle and increase urinary excretion of potassium, calcium, and phosphorus, with decreased excretion of sodium and subsequent fluid retention. Impaired glucose tolerance, and suppressed cellular immunity with an increased risk of infection also occurs. Chronic (over a period of weeks) excess glucocorticoid therapy will elevate blood pressure and cause truncal obesity, osteoporosis, muscle and cutaneous atrophy, vascular fragility, and poor wound healing.

SECONDARY ADRENAL INSUFFICIENCY

When the pituitary or hypothalamic lesion is permanent, these patients can be placed on maintenance doses of glucocorticoid as described for patients with primary adrenal insufficiency. There is usually no need for mineralocorticoid replacement, as minor abnormalities in aldosterone secretion can usually be met by high dietary sodium intake. Of course, these patients often need replacement of other hormones as determined by the pituitary function tests and clinical situation.

HYPOTHALAMIC-PITUITARY-ADRENAL AXIS SUPPRESSION

Ingestion of pharmacologic doses of glucocorticoids administered for nonendocrine diseases is the most common cause of adrenocortical insufficiency today and the area in which treatment modalities are the most varied and most controversial.

When supraphysiologic doses of glucocorticoid are administered, inhibition of the adrenal gland's ability to respond to ACTH occurs early, within days. Suppression of the hypothalamic-pituitary axis occurs with more prolonged therapy (weeks). Recovery from prolonged supraphysiologic glucocorticoid therapy occurs in the reverse order, with the return of hypothalamic-pituitary responsiveness preceding adrenal recovery (see Chapter 64).

The risk of suppressing the hypothalamic-pituitary-adrenal axis varies widely with the dosage and duration of therapy as well as probable individual variability. Potential suppression of the axis is minimized by alternate-day glucocorticoid therapy. There is little agreement as to when the patient should be considered to be at risk for impaired adrenal reserve. There have been reports in the literature of patients dying in shock following surgery after having received glucocorticoids preoperatively for as short a time as five weeks. A conservative approach is recommended even though many patients may receive treatment during severe stress who do not require it. As a general rule, patients who have been on daily glucocorticoid therapy for longer than two weeks should be considered to have adrenal insufficiency. Glucocorticoids should be administered during stressful situations if endocrine testing has not been performed to document an intact axis. Recovery of the pituitary-adrenal axis may take up to 12 months in patients who have been on prolonged glucocorticoid therapy.

ACTH has been administered to hasten hypothalamic-pituitary-adrenal recovery. This therapy will restore adrenal responsiveness but does not improve and may further impair hypothalamic-pituitary recovery. Because the hypothalamus and pituitary must recover first, there is no benefit to ACTH stimulation of the adrenal gland, as discontinuation of the ACTH therapy will be followed by a prompt decrease in glucocorticoid production.

If the glucocorticoid therapy is of less than two weeks' duration and there is no further indication for its use, we would discontinue therapy abruptly. There is little need to taper the dosage because the axis would not be suppressed, but many people do report feeling tired and weak when high-dose glucocorticoids are discontinued. If a tapering of the dosage is done it should be over only a few days.

If the glucocorticoid therapy is no longer indicated but has lasted longer than two weeks, the patient should be considered to have suppression of the hypothalamic-pituitary-adrenal axis and the glucocorticoid should not be discontinued suddenly. Our first step in management of these patients is to taper the dosage to replacement levels over several days.

Once the patient is stable on a replacement dosage we prescribe 20 mg of hydrocortisone once daily in the morning, around 10:00 A.M. This dosage regimen allows the patient to feel well but does not cause hypercortisolism. However, its main purpose is to allow the normal early morning surge of ACTH secretion and thus permit recovery of the hypothalamic-pituitary-adrenal axis.

We assess recovery by the short ACTH, or Cortrosyn, test. This can easily be done in the office at virtually no risk to the patient. A normal 1-hour plasma cortisol response to an intravenous or intramuscular injection of ACTH (cosyntropin, 250 μg) correlates with recovery of the hypothalamic-pituitary-adrenal axis. The reason is that the adrenal gland requires previous stimulation by endogenous ACTH to be able to respond acutely to a bolus of administered ACTH. The normal response at 60 minutes after ACTH administration is an increment of the plasma cortisol of greater than 6 μg/100 ml, with the absolute value being greater than 20 μg/100 ml.

CONCLUSION

Adrenocortical insufficiency is the result of primary adrenal disease, pituitary or hypothalamic disorders, or administration of supraphysiologic doses of glucocorticoids. Treatment regimens are summarized in Table 2.

TABLE 2   Adrenal Insufficiency

Maintenance Therapy

Glucocorticoid
12–15 mg/m^2 per day of hydrocortisone equivalent (the usual adult dose is 30 mg per day with ⅔ in the morning and ⅓ in the afternoon)
Monitor clinical response

Mineralocorticoid
Florinef, 0.05–0.2 mg per day
Liberal sodium intake
Monitor weight, blood pressure, and serum potassium level

Patient education
Adjusting glucocorticoids for stress
Medic-Alert bracelet

Treatment of Stress

Minor
Double dose of glucocorticoids until illness resolves
High salt intake

Major
300 mg of parenteral hydrocortisone daily
Intravenous fluids and electrolytes

CUSHING'S SYNDROME

DAVID N. ORTH, M.D.

Cushing's syndrome is caused by a chronic excess of glucocorticoids. There are three major causes of endogenous Cushing's syndrome, in which the glucocorticoid is cortisol: Cushing's disease, which is bilateral adrenal hyperplasia caused by hypersecretion of ACTH by the pituitary gland; ectopic ACTH syndrome, caused by inappropriate secretion of ACTH by nonpituitary tumors that are usually malignant; and hypersecretion of cortisol by benign or malignant tumors of the adrenal cortex. Since the primary abnormality is different for each of these three forms of Cushing's syndrome, the rationale for treating each is also different.

Ideal therapy for any form of Cushing's syndrome should achieve four objectives:

1. to correct Cushing's syndrome by lowering daily cortisol secretion to normal;

2. to eradicate or prevent any tumor that might threaten the health of the patient;

3. to avoid permanent endocrine deficiency; and

4. to avoid permanent dependence on medications.

In practice, it is sometimes necessary to compromise the last two of these objectives in order to realize the first two.

CUSHING'S DISEASE (PITUITARY ACTH DEPENDENT BILATERAL ADRENOCORTICAL HYPERPLASIA)

The hypercortisolemia of Cushing's disease is a curable condition. However, it is sometimes necessary to employ more than one mode of therapy before the cure is achieved. The patient should be aware of these facts before therapy is begun.

Since the primary observable abnormality in Cushing's disease is pituitary hypersecretion of ACTH, rational therapy should first be directed at the pituitary gland, not at the adrenal glands. In the adult, transphenoidal pituitary microadenomectomy is my usual first therapy. In a patient 18 years of age or younger, it is conventional external pituitary irradiation. However, therapy must be appropriate to the individual patient and clinical situation. In a young adult with very mild, uncomplicated Cushing's disease and no radiographic evidence of a pituitary microadenoma, for example, one might select pituitary irradiation as the initial treatment.

Pituitary Surgery

Transcranial pituitary surgery was not a very successful form of therapy. Over the last several years, however, transphenoidal microsurgery has become the treatment of choice for most adult patients with Cushing's disease. The rationale for this treatment is that an ACTH secreting anterior pituitary microadenoma is the primary cause of the disease. As discussed later, this may not necessarily be correct. When successful, transsphenoidal microadenomectomy provides a prompt cure for the cause of the Cushing's syndrome and achieves the ideal objectives of therapy.

The surgical approach is via a gingival incision above the roots of the upper incisors and leaves no external scar. The objective is to remove all ACTH secreting adenoma tissue and leave as much normal pituitary tissue as possible. The latter objective should be sacrificed, if necessary, to achieve the former in older patients who do not desire continued fertility. Morbidity is very low when the operation is performed by a neurosurgeon experienced in transsphenoidal surgery. Most patients have transient diabetes insipidus, usually lasting only a few days; it may persist several weeks in some patients, but is rarely permanent. Other pituitary function is usually left intact. Significant intraoperative hemorrhage is sometimes encountered owing to anatomic variations in venous drainage, such as anterior communication between the cavernous sinuses, but it is rarely life-threatening. Less dramatic oozing of blood is the rule in patients with Cushing's disease, in contrast to patients with other pituitary tumors. It may result in loss of a few hundred milliliters of blood and may interfere with adequate identification and resection of small microadenomas. Cerebrospinal fluid rhinorrhea occurs less frequently as the neurosurgeon gains experience. When a significant amount of tissue is removed, a piece of thigh muscle of equal size is inserted in the sella to prevent prolapse of the arachnoid. When less tissue is removed, no packing or only a small piece of gelfoam may be required. Persistent rhinorrhea occasionally requires repair. Meningitis has also become much less frequent as the result of refined surgical technique and use of preoperative nasal decongestant and antibiotic prophylaxis. Patients may be bothered in the immediate postoperative period by the nasal packing, which can produce a severe sinuslike headache. Mucosal edema may cause transient tearing and middle ear discomfort from occlusion of the lacrimal ducts and eustachian tubes, respectively. Postoperative ecchymoses around the orbits, nose, and upper lip are common in patients with Cushing's disease. Within a very few days, most patients feel quite well.

When supraphysiologic dosage of steroids is withdrawn by the neurosurgeon, one can determine if the patient is cured by measuring the morning plasma cortisol or ACTH levels, or both. Prior to this time, glucocorticoids may suppress ACTH secretion by residual adenoma tissue and give the erroneous impression that the tumor has been completely resected. Actually, there is no evidence that high dosage of steroids, routinely administered to reduce postoperative cerebral edema after intracranial surgery, are of benefit after transsphenoidal surgery. Preoperative steroid administration is certainly unnecessary. Four times the usual maintenance dose of cortisol (that is, 80–120 mg of hydrocortisone hemisuccinate—Solu-Cortef) can be given as a continuous intravenous infusion in the recovery room on the day of surgery, when the patient, if cured, will be ACTH deficient and may require additional steroid. The day after surgery, twice the maintenance dose (20–30 mg every 12 hours) can be given, and a maintenance dose thereafter. In any case, the dose should at least be halved every day until a single morning maintenance dose of 20–30 mg is reached. Hydrocortisone, a short-acting steroid, is preferable to long-acting dexamethasone, since virtually no cortisol from the previous morning's dose will remain in the circulating plasma the next morning. In patients who are cured, the morning plasma cortisol level is usually less than 5μg/dl, and the plasma immunoreactive ACTH level is low or undetectable.

With the source of excessive ACTH secretion removed, the patient now has isolated ACTH insufficiency and will quickly develop bilateral adrenocortical atrophy and unresponsiveness to exogenous ACTH. The reason is that the chronic hypercortisolemia caused by ACTH hypersecretion by the microadenoma suppressed ACTH secretion by the normal corticotrophs in the remaining anterior pituitary. There may be actual loss of identifiable, mature corticotrophs. Thus, once the microadenoma is removed, the patient is no different than one who has suddenly had his chronic pharmacologic dosages of exogenous steroids stopped or who has just had his cortisol producing adrenal tumor removed: It will take several weeks to several months to recover normal pituitary-adrenal function.

During this recovery phase, the patient must be treated for secondary adrenocortical insufficiency. Mineralocorticoid is unnecessary, since the renin-angiotensin-aldosterone system is intact. The patient should wear a medical identification bracelet or necklace with "Addison's disease" or "adrenal insufficiency" on it and should carry an identification card that lists his name, medications, instructions for emergency use of injectable dexamethasone phosphate (Decadron) and the name and telephone number of his physician. He should carry a preloaded syringe containing 4 mg of dexamethasone in 1 ml of solution with him at all times and should be instructed how to deal with stressful situations, such as surgical or accidental trauma, sudden fluid loss from hemorrhage or diarrhea, or vomiting resulting in inability to take his steroid medication. The threshold for injecting the dexamethasone must be low, since it can cause no harm, whereas delay is potentially harmful. The medication should be used in any stressful situation, after which the patient should consult a physician. For febrile illnesses associated with malaise, the patient should increase his glucocorticoid dosage two- or threefold for no longer than three or four days. If he gets worse during that period or is not well enough to return to his usual steroid dose at the end of it, he should consult a physician.

The length of time the patient has ACTH insufficiency varies from as little as several weeks to as long as two years or more and seems to depend upon two factors. The first is the severity and duration of his prior hypercortisolemia. As with exogenous steroid administration, the more glucocorticoid to which the patient is exposed and the longer he is exposed to it, the more profound will be his pituitary ACTH secretory suppression. The second factor is the nature of his postoperative maintenance glucocorticoid therapy, which should be adequate but not excessive. Most patients do very well taking 20 mg of cortisol (hydrocortisone, Cortef) each morning. Some patients tolerate less; other patients may require 25 or, occasionally, 30 mg. Long-acting synthetic steroids, such as dexamethasone, prednisone, and prednisolone, should be avoided. The cortisol should be given in the morning or, if an evening dose seems absolutely necessary, only a small fraction of the total daily dosage should be given in late afternoon or early evening. These measures are aimed at reducing the level of exogenous steroid still in the plasma when the maximum stimulus for ACTH secretion occurs, between about 3 A.M. and 8 A.M. Recovery can easily be tested at intervals of three months or so by delaying the morning dose of cortisol and performing a standard intravenous ACTH (Cortrosyn) stimulation test. When the patient's morning basal plasma cortisol level increases to 10 μg/dl or more, maintenance steroids are no longer required. When ACTH causes an increment in plasma cortisol of 6 μg/dl above baseline and a value of 20 μg/dl or more 60 minutes after the drug is given, steroid cover during stressful situations is no longer necessary.

The cure rate with transsphenoidal pituitary microadenomectomy for Cushing's disease probably depends on several factors, first and foremost the correctness of the diagnosis. Some patients with ectopic ACTH syndrome, particularly those with bronchial or thymic carcinoid adenomas, may suppress during the standard high-dose dexamethasone test and, like most patients with ectopic ACTH syndrome, respond to metyrapone. They may thus be difficult to distinguish from patients with Cushing's disease. In the absence of a demonstrable pituitary lesion by CT scanning or of a significant central-to-peripheral plasma ACTH gradient during catheterization of the petrosal venous sinus—a variable finding even in patients with proven Cushing's disease—exclusion of an ectopic source of ACTH may be the only alternative.

A second factor may be the stringency of the radiologic criteria required by the neurosurgeon in order to operate. Thus, in patients in whom a pituitary lesion is demonstrated by CT scan, microangiography, or both, microadenomectomy will be successful more often than in patients who fail to meet this criterion.

A third factor may be the criteria used for determining cure. If the patient does not have hypocortisolemia and low ACTH levels after steroids are withdrawn, he is probably not cured. Even if morning plasma cortisol and ACTH levels and daily steroid excretion are perfectly normal, diurnal rhythmicity and suppressibility with low-dose dexamethasone should be demonstrated. Even then, such patients should be re-evaluated periodically for recurrent Cushing's syndrome.

Fourth, the assumption that the individual patient with Cushing's disease has a single ACTH secreting microadenoma as the primary cause of his disease may not be correct. The evidence supporting this assumption is: (1) that a pituitary microadenoma is found in most patients; (2) that microadenomectomy results in cure of the Cushing's disease; (3) that transient pituitary ACTH deficiency follows surgery, and (4) perhaps most importantly, that diurnal rhythm and dexamethasone suppressibility are normal when pituitary-adrenal function recovers, several weeks to months later. This assumption is probably valid for many patients with Cushing's disease, but it may not be true for all of them. In some patients, the primary abnormality may be hypothalamic hypersecretion of corticotropin releasing factor (CRF) or hyposecretion of some as yet undefined hypothalamic tonic inhibitory factor. Several cases of recurrent Cushing's disease have occurred in patients apparently cured and fulfilling the criteria above; in one of these patients corticotroph hyperplasia, not a recurrent or second microadenoma, was found during a second exploration. Cushing's disease may represent a continuum, ranging from mild hyperplasia without demonstrable alteration in pituitary-adrenal function at one end of the spectrum to a microadenoma causing hypercortisolism and suppression of normal corticotroph differentiation and secretion at the other. This continuum may represent different disease processes in different patients, or different stages of the same disease process in the same patient. The length of time required to develop Cushing's disease is not known, and transsphenoidal surgery is a relatively recent development. Thus it may be too early to determine how many patients will develop recurrent Cushing's disease after apparently successful microadenomectomy.

Fifth, a group of patients with Cushing's disease has recently been described who had: (1) greater resistance to dexamethasone suppression, (2) significant suppression with a dopaminergic agonist, bromocriptine, (3) a pituitary adenoma adjacent to the pars nervosa, (4) nerve fibers in the microdenoma, which are not found in normal pars distalis or in the microadenomas that usually cause Cushing's disease, and (5) a much lower cure rate with transsphenoidal microadenomectomy. These patients were thought to have pars intermedia-type microadenomas, as contrasted with the presumably more common pars distalis-type microadenomas. The surgical failures were thought to result, at least in part, from adenomatous hyperplasia in grossly normal tissue adjacent to the visible microadenoma that remained after surgery.

Finally, the experience of the surgeon with these tumors and his or her ability to identify and resect them completely is extremely important. The success rate of experienced neurosurgeons varies from about 60 to 80 percent, with the lower figure probably more nearly representing the general experience. If it were possible to identify in advance those patients for whom conventional microadenomectomy was likely to be unsuccessful, one might consider more aggressive pituitary resection or alternative forms of therapy.

If transsphenoidal surgery is unsuccessful, there are several options. One should first review the data to be sure the diagnosis was correct. If there is any doubt, additional tests should be performed. If there is no doubt, the options are: Repeat transsphenoidal surgery, external pituitary irradiation, and medical or surgical adrenalectomy, with or without pituitary irradiation.

In adult patients who do not desire additional children, I usually prefer a second transphenoidal operation, with more radical resection of the pituitary gland. Little is known about the results of repeat transsphenoidal surgery. The cure rate is probably considerably lower than with the first procedure, but we have achieved cures after a second and, in one case, a third operation. Technically, repeat surgery presents no problem and takes much less time, since the approach through the nasal septum and posterior wall of the sphenoid sinus has already been prepared. Postoperative morbidity is certainly no greater than after the first operation and is often much less. The patient should understand that pituitary tissue will be removed until a microadenoma is clearly identified or until no pituitary tissue remains in the sella turcica. He should be told that, if the surgeon performs a complete hypophysectomy, replacement sex steroids and thyroid hormone will be required, and, if the Cushing's disease is cured, permanent daily replacement glucocorticoid therapy will be required. He should also be warned about more prolonged diabetes insipidus; permanent diabetes insipidus is unusual, even after total hypophysectomy. I prefer that the neurosurgeon be aggressive, rather than conservative, during the second procedure in order that I can be assured that no further benefit can be gained from additional pituitary surgery and can direct my attention elsewhere in the event of failure.

Pituitary Irradiation

External pituitary irradiation can be given either as conventional megavoltage (^{60}Co or linear accelerator) or heavy particle (alpha particle, proton beam, Bragg peak) irradiation. Conventional irradiation is given via multiple opposed ports at a fractional rate of no more than 200 rads per day, 5 days per week, for a total tumor dosage of 4200–4500 rads. Lower dosage is less effective; dosage greater than 4800 rads is associated with complications we have not encountered with the recommended dosage. Complications also increase significantly if the recommended fractional dose rate is exceeded. Heavy particle irradiation is usually given in a single sitting via multiple ports, and total tumor dosage may exceed 10,000 rads. The advantages of heavy particle irradiation are the relatively high cure rate and the short length of time required for therapy. Its disadvantages are that it can be delivered at only two centers in the United States, the Donner Laboratory in Berkeley and the Massachusetts General Hospital in Boston, and that the incidence of complications, such as panhypopituitarism and ocular nerve palsies, is much higher than with conventional irradiation (with which they are very rarely seen). Conventional pituitary irradiation is my preferred form of therapy.

Primary Therapy. In children 18 years of age or less, irrespective of the duration of their disease, pituitary irradiation is my first choice of therapy, since 80 to 85 percent of such patients will be cured. Response is usually rapid, with 20 percent cured within two months after beginning irradiation and 50 percent cured within six months. Occasional patients may require 12 or even 18 months before cure is obtained, but they usually show earlier improvement in basal steroid secretion and dexamethasone suppression. Conventional irradiation in children, as in adults, very rarely results in loss of other pituitary function. Basal hormone levels are usually normal. Responses to provocative tests, such as growth hormone response to hypoglycemia, may be subnormal in some subjects, but this is not associated with clinical manifestations: Growth resumes, sexual development proceeds normally, and hormone replacement is unnecessary. However, children cured of any form of Cushing's syndrome by any means do not demonstrate catch-up growth; every inch lost prior to cure is permanently lost. Therefore, prompt diagnosis and treatment are mandatory. The medial temporal cerebral cortex receives significant irradiation, but we have seen no impairment of intellectual or psychologic function. In very young children, one might be concerned about irradiation of the carotid siphon, since postirradiation hypoplasia might occur, causing relative carotid stenosis in adulthood. However, Cushing's disease is distinctly unusual in children less than 7 years of age, and we have found no evidence of this complication in older children. Occasional patients will have transient hypoadrenocorticism, similar to that observed after successful transsphenoidal microadenomectomy, and should be treated in a similar manner. If one wished to reduce cortisol secretion more rapidly, metyrapone (Metopirone) or aminoglutethimide (Cytadren), inhibitors of adrenal steroidogenesis, can be used while awaiting the full effect of irradiation. In children who are not cured, I usually recommend surgical total bilateral adrenalectomy. In patients with radiographic evidence of a pituitary mass, transsphenoidal surgery might be preferred. However, the neurosurgeon should understand that normal anterior pituitary function must be preserved, unless the tumor itself poses a threat to health.

In adults, conventional pituitary irradiation is not nearly so successful. Based on our experience with about 130 patients, approximately 15 percent of adults over the age of 20 will be cured by this therapy, and an additional 30 percent will be sufficiently improved that no other therapy, except perhaps small doses of metyrapone or aminoglutethimide, will be required. Others report cure rates of up to 30 percent and similar rates of improvement. It is age at the time of therapy, not at the onset of disease, that appears to result in this difference in response to therapy. Adults also respond somewhat more slowly than children, often taking 6 to 12 months to respond fully to therapy. I reserve pituitary irradiation as primary treatment for young adults who have mild Cushing's disease and no radiographic evidence of a pituitary tumor or for patients in whom surgery is contraindicated.

Adjunctive Therapy. I recommend conventional pituitary irradiation for all patients who undergo total adrenalectomy. Other than intraoperative death and lifelong dependence on daily steroid replacement, the most serious complication of adrenalectomy is Nelson's syndrome, manifested by progressive sellar enlargement, hyperpigmentation, ocular nerve palsies, visual field defects, severe headaches, and extreme elevations of plasma ACTH and ACTH related peptides. This complication occurs in 5 to 20 percent of adults and 25 to 35 percent of children, yet we have not observed Nelson's syndrome in the 5 children and 35 adults we have treated with pituitary irradiation prior to or soon after bilateral adrenalectomy. Although there are reports of occasional patients who have developed this disorder despite prior pituitary irradiation, we conclude from our experience that

pituitary irradiation may have a role in preventing Nelson's syndrome. The exact mechanism is not clear, but patients who have had pituitary irradiation plus bilateral adrenalectomy have lower plasma ACTH levels while taking replacement steroid medication than do patients who have had adrenalectomy alone. This could result either from reduction in the number and/or functional capacity of pituitary ACTH secreting cells, or from reduction in CRF secretion by the hypothalamus, which receives significant irradiation, or both.

For adults not cured by transsphenoidal hypophysectomy, I recommend pituitary irradiation, administering o,p'DDD (mitotane, Lysodren) or adrenal enzyme inhibitors or both during irradiation to control the hypercortisolemia and evaluating the patient at intervals for response. If the patient is cured, obviously no further therapy is required. If he shows no response within 6 to 12 months, medical or surgical adrenalectomy should be undertaken. In this way, the patient has a chance for cure without operative risk or permanent adrenal insufficiency and has received preventive therapy for Nelson's syndrome should medical or surgical adrenalectomy be required. As noted below, administration of o,p'DDD for periods of as little as four to six months may result in permanent adrenal insufficiency. I use this drug only if hypercortisolism is not adequately controlled by the enzyme inhibitors.

An 80 percent cure rate has been reported in adult patients treated with conventional pituitary irradiation in combination with o,p'DDD. The initial dosage was 4 gm daily in divided doses, the largest taken in the evening to minimize unpleasant side effects; the maintenance dosage was 1.5–2 gm per day for 6 months to 7 years. Over half of the patients responded within four months and remained in remission after the drug was discontinued; several required cortisol replacement therapy. The late responders had recurrent Cushing's disease when o,p'DDD was discontinued and probably should be considered candidates for surgical adrenalectomy. I have had no personal experience with this treatment or with conventional pituitary irradiation and subtotal adrenalectomy (total adrenalectomy on one side and 50 to 75 percent resection on the other), for which a similar success rate has been reported.

Finally, one might reasonably consider giving conventional pituitary irradiation after successful transphenoidal surgery to reduce the risk of recurrent Cushing's disease. This would be especially relevant in patients whose daily cortisol secretion was reduced to normal and who were therefore cured of Cushing's syndrome, but who were not hypoadrenal immediately after transphenoidal surgery.

Adrenalectomy

Surgical Adrenalectomy. Total bilateral adrenalectomy can be performed either via bilateral back incisions or transabdominally. The former approach is technically more difficult, but the exploration is limited to the retroperitoneal space and causes much less postoperative morbidity. It is not uncommon to transect the posterior reflection of the pleura during the back approach, especially on the left, causing a pneumothorax that must be treated with suction. Major complications include intraoperative hemorrhage and postoperative wound dehiscence and infection, but these have become increasingly infrequent as the diagnosis of Cushing's syndrome has been made earlier, when its manifestations are less severe. It is imperative that the adrenals be removed en bloc with the surrounding adipose tissue, since rupture of the adrenal capsule and spillage of adrenocortical cells into the operative bed can result in recurrent Cushing's syndrome.

As is the case for patients having transsphenoidal surgery, preoperative steroid medication is unnecessary. Steroid administration can be begun during induction of anesthesia or when the adrenal glands are removed. The dosage of steroids should be similar to or greater than that given after transsphenoidal hypophysectomy: 100–200 mg of hydrocortisone hemisuccinate the day of surgery, at least halving the dose each day until the maintenance dosage is reached. Many physicians are more comfortable giving larger doses of steroids for longer periods of time. There is no evidence that this is necessary. However, as long as the total dosage is not more than about two or three times what I have recommended and is at least halved each day postoperatively, it is unlikely to cause any problems. High dosage of glucocorticoids will mask the fever resulting from infection and should not be used for the treatment of hypotension in lieu of investigating possible causes, such as internal hemorrhage. It is not uncommon for the Cushing's patient to have a chronic urinary tract infection, symptoms and signs of which become manifest only after he is eucortisolemic.

The patient is now an Addison's patient and must be given daily replacement doses of both glucocorticoid (hydrocortisone 20–30 mg per day,

prednisone 5 mg per day, or dexamethasone 0.5 mg per day) and mineralocorticoid (9α-fluorohydrocortisone, fludrocortisone, Florinef). He must always wear an identification bracelet and carry a syringe filled with dexamethasone, and should be instructed in dealing with emergencies as discussed above. Some surgeons have taken an interesting approach for avoiding adrenal insufficiency: Part of one of the resected adrenals is implanted subcutaneously, where it continues to function. If it secretes too much cortisol, an additional portion can be resected during a minor surgical procedure. It is an attractive approach, but one with which I have had no personal experience.

Medical Adrenalectomy. Adrenalectomy can also be performed by chronic administration of o,p′DDD, alone or in conjunction with pituitary irradiation, as discussed above. O,p′DDD affects mostly the zona fasciculata, tending to spare the zona glomerulosa; plasma aldosterone and plasma renin activity remain normal with low doses of o,p′DDD. However, higher doses and chronic administration can cause aldosterone deficiency as well. It is thought that oxidation or hydroxylation of o,p′DDD by cytochrome P-450 dependent enzymes in the adrenocortical cell is necessary for its cytotoxic effect. In this regard, it is important to recognize that spironolactone (Aldactone), which may be used as a diuretic or antihypertensive in patients with Cushing's syndrome, depletes the level of cytochrome P-450 dependent enzymes in the adrenal cortex and thereby blocks the effect of o,p′DDD. O,p′DDD also has extra-adrenal effects, altering the metabolism of a variety of steroids, including cortisol and aldosterone, and making measurement of urinary steroid metabolites an unreliable index of secretion. In addition, plasma ACTH has also been observed to remain the same or actually decrease in patients receiving o,p′DDD, without pituitary therapy. This suggests that there may be an effect of o,p′DDD on the hypothalamus and/or the pituitary itself.

This drug is best used as an adjunct to pituitary irradiation to control cortisol secretion or to perform medical adrenalectomy in patients who do not respond adequately to irradiation. It can also be used in selected patients in whom pituitary and adrenal surgery is contraindicated. It is not an easy drug to use. Patient acceptance varies, it takes several weeks to achieve significant reduction in cortisol secretion when the drug is used alone, there is the risk of developing adrenal insufficiency, the effects of the drug persist long after it is discontinued, and therapy must be monitored with plasma, rather than with urine steroids. For these reasons, I do not use this drug for primary therapy. The dosage and timing of administration have already been discussed. As in patients who have had surgical adrenalectomy, I believe that patients who have had medical adrenalectomy should have conventional external pituitary irradiation as well.

Other Treatments

Adrenal Enzyme Inhibitors. It has been suggested that metyrapone or aminoglutethimide alone may be used for the control of otherwise untreated Cushing's disease. This is not my experience. Plasma ACTH levels rise impressively after the administration of these drugs, effectively overcoming the pharmacologic blockade within a few days. Although very large doses of the drugs, especially when given in combination, may be effective in controlling hypercortisolemia, they have several drawbacks: (1) they do not address the primary cause of the disease, (2) they do not cure the disease, they only control it and must therefore be given permanently, (3) they have significant gastrointestinal, central nervous system, and endocrinologic side effects, and (4) continued therapy with these drugs is inordinately expensive. On the other hand, they are useful, alone or in conjunction with o,p'DDD, for lowering cortisol production and improving the patient's condition prior to surgery, for controlling cortisol secretion while awaiting the full effects of pituitary irradiation, or for reducing cortisol secretion to normal in patients who are improved but not completely cured by pituitary irradiation. In addition, their important use in the treatment of ectopic ACTH syndrome and adrenal tumors is discussed below.

Centrally Active Drugs. Cyproheptadine HCl (Periactin) is a serotonergic antagonist that also has antihistaminic, anticholinergic, and sedative effects. This drug has been reported to induce remissions of Cushing's disease and Nelson's syndrome. Its mechanism of action is not clear, but it may exert its effect directly on the microadenoma cell. The number of patients whose Cushing's disease is controlled with this drug is also unclear; in our experience not more than 10 percent have a sustained adequate response, although another group has had a 40 percent response rate. As with adrenal enzyme inhibitors, cyproheptadine controls but does not cure Cushing's disease. Therefore, it must be continued indefinitely. Its

most unusual side effect is marked stimulation of the appetite of many patients taking the drug. Some are unable to control their appetite and experience a rapid weight gain which, if their Cushing's disease is uncontrolled, is superimposed upon their existing Cushingoid obesity. The drug is usually started in divided doses totaling about 4 mg per day and increased as tolerated to approximately 24 mg per day before one concludes there will be no therapeutic benefit. I would reserve it for unusual patients in whom other measures have failed.

Bromocriptine mesylate (Parlodel) is a dopaminergic agonist that appears to exert its effect at the level of the pituitary. Although it lowers plasma ACTH levels significantly in some patients with Cushing's disease, it rarely, if ever, lowers ACTH and cortisol secretion to normal. Thus, although bromocriptine, like cyproheptadine, may be a useful investigative tool for elucidating the derangements in hypothalamic-pituitary function in Cushing's disease, one should not delay effective therapy by testing the response to these drugs.

ECTOPIC ACTH SYNDROME

Optimal treatment for this disorder is to remove the ACTH secreting tumor. However, most of these tumors are malignant and cannot be resected completely at the time of their discovery. In fact, secretion of ACTH by these neoplasms has been cited by some oncologists as an unfavorable prognostic sign. Even if the tumor cannot be eradicated, the hypercortisolism can be controlled. This is important, since the metabolic abnormalities often present a more acute threat to the patient's life than the tumor itself. Reducing cortisol secretion to normal can prolong the useful life of the patient, permit his immune system to operate optimally, and give the oncologist time and favorable metabolic conditions in which to provide specific antitumor therapy. The two means for controlling hypercortisolism are the use of inhibitors of adrenal steroidogenesis and medical or surgical adrenalectomy.

Adrenal Enzyme Inhibitors

Two drugs are currently available for this purpose. Aminoglutethimide blocks the conversion of cholesterol to Δ^5-pregnenolone, the first step in the synthesis of both adrenal and sex steroids. Metyrapone blocks the conversion of 11-deoxycortisol to cortisol, the last step in cortisol biosynthesis. The reason they are effective in ectopic ACTH syndrome, but not in otherwise untreated Cushing's disease, is that ACTH production by the non-pituitary tumor does not rise to compensate for a falling plasma cortisol level and thereby override the biosynthetic blockade. These drugs may be effective alone or can be used in combination to enhance effectiveness and minimize side effects. The dose is similar to that used as adjunctive therapy in Cushing's disease. In patients with ectopic ACTH syndrome, they may produce hypoadrenocorticism within two days. Aminoglutethimide inhibits the synthesis of aldosterone as well as cortisol and is more likely to produce symptoms of adrenocortical insufficiency. Metyrapone also inhibits aldosterone secretion, but it leads to increased production of deoxycorticosterone, a precursor that is itself a potent mineralocorticoid. Thus metyrapone does not usually cause clinically significant mineralocorticoid deficiency. Oral or intravenous potassium supplementation or both may be required acutely to treat the profound hypokalemia encountered in some patients. Potassium sparing diuretics may be required to induce natriuresis to correct the hypertension and edema secondary to the sodium retention caused by severe hypercortisolemia. Insulin may be required to control diabetes mellitus. However, these measures can often be discontinued within a few days. Until recently, aminoglutethimide was an investigational drug. Therefore, my experience has mostly been with metyrapone, which I have found to be effective when used alone in most patients. With moderate dosages (250–500 mg 3 times a day), replacement glucocorticoid therapy is usually not required. In rare patients given aminoglutethimide alone, and in a somewhat higher percentage of patients taking aminoglutethimide in combination with metyrapone, adrenal insufficiency may occur. One can either reduce the dosage of the drug(s) or add replacement steroids; I prefer the former.

Therapy must be monitored by measuring plasma cortisol or urinary free cortisol levels in patients receiving metyrapone. Although biologically inactive, 11-deoxycortisol is a 17-hydroxycorticosteroid and is measured as such in the urine. It should be noted, in this regard, that some radioimmunoassays for cortisol have significant cross-reaction with 11-deoxycortisol, so that an extraction or fractionation step may be necessary prior to measurement. Treatment should be continued as long as necessary, which is usually as long as the patient survives his tumor and has his adrenal glands intact.

Adrenalectomy

As discussed previously, adrenalectomy can be achieved either surgically or medically. Patients with inoperable but indolent ectopic ACTH secreting tumors, such as medullary carcinoma of the thyroid, should be considered candidates for adrenalectomy, rather than for the use of adrenal enzyme inhibitors. The principles are the same as those discussed above. O,p′DDD can also be used in conjunction with aminoglutethimide or metyrapone in patients whose hypercortisolemia is difficult to control or in whom very rapid control is desired.

ADRENOCORTICAL TUMORS

Surgery

The treatment of choice for adrenal tumor is complete surgical resection of the neoplasm, which usually requires removal of the involved adrenal gland and may require unilateral nephrectomy in patients with adrenal carcinoma. The surgeon should be aggressive with these tumors, since their size, gross appearance, and histologic characteristics are not accurate predictors of their subsequent benign or malignant behavior. A transabdominal approach is usually required to obtain sufficient exposure and to explore the contralateral adrenal gland adequately. If the patient has severe Cushing's syndrome, the risk of intraoperative and postoperative complications is greatly increased. Since these patients are exquisitely sensitive to the action of adrenal enzyme inhibitors, it may be wise to treat patients with severe Cushing's syndrome with metyrapone or aminoglutethimide for several weeks prior to surgery. The risk of delay must be weighed against the risk of immediate surgery. Our experience with adrenal adenomas is excellent. Surgical complications are infrequent, and all of our 30 patients have been cured. They have prolonged postoperative pituitary-adrenal insufficiency and must be treated with replacement dosage of glucocorticoid as discussed above. Our experience with surgical treatment of adrenal carcinoma is much less gratifying. Eighty-five percent of the patients we treated at Vanderbilt have died, 50 percent within three years and the rest within eight years. Metastasis to the liver and lungs is the rule.

O,p'DDD

Mitotane has long been used as a chemotherapeutic agent in patients with adrenal crcinoma. It is more or less selectively toxic for adrenocortical cells, inhibiting both their growth and steroid secretion. There is little or no evidence that the drug prolongs life, however. We have observed objective remissions of adrenal carcinoma in a few patients, but have seen the tumor recur in the same patients while they were still taking o,p'DDD. Thus o,p'DDD must be considered a palliative drug only, and one with unpleasant side effects. Since neither radiotherapy nor other chemotherapy has proved useful with these tumors, however, it is the only agent that may be of value in the patient with inoperable disease. Mitotane should be given with milk or food; late evening doses are best tolerated in terms of side effects. The drug should be given orally in divided doses, starting with 1 gm or less per day and increasing the dose every few days to maximum tolerance level up to 24 gm or more per day. This dosage should be maintained for as long as the patient tolerates it and there is objective remission. O,p'DDD interferes in the extra-adrenal metabolism of cortisol, so that urinary 17-hydroxycorticosteroid levels cannot be used as an accurate index of steroidogenesis; plasma cortisol or urinary free cortisol levels can be used for this purpose. Since o,p'DDD affects the normal adrenal glands as well as the tumor, there is the risk of inducing hypoadrenocorticism, which should be looked for and treated if necessary. The drug is stored in fat, such as adipose and nervous tissue. Therefore its effect persists for extended periods of time after the drug is discontinued.

Adrenal Enzyme Inhibitors

These drugs are useful in preparing patients with severe Cushing's syndrome for surgery and for controlling steroidogenesis in patients with inoperable adrenal carcinoma. They should be used in preference to o,p'DDD for these purposes. In carcinoma patients in whom virilization is a major complication, aminoglutethimide, which blocks the cortisol biosynthetic pathway before adrenal androgens are produced, may be more effective. However, it should be remembered that it will also block ovarian estrogen synthesis.

PRIMARY ALDOSTERONISM

RICHARD HORTON, M.D., and WILLA A. HSUEH, M.D.

First described by Conn in 1955 as producing hypertension, hypokalemia, renal potassium wasting, and striking neuromuscular symptoms in association with an adrenal adenoma, this disorder is now recognized to have multiple etiologic agents. It usually presents as a subtle cause of hypertension, making it mandatory to screen all hypertensive patients for unexplained hypokalemia before initiating diuretic therapy. The classic disorder and still the most common (80 to 90 percent) is the single adenoma. This benign neoplasm secretes considerable aldosterone and aldosterone precursor, 18 OH–corticosterone (18 OH B), which completely suppresses renin release and typically induces rather severe renal potassium wasting and hypokalemic alkalosis. The tumor is small (0.5 to 2 cm) but is only relatively autonomous (no response to changes in sodium balance and angiotensin II) but exaggerated response to exogenous or endogenous (circadian) ACTH while supine or standing).

Next in frequency is the so-called idiopathic or bilateral hyperplasia with or without micronodular hyperplasia. This entity continues to defy our understanding, since studies suggest a primary disorder of the adrenal itself. Despite the hyperplasia, the adrenals generally secrete less aldosterone than does an adenoma, without releasing precursor steroids. The electrolyte picture is less severe and there is a response (often exaggerated) to upright posture. Renin levels are not totally suppressed and there is a response to exogenous angiotensin II.

Rarely, an isolated case or family is described with the glucocorticoid remediable type. Some investigators have suggested testing all patients with primary aldosteronism for this entity. However, in the absence of a family history, the authors have not found this necessary or practical. There have also been reports of a few families with congenital aldosteronism. The syndrome may also be associated with adrenal cancers producing aldosterone (rare), or a mixed type secreting aldosterone, cortisol, and androgens which can be identified by the presence of Cushing's syndrome with associated virilization and hypertension. (In the usual patient with Cushing's syndrome, the mineralocorticoid excess is due to the combined activity of cortisol, desoxycorticosteroid, and corticosterone, while aldosterone levels are reduced.)

The diagnosis of primary aldosteronism is confirmed by demonstrating inappropriate aldosterone levels in the face of hypokalemia, a low renin value (PRA < 1 ng/ml/hr), and a lack of suppression of aldosterone in plasma after Florinef administration (0.2 mg every 12 hours for 3 days). This occurs in all types of hyperaldosteronism. We also follow body weight, since patients in an escape phase of this disease will not gain weight on this regimen, while normal subjects and most hypertensive patients will gain 2 to 4 pounds.

Once aldosteronism is confirmed, differential diagnosis is important and challenging, because choice of therapy depends on etiologic factors (Table 1). Although the plasma aldosterone response to various agents or posture has been proposed, to distinguish adenoma from hyperplasia, it is our opinion that localizing techniques are the most reliable. The clinician currently has available the iodocholesterol scan, the adrenal CT scan—particularly the newest generation scanner—and direct invasive simultaneous bilateral adrenal vein catheterization. A recent study also indicates that elevation of both plasma aldosterone and 18 hydroxy B levels indicates the presence of an adenoma, while the 18 hydroxy B level is normal in the presence of hyperplasia. In addition, a disturbance in dopaminergic inhibition of aldosterone secretion in hyperplasia has also been suggested because the aldosterone response to metaclopromide was decreased. If 18 OH B values and an adrenal CT scan are not diagnostic, simultaneous adrenal vein catheterization and comparison with caval or peripheral blood is indicated. Lack of a gradient on one side points to a tumor on the contralateral side, and a clear-cut gradient contralaterally confirms this impression. Adrenal vein cortisol values are very helpful, since values of > 50 ug/dl indicate successful entry into the adrenal vein. Our experience is that other maneuvers and test procedures are less definitive in differential diagnosis.

MANAGEMENT AND TREATMENT DURING THE PERIOD OF DIAGNOSIS

The treatment of primary aldosteronism is directed toward reducing the hypertension and reversing the potassium depletion. During the periods of diagnosis and of therapy and management, these two aspects may be approached differently. For example, when the diagnosis is first suspected, the hypertension must be managed without use of diuretics, since these agents would markedly alter the renin-angiotensin system as well as further change the potassium status. Our approach is to control blood pressure, possibly only partially, with alpha methyl dopa (Aldomet), 500 mg b.i.d. or t.i.d., or other sympatholytic agents. If the patient is already taking various antihypertensive drugs and diuretics and possibly on a low-sodium diet as well, we stop all these procedures with the permission and monitoring of the referring physician for three weeks prior to initiating any studies. Potassium depletion from diuretics will take as long as three to four weeks to be reversed with a normal potassium intake. We do not use potassium supplements during this initial period, since K^+ can directly stimulate aldosterone.

TREATMENT OF AN ADENOMA

Demonstration of an adenoma that has been localized by iodocholesterol scan, CT, or adrenal vein analysis and radiopaque dye injection is an

TABLE 1   Treatment of Primary Aldosteronism

Etiologic Factor	Preferred Therapy
Adenoma	Unilateral adrenalectomy
Hyperplasia	Spironolactone (Aldactone), 100–400 mg daily
Carcinoma	Unilateral adrenalectomy
Glucocorticoid responsive	Dexamethasone, 0.5–0.75 mg daily
Indeterminate	Thiazide diuretics

indication for surgery. The response to surgery can be predicted by the medical use of spironolactone (Aldactone). This synthetic steroid lactone is a competitive antagonist of aldosterone and other mineralocorticoids in the distal nephron and other target cells. Large doses are administered (300–600 mg daily, that is, 100 mg q.i.d.) for 3 to 4 weeks prior to surgery. Weight loss occurs within the first seven to ten days with a slow blood pressure decline. Normalization of blood pressure is a good predictor of a successful adrenal removal. This response is not diagnostic of an adenoma, however, since patients with other types of primary aldosteronism, as well as patients with low renin essential hypertension, are also somewhat responsive.

Hypokalemic alkalosis is a cardinal feature of the syndrome and tends to be more severe when the etiologic factor involves a functioning adenoma. Potassium depletion would pose a significant risk factor during anesthesia and the surgical period itself, via problems in cardiac rhythmicity, voluntary and involuntary muscle activity, and paralytic ileus. Potassium repletion must therefore be accomplished prior to surgery, usually with spironolactone and a low-sodium diet alone. Some endocrinologists add 4–6 gm of potassium chloride to the diet in the week prior to surgery.

Surgical Period

Most experienced adrenal surgeons now prefer the posterior flank approach because of ease of exposure of the adrenal gland. The adenomas are usually small, discrete, smooth, and rounded, and the entire gland is removed. The availability of the various scans and, when necessary, direct catheterization procedure allows us to operate with a high degree of assurance. If a discrete tumor is not found in the gland, the removed adrenal should be meticulously sectioned to look for a microscopic adenoma. In addition, we insist that the surgeon explore the other side with a second flank incision and carefully palpate the opposite adrenal.

Postoperative Period

Increased aldosterone secretion with sodium retention has chronically suppressed the secretion of renin. It is therefore not surprising that removal of the functioning adrenal adenoma and remainder

of the adrenal should precipitate a state of hypo-aldosteronism. This will persist until the renin-angiotensin system becomes functional again and the suppression of zona glomerulosa cells is reversed. Preoperative treatment with spironolactone should lower blood pressure, reverse the electrolyte disorder, and, at least in some patients, reactivate the renin-angiotensin system, perhaps reducing the later period of hypoaldosteronism. In any event, following the removal of the adenoma, the patient has lost a major regulator of potassium. If the serum potassium level was normal at the time of surgery, it is our approach to monitor serum potassium levels in the recovery room and replace it only if needed. The surgeons must be aware that routine intravenous use of 40–60 mEq per day of potassium could potentially induce hyperkalemia, and intravenous use of K^+ must be carefully monitored.

In the ensuing weeks only a rare patient will not recover from renin suppression. Happily, more than 70 percent of patients will be cured of their hypertension, and all patients will have improvement of their hypertension. Despite potential cure, an occasional patient will refuse surgery or may not be a surgical candidate. It may be necessary to use diuretics with potassium supplementation or aldosterone antagonists as long-term medical therapy. Spironolactone is of course the treatment of choice in this situation; however, side effects can ensue, limiting their use. These are discussed below.

MANAGEMENT AND TREATMENT OF PRIMARY ALDOSTERONISM DUE TO BILATERAL HYPERPLASIA

Primary aldosteronism due to adenoma and that due to hyperplasia has distinctly different courses. When bilateral adrenalectomy was utilized as definitive therapy for aldosteronism secondary to hyperplasia, the electrolyte disorder was cured; however, less than 20 percent of patients were cured or noted significant improvement of their hypertension. This has led to considerable discussion that the bilateral adrenal disorder is secondary to the basic hypertensive process or that these patients suffer from an extension or extreme phase of the common disorder known as low renin hypertension, in which aldosterone secretion is normal. However, even in low renin hypertension, there is hypersensitivity to exogenous angiotensin

II. The general agreement in the field is that patients in whom an adenoma cannot be demonstrated should be treated medically instead of undergoing bilateral adrenalectomy with the resultant necessity for lifelong glucocorticoid replacement.

Spironolactone therapy, therefore, is the treatment of choice. This compound is a pure antagonist to aldosterone action and is effective initially in doses of 200–400 mg daily. Although most patients with idiopathic adrenal hyperplasia have a decrease in blood pressure in response to spironolactone, many will require further treatment with additional antihypertensive agents. The serum potassium level increases to the normal range within one to two weeks of starting spironolactone therapy, and plasma renin activity can continue to increase for up to six months. Within the first few months of treatment, little change in plasma or urinary aldosterone levels occurs, despite the marked increases in renin activity. This would suggest that in addition to its mineralocorticoid receptor effects, spironolactone also acts directly to reduce aldosterone biosynthesis and secretion. This effect is seen in both adenoma and hyperplasia patients during long-term therapy. The advantage here is the possible reduction in dosage, and we and others have had occasional patients in whom the therapeutic dose gradually fell from 300 to 75–100 mg daily. Spironolactone inhibits various steroid hydroxylation steps, not only in the adrenal cortex but also in the gonad, which results in distinctly unfavorable side effects. At doses exceeding 100 mg daily, it tends to block testosterone biosynthesis, and in the periphery it can block androgen action. In some series as many as 50 percent of men ingesting spironolactone complained of tenderness and enlargement of the breasts and decreased libido. In women fewer side effects are noted, although reports of breast tenderness and menstrual irregularities have appeared. Therefore, in men the use of spironolactone may be unacceptable for the long term. Other side effects include diarrhea, rash, and mental confusion.

Alternatively, triamterene (Dyrenium) can be used in doses of 100–300 mg daily. It is a distal potassium sparing diuretic that has a direct effect on the renal tubule by inhibiting sodium reabsorption independent of aldosterone. However, spironolactone appears to be more effective in controlling blood pressure and potassium than triamterene. Reported side effects of triamterene include blood dyscrasia, liver damage, and gastrointestinal disturbances. Triamterene and spironolactone should not be given together, and neither should be given with potassium supplementation. Both drugs should be used cautiously in the face of renal disease because of increased problems with hyperkalemia. When used in combination with more proximally acting diuretics that increase distal tubular sodium delivery, both drugs increase the degree of diuresis. In Europe, amiloride, a drug that blocks entry of sodium ions into a transport mechanism in the distal tubule, is also available.

Recent studies indicate that aldosterone secretion may also be influenced by dopamine locally, which inhibits production. A few patients with hyperplasia have secreted inappropriate amounts of aldosterone during cyclic changes (nadir) in plasma dopamine. There have also been reports that some patients respond to dopaminergic agents, such as bromocriptine (Parlodel). Side effects such as nausea and dizziness may occur. These studies are cited to indicate that progress is being made which may provide new insights into this disorder.

OTHER TYPES OF PRIMARY ALDOSTERONISM

Management of primary aldosteronism resulting from a carcinoma of the adrenal cortex involves surgical excision with preoperative potassium replacement, usually with spironolactone. If the tumor also secretes glucocorticoids, glucocorticoid replacement may be necessary until the remaining adrenal functions normally (see Chapter 27).

Glucocorticoid suppressible hyperaldosteronism is very rare and usually familial. Affected family members are treated with dexamethasone, 0.5–0.75 mg daily. The mechanism is quite unclear, but aldosterone secretion appears to be chronically driven by normal levels of ACTH and cortisol.

Indeterminate hyperaldosteronism has been defined by some as involving hypertension and elevated aldosterone and normal serum potassium levels without renal K^+ wasting. Since the hypertension is mild and aldosterone is suppressible, it is our advice that these people be treated as low renin hypertensive patients by therapeutically controlling the blood pressure elevation per se. We and others have seen a few such cases evolve into definable types of primary aldosteronism, but this experience is limited and surgical intervention is not warranted until the cardinal manifestations of primary aldosteronism appear.

ISOLATED HYPOALDOSTERONISM

JAMES C. MELBY, M.D.,
and GEORGE T. GRIFFING, M.D.

Despite the relatively late recognition of hypoaldosteronism, this entity has become increasingly recognized in many medical centers as the major cause of hyperkalemia. The hallmark of hypoaldosteronism is hyperkalemia, which is usually asymptomatic but may be associated with neuromuscular symptoms, cardiac arrythmias, syncope, and death. There are two principal forms of isolated hypoaldosteronism: congenital aldosteronism due to primary mineralocorticoid resistance (pseudoaldosteronism) or to an inborn error in aldosterone biosynthesis—corticosterone methyloxidase types I and II deficiencies; and in adults, the syndrome of hyporeninemic hypoaldosteronism, which is due to alterations in the function of the renin-angiotensin system. Congenital aldosteronism is extremely rare, and most of this chapter is therefore limited to the syndrome of hyporeninemic hypoaldosteronism (SHH). The most common form of congenital aldosteronism is corticosterone methyloxidase type II deficiency, which is inherited as an autosomal recessive trait and has its onset at 1 to 3 weeks of age with manifestations of dehydration, vomiting, and failure to grow and thrive. All of the patients are hyponatremic and hyperkalemic and exhibit a metabolic acidosis. Plasma renin activity is actually elevated. Plasma levels of aldosterone are low and plasma levels of 18-hydroxy-corticosterone are elevated. These patients are treated with synthetic mineralocorticoids, namely, 9α-fluorocortisol (usually 0.1 mg mg/day, never less than 0.05 mg./day), for a variable duration of time, since the defect tends to ebb with age.

The incidence of diagnosis of SHH in the general population is increasing yearly. The median age of onset is in the last sixties and males outnumber females. Nearly 80 percent of patients exhibit chronic renal insufficiency and more than half have diabetes mellitus. All of the patients are hyperkalemic and most exhibit a hyperchloremic metabolic acidosis with a mild to moderate hyponatremia. The plasma renin activity is low, both basal and stimulated, as is the plasma aldosterone level.

PREVENTION AND ANCILLARY TREATMENT

Once the diagnosis of SHH has been made, factors that precipitate or perpetuate suppression of renin and/or aldosterone biogenesis should be avoided. Diabetes mellitus is the most common cause of SHH in the United States, and the successful treatment of diabetes mellitus improves nearly every level of the renin-aldosterone axis. It is also the most treatable cause.

AVOIDANCE OF FACTORS TENDING TO SUPPRESS RENIN AND/OR ALDOSTERONE SECRETION

Volume Expansion

Chronic volume expansion is a well-known cause of renin suppression. This results in hypoaldosteronism and, in some clinical situations, hyperkalemia. Hypoaldosteronism from volume expansion occurs in postadrenalectomy patients following surgical excision of an aldosterone-producing adenoma. These patients can develop severe hyperkalemia and hypotension lasting several days to weeks after surgery. This also occurs in patients chronically ingesting sodium bicarbonate (baking soda), usually to treat gastrointestinal ulcer disease. Another rare cause of hypoaldosteronism is Gordon's syndrome. This is associated with renin suppression, hypoaldosteronism, hyperkalemia, and is believed to be due to excessive sodium reabsorption at the distal tubule.

Medications

Many medications can interfere at multiple points in the renin-aldosterone axis. Avoidance of these drugs can be of major importance in the clinical management of hypoaldosteronism.

Beta-Blocking Adrenergic Drugs. These drugs interfere with renin secretion and are associated with hyporeninemic hypoaldosteronism. Juxtaglomerular cells that synthesize and secrete renin contain β1-adrenergic receptors. Either intrinsic neuronal or extrinsic adrenergic stimuli trigger these receptors, resulting in an immediate release of renin. Propranolol and similar agents are β-adrenergic receptor blockers which prevent

131

renin release and produce hyporeninemic hypoaldosteronism. These drugs should be avoided in patients with known hypoaldosteronism or in diabetic patients with latent hypoaldosteronism.

Prostaglandin Synthetase Inhibitors. These drugs, which specifically inhibit cyclo-oxygenase, block renin release and have been associated with severe hyperkalemia due to hyporeninemic hypoaldosterone. Prostaglandin E_2 directly stimulates renin release, probably by a direct action on the juxtaglomerular apparatus. Furosemide-induced renin release is blunted by indomethacin and other prostaglandin synthetase inhibitors. Use of indomethacin and similar prostaglandin inhibitors is widespread in clinical therapeutics. These drugs should be avoided in patients with hypoaldosteronism and in diabetic patients with subclinical aldosterone insufficiency.

Converting Enzyme Inhibitors. Captopril (Capoten), MK-421 (Enalapril), and other converting enzyme inhibitors act by inactivating angiotensin-converting enzyme. This interrupts the renin-aldosterone axis, resulting in iatrogenic hypoaldosteronism. These drugs have been introduced only recently to the medical community and the clinical significance of hypoaldosteronism is unknown. Because of these unknown risks, it behooves the clinician to monitor high-risk patients on converting-enzyme inhibitors closely for hyperkalemia.

Heparin. Polysulfated glucosaminoglycans, like heparin, impair aldosterone biosynthesis from the zona glomerulosa. With prolonged administration, heparin can produce significant hypoaldosteronism with severe hyperkalemia. This is due to a direct toxic effect on the zona glomerulosa, evidenced by hyper-reninemic hypoaldosteronism and zona glomerulosa atrophy. The least toxic dose of heparin is unknown, but a dose as small as 20,000 U per day for five days has been observed to reduce aldosterone secretion. This is an uncommon cause of hypoaldosteronism, but it is important because it is reversible and has been associated with lethal hyperkalemia.

Potassium-Sparing Diuretics. Diuretics that conserve potassium include spironolactone, triamterene, and amiloride. These drugs should be avoided in patients with hypoaldosteronism and are relatively contraindicated in patients with diabetes mellitus and chronic renal failure. Each of these drugs has a different mode of potassium conservation. Spironolactone has two effects: It is a mineralocorticoid receptor antagonist, and it inhibits aldosterone biosynthesis, presumably by competing with intermediates in corticosteroid biogenesis. Triamterene produces potassium retention by a direct action on non–aldosterone-mediated distal tubular exchange sites. Amiloride acts on the luminal surfaces of epithelial membranes to block sodium channels, resulting in less sodium resorption and potassium secretion.

Adrenolytic Therapy. Drugs that impair adrenal function are increasingly used for the hormonal treatment of breast cancer and medical management of Cushing's syndrome. These drugs include aminoglutethimide (Cytadren), o,p′-DDD (mitotane), metyrapone (Metopirone), and trilostane. They block various enzymatic steps in the biosynthesis of corticosteroids. This usually results in impaired secretion of all classes of the corticosteroids: mineralocorticoids, glucocorticoids, and adrenal sex steroids. Lower doses of these drugs may not be associated with hyperkalemia, since secretion of aldosterone precursors may confer significant mineralocorticoid activity (deoxycorticosterone).

Other Drugs. As our understanding of the pathophysiology of the renin-aldosterone system enlarges, some of the currently available and investigational drugs may be found to have adverse effects on the renin-aldosterone system. For example, drugs affecting the dopaminergic system have been shown to produce significant alterations in aldosterone secretion. It is believed at the present time that aldosterone is under tonic dopamine inhibition, and it is possible that administration of dopaminergic agonists, such as bromocriptine, could impair aldosterone secretion in certain physiologic situations. These hypothetic effects are at present only speculative, and the dopamine-aldosterone inter-relationship is currently under investigation.

Reduced Potassium Load

Reduction of extracellular potassium load can be the single most effective preventive measure in controlling hyperkalemia. Reducing dietary intake of potassium can be extremely helpful in avoiding hyperkalemia. Patients—and many physicians—have little awareness of the potassium content of many foods. Low-salt foods and salt substitutes often contain potassium as the alternative cation. For example, low-salt milk contains 60 mEq/L of potassium. Other foods high in potassium include dried fruits (30 mEq/cup), meat (60 mEq/pound), decaffeinated coffee (4 mEq/cup), and a variety of other foods. Other sources of potassium include transfusions of bank blood (30 mEq/L) and high-dose penicillin (1.7 mEq/10^6 U).

Control of Diabetes Mellitus

As mentioned previously, this disorder is commonly associated with hyperkalemia and hypoaldosteronism due to multiple defects in the renin-aldosterone system. In addition to these factors, diabetic patients are predisposed to hyperkalemia because of insulin deficiency and hyperglycemia. Both insulin deficiency and hyperglycemia can independently produce a maldistribution of total body potassium. Hyperglycemia results in extracellular hyperosmolality, resulting in an extracellular flux of potassium. Furthermore, insulin deficiency prevents cellular uptake of potassium, presumably related to the metabolic actions of this hormone. Both of these adverse effects, insulin deficiency and hyperglycemia, can be prevented by judicious control of the diabetes. Type II adult-onset, non–insulin-dependent diabetics should be encouraged to lose weight if obese, abstain from alcohol, and use oral hypoglycemic agents if necessary. Type I juvenile-onset, insulin-dependent diabetics may benefit from home glucose monitoring and split-dose insulin regimens.

Whatever the method of diabetic control, the level of blood sugar and normality of carbohydrate metabolism correlate directly with potassium homeostasis. Patients who are chronically hyperglycemic experience more hyperkalemia; and conversely, better controlled diabetics have more normal potassium balance. Furthermore, the long-term control of glucose homeostasis in diabetes mellitus can reduce the risk of hypoaldosteronism. Autonomic insufficiency results in hyporeninemic hypoaldosteronism, and this is a potentially avoidable risk in well-controlled diabetes mellitus. The degree of autonomic neuropathy correlates with the extent and duration of hyperglycemia. If this can be prevented, it would remove an additional potential cause of hyporeninemic hypoaldosteronism in the diabetic patient.

Interstitial Nephritis

In interstitial nephritis, hyperkalemia occurs early, before chronic renal failure. This disease is associated with a high frequency of hyporeninemic hypoaldosteronism, presumably owing to juxtaglomerular damage and impairment of renal synthesis and secretion. Early recognition of this disease is important because it is preventable and, in some cases, reversible. The leading causes of interstitial nephritis in many series are anatomic genitourinary abnormalities which, following early identification, are surgically correctable. Analgesic abuse with aspirin or phenacetin (>2 kg) is a potentially reversible cause of interstitial nephritis. Other treatable causes of this disease include hyperuricemia, nephrocalcinosis, nephrolithiasis, and sickle cell disease.

TREATMENT OF HYPOALDOSTERONISM

There is no ideal medical therapy for hypoaldosteronism. Many of the therapeutic modalities have limited benefits and are a calculated risk to selected patients. The majority of patients with mild selective hypoaldosteronism may require no therapy at all. When preventive measures are employed and patients are educated concerning their disease, specific therapy can be avoided. The decision to treat hypoaldosteronism and selection of a specific therapeutic agent depends on a number of factors, including the presence of diabetes mellitus, the degree of hyperkalemia, the age of the patient, blood pressure, sodium balance, and renal function.

Mineralocorticoid Therapy

This is the mainstay of therapy for mineralocorticoid deficiency states. 9α-fluorocortisol (fludrocortisone acetate, or Florinef) is the most potent synthetic mineralocorticoid. It also has glucocorticoid activity but is not used as a systemic anti-inflammatory agent because of its salt-retaining qualities. It is absorbable from the gastrointestinal tract and can be administered as oral tablets (0.1 mg). 9α-fluorocortisol is used in dosages of 0.1–1.0 mg per day, which is equivalent to between 200–2000 μg of aldosterone. Ninety percent of patients become normokalemic in this dosage range of 9α-fluorocortisol. Many patients with hypoaldosteronism have hypertension, mild renal failure, or incipient congestive heart failure. These patients cannot excrete a sodium load and are prone to excessive blood volume expansion. The use of 9α-fluorocortisol in these patients would correct the hypokalemia but could lead to hazardous fluid accumulation. It is thus often wise either to avoid 9α-fluorocortisol therapy or combine it with a diuretic.

Diuretics

Diuretics may be the cardinal therapy for patients with hypoaldosteronism and coexisting diseases associated with sodium retention. Older patients with hypertension, mild renal impairment, and congestive heart failure in general respond better to diuretic therapy than mineralocorticoid replacements. Since kaliuresis is the goal of diuretic therapy, the choice of a potent kaliuretic drug is of the utmost importance.

Chlorthalidone meets this requirement and may be administered in once daily doses (25 mg per day). A cheaper but slightly less kaliuretic agent is hydrochlorothiazide. This drug has a shorter duration of action and should usually be administered in twice daily doses (50–100 mg per day). The "loop" diuretics, such as furosemide or ethacrynic acid, are less potent kaliuretic agents but induce a greater degree of natriuresis. These are short-acting drugs and should be administered in twice daily doses (80 mg per day).

Although these drugs can correct the hyperkalemia associated with hypoaldosteronism, they are associated with side effects that may obviate their use. Both diabetes mellitus and hyperuricemia are frequently asociated with hypoaldosteronism, and diuretics exacerbate both of these conditions. Thiazide drugs in particular impair insulin secretion and can necessitate initiation or increase of insulin therapy in some patients. Furthermore, thiazides are sometimes associated with precipitation of gout in hyperuricemic patients, which is a common coexisting problem in hypoaldosteronism. A potential benefit of diuretic therapy is stimulation of residual renin release in otherwise hyporeninemic patients. Patients with hyporeninism due to autonomic insufficiency could be cured, or at least experience improvement, of their hyporeninism following the use of diuretics.

Sodium Bicarbonate Therapy

Sodium bicarbonate cannot be recommended as routine therapy in the treatment of SHH. This treatment is especially hazardous in elderly patients with coexisting renal impairment, congestive heart failure, and hypertension, because of the increased sodium load. Children with defects in aldosterone biosynthesis may require sodium bicarbonate during the acute onset of the illness.

Kayexalate (Polystyrene Sulfonate)

This is a cation exchange resin that can be given orally or via the rectum to correct hyperkalemia. Kayexlate removes approximately 1 mEq/g resin by exchanging sodium for potassium in a

1:1 ratio. Administration of kayexlate therefore increases sodium load and may be contraindicated in patients unable to tolerate an increase in sodium intake. Calcium-exchange resins have been under investigation for this problem, but they are not currently available for clinical use. The most efficient way of administering kayexlate is by rectal enema. Approximately 50 gm kayexlate (2 teaspoons = 10 gm) is combined in solution with 25 percent sorbitol or 20 percent dextrose. The enema is retained for 60 minutes, and several enemas can be instituted if necessary. One enema can reduce the plasma potassium concentration by approximately 0.5 mEq/l.

Patients often prefer oral kayexlate, but this frequently produces nausea and constipation. Therefore diarrhea should be induced by cathartics prior to administration of kayexlate. Fifty grams of kayexlate are combined in a 20 percent sorbitol solution and given two to four times a day. The major problems with this therapy are the poor patient acceptance and the excessive sodium load administered. Thus, this agent is rarely used by clinicians treating hypoaldosteronism.

SUMMARY

In conclusion, SHH is a common cause of hyperkalemia in the general population. It is best treated by prevention, but specific and effective therapy is available. The choice of therapy frequently depends on a number of clinical variables, including the age of the patient, the presence of diabetes mellitus, blood pressure, salt balance, and renal function. Older patients with hypertension, renal impairment, or incipient congestive heart failure are often best treated by either diuretics or combined diuretics and mineralocorticoid replacement therapy. Younger patients respond best to combinations of salt and mineralocorticoid replacement therapy.

Despite the broad range of therapeutic agents, many patients with hypoaldosteronism have difficulty in maintaining normal sodium and potassium homeostasis. It therefore behooves the clinician to educate the patient regarding his disease and to employ measures to prevent life-threatening hyperkalemia. In the future, new forms of therapy, especially for hyporeninemic hypoaldosteronism may become available.

This chapter was supported in part by USPHS grants 1-T30-AM21683, 5-T32-AM07201, 5-P0-HL18318, and 5-RO1-HL18318 from the National Institutes of Health.

CONGENITAL ADRENAL HYPERPLASIA

CLAUDE J. MIGEON, M.D.

VARIOUS FORMS OF CONGENITAL ADRENAL HYPERPLASIA

Congenital adrenal hyperplasia is a disorder related to a deficiency of one of the enzymes necessary for the biosynthesis of cortisol by the adrenal cortex. This deficiency results in a decreased cortisol secretion, a compensatory increase in ACTH output with hyperplasia of the adrenal cortex, and increased secretion of cortisol precursors. As shown in Table 1, each enzyme deficiency results in a specific pattern of steroid secretion characterized in each case by a decreased secretion of the steroids located after the deficient enzyme in the biosynthetic pathway and an increase of the steroids prior to that deficiency. By far the most frequent form is the 21-hydroxylase deficiency, and its treatment will therefore be the main object of this discussion. Specific treatment of the other forms will be discussed at the end of this chapter.

In 21-hydroxylase deficiency the cortisol precursors that are secreted in large amounts include androstenedione and 17-hydroxyprogesterone. About 10 percent of androstenedione is metabolized peripherally into testosterone, which causes masculinization of the female fetus as well as virilization postnatally. The metabolites of androstenedione are excreted in urine as 17-ketosteroids. The increased secretion of 17-hydroxyprogesterone produces a salt-losing tendency that will be compensated by an increase in aldosterone secretion if the 21-hydroxylase deficiency is moderate (*simple virilizing form*). However, if the deficiency is more severe, aldosterone cannot be secreted and the salt-losing tendency cannot be compensated, resulting in the *salt-losing form*.

The overall goal of the treatment of 21-hydroxylase deficiency is to administer an amount of cortisol that will result in the suppression of ACTH secretion by the anterior pituitary, which is turn will result in cessation of secretion of adrenal corticosteroids. In additi.n, if the salt-losing tendency is not compensated, mineralocorticoid replacement will be needed. Therapy should be started as early as possible because of the untoward influence of the untreated syndrome on growth and on the psychologic adjustment of patients. Furthermore, the treatment of the salt-losing form in the newborn period is an emergency.

TABLE 1 Various Forms of Congenital Adrenal Hyperplasia and Their Respective Patterns of Steroid Secretion

Enzyme Deficiency	Clinical Form	Cortisol	Other Gluco-corticoid	Aldoste-rone	Other Salt-retaining H	Androgens	Renin
Severe 21-OH	Salt-losing	−		−		+ +	+
Moderate 21-OH	Simple virilizing	N		+		+ +	+
Mild 21-OH	"Attenuated"	N		±		+	±
11-OH	Hypertensive	−	S + +	−	DOC + +	+ +	−
17-OH	Hypertensive	−	B + +	−	DOC + +	−	−
3β-ol-dehydrogenase	−	−		−		− (DHA + +)	+
20-OH/22-OH 20,22-desmolase	−	−		−		−	+
Abnormal cholesterol ester	Adrenoleuko-dystrophy	−		−		N or −	+
Esterase	Xanthomatosis	−		−			+

Note: N, normal secretion; +, increased secretion; −, decreased secretion; S, 11-deoxycortisol; B, 17-deoxycortisol; DOC, 11,17-deoxycortisol; DHA, dehydroisoandrosterone.

TREATMENT OF THE ACUTE ADRENAL CRISIS

This occurs usually between the third and tenth day of life. In somewhat less severe cases it can occur later on in life. The deficiency of both cortisol and aldosterone results in salt loss with dehydration and hypoglycemia.

After a prompt evaluation of the patient and collection of blood for complete blood cell count, serum chemistry, and steroid measurement (17-hydroxyprogesterone and androstenedione), intravenous fluid therapy must be started immediately.

First Hour of Treatment

Isotonic saline in 5 percent glucose (20 ml/kg of body weight, up to 500 ml) is given. This fluid therapy is classic and accepted by most specialists in the field. However, it will usually not correct the acidosis, and for this reason the following intravenous fluid mixture is preferable: one-third: 1/6 M sodium lactate; two-thirds, 0.85 percent sodium chloride; plus addition of dextrose to make a 5 percent solution. This mixture can be used throughout the first 24 hours of intravenous fluid therapy.

Using the intravenous set, 50–100 mg of Solu-Cortef (depending upon the size of the patient) is given over a 1-minute period, while an additional 50–100 mg of Solu-Cortef is mixed in the intravenous fluid. Intramuscular cortisol or cortisone acetate ($37.5mg/m^2$ per 24 hours) and DCA (1 mg per 24 hours) are also administered.

At End of First Hour

If blood pressure has not improved, plasma (10 ml/kg up to a maximum of 500 ml) with addition of 50–100 mg of Solu-Cortef is infused during the second hour.

If the blood pressure is satisfactory, isotonic saline in 5 percent glucose (60 ml kg up to 2500 ml) with the addition of 100–200 mg of Solu-Cortef will be infused over the next 24 hours.

After 2 Hours of Intensive Treatment

Most patients are under control by this time. The intravenous infusion of isotonic saline in 5 percent glucose is continued (or resumed if it was interrupted by the administration of plasma) for the rest of the day. Generally speaking, the total intravenous fluid during the first 24 hours should be 80 ml/kg of body weight, but not exceeding 3000 ml in adult subjects. Young infants may require up to 120 ml/kg. The total amount of Solu-Cortef will range from 250 to 500 mg per 24 hours, depending on patient size.

A few patients may remain in shock after 2 hours of intensive treatment. Prognosis in these cases is not good, and additional therapeutic measures may be necessary. Several sympathomimetic drugs, such as phenylephrine hydrochloride (Neo-Synephrine), L-norepinephrine bitartrate (Levophed) or epinephrine, are quite effective in improving peripheral blood pressure. However, they tend to decrease renal and cerebral blood flow. Another synthetic sympathomimetic amine, isoproterenol hydrochloride (Isuprel), may be preferable; it is given diluted 1:500,000 with intravenous fluid at the rate of 0.5–5 mcg per minute. Heart rate, blood pressure, and urine flow must be monitored carefully for adjustment of the rate of administration of the drug. Metaraminol bitartrate (Aramine) (25 mg diluted in 250–500 ml of intravenous fluid) can be used with constant monitoring of the blood pressure as a guide for the rate of infusion. Another approach has been the administration of massive amounts of intravenous glucocorticoids (Solu-Cortef, 50 mg/kg of body weight) during the first 24 hours of treatment. It must be emphasized that the evaluation of the efficacy of any of these therapeutic measures is difficult. A scientific appreciation is practically impossible, since no patient can be his own control for a specific therapeutic regimen, and accurate comparison of the results with the various drugs in large enough groups of patients has not been made systematically.

It is important to note that *morphine, barbiturates* and *other sedatives* are contraindicated. *Potassium* must also be avoided.

When the acute adrenal crisis occurs later in life, it has been precipitated by an acute infection. The treatment of such infection must be carried out with the specific antibiotics as required.

During the whole period of intensive treatment there must be frequent evaluation of the vital signs as well as serial determinations of the serum chemistry values and blood hematocrits. The treatment should be adjusted as these clinical and laboratory data dictate. It must be remembered that administration of too much intravenous fluid and/or too much NaCl concomitantly with large amounts of salt-retaining hormone can result in pulmonary edema, cardiac failure, or hypernatremia.

MAINTENANCE THERAPY

Replacement of Glucocorticoids (Table 2)

Cortisol is the drug of choice for the treatment of adrenocortical insufficiency for the following reasons: (1) It is the main glucocorticoid secreted physiologically by the human adrenal cortex; (2) it contributes to sodium retention, whereas many of the synthetic preparations have little or no effect; and (3) its dosage is more easily adjusted to the needs of the patients than that of synthetic preparations with very high potency, such as dexamethasone. However, prednisolone (or prednisone) can be used in adolescents and adults who may find it difficult to comply with the need to distribute the total 24-hour dose of cortisol throughout the day.

The rate of secretion of cortisol in normal subjects of both sexes, from the age of 20 days to adulthood, is related to body size: *The mean and one standard deviation are 12 + 2 mg per m^2 of body surface area per 24 hours.* During the first 5 to 10 days of life, the value is 18 mg per m^2 per 24 hours. Hence, maintenance dosage based on production rate will be an intramuscular injection of cortisol of 12 mg per m^2 per 24 hours (or 16 mg if cortisone acetate is used). Instead of an intramuscular injection each day, three times the daily dosage can be administered every third day,

TABLE 2   Treatment of 21-Hydroxylase Deficiency During Maintenance and Stress

	Maintenance (mg/day)	Stress (mg/day)
Cortisol Replacement		
Oral cortisol (⅓ dose, t.i.d.)	25/m^2	75/m^2
Intramuscular cortisol	12.5/m^2	37.5/m^2*
Intravenous cortisol sodium succinate (Solu-Cortef)	—	100–200†
Aldosterone Replacement		
Subcutaneous Doca pellets	125–250 every 9 to 12 months	If pellets present, no additional therapy
Oral 9α-Fluorocortisol acetate	0.05–0.10	0.05–0.10
Intramuscular Dopa	—	1*

*Intramuscular therapy is given if patient cannot retain oral preparations.

†If oral therapy has not been retained for more than 12 hours, give about half of dose stat and the other half along with isotonic saline in 5 percent glucose.

since this preparation tends to be reabsorbed slowly. However, many patients find it difficult to submit to intramuscular injections for a lifetime and therefore prefer oral preparations. The oral daily dose of cortisol is twice the intramuscular dose (25 mg per m^2 per 24 hours), and one-third of this daily dose is given every 8 hours. Often one elects to give an amount in the evening that is greater than the two others, to suppress the ACTH surge of the early morning hours.

If prednisolone is used, the dosage is 5 mg per m^2 per 24 hours, one-half of this daily dose being given every 12 hours. Other synthetic compounds, such as triamcinolone, are not recommended. Overtreatment with any glucocorticoid may result in pseudotumor cerebri. It seems, however, that the synthetic products may have a greater tendency to bring about this side effect.

Replacement of Salt-retaining Hormone (Table 2)

Infants over 2 weeks of age and children have an aldosterone secretion rate that is not significantly different from that of adult subjects. The values range from 25 to 160 mcg per 24 hours, with a mean of 80 mcg. Replacement dosage will thus be similar at all ages.

Aldosterone is not available as a drug. However, the acetate of desoxycorticosterone (DOCA), a normal precursor of aldosterone, can be used successfully at a daily dose of 1–2 mg i.m., as can 9α-fluorocortisol (Florinef), a synthetic compound with marked salt-retaining activity, in a daily dose of 0.05–0.15 mg orally.

Desoxycorticosterone acetate used to be also commercially available as 125-mg pellets for subcutaneous implantation. Pellets are slowly absorbed and two of them can last for a period of 9 to 12 months. In my opinion, DOCA pellets and intramuscular cortisol are the choice preparations for the first two years of life, as it is often difficult to determine whether oral therapy is retained in infants who tend to regurgitate or vomit. Unfortunately, pharmaceutical companies have not seen fit to continue producing pellet preparations because of their limited usage and consequent lack of profit.

THERAPY UNDER CONDITIONS OF MEDICAL STRESS

It is well known that the rate of cortisol secretion increases markedly during any type of stress, including infection with fever, burns, or surgery. It has also been well documented that in some patients with adrenal insufficiency the inability to increase the secretion of glucocorticoid can result in grave disorders and even death. For these reasons it is of great importance that the dosage of cortisol be carefully adjusted under conditions of stress.

Minor infections with very low grade fever may not necessarily require a change in treatment, whereas moderate stresses may be covered by doubling the maintenance dose. Dosage should be tripled for major infections and high grade fever (Table 2). The modification in therapy should last only for the period of stress in order to avoid the problems related to overtreatment.

It must be noted that during medical stress there is need for an increase in cortisol replacement but not in salt-retaining hormone. If for any reason the patient cannot retain oral therapy during stress, intramuscular preparations must be administered (Table 2). If the patient has been without therapy for more than 12 hours, it is necessary to administer intravenous cortisol (Solu-Cortef) along with replacement fluid therapy. In some patients with hypoglycemic unresponsiveness it is difficult to establish an intravenous line, in which case Solu-Cortef can be given intramuscularly, plus glucose.

THERAPY AT THE TIME OF SURGERY

As already noted, anesthesia and surgery result in a marked increase in cortisol secretion rate. To mimic this effect in patients with adrenal insufficiency, intramuscular cortisol (35.5–50 mg per m^2 per 24 hours) and DOCA (1 mg per 24 hours) are substituted for the maintenance therapy. This treatment (Table 3) is started two days prior to surgery to establish proper levels of steroids during the surgery itself. The same treatment is continued for the first few postoperative days. In the absence of any complications the treatment may be slightly decreased on the fifth day, and replacement therapy can be resumed on the sixth postoperative day.

In case of emergency surgery it is obviously impossible to prepare the patient ahead of time (Table 3). For this reason, it is important to supplement the intramuscular therapy with an immediate dose of 100 mg of Solu-Cortef prior to anesthesia, followed by 100–200 mg of the same intravenous preparation given as a continuous infusion during surgery and recovery. This intravenous therapy can be stopped 24 to 48 hours after surgery, and the rules for elective surgery will then apply.

If the patient is a salt loser, oral Florinef is replaced by intramuscular DOCA (1 mg daily). It must be noted that requirements for fluid therapy in these patients will be similar to those of normal subjects.

THERAPY DURING PREGNANCY

Women receiving normal replacement therapy will usually have normal gonadal function and can become pregnant.

It is well known that during pregnancy plasma cortisol levels increase markedly. This is due in a large part to an increase of the plasma protein that binds the steroid. However, there is no definite change in cortisol secretion rate. For these reasons, therapy during pregnancy should remain at the maintenance level. If the patient is on oral therapy, and if repeated vomiting occurs, it is evident that the treatment must be shifted to intramuscular preparations.

Labor and delivery are known to increase the secretion of cortisol markedly. To mimic these physiologic conditions, stress therapy should be initiated at the beginning of labor. Barring complications, maintenance levels can be resumed 12 hours after delivery.

GENERAL RULES FOR THE TREATMENT OF 21-HYDROXYLASE DEFICIENCY

1. Therapy must be initiated as early as possible. In the forms accompanied by salt loss, an acute adrenal crisis occurs shortly after birth, requiring immediate treatment. Early treatment is also important in the non–salt-losing forms to prevent progressive virilization and rapid growth in early childhood but short stature in adulthood.

2. Cortisol is the glucocorticoid of choice. Its dosage is related to body size but must be adjusted to the specific requirement of each patient. In contrast, the mineralocorticoid replacement (intramuscular Doca or oral Florinef) is not related to body size but must also be adjusted individually.

3. Requirements are determined by close follow-up of clinical symptoms (blood pressure, statural growth, bone age) and of laboratory measurements. The best laboratory indices are urinary 17-ketosteroid excretion and plasma androstenedione levels; the values of urinary pregnanetriol and plasma 17-hydroxyprogesterone are much less

TABLE 3   Treatment of 21-Hydroxylase Deficiency at Time of Surgery

Days to Surgery	Elective Surgery		Emergency Surgery		
	Intramuscular Cortisone (mg/m²/day)	Intramuscular Doca* (mg/day)	Intramuscular Cortisone (mg/m²/day)	Intravenous Solu-Cortef (mg/day)	Intramuscular Doca* (mg/day)
−2	37.5–50.0	1			
−1	37.5–50.0	1			
Preanesthesia	37.5–50.0	1	37.5–50.0	100 (stat)	1
During surgery	—	—	—	100–200 (continuous infusion during surgery and recovery)	
+1	37.5–50.0	1	37.5–50.0		1
+2	37.5–50.0	1	37.5–50.0		1
+3	37.5–50.0	1	37.5–50.0		1
+4	25.0–37.5	1	25–37.5		1
+5	Resume replacement therapy		Resume replacement therapy		

*In salt-losing patients

reliable. In patients with salt loss, serum electrolytes and plasma renin activity will be helpful guides to mineralocorticoid replacement therapy.

4. Patients and their parents must be properly educated so that they will understand the need for lifetime treatment. They also must understand the importance of adjusting therapy during stress.

5. It is advisable that patients undergoing cortisol and salt-retaining therapy wear either dog tags or a bracelet or carry an identification card in their wallet, so that in case of accident with loss of consciousness they may receive proper stress treatment.

6. Abnormalities of the external genitalia must receive proper surgical correction, if possible before 1 year of age.

ADJUSTMENT OF THERAPY TO THE ENZYME DEFICIENCY CAUSING THE ADRENAL HYPERPLASIA

As shown in Table 1, there are several other forms of congenital adrenal hyperplasia besides the salt-losing and simple virilizing forms.

In the "attenuated" form of 21-hydroxylase deficiency (previously called "acquired" adrenal hyperplasia), symptomatology is noted at the time of puberty and only in females. It includes virilism and oligo- or amenorrhea. The treatment consists of cortisol replacement therapy as described for the moderate and more severe forms of 21-hy-

droxylase deficiency. However, there is no need for mineralocorticoid replacement.

The hypertensive form due to *11-hydroxylase deficiency* also requires cortisol replacement therapy without mineralocorticoid replacement. The adequacy of therapy in this form will be based on the measurement of 11-desoxycortisol (Compound S) in blood or its metabolites in urine, which are measured as 17-hydroxycorticosteroids.

The *17-hydroxylase deficiency*, like the 11-hydroxylase deficiency, results in hypertension. In addition, patients with this form of enzyme deficiency are unable to produce gonadal steroids, which results in an absence of masculinization of the external genitalia in male infants. The hypertension will be corrected by the administration of cortisol replacement therapy. In addition, males and females will require gonadal replacement at the time of puberty. Most male patients present female external genitalia at birth, are raised in the female gender, and therefore receive estrogens at puberty.

The rare cases of deficiency of *3β-hydroxysteroid dehydrogenase* or of one of the enzymes necessary for pregnenolone synthesis (20-hydroxylase, 22-hydroxylase, 20, 22-desmolase) present a salt-losing syndrome that requires treatment with cortisol and aldosterone replacement. However, many of these patients die early in life despite adequate therapy. Those with a partial form may survive and will also present with abnormalities of the secretion of gonadal steroids.

Patients with *familial xanthomatosis* present a rapidly progressive neurologic syndrome and extensive calcification of the adrenal glands. Theoretically these patients require both cortisol and aldosterone replacement therapy. Unfortunately, most patients die early in life because of the neurologic disorder.

Adrenoleukodystrophy is an X-linked recessive disorder characterized by an accumulation of cholesterol esters with long chain fatty acid. This results in diffuse cerebral sclerosis and adrenal insufficiency. The latter usually procedes the neurologic syndrome by several years. The adrenocortical dysfunction requires both cortisol and aldosterone replacement treatment. Although the adrenal dysfunction can be treated adequately, most patients die early in adolescence of the neurologic abnormalities.

LATE-ONSET VIRILIZING CONGENITAL ADRENAL HYPERPLASIA

FREDERIC C. BARTTER, M.D.

Late-onset virilizing congenital adrenal hyperplasia (CAH), sometimes misnamed "acquired" CAH, has been reported to be caused by adrenal cortical 11-hydroxylase deficiency and 21-hydroxylase deficiency and, rarely, by the coexistence of the two defects in the same patient. The symptomatology in late-onset cases ranges from the presence of unexplained hirsutism with menstrual irregularities and acne in females, to the full-blown syndrome, with clitoral hypertrophy, deepening of the voice, and early epiphyseal closure in female patients at about the time of puberty. Rarely hypertension, and even more rarely hypokalemia, has been observed in late-onset CAH. The syndrome of salt-losing CAH has not been reported to appear as late as the age of puberty. A special form of late-onset CAH, observed before any signs are noted and termed "cryptic" CAH, has been identified through histocompatibility leukocyte antigen (HLA) typing. This is possible because the 21-hydroxylase deficiency (but not 11-hydroxylase deficiency) is linked to the HLA gene on chromosome 6. Late-onset CAH frequently coexists with, or is wrongly diagnosed in, the polycystic ovary or Stein-Leventhal syndromes.

11-HYDROXYLASE DEFICIENCY

This disorder has been reported in women with polycystic ovary disease and in those with apparently normal ovarian function. The cases are generally detected because of hirsutism appearing prior to or at the time of puberty in female patients. Because the enzymatic deficiency leads to overproduction of desoxycorticosterone as well as of Δ-4-androstenedione and testosterone, a few cases also have hypertension, and a few of these may have hypokalemia in addition. Specific tests are required to establish late-onset CAH in hirsute women when other signs of virilization are absent. This syndrome may go undetected in males if hirsutism is delayed until puberty; it must be suspected if hypertension, especially with hypokalemia, appears early in males without evident cause. The diagnosis is based upon the determination of plasma 11-deoxycortisol (compound S) or of urinary tetrahydro-compound S (H_4S). Whereas these steroids may appear to be merely high-normal in the basal state, their response to ACTH in late-onset CAH generally includes a rise to values much above normal.

LATE-ONSET CAH ATTRIBUTED TO 21-HYDROXYLASE DEFICIENCY

This syndrome, like that attributed to 11-hydroxylase deficiency, has been reported in women with and without polycystic ovary disease. With this syndrome, as with the 11-hydroxylase defect, hirsutism, acne, and even virilism with clitoral hypertrophy may first appear in childhood and early youth; hypertension and hypokalemia do not occur. This syndrome also may be undetected in males close to puberty.

The diagnosis is based upon determination of plasma 17-hydroxyprogesterone or of urinary pregnanetriol. These steroids also may show high-normal values in the basal state, but rise to very high levels after injection of exogenous ACTH. In addition, observations made when plasma ACTH is at its 24-hour circadian acrophase (for example, 12:00 M. to 8:00 A.M.) may show diagnostically high values for plasma 17-hydroxyprogesterone. With ACTH stimulation, heterozygotes for CAH (21-hydroxylase) show values above normal for plasma 17-hydroxyprogesterone but below those of homozygotes.

Since the gene for 21-hydroxylase is linked to HLA antigens on chromosome 6, HLA typing of families, together with ACTH stimulation, may allow the identification of a clinically mild ("cryptic") form of late-onset 21-hydroxylase deficiency, which presumably results from the combination of a defective allele (severe form) with a defective allele (mild form).

PRINCIPLES OF TREATMENT

The therapeutic implications of late-onset CAH involve three areas: genetic counseling, the treatment of polycystic ovary syndrome if present, and partial suppression of adrenal androgen secretion by suppression of ACTH secretion.

With regard to genetic counseling, the classic syndromes of CAH are inherited as Mendelian recessive traits, so the expected frequency of haplotype transmission can be foretold with confidence. The parents of the affected child must be told that statistically, one-quarter of their offspring may have CAH, one-half of them may carry one haplotype for the disorder, and one-quarter of them may be unaffected. The affected child should be informed that all of his offspring will carry one haplotype for the disorder.

Treatment of the polycystic ovary syndromes found with late-onset CAH is necessary to reverse and prevent further virilization—and to restore normal menstrual cycles and prevent or treat sterility. Although adrenal suppression often lowers ovarian production of testosterone and androstenedione, additional treatment is required for the polycystic ovary disease.

Partial suppression of ACTH, and thus of adrenal secretion, should be undertaken in all patients diagnosed as having CAH. Failure to do so before puberty may result in premature closure of the epiphyses and consequent limitation of linear growth. Failure to suppress ACTH may also result

in major hypertrophy of the adrenal cortex, even to a degree requiring surgical correction. Furthermore, the patient with CAH is always at risk for the severe—or even fatal—complications of intercurrent infections or of nonrelated surgical procedures. This risk results from the inability of the adrenal cortex to respond to such events with an adequate secretion of extra amounts of cortisol. In addition, males with untreated (or even undertreated) CAH may develop painful, swollen, tender testes that must be treated by partial suppression of ACTH secretion.

The Preferred Approach

The treatment of coexisting polycystic ovary disease, generally requiring partial suppression of pituitary secretion of follicle stimulating hormone and luteinizing hormone with estrogen and progesterone, is beyond the scope of this chapter. "Wedge" resection of the ovaries, formerly done frequently, is now seldom used except to hasten pregnancy. This is discussed in Chapter 83.

Partial suppression of ACTH secretion is accomplished with cortisol; use of a long-acting analogue of cortisol is even better. Normal cortisol secretion is about 25 mg/M^2 body surface area per day; this "physiologic" suppression in a 1.7-M^2 subject can generally be achieved with 12.5 mg given orally in the mornings and 25 mg in the evenings. The larger evening dose is important to avoid excessive nocturnal rise in the concentration of plasma androgens—androstenedione and testosterone—which may promote early closure of the epiphyses even if other signs of virilization are prevented. With the 21-hydroxylase defect in patients with late-onset CAH, it has been shown that the greatest circadian rise in plasma 17-hydroxyprogesterone occurs during the hours between midnight and 8:00 A.M., when plasma ACTH is at its peak.

Longer-acting steroids are generally more effective. For example, prednisone (2.5 mg in the morning and 5.0 mg in the evening) is sufficient in most children. Alternatively, dexamethasone, 0.5 mg per day, p.o. in children, and 1.0 mg per day, p.o., in adults—given in the evening—may be used. Since the salt-losing form of CAH (a form of 21-hydroxylase deficiency in which aldosterone secretion by the zona glomerulosa is deficient) has not been seen in late-onset CAH, sodium retaining steroids have no place in the therapeutic armamentarium. In patients who cannot take or retain oral medications, cortisone, 50 mg per day i.m. may be substituted.

Side effects of treatment are those of excessive secretion of cortisol, which produces the plethora, thinning of the skin, truncal obesity, and osteoporosis of Cushing's syndrome. These should not appear when the recommended dosages are used. Assessment of the effectiveness of treatment may be made from 24-hour urinary pregnanetriol, H_4S, or both, or from estimates of plasma androstenedione, compound S (11-deoxycortisol), or 17-hydroxyprogesterone. Measurements at expected acrophase in the circadian rhythms of the plasma steroids are of much greater value than the usual morning values alone, as the greatest rise in the undertreated patient may be expected in the very early morning before 6:00 A.M.

The Pros and Cons of Treatment

It is worthy of repetition that patients known to have CAH should always be treated. One may thus avoid the risk of massive hypertrophy of the adrenals in all patients and of the development of enlarged testes in males. In addition, if the CAH results from 11-hydroxylase deficiency, the development of hypertension and potassium depletion attributable to desoxycorticosterone overproduction can be avoided.

HIRSUTISM

HIRSUTISM

JAMES R. GIVENS, M.D.

Hirsutism is defined as excessive growth of hair in the female in the androgen-responsive skin zones located in the center of the body, namely, the upper lip, chin, neck, chest, lower abdomen, and the perineum. The hair on the back, upper arms, and thighs is also androgen-responsive. Androgens stimulate the secretion of oil from sebaceous glands (seborrhea) and increase the diameter, pigmentation, as well as the linear growth of hair in the responsive zones.

Hyperandrogenism is one of the most common endocrinopathies encountered in women. The measurement of testosterone (T) production rates in hirsute women has established that most (at least 90 percent) are hyperandrogenic. Approximately 10 percent of women in the reproductive years in this country are hirsute. The incidence is even greater in postmenopausal females. While the hirsutism per se may seem to have little medical consequence, it may cause significant psychologic disturbance. The physician should have a positive rather than a cavalier attitude toward treatment of the hirsute patient, since the associated androgen excess will respond to medical therapy or surgery. A caring, sympathetic, positive attitude on the part of the physician is essential to the overall management of this common medical problem.

From a practical standpoint, the major decision necessary for appropriate treatment of a hirsute female is whether the hyperandrogenism is (1) LH-dependent; (2) ACTH-dependent; (3) a combination of these two; (4) related to hyperprolactinemia; (5) due to an androgen-secreting tumor of the adrenals or ovaries; or (6) drug related.

The first step toward making a decision as to the type of treatment for the hyperandrogenism of a hirsute female is to obtain an accurate history and perform a thorough physical examination. The age of adrenarche, thelarche, and menarche and the character and frequency of menses are deter-mined. An early adrenarche and/or hirsutism associated with regular menstruation are usually associated with ACTH-dependent hyperandrogenism of adrenal origin, whereas hirsutism associated with oligoamenorrhea is usually due to an LH-dependent ovarian source or a combination of the two. Careful inquiry is made concerning any drugs the patient is taking that may cause hirsutism, such as phenytoin, diazoxide, minoxidil, androgens, and corticosteroids.

Knowledge of the dynamics of the development of the hirsutism is important in identifying those who are at risk for having an androgen secreting adrenal or ovarian tumor. Sudden development of hirsutism in a female in her mid-thirties with rapid progression suggests an androgen secreting tumor, whereas slow progression beginning at puberty is more likely to be the result of a nontumorous, hyperplastic, LH- or ACTH-dependent condition.

The family history is important in identifying familial endocrinopathies that cause hirsutism. The polycystic ovary syndrome is frequently familial and is usually dominantly inherited. In my experience, a high incidence of oligoamenorrhea and/or hirsutism in a family is usually due to familial polycystic ovarian disease or hyperthecosis. Inquiry is made concerning pelvic surgery in family members, particularly wedge resection of cystic ovaries, to identify those who have the polycystic ovary syndrome. There is a high incidence of glucose intolerance, obesity, hypertension, and hyperlipidemia associated with familial hyperthecosis.

The physical examination should determine whether the patient has simple hirsutism or if she is virilized. In addition to hirsutism, the virilized female has temporal recession of the scalp hairline, clitoromegaly, a deep voice and an android physique. To serve as a basis for judging the effectiveness of therapy, the distribution of hair is carefully recorded according to the following scale: 1 +, hair on the upper lip; 2 +, hair on the upper lip and sideburns; 3 +, hair on the upper lip, sideburns, and chin; and 4 +, a male-type beard. The character of the hair should also be noted; that is, whether it is terminal (dark and coarse) or villous (downy and light in color). A close-up photograph of a specified involved area after one to two weeks of growth is valuable in documenting the degree and type of hirsutism.

The presence of galactorrhea is a significant finding, since the amenorrhea-galactorrhea syndrome may be associated with hyperandrogenism. Any stigmata of Cushing's syndrome, acromegaly, hypothyroidism, hyperthyroidism, and liver disease is noted. The pelvic examination is of special importance. The type of escutcheon (male or female) is described and any abnormality of the external genitalia noted. The size and character of the uterus and ovaries are assessed and recorded. If obesity prevents an accurate evaluation of the size and nature of the uterus and the ovaries, pelvic ultrasonography is done.

LABORATORY TESTS

If the history and physical examination suggest the patient may have Cushing's syndrome, acromegaly, or liver or thyroid disease, the appropriate tests are obtained to exclude or include the suspected diagnosis.

The following assays are obtained to assess the degree and type of hyperandrogenism: total T, TeBG binding capacity (TeBG-BC), free T, LH, FSH, prolactin, and dehydroepiandrosterone sulfate (DHEAS). Owing to the marked variability of the circulating levels of most of these hormones, three separate blood specimens are obtained every 30 minutes or every hour and the plasma pooled for one assay. A SMAC-12 screening battery of tests, which includes a fasting blood sugar and liver and renal function tests, is obtained to serve as a basis for comparison during therapy.

ANDROGEN SECRETING TUMORS

If the total T is greater than 200 ng/dl or the DHEAS level is greater than 800 μg/dl, there is a high probability of an ovarian or adrenal androgen-secreting tumor. Since hormone provocation and suppressive tests are not reliable in identifying the glandular site of androgen secreting tumors, other methods of detection are used. CT scanning of the adrenals is requested first, and, if a tumor is identified, surgical excision is accomplished. If an adrenal tumor is not identified, ultrasonography of the ovaries is performed. The appropriate surgery is performed if an ovarian tumor is identified.

If a tumor is not observed in either the adrenals or ovaries and the elevated level of T or DHEAS persists, catheterization of the adrenal and ovarian veins is performed with measurement of the androgen levels in the effluent blood of each gland.

GALACTORRHEA AND/OR HYPERPROLACTINEMIA

If the total T level is less than 200 ng/dl and the DHEAS level is less than 800 μg/dl, there is an LH-dependent and/or ACTH-dependent, nontumorous source of the excess androgens. When there is galactorrhea or if the prolactin level is elevated, the hyperandrogenism may be part of the amenorrhea-galactorrhea syndrome, which includes polycystic ovaries and overproduction of adrenal androgens. The pathophysiology of the development of polycystic ovaries in patients with prolactin excess is not understood. If the hyperandrogenism is related to the hyperprolactinemia, a dramatic decrease in the hyperandrogenic state occurs with bromocryptine* therapy or with removal of a prolactinoma, but not all respond. The improvement is impressive when it occurs, not only in the androgen related signs and symptoms, but also in other aspects of the syndrome, such as hypertension, obesity, and fluid and salt retention.

LH-DEPENDENT ANDROGENIC OVARIES

If the patient does not have galactorrhea and/or hyperprolactinemia, the size of the ovaries and/or the LH/FSH ratio must be taken into account. Those patients who have bilaterally enlarged ovaries and/or an increased LH/FSH ratio greater than three are given a combination-type oral contraceptive, norethindrone†, 2 mg, with mestranol, 0.1 mg (N+M 2 mg), for 21 days. Total T, free T, and DHEAS are repeated at the end of the 21 days. In LH-dependent ovarian hyperandrogenism, such as the polycystic ovary syndrome, total T and free T are reduced to well within the normal range; that is, the total T is less than 50 ng/dl and the free T less than 0.5 ng/dl. If the androgen levels are suppressed within the normal range after 21 days, the patient is continued on N+M 2 mg as suppressive therapy, assuming she does not desire pregnancy.

*Parlodel, Sandoz Pharmaceuticals
†Ortho Novum 2 mg, Ortho Pharmaceuticals

If the total T and/or free T are elevated at the end of 21 days, N + M 2 mg is repeated for another cycle and the tests repeated at the end of the second cycle. If total T and/or free T are still elevated and DHEAS is elevated at the end of the second cycle, dexamethasone*, 0.5 mg at bedtime, is added and the tests repeated at the end of the third cycle. If the levels are now suppressed to normal with the addition of dexamethasone, it is assumed the patient has a combined ovarian and adrenal source of excess androgens requiring both LH and ACTH suppression.

ACTH-DEPENDENT EUCORTISOL ADRENAL HYPERANDROGENISM

Hirsute women who have normal cortisol levels, an elevated DHEAS level with normal-sized ovaries, and a normal LH/FSH ratio have adrenal hyperandrogenism and dexamethasone therapy, 0.5 mg at bedtime is begun. The androgen assays are repeated in one month to determine the degree of suppression. The therapeutic goal is to suppress the DHEAS level to less than 100 µg/dl and maintain a serum cortisol level of 3–5 µg/dl. If these criteria are followed, the patient will retain the ability to respond to stress without requiring increased glucocorticoid replacement. If at the end of one month the DHEAS and free T levels are not reduced to within the normal range, N + M 2 mg may be added, since there may also be an LH-dependent component to the hyperandrogenism. If the DHEAS and free T levels are suppressed to normal with both agents, then a dual source of androgens is implied and continued therapy utilizing both agents is advised.

IDIOPATHIC HIRSUTISM

If the hirsute woman has normal-sized ovaries, a normal LH/FSH ratio, and a normal DHEAS level, she is considered to have idiopathic hirsutism. In our experience, most of these women have androgenic polycystic ovaries and respond favorably to LH suppression using N + M 2 mg. Some 80 percent of these hirsute women require only N + M 2 mg to correct their hyperandrogenism. However, suppression of the androgen levels by N + M 2 mg should not be interpreted to mean

the patient has a pure LH-dependent ovarian source of androgens, since this agent also decreases the DHEAS level by approximately 30 percent. Only 20 percent require the addition of dexamethasone to N + M 2 mg to normalize completely their free T and DHEAS levels.

N + M 2 mg not only decreases the androgen production from the ovaries but also increases the TeBG-BC, which decreases the amount of T available as free T for distribution to androgen responsive tissues. N + M 2 mg may also diminish 5-α reductase activity intracellularly, which is necessary for the expression of androgenicity through transformation of T to dihydrotestosterone.

OBESITY

Obesity is common among hyperandrogenic hirsute females. The relationship of obesity to hyperandrogenism remains largely undefined. However, weight reduction alone may decrease the hyperandrogenemia to a significant degree. Therefore, weight reduction through reduced caloric intake is an important adjunct to hormonal suppressive therapy for the hyperandrogenic, obese, hirsute female.

EXTENDED TREATMENT PROGRAM

The patient is seen again in the office at the end of 3, 6, and 12 months of therapy. At each visit, blood is obtained for free T and DHEAS assays and careful inquiry made concerning possible side effects of therapy. For those receiving N + M 2 mg, side effects may include nausea, headaches, increased blood pressure, or leg pains. The most common of these is nausea, which is reduced by having the patients take their medication at bedtime; they gradually become used to the medication and the nausea disappears. For those patients receiving dexamethasone, insomnia, fluid retention, weight gain, increased appetite, and nervousness are common.

If DHEAS and/or free T are normal at the third month office visit, the dose of N + M and/or dexamethasone is reduced by one-half to norethindrone*, 1 mg, and mestranol, 0.5 mg (N + M 1/50), and dexamethasone, 0.25 mg h.s., to arrive at the smallest dosage of steroids necessary to ac-

---

*Decadron, Merck, Sharp & Dohme

*Ortho Novum 1/50, Ortho Pharmaceuticals

complish continued suppression. Massively over-weight women frequently cannot shift to the lower dose because they do not have the same degree of androgen suppression and freedom from menstrual problems with the half-dose as they did with the full dose of N + M and/or dexamethasone.

Dexamethasone is stopped at the end of one year because (for reasons that are unclear) some hirsute women do not have a return of the adrenal hyperandrogenism after this period of suppression. The hirsute women receiving N + M 2 mg may also interrupt their therapy at the end of one year to determine if the hyperandrogenism recurs. Most require long-term suppressive therapy.

The hirsute women with LH-dependent ovarian hyperandrogenism who cannot take N + M 2 mg because of a contraindication are given medroxyprogesterone*, 10 mg 3 times a day, as a suppressive dosage. The dosage is adjusted downward at the end of one month for continued suppression of LH and the hyperandrogenism. The beneficial effect of this agent is due to increased clearance rate of T as well as suppression of LH.

During the past year we have utilized spiro-nolactone†, 25 mg 3 times a day on days 5–21 of the menstrual cycle, in women who could not take sex steroids. This is a particularly effective agent because it reduces ovarian hyperandrogenism through blockade of 17,21-lyase activity and func-

*Provera, Upjohn
†Aldactone, Searle & Co.

tions as an antiandrogen by blocking the intracell-ular androgen receptor sites. Spironolactone is also beneficial as an adjunct agent to oral contraceptive therapy, particularly in those who develop fluid retention and peripheral edema.

RESPONSE OF HIRSUTISM

The response of hirsutism to medical sup-pressive therapy of the hyperandrogenism is grad-ual rather than immediate. Decreased oiliness of the skin with clearing of the acne usually occurs with one to three months of suppressive therapy. The first observed change in the hirsutism is a de-creased growth rate, and later the hair shaft di-ameter decreases and the hair becomes lighter in color. These changes are detectable after 6 to 12 months of suppressive therapy. The response of hirsutism is more dramatic with oral contraceptive suppression than with dexamethasone suppression alone. A decrease in the hair density is not as im-pressive as the change in the character of the hair (terminal, dark hair changes to villous, downy hair). Electrolysis is frequently necessary to re-move the acquired hair. The earlier therapy is be-gun, the better the response. Medical suppressive therapy prevents acquisition of new hair. Objective documentation of the effectiveness of therapy can be accomplished by following ovary size by ultra-sonography and the hair density and character by a close-up black-and-white photograph of the in-volved area.

BARTTER'S SYNDROME

BARTTER'S SYNDROME

FREDERIC C. BARTTER, M.D.

Bartter's syndrome is a condition characterized by hypokalemia and metabolic alkalosis, hyper-reninemia with secondary aldosteronism, increased prostaglandins E_2 and I_2, and normal blood pressure, with pressor resistance to angiotensin II and norepinephrine. The histopathologic findings in the kidney include hyperplasia of the juxtaglomerular apparatus. Recently a defect in chloride (and sodium) reabsorption in the thick ascending limb of Henle's loop has been considered as the "proximate" cause, and it appears to provide a reasonable explanation for the chain of events that characterizes the syndrome. Since this defect in chloride reabsorption has been found in the patients originally described, and in all subsequently described patients who satisfy all the other criteria and were adequately studied with renal clearance techniques, it seems logical to give the name Bartter's syndrome to those with this constellation of clinical and pathologic features. Also included will be those patients who may have hypomagnesemia in addition.

Since the rationale of therapy must depend upon the correct sequence in the pathophysiology, previous and present modes of therapy are discussed in the light of current concepts of pathophysiology. In addition, since many of the patients who originally present with this disorder are children, the effect of treatment on physical development is assessed.

PATHOPHYSIOLOGY

The current hypothesis suggests that a defect in chloride (and sodium) reabsorption in the thick ascending limb of Henle's loop can result immediately in increased distal flow, which increases secretion of potassium and thus its excretion in the urine. The resultant lowering of potassium concentration in plasma and intersitial fluid causes increased production of PGE_2 by renal cells and of PGI_2 by blood vessels. The increases in PGE_2 and PGI_2 stimulate renin secretion, with resulting increased angiotensin II production, which in turn stimulates increased aldosterone secretion. Aldosterone secretion is not as high as might be expected from the corresponding elevation of plasma renin activity, since the hypokalemia that increases renin release can independently lower the plasma aldosterone concentration, and thus the urinary excretion of aldosterone.

The blood pressure, which is normal in patient's with Bartter's syndrome, appears to be the result of four agents, all found in excess. Two are pressor—angiotensin II and norepinephrine, and two are depressor—prostaglandin I_2 and bradykinin.

TREATMENT

Since urinary potassium loss and resultant hypokalemia are major features of the syndrome, treatment must always include measures effective in restoring and maintaining normal body potassium. Body potassium can be increased wth dietary intake, but few patients can eat enough potassium-containing foods to maintain plasma potassium in the normal range (3.5–5.0 mEq/1). Almost all patients require potassium supplements in the course of treatment. The supplements are usually given as 10 percent potassium chloride solution (1.3 mEq/ml), potassium gluconate, or potassium citrate. Powder that can be mixed with water, orange juice, or tomato juice is also available in packets of 20 mEq. Usually 120 to 240 additional mEq are needed each day to maintain potassium stores. The mode of administration will depend on the patient's preference.

Since the majority of the potassium in the urine enters the tubular lumen as a result of distal tubular secretion rather than by filtration, measures designed to decrease secretion are required. The known stimuli to distal tubular secretion include sodium-retaining steroids, distal tubular solute flow, and processes that increase the electronegativity of the distal tubular lumen. Accordingly, therapeutic measures are directed toward some or all of these processes.

Restoration of plasma and body potassium with oral potassium loads will increase both aldosterone secretion and plasma aldosterone concentration and will lower plasma renin activity. Therefore, measures designed to lower both plasma renin and aldosterone secretion are required with the potassium loading.

The use of spironolactone, which blocks the distal tubular action of aldosterone, is often beneficial in raising plasma potassium concentration and restoring body stores. One hundred to 300 mg (1.5–4 mg/kg) are frequently needed to bring about the desired result. The patient's plasma potassium level must be monitored frequently to prevent transient hyperkalemia that can occur if this drug is given with supplemental potassium.

The renal defect that is always present in Bartter's syndrome can increase renal potassium loss by purely renal mechanisms. Thus the defect in chloride reabsorption in the loop of Henle can, by increasing distal flow, stimulate distal secretion of potassium by a mechanism not dependent upon aldosterone or prostaglandins. Drugs that inhibit non–aldosterone-dependent renal tubular secretion of potassium, such as triamterene (Dyrenium, S.K.F.) and amiloride (Moduretic, MSD) offer an additional mode of therapy. It may be possible to achieve complete control of potassium metabolism in patients with Bartter's syndrome with a combination of agents.

Most patients with Bartter's syndrome can lower urinary sodium to intake and thus do not have "obligatory" renal sodium loss. A low-sodium intake results in minimal distal tubular sodium flow, and thus renal secretion of potassium is decreased, pari passu. In some patients, sodium restriction together with potassium supplements suffices to control serum and body potassium concentration.

A high-sodium intake has been recommended by some investigators for patients with renal sodium-losing disease thought to suffer from Bartter's syndrome. In this disorder the high sodium intake lowers plasma renin activity and aldosterone secretion. In patients with Bartter's syndrome, possessing the chloride reabsorption defect, however, a sodium load invariably lowers serum potassium even farther. This occurs even in patients who achieve some lowering of plasma renin activity with saline expansion. In some patients who

cannot restrict their sodium intake (such as adolescents who are addicted to potato chips, french fries, and other high-salt foods), it is necessary to give a drug such as spironolactone designed to block distal potassium secretion.

It has been suggested that plasma renin activity could be lowered by beta-adrenergic inhibitors, in view of the partial control of renin release via beta-adrenergic receptors. We have found little clinical value in such agents.

In light of the regular elevation of renal (and probably vascular) prostaglandins in the untreated patient with Bartter's syndrome, a variety of drugs that block prostaglandin synthesis at various sites in the biosynthetic pathway have been considered for treatment. Bourke and associates attempted to use mepacrine (quinacrine dihydrochloride), which has been shown to block the release of arachidonic acid from membranes and thus to inhibit production of prostaglandins such as PGE_2 and PGI_2. Unfortunately, this drug, in the dosage given, did not appear to be clinically valuable.

When the biosynthetic pathway of prostaglandins is inhibited with cyclo-oxygenase inhibitors, the production of PGE_2 and PGI_2 is suppressed, plasma renin and angiotensin II decrease, aldosterone secretion decreases, and plasma potasium concentration rises. It has regularly been observed, however, that the plasma potassium does not rise to or stay at a normal figure. We therefore believe that although the potassium loss which depends on aldosterone is ameliorated, that which depends on the renal defect is unchanged.

The cyclo-oxygenase inhibitors that have frequently been used include indomethacin (Indocin, MSD), ibuprofen (Motrin), and aspirin. The dosages range from 75 to 150 mg of indomethacin a day (1–2 mg/kg) or from 400 to 1200 mg per day (6–20 mg/kg) of ibuprofen. Aspirin, 600 mg to 6 gm a day (100 mg/kg/day), has also been of benefit. Those patients who cannot take indomethacin because of its ulcer-potentiating properties can frequently be managed on ibuprofen or aspirin.

Hypomagnesemia has been found occasionally in patients with Bartter's syndrome. Persistent hypomagnesemia—such as that found in the patients studied by Gitelman and associates in 1966, who suffered from a syndrome closely resembling Bartter's syndrome but were never definitely shown to have it—is rarely found in patients meeting all other criteria. Although magnesium depletion has not been shown to play an essential part in Bartter's syndrome, restoration of the serum magnesium to normal with magnesium (as the chloride or gluconate) frequently helps correct the hypokalemia. Dosages required to restore plasma magnesium concentration to normal vary from 10 to 20 mEq per day and must be adjusted on an individual basis.

The vascular insensitivity to angiotensin II and to norepinephrine, which has been a feature of the syndrome, has been unresponsive to any treatment except that of the cyclo-oxygenase inhibitors. After the prostaglandins are suppressed in this manner, the patients' blood pressure can be elevated with smaller amounts of angiotensin. It was thought that continued treatment with the prostaglandin synthetase inhibitors might result, with time, in a rise in blood pressure. However, no case has been reported in the literature, although patients have been treated with indomethacin and ibuprofen for over three years. This can probably be attributed to the fact that the pressors—renin, angiotensin, and aldosterone—are originally elevated in response to elevated quantities of depressors—bradykinin and PGI_2—and that the "feedback loop" was interrupted with the PG synthetase inhibitors.

Children with Bartter's syndrome frequently present with height and weight in the third to fifth percentile. The rate of growth in early childhood increases with treatment. This effect is doubtless related to partial restoration of potassium stores. This relationship of growth to therapy, however, is not well understood. Adolescents frequently show acceleration of growth despite noncompliance with therapy and resulting persistence of hypokalemia. In addition, a number of adults of normal stature with the disorder may have had it since early childhood.

Side Effects

The side effects of the treatment outlined here include hyperkalemia, with its potential effects on the heart. A combination of potassium supplements with a drug that inhibits tubular potassium secretion, such as aldactone, triamterene, or amiloride, requires careful monitoring of the serum potassium concentration, the electrocardiogram, or both. Such caution applies not only to drugs that inhibit potassium transport, but also to the inhibitors of prostaglandin synthesis, since their use lowers plasma renin activity and thus plasma aldosterone concentration.

The prostaglandin synthetase inhibitors also produce retention of sodium directly, probably by lowering glomerular filtration rate. This side effect is always reversible and does not represent permanent renal damage.

Preferred Approach

Since each patient with Bartter's syndrome has a different degree of renal damage, it is difficult to cite a preferred approach for all patients. Prostaglandin synthetase inhibitors, together with aldactone or triamterene, will often push the serum potassium concentration towards normal. The persisting hypokalemia generally requires potassium supplements, preferably with the patient restricted to a low sodium intake. The plasma potassium concentration is the best index for the effectiveness of treatment.

IDIOPATHIC EDEMA

IDIOPATHIC EDEMA

DAVID H. P. STREETEN, M.B.,
D.Phil., F.R.C.P.

In the present era, despite the profusion of diuretics available for the treatment of most types of fluid accumulation, there are still reasons why most patients with idiopathic edema frequently become resistant to conventional diuretic therapy. A short summary of what is known about the pathogenesis of this group of disorders is essential to an understanding of their most effective treatment.

PATHOGENESIS

When one has excluded the many known causes of edema, ranging from such common conditions as congestive heart failure, intrinsic renal diseases, and cirrhosis, to more unusual causes, such as hypothyroidism, hyperthyroidism, Cushing's syndrome, protein-losing enteropathy, other types of hypoproteinemia, and many others, there remains a group of patients whose edema is of unknown origin. In most of these patients, perhaps 80 percent of them in the United States, a strong orthostatic component of the pathogenesis of their edema can easily be demonstrated. When these patients remain on their feet or in the seated position for several hours, their excretion of sodium and water or of water alone falls to a greater extent than it does in healthy, nonedematous subjects. The excessive fall in excretion appears to result from a disorder of the vasculature causing undue transudation of fluid from the capillaries in the dependent limbs, since the pathogenetic sequence that follows can be largely prevented by application of external pressure to the legs and pelvis. In the absence of such external pressure, continuing transudation leads to a greater orthostatic fall in plasma volume than in normal subjects. Presumably in consequence of this hypovolemia, there

follows (1) an excessive stimulation of vasopressin release resulting in *orthostatic water retention,* or (2) an excessive production of aldosterone, perhaps via renin release, and an abnormally profound fall in glomerular filtration rate, together leading to *orthostatic sodium* (and water) *retention.* The fluid retained by these mechanisms replenishes the depleted plasma volume and permits continuing transudation and measurably excessive swelling of the legs while the upright posture is maintained. When recumbency is resumed, the described chain of events is broken by the fall in hydrostatic pressure in the legs. Thus, the accumulated fluid is redistributed to the upper parts of the body, often causing edema of the eyelids, the face, and the hands the following morning and allowing at least some of the retained fluid to diffuse back into the vascular compartment where it is excreted as the orthostatic hyperaldosteronism, hypervasopressinism, or both subside.

It is not known why patients with these types of orthostatic edema transude excessively from the capillaries in their dependent limbs in the upright posture. Whether it results from a thickening of the capillary basement membrane or from the action of a local dilator of the precapillary sphincter (bradykinin? prostaglandin?) or from deficiency of a specific vasoconstrictor, such as dopamine, or from some other cause, remains to be determined.

It should be added that, since there is no clear evidence of the pathogenic mechanism(s) of fluid retention in the minority of patients whose idiopathic edema is of the nonorthostatic type, no special therapeutic measures can be recommended for these patients.

TREATMENT

General Considerations

Since idiopathic edema is a chronic disorder that seldom remits, it is important for both the physician and the patient to appreciate that all medications are capable of doing harm as well as good and that the smallest amount of medication compatible with reasonable comfort should be used. A few patients with idiopathic edema have a tendency to escalate the dosage of their drugs in a compulsive desire to get rid of any vestige of excess fluid. This tendency should, of course, be resisted when it becomes apparent.

A good general principle is to prescribe medications one at a time, monitoring the effects of each addition to the therapeutic program on measurements of body weight. These measurements should be made and recorded each morning on arising and each evening before retiring, always after emptying the bladder, for at least two weeks, preferably four weeks, before the commencement of any medications. These records serve to determine whether mean weight gain from the beginning to the end of orthostasis (usually from morning to evening) is excessive—more than 1.5 lb (0.7 kg)—since such excessive weight gain is the hallmark of orthostatic fluid retention. They also serve to document the presence of any premenstrual increment in body weight. Continued measurements during successive changes or additions to therapy indicate whether the treatment is or is not effective in producing a gradual downward trend in morning weight and/or a consistent reduction in mean weight gain *intra diem to less than* 0.7 kg and preferably less than 0.5 kg. Therapy that fails to produce improvement in at least one of these respects during a trial lasting four weeks or more should clearly be abandoned.

Posture

Since by definition orthostatic edema accumulates exclusively when the patient is in the upright posture, the patient should be made aware of this fact and encouraged to reduce the length of time spent sitting and standing each day as much as is compatible with a reasonable life style. Whenever the opportunity is available, the patient should sit or lie down with the legs elevated. This often requires minor adjustments of social habits. It may be advisable for some severely affected patients to lie down on a couch for 2 or 3 hours after lunch each day and/or after dinner each evening to reduce the total duration of orthostatic fluid retention and to promote its excretion in recumbency.

Food and Fluid Intake

When these patients are obese, caloric restriction is required. In the majority of instances in which there is orthostatic sodium retention, reduc-tion of sodium intake is helpful and should be prescribed to an extent compatible with individual needs. Some patients are able, by purchasing low-salt foods, to restrict sodium intake to 10–30 mEq daily, with benefit. In others, it may be possible only to exclude obviously salty foods, such as ham, pickles, salted potatoes or peanuts, either because low-salt foods are too expensive or unavailable, or because of noncompliance with recommendations. Requirements for diuretic drugs are obviously reduced or obviated if sodium intake can be sufficiently restricted, and in this way, diuretic-induced potassium losses can be minimized.

Some patients consume unusually large volumes of fluids either because of habit or because of an excessive thirst. It is worthwhile to estimate average daily fluid intake, and when this exceeds a reasonable amount (about 1000–1200 ml daily) to recommend a reduction in the volume of liquids inbibed. The possibility of reducing excessive thirst by drug therapy is not practicable at present but might be a useful therapeutic adjuvant in the future.

Conventional Diuretic Drugs

In patients whose fluid retention is mild or intermittent, a thiazide diuretic (for example hydrochlorothiazide, 50 mg) may be all that is required. Frequently, however, such therapy loses its initial effectiveness when administered at the beginning of the active part of the day (the morning in most people, or the evening in workers on night shifts). When this happens, it is almost invariably helpful to recommend that the patient try to elevate the legs and to take the diuretic after the daily chores have been completed. In this way, a brisk diuresis will almost always ensue, facilitating rapid excretion of fluid retained during the preceding hours of orthostasis, so that diuretic action is complete before the patient goes to bed and nocturia (often a troublesome complaint even before treatment of orthostatic edema) can be reduced or prevented. Chlorthalidone has been particularly useful in my experience, but there is no objective evidence of its superiority to other diuretics in these patients. The rapidity and effectiveness of furosemide might commend its use during the few recumbent hours before sleep. Occasional or more frequent measurement of serum potassium concentration is advisable. If and when hypokalemia occurs, it should be treated either with potassium supplements or by changing to a potassium-sparing diuretic. Spironolactone has been widely employed for this purpose and its use is appropriate, a priori, as a direct means of preventing the effects of the secondary hyperaldosteronism so many of these patients manifest. Since spironolactone has prolonged action it may be given at any time of the day. Dosages less than 100 mg daily are preferred, since higher doses may cause breast tenderness, menstrual irregularities, amenorrhea, or occasionally mild hirsutism. Triamterene may also be used in doses of 100 mg daily. Amiloride, recently made available in the U.S., holds promise as a potassium-sparing diuretic. The use of such proprietary combinations as Aldactazide, Dyazide, and Moduretic is not generally recommended, since they often have insufficient potassium-sparing activity to prevent the occurrence of hypokalemia. However, their use in a dose of two tablets each evening does simplify therapy in those individuals in whom hypokalemia does not supervene during a trial of their use.

Drugs to Reduce Orthostatic Weight Gain

Diuretics often become ineffective in reducing the accumulation of fluid during the time of the day spent in the upright posture. This can be shown by measuring mean weight gain from the beginning to the end of orthostasis on successive days. The only medications that are effective in reducing orthostatic weight gain are sympathomimetic amines. Of these ephedrine is the simplest to administer and should be prescribed if the treatment described above fails to reduce the discomfort resulting from edema formation. A dose of 25 mg 3 times daily is often beneficial, as evidenced by a reduction of weight gain intra diem toward normal limits. When ephedrine causes palpitations or fails to reduce weight gain from morning to evening, its use should be abandoned. In such circumstances dextroamphetamine is frequently effective and often restores weight gain intra diem to about 0.5 kg without other therapy. It should be prescribed in a dose of 10 mg as a sustained-release capsule or Spansule each morning. If there is slight but inadequate reduction in weight gain from morning to evening, a dose of 15 mg in the morning or 10 mg upon awakening and again at noon may be more effective. Occasionally 25 mg daily may be needed. If there is no improvement in weight gain intra diem, the amphetamine should be discontinued. Some patients become unduly tense, nervous, or excitable for the first few days of amphetamine therapy. If these symptoms persist, the treatment should be combined with a barbiturate or stopped. Usually any initial excitement or garrulousness will subside in a few days and the dextroamphetamine appears almost to have a tranquilizing action after several weeks. As long as the drug is taken for its action on fluid accumulation and not for its psychic, mood-elevating effects—which are relatively transient unless dosage is progressively escalated—addiction, dependence, and any other serious side effects have not been observed by us to result from the use of dextroamphetamine in more than 100 patients with idiopathic edema over the past 25 years. In many patients we have stopped the administration of dextroamphetamine abruptly without withdrawal effects except for some sleepiness for a day or two. The most valuable aspects of its use are its safety in the doses prescribed and its continued effectiveness in reducing weight gain from morning to evening as long as it is administered—for up to 18 years in some patients whom we have studied repeatedly.

Other Drugs

Kuchel and associates showed that dopamine excretion in the urine was subnormal in a group of patients with idiopathic edema in the recumbent, albeit not in the upright, posture. The finding suggested that deficiency of this natriuretic catecholamine might actually be the cause of orthostatic edema in some patients. For this reason, the dopamine agonist bromocriptine has been used for the treatment of idiopathic edema. Unfortunately, our own observations and those of others have cast doubt on the usefulness of this form of therapy in more than a small minority of patients. A similar rationale has led to a trial of L-dopa in a few patients with idiopathic edema. This too has been transiently effective in a few but not in most patients. It is of interest to note that, unlike dopamine, bromocriptine has relatively slight natriuretic action. It is possible that the efficacy of dextroamphetamine may depend on endogenous dopamine release, which the amphetamine probably induces. For these reasons, the usefulness of dopamine agonists that might be developed in the future will be worthy of full investigation.

Propranolol has been prescribed by some clinicians, but its effectiveness in idiopathic edema has not been convincingly documented.

Special Stockings

Since elastic bandages and pressure garments (for example, MAST suits) have been shown to reduce edema and to promote normal excretion of sodium and water in the upright posture, it seemed obvious that elastic stockings or individually fitted Jobst garments might be therapeutically useful. On some patients they can be used to advantage and will reduce or obviate the need for medications. Unfortunately, most patients stop using stockings or garments after a disappointingly short period because they are uncomfortable, or difficult to put on, or tend to aggravate swelling by raising the temperature of the legs, particularly on hot days when orthostatic edema tends to be most severe.

RESULTS OF TREATMENT

It is usually possible to reduce morning weight by at least 2–4 kg and to decrease the mean weight gain during the orthostatic portion of each day to or toward the normal range of 0.7 kg or less, with the therapeutic program described above. Patients almost always experience symptomatic improvement, including reduction of discomfort in the legs and abdomen; loss of numbness and tingling in the hands and fingers (thus occasionally obviating the need for surgical relief of the carpal tunnel syndrome); and disappearance of headaches, periorbital edema, and the impaired cerebration of which they frequently complain. Irritability and depression are diminished and should not be treated with tranquilizers, some of which aggravate fluid retention. Weight records serve to document the improvement in fluid retention objectively, and pitting edema of the legs or ankles, which is demonstrable at the end of the day, before therapy, should be reduced or completely overcome. The extent to which these desirable results are accomplished should dictate the vigor with which the suggested therapeutic measures are applied.

DIABETES

CHILDHOOD DIABETES MELLITUS

KENNETH H. GABBAY, M.D.

Diabetes mellitus in children occurs in two distinct forms, an acute insulin deficiency state (type I, or juvenile-onset diabetes mellitus—JODM), and a far less common form (maturity-onset diabetes in youth—(MODY), which is usually associated with obesity and either normal or elevated insulin levels. Type I diabetes mellitus, by far the most common type of diabetes in children, is a lifelong disease that has an abrupt onset. In addition to its metabolic derangements, it is frequently associated with psychologic and social stresses for the patients and their families. Successful management of these acute disturbances draws heavily upon the resources and abilities of the physician and the treatment team. In addition to understanding the biochemistry and physiology of the acute and long-term insulin deficiency state, the physician has to be a sensitive observer of patient and family interactions, a master dissipator of guilt feelings, a trusted advisor, and, within realistic limits, a social engineer. In contrast to families of patients with adult-onset diabetes, the family of the child with diabetes must be treated as a unit for therapy to be successful.

The therapy of childhood diabetes encompasses three phases, each of which is associated with distinct types of problems and therapeutic concerns. These phases are:

1. *The discovery phase* (first two weeks). The period with the discovery and diagnosis of diabetes and includes the initial therapy of acute insulin deficient state and associated ketoacidosis, and the one- to two-week period of patient and family education and the beginning of their adjustment to the disease.

2. *The formative phase* (two years), The long-term pattern of patient and family behavior and the adjustments to diabetes, to the environment, and to each other are established during this formative phase. This period encompasses the "remission" period and frequently occurs during adolescence. It may be fraught with considerable turmoil, disease denial, testing, and manipulative behavior by the patient, the family unit, or both.

3. *The outcome phase* (lifelong). This phase usually extends from the postadolescent period and through adult life and old age. It is during this phase that the outcome of the disease and the effects of various treatment regimens manifest themselves. Of primary therapeutic concern during this period is the prevention and amelioration of a variety of diabetic manifestations that can adversely affect the eyes, kidneys, and the nervous and cardiovascular systems.

THE DISCOVERY PHASE

Diagnosis

More than 75 percent of the new cases today are diagnosed or suspected of having diabetes mellitus by their *families* or local physician before coming to the hospital. Approximately 80 percent of the remaining 25 percent will have been seen by a physician or at an Emergency Room at least once in the previous two weeks, and the diagnosis missed. Table 1 lists the incidence of various symptoms reported by 167 patients newly diagnosed as having diabetes mellitus admitted to the Children's Hospital between 1977 and early 1981. The new cases cluster in the early fall and winter with relatively few cases during the summer. However, the seasonal pattern differs from year to year.

TABLE 1 Frequency of Symptoms at Admission in Newly Diagnosed Juvenile Diabetics

Cardinal Symptoms (%)		Associated Symptoms (%)	
Polydipsia	87	Fatigue	55
Polyuria	87	Anorexia	29
Weight Loss	50	Nausea, vomiting	29
Nocturia	42	Abdominal pain	21
Enuresis (2°)	20	Polyphagia	20

154

Headache, bacterial infection, and irritability were each reported by 12 percent of the patients, while fever, blurred vision, vaginal moniliasis, and viral infections were reported by less than 7 percent of the patients. Kussmaul's respiration and coma were present in only 8 and 2 percent of the subjects respectively. Polyphagia is an uncommon symptom of juvenile diabetes, which is not the case in adult diabetes.

The task of making the diagnosis can occasionally be very difficult, particularly in most severe cases (that is, they *become* severe because the diagnosis is repeatedly missed). The only safety is in having a well-developed index of suspicion for diabetes and its protean manifestations. I have seen a case of "vaginal discharge" treated for 3 months by the mother's gynecologist, a case of "psychogenic polydispsia" treated for 4 months by the family physician, and a case of "blurred vision" and fatigue with a documented 1-diopter change in refraction over a six month period which was followed by an optometrist, all these patients presented in severe ketoacidotic coma with malignant consequences.

Management of Diabetic Ketoacidosis (DKA)

It should be remembered that acute DKA is only a short moment in a diabetic patient's life. It is dramatic, it gives the physician an opportunity to exercise his or her diagnostic, technical, and therapeutic skills (and some anxious moments), it is life-threatening to the patient, but all in all it is a fleeting moment in the overall disease process to the patient and his family. As specialized intensive care units become more prevalent, we as physicians should eschew the tendency to think that our job is complete when the patient is out of ketoacidosis. We should think about what happens *after* the successful conclusion and resolution of DKA, even as we are dealing with it.

DKA is diagnosed when the blood glucose level is greater than 300 mg percent serum bicarbonate level is less than 15 mEq/l, blood pH is less than 7.30, and the plasma acetone is positive at a 1:2 dilution. A strongly positive reaction for acetone in serum, an arterial pH of less than 7.25, and 4 plus glycosuria is almost certainly diagnostic of DKA, and therapy should be embarked upon without waiting for additional laboratory results. Table 2 lists the sequence of steps in caring for the young diabetic in ketoacidosis.

TABLE 2 Sequence of Care on Admission of Child in Diabetic Acidosis and Coma (the First 30 Minutes)

History and physical examination
Diagnostic phase: Draw blood for laboratory studies, start intravenous line, and catheterize if needed
Begin fluid therapy
Administer insulin
Begin flow sheet
Calculate fluid-electrolyte deficits and maintenance requirements
Follow-up on diagnostic and therapeutic steps

History and Physical Examination

Evaluate acute status, paying particular attention to the state of consciousness (for example, coma, agitation), respirations (Kussmaul's), vital signs (shock, core and peripheral temperatures), dehydration (sunken eyes, skin tenting), and acute abdomen. Agitation and a rapidly changing state of alertness on admission are particularly worrisome signs in a child with diabetic ketoacidosis. They suggest a longstanding metabolic disturbance and are usually found in patients in whom the diagnosis was previously missed. This combination of symptoms and history should elicit particular concern for impending cardiorespiratory arrest and possible brain herniation. I have also seen a number of cases of severe ketoacidosis that presented as "an acute abdomen" and resolved shortly after rehydration, but a few cases were truly acute appendicitis. It is important to note that skin temperatures in patients who are severely dehydrated and in shock do not necessarily reflect the true core temperature. Since insulin administration will restore glucose metabolism as a fuel, the core temperature may rise drastically particularly in a patient who has not yet had adequate peripheral circulation established.

In known diabetic cases, it is important to find out why the patient developed ketaocidosis (for example, infection, insulin injection error, recidivism) to determine the presence of hidden underlying causes.

Diagnostic Phase

Obtain blood for laboratory studies, and establish an intervenous line at the same time. A good intravenous route is essential, and if the patient is in shock or has a compromised circulation, one should have no hesitation whatsoever in putting in a surgical cutdown. The essential laboratory work should include the determination of glucose, bicarbonate, pH, and electrolytes, including K, NA, Cl, Ca, Mg, and P. The blood glucose level can and should be determined immediately at the bedside by the physician using Chemstrips or Dextrostix (the answer is available in a few minutes—SuperSTAT), as should the serum acetone level, using Acetest tablets (with serial serum dilutions). The latter is of use only in the acute management of the patient and should be done on the premises. If the patient is severely obtunded (also usually dehydrated and shocky), it is wise to send blood to the blood bank for typing and cross-matching, and to place on hold one unit of the *freshest* blood available. This can be used for expansion of blood volume and to improve tissue oxygenation in some instances.

If the patient is comatose, a urinary catheter should be inserted and the urine tested for glucose and acetone. The diagnosis of diabetes can be readily and immediately made at this point and therapy initiated without the need to wait for all the results. Urine output should be recorded on the I + O flow sheet.

Fluid and Electrolyte Therapy

Fluid therapy should begin immediately upon insertion of the intravenous line. There is no need to wait for laboratory results before starting fluid replacement in a dehydrated patient. The patient's degree of dehydration should be assessed (5, 10, 15 percent). Most patients with ketoacidosis are at least 10 percent dehydrated, and the most severely affected are usually 15 percent. About one-half of the replacement fluid may be given in the first 8 hours and the remaining one-half over the next 16 to 24 hours. Maintenance fluid has two components: insensible water loss via perspiration and lung water (approximately 300 to 400 ml/m^2 per day) and urine output. The first component is relatively unaffected by DKA; however, the urine output can be prodigious as a result of osmotic diuresis and should be replaced hourly with one-half normal saline, with added 40 mEq K$^+$ (20 mEq KCl plus 20 mEq K phosphate/l). Urinary output should continually be replaced, in addition to the replacement and maintenance fluids listed above. When blood glucose levels fall toward the renal threshold, the osmotic diuresis slows and conventional formulae (for example, 1500–200 ml/m^2 per day) may be resorted to for calculating maintenance fluid requirements.

In a 30-kg child with 10 percent dehydration, fluids may be given as follows over the first 24 hours:

First 30 to 60 minutes: Run normal saline (or fresh frozen plasma) as rapidly as possible at 20 ml/kg to expand the vascular compartment rapidly and treat shock.

Hours 2 to 24: One-half normal saline with potassium supplementation (20–40 mEq/l depending on serum K$^+$) is given. Potassium should be added to intravenous fluids as soon as insulin is given and urine output is established, and may be given as 1/2 KCl + 1/2 KPO$_4$. Dextrose (5 percent) is added when the blood glucose level reaches 250 to 300 mg percent.

*Hyper*natremic dehydration must be treated as such even with concomitant ketoacidosis—that is, aim to replace fluid deficit less vigorously over a 48-hour period.

Bicarbonate. I do not recommend giving bicarbonate to correct the acidosis unless the blood pH is below 7.0. If given, it should not be administered as a bolus but slowly infused over a 1-hour period at about a 1 mEq/kg dose. When given, it should be added to one-half normal saline rather than normal saline, as it will convert the latter to a hypertonic solution.

Potassium and Phosphate Replacement. The patients may present with normo- or hyperkalemia because of acidosis, while in fact they are total body potassium depleted (5–10 mEq/kg). Successful insulin action will result in a shift of K$^+$ to the intracellular compartment, resulting in hypokalemia with its attendant severe consequences. Thus patients will always need potassium supplementation, which should be given in the intravenous fluids at a concentration not exceeding 40 mEq/l. The inorganic phosphate story is similar, and hypoposphatemia can also have severe consequences. It is therefore recommended to give the K$^+$ supplement as one-half KCl and one-half K phosphate. The EKG leads may be used to monitor for hypo- and hyperkalemia.

Insulin Administration

The only way to resolve diabetic ketoacidosis is to give insulin. Insulin is needed to restore normal glucose oxidation and to turn off lipolysis and the consequent ketone body formation and associated metabolic acidosis. There are many methods and regimens for giving insulin—all will work. The key determinant of success is intensive hourly monitoring of the patient's status and cognizance of the results of prior therapeutic moves. It should be noted that since the half-life of insulin in the *circulation* is approximately 5 minutes, the patient will be nearly insulin deficient within one-half hour after intravenous insulin infusion is discontinued. The consequent and usually more severe ketoacidosis can be detrimental to the patient. It should be emphasized that a decrease in glucose to a level of 200–250 mg percent in a patient being treated by intravenous insulin infusion should be treated by the addition of 5 percent dextrose to the intravenous fluids *rather* than by discontinuation of insulin. The cessation of intravenous insulin infusion should always be preceded by a subcutaneous or intramuscular dose to provide continuing insulin levels to the patient.

Numerous studies have shown that the route of insulin administration (intravenous, subcutaneous, or intramuscular) is immaterial as long as the patient monitoring and the decision-making process are adequate, and that ''low''-dose insulin gives as good results as ''high''-dose, albeit with fewer consequences. One suggested protocol for insulin therapy is to give to a total initial regular insulin dose of 0.5 U/kg body weight as follows: half as an intravenous loading bolus (0.25 U/kg), and half to be given either subcutaneously or intramuscularly. It is important to draw blood for glucose and bicarbonate level measurements in 1 hour to assess the insulin action. A repeat subcutaneous or intramuscular dose of insulin should be given at 2 hours, if needed. The additional dose of insulin (U/kg) depends on the assessment of the effect of the prior dose. The initial decrease in glucose level is in large part attributable to better hydration and is not necessarily an indication of insulin action. An increase in bicarbonate generally indicates that normal glucose oxidation is being restored and lipolysis is being turned off.

Diabetes Education and Adjustment

The resolution of diabetic ketoacidosis signals the beginning of a different emphasis in therapy. During this period we attempt to (1) stabilize the patient on an insulin injection routine, (2) educate the patient and family about diabetes and its care, (3) allay any fears or guilt feelings on the part of family members, (4) support the family unit in building confidence in their current and future ability to care for the patient, and (5) plan an individualized program for care after discharge and support activities. It is emphasized that *all* new childhood diabetes patients should be hospitalized and put through this type of program, regardless of whether their metabolic abnormalities are mild enough to be treated on an outpatient basis. This initial period of disease discovery and adjustment is crucial in establishing a comfortable, healthy attitude in dealing with diabetes.

Establishing Insulin Dose Routine

After resolution of diabetic ketoacidosis, I immediately place the patient on an appropriate dose of NPH insulin (0.25–0.5 U/kg) in the morning, and supplement it with regular insulin at noon, before supper, and at bedtime if needed. The total insulin dosage, and blood glucose levels monitored at the above time periods on day one and in the fasting state on the following morning, determine the nature and the amount of the insulin dose on day two. The NPH dose is adjusted, and a small amount of regular insulin is usually added in the morning. I will frequently add a small NPH and regular dose to be given just before supper, to obtain better bedtime and nocturnal glucose levels. The total dosage of insulin in my patients averages 0.78 U/kg/day, and about 90 percent of them will be discharged on a regimen consisting of 2 insulin shots given in the morning and before supper. Regular insulin usually constitutes one-fourth to one-third of the total morning dose (for example 10 U NPH/3 U regular insulin), and the presupper dose (NPH and regular) is usually one-fourth of the total daily dosage.

Although other types of long-acting insulins may be used, I have a distinct preference for NPH insulin because of a more predictable duration of action and greater familiarity with its use. Unlike other long-acting insulins, NPH can be mixed with regular insulin in the same syringe without altering the characteristics of either. I generally use single peak insulin, which is purified by size chromatography, rather than the more expensive monocomponent insulin, which is additionally purified by ion exchange chromatography. With the exception of specialized use (such as allergy and lipoatrophy), there is no demonstrated convincing reason to use the more expensive insulins.

Insulin Administration and Blood and Urine Testing

I teach all patients, regardless of their age, and their families to embark immediately on their own blood glucose and urine testing, with explanation and discussion of the results and the rationale for insulin dose adjustment. Patients and families are encouraged to give their own insulin injections, and patient age is not necessarily an impediment. I feel that a properly prepared 8-year-old can easily handle insulin injections with parental supervision (an unusual exception is a girl who has been administering her own insulin twice daily since becoming diabetic at the age of 5 years). Children 4 years of age are encouraged to assist the parent in urine testing.

During this five- to seven-day period, the educational efforts are time-consuming and require individualized sessions with the patient and the parents. During this time the patient dresses in regular clothes, and every effort is made to simulate a "home" outpatient situation. During these sessions the patient and family are patiently and comprehensively instructed by the diabetes team (physicians, diabetes resource nurse, nutritionist, and physiotherapist) to develop a basic understanding of diabetes mellitus as a condition of insulin deficiency that can be controlled but not cured at the present time. They are told that it will not go away or be outgrown, and they are taught to differentiate between adult- and juvenile-onset diabetes. The normal values for fasting and postprandial blood glucose levels and the normal pancreatic response to food are explained. I stress that the main objective of therapy is to normalize blood glucose levels and restore normal metabolism as much as possible *without* the effort becoming detrimental to the continued growth and overall well-being of the patient. I emphasize that normalization of blood glucose levels is our best current indicator of "diabetes disease control" and is achieved by a combination of (1) insulin replacement, (2) dietary planning, and (3) exercise. The role of illness and infections in influencing diabetes control is explained.

It is during these sessions that significant guilt feelings on the part of the parents emerge. Usually the emphasis is on which parent's ancestors had or have diabetes. I allow complete venting of these strong feelings of guilt, anxiety, and aggression, and eventually I contribute an explanation of juvenile diabetes as an inherited disease, almost certainly contributed to by genes inherited from *both* parental sides, with a probable major additional contribution by the environment. In virtually all cases, the venting of tensions and explanations of our current knowledge of diabetes allow the parents to redirect their anxieties and rechannel their energy into more pertinent, constructive learning. In some families the development of diabetes in a child reinforces family unity, while it can be extremely disruptive in others with pre-existing difficulties.

The sessions also have some very specific practical goals that must be achieved before discharge from the hospital. These are as follows:

1. Urine testing for glucose (Clinitest tabs) and acetone (Acetest tabs), and the rationale for testing.

2. Blood glucose monitoring with fingersticks using the Monolet and Chemstrips. The patient is instructed to do at least one test a day at home, each day at a different time.

3. Correct technique for drawing insulin and injection, including instructions for site rotation. The patient practices saline injection on a "Sugar Baby" doll (developed by Bell Telephone), and more often than not on our diabetes resource nurse.

4. Recording of results of tests and insulin dosage in Clinilog book.

5. Sessions with the nutritionist to devise and explain an appropriate diet and the importance of the diet in the management of diabetes. Our basic aim is to incorporate the family's diet and life style into the diet planning. Insofar as possible, the patient is urged to eat with the family, at approximately the same time every day, and to eat the same meals as the family, with the exception of avoidance of refined concentrated carbohydrates. The patient is allowed one sweet per week and is advised to celebrate birthdays and holidays normally but prudently.

6. Sessions with the physiotherapist to plan a program of exercise and activity appropriate to the child. The patient is scheduled for daily exercise while in the hospital. The interaction of exercise with insulin and diet is carefully explained, as are methods to deal with vigorous sport activities (for example extra snack, reduced insulin dose in some patients).

7. Recognition of hypoglycemia and its premonitory signs and symptoms. A glucagon kit and indications for its use are given. The family is instructed to carry a small tube of cake frosting (such as Pillsbury—this pastelike sugar sells for a few pennies and is just as useful as the far more expensive pharmaceutical "diabetic" sugar gels).

8. While in the hospital, collections of 24-hour block urines (8:00 AM-noon, noon-4:00 PM, 8:00 PM-8:00 AM) are performed, and kits and instructions for home collections are given. These block urines are used to quantitate the amount of glycosuria at each time period, and to assist in the planning of better insulin dosage (amount, long- or short-acting, and timing).

9. The use, significance, and irrefutable

meaning of glycosylated hemoglobin levels in the assessment of glycemia are explained. The patient is urged to consider low levels of these indicators of "diabetic control" as challenging targets for therapy.

10. An application form for a Medic Alert bracelet is completed and sent.

The intense program described above is nevertheless carried out in a low key, with emphasis on achieving confidence and security. One should try to involve the patient and family as much as possible in these efforts. Before discharge, the patient visits the outpatient Diabetic Clinic in order to be familiar with the routine. The patient and family are instructed to call the physician every morning for a week or until they feel comfortable with the management of diabetes. Finally, they have a trial "Independence Day" in the hospital, where the child and parent manage every detail of care and function as they would at home. These efforts form a solid basis on which to build during future clinic visits.

THE FORMATIVE PHASE

After discharge from the hospital, daily telephone contact continues with the patient and family. Usually this is necessary for about one week. They are instructed to return to the clinic two weeks after discharge, at which point the progress of the patient and previously identified problem areas are reviewed. Previous teaching is reinforced and any questions are answered. Clinic visits continue at one-month intervals for about six months, after which the patients are seen at two- to three-month intervals. The frequency of clinic visits necessarily varies and depends on many factors. A physician and a diabetes nurse are constantly on call and accessible to the patients and families (via page devices and telephone).

The "remission" period frequently begins shortly after discharge from the hospital. I explain my belief that "remission" merely represents a temporary and partial restoration of balance between residual insulin production and body requirements, and hence is not a lasting phenomenon. Although I have seen remission periods characterized by significant reduction in insulin requirements lasting 1–1½ years, I have never seen permanent remissions. During this phase, insulin injections are continued even if the requirements are as low as 2 per day. Temporary elimi-

nation of insulin injections frequently leads to unjustified and unrealistic expectations.

The key to successful outpatient management of diabetes is the continuity of medical care available to the patient and family. There is nothing more frustrating and unrewarding for a patient with a chronic process than to have a different physician of nurse every visit. One should attempt to have each patient see the same physician at the clinic visit for examination and instructions.

The patient is asked to collect at home and bring to the clinic a fractional 24-hour urine collection for glucose estimation. Random blood sugar and glycosylated hemoglobin levels are obtained at each visit. In addition, each patient has the meal plan diet reviewed and revised by the nutritionist, who gives diet instructions to the patient on an individual basis. Each patient has the diet plan adjusted annually. Particular attention should be paid to the increasing requirements for calories of a growing adolescent patient. The diabetes nurse will usually review and instruct patients in all aspects of diabetes mellitus and self-care. An assessment of knowledge and skills is performed annually. Group discussions are held before the clinic meetings to allow youngsters and their siblings an opportunity to share thoughts, fears, and questions relative to diabetes mellitus and its management. The basic attitude that we attempt to communicate is that diabetes is common, shared by many children who are indeed able to lead happy, successful, and well adjusted lives, with virtually no activity barred.

Finally, the clinic visit and the results of the 24-hour urine glucose analysis and glycosylated hemoglobin and other data are reviewed by the entire clinic staff 10 days later. Any therapeutic alterations or unexpected results are immediately communicated by telephone to the patient and family. These staff meetings serve the dual purpose of familiarizing everyone with all the patients, as well as providing an opportunity to discuss difficult problem cases.

THE OUTCOME PHASE

This lifelong phase essentially deals with the adult course of juvenile diabetes. It is during this time that the effects of diabetes and the results of therapy described above are manifested. At the present time, despite circumstantial evidence, there is no clear-cut consensus that attempts to "control" diabetes by attaining normoglycemia are helpful in the prevention of diabetic manifestations. My own belief is that the goal of achieving normoglycemia is important and indeed must be strenuously attempted, but in a humane and enlightened approach that is cognizant of the development of the individual and the limitations of our knowledge of the pathogenetic mechanisms of the complications. We simply do not know whether these complications are independent manifestations of the disease process which are exacerbated by hyperglycemia, or entirely secondary to hyperglycemia. Nevertheless, it is possible today to delay and ameliorate many of the complications of diabetes mellitus and permit the diabetic patient to lead a useful, happy, and productive life.

THE ADULT DIABETIC PATIENT

CHARLES R. SHUMAN, M.D.

Treatment goals for both type I and type II diabetes mellitus involve comprehensive programs to correct hyperglycemia, maintain normal nutrition, achieve psychosocial adjustment, and deter disease-related complicatons of both acute and chronic nature. The equilibration of insulin requirements and insulin supply is necessary for regulation of carbohydrate, lipid, and protein metabolism. This is achieved through dietary planning, exercise, administration of exogenous insulin or oral agents, and educational programs elucidating the nature of the disease and benefits of its control, which will lead to a long and useful life.

PRINCIPLES OF MODERN DIABETES MANAGEMENT

Therapeutic programs must be individualized to accommodate the needs of each patient because of the variability in blood glucose responses to daily stresses, activity, illness, insulin administra-

tion, and drugs. Among the basic elements for successful treatment are these:
1. realistic goals of health maintenance;
2. specific therapeutic programs;
3. psychologic support and reassurance; and
4. patient education, motivation, and understanding.

HEALTH MAINTENANCE

Information concerning the nature of diabetes and its control must be provided, and criteria must be developed for blood and urine glucose concentrations which permit sufficient latitude to avoid extremes of hypoglycemia and ketosis (FBS, 80–130 mg/dl; postprandial, 120–180 mg/dl). Physical training and exercise programs must be maintained, and active psychosocial balance in daily living should be encouraged. The physician should also schedule periodic examinations.

THERAPEUTIC PROGRAMS

Meal-planning is a basic requirement for all patients, and exercise must be programed to the capabilities and habits of the individual. Oral agents are selected for type II patients unresponsive to diet despite compliance. Insulin is required for type I patients, during pregnancy and acute stress, and for some type II patients with hyperglycemia.

PSYCHOLOGIC SUPPORT

The emotional impact of the diagnosis is alleviated by a confident, reassuring approach by the trained professional. An atmosphere of trust is established by the provision of information required for an understanding of the patient's role in his care. This relationship is essential for successful treatment.

EDUCATIONAL PROGRAMS

The following areas are vital to patient education:
1. Acquiring knowledge of diabetes and the importance of its control.
2. Self-monitoring of blood glucose and of urine glucose and ketones.
3. Recognition of hypoglycemia, its causes, and prevention.
4. Correction of hyperglycemia and threatened ketoacidosis. Treatment during "sick days."

5. Use of insulin injection techniques and rotation of sites.

6. Foot care and personal hygiene.

7. Identification bracelet and card; membership in organizations devoted to diabetes. Provision of educational material and discussion of specific points involved in treatment and health maintenance program.

DIETARY PLANNING FOR ADULT DIABETIC PATIENTS

Instructions in basic nutritional needs and meal-planning are required for all diabetic patients. Selections of foods are made which satisfy the dietary habits and preferences of most patients. Emphasis is placed on regularity of meals; constancy of caloric intake; partitioning of protein, fat, and carbohydrate; and the qualitative aspects of foods, that is, type of fats, protein sources, fiber content, and avoidance of sugar enrichment. Thus a degree of regimentation and discipline is required which will not detract from the enjoyment of eating.

Type I patients must eat regularly and time the caloric intake to the time-activity course of their insulin. Catabolic effects of insulin deprivation require nutritional rehabilitation to replace lean body mass and fat. Dietary patterns are devised to fit the daily activity and exercise schedules. Added calories are provided (about 20 gm of carbohydrate per hour) for strenuous exercise.

Type II patients, many of whom are overweight, are given hypocaloric diets that result in marked improvement in fasting and postcibal blood sugar even before significant weight reduction occurs. These patients are not challenged by the dangers of hypoglycemia but require intensive dietary counseling to achieve and maintain normal weight and improved glucose tolerance. A loss of 1.5 to 2.0 pounds weekly is desirable. Short-term fasts (seven to ten days) may be required for selected patients with an unfavorable response to a mixed hypocaloric diet.

Calories

Current evidence demonstrates that control of caloric intake is the most essential objective in the dietary management of diabetes. Previous concerns with carbohydrate and fat content of the diet have been relegated to a secondary role in view of the observations that higher levels of carbohydrate feeding with reduction of fats provide a palatable

TABLE 1   Caloric Requirements Related to Ideal Body Weight

| | Calories per Kilogram (IBW) per Day | | |
If Patient Is	Sedentary	Moderately Active	Very Active
obese	20–25	30	35
normal	30	35	40
underweight	35	40	45–50

diet with no effect upon plasma glucose concentrations or on insulin or sulfonylurea requirements compared with isocaloric diets of lower carbohydrate content.

To determine caloric intake, estimate ideal body weight (IBW):

1. Male: 106 lb for first 5 ft in height; add 6 lb for each additional inch.
2. Female: 100 lb for first 5 ft in height; add 5 lb for each additional inch.
   (Add 5 to 15 lb for medium and/or heavy frame.)

Convert pounds to kilograms: Divide pounds by 2.2 (Example: 132 lb ÷ 2.2 = 60 kg.)

Determine total daily caloric requirement: Multiply IBW in kilograms by calories per kilogram per day (Table 1).

Example: A 5'10" male, 36 years old, weighing 140 pounds, works as a tool and die maker:

$$106 \text{ lb (5 ft)} + 60 \text{ lb (10 in)} = \frac{166 \text{ lb}}{2.2} = 75 \text{ kg.}$$

IBW − 75 kg × 40 calories/kg (moderate activity) = 3000 calories daily

Convert 3000 calories into protein, fat, and carbohydrates.

Protein: 20 percent of total calories. 1 gm protein = 4 calories

$$3000 \text{ calories} \times 20 \text{ percent} - \frac{600}{4} = 150 \text{ gm}$$

CHO: 50 percent of total calories. 1 gm CHO = 4 calories

$$3000 \text{ calories} \times 50 \text{ percent} - \frac{1500}{4} = 375 \text{ gm}$$

Fat: 30 percent of total calories. 1 gm fat = 9 calories

$$3000 \text{ calories} \times 30 \text{ percent} - \frac{900}{9} = 100 \text{ gm}$$

Diet #1: 3000 calories. Protein 150, CHO 375, fat 100 gm.

This level of caloric intake is needed to increase body weight during relatively high energy expenditure.

Example: A 5'6" housewife, 40 years old, weighing 175 pounds has been inactive:

$$100 \text{ lb (5 ft)} + 30 \text{ lb (6 in)} = \frac{130 \text{ lb}}{2.2} = 60 \text{ kg.}$$

$$\text{IBW} - 60 \text{ kg} \times 20 \text{ calories/kg (sedentary activity)} = 1200 \text{ calories/kg}$$

Convert 1200 calories into protein, fat, and carbohydrates.

Protein: 20 percent of total calories

$$1200 \text{ calories} \times 20 \text{ percent} = \frac{240}{4} = 60 \text{ gm}$$

CHO: 50 percent of total calories

$$1200 \text{ calories} \times 50 \text{ percent} = \frac{600}{4} = 150 \text{ gm}$$

Fat: 30 percent of total calories

$$1200 \text{ calories} \times 30 \text{ percent} = \frac{360}{9} = 40 \text{ gm}$$

Division of Foods into Meals

Carbohydrate ration is divided into three meals and a bedtime snack.

Breakfast	Lunch	Dinner	Bedtime
2/7	2/7	2/7	1/7

For some Type I actively working patients and children, a midmorning and midafternoon snack are required.

Breakfast	Mid A.M.	Lunch	Mid P.M.	Dinner	Bedtime
2/10	1/10	2/10	1/10	3/10	1/10

When converting the diet prescription into foods for meal planning, one may round off to the nearest value for a complete exchange. Bread and milk exchanges may be given as one-half an exchange, for example, one-half cup milk or one-half slice of bread. The caloric content may vary by 10 percent in some instances. Variations in amounts of meat and fat exchanges which occur with the use of household measurements will not significantly influence blood glucose concentration but will affect the caloric value of the diet.

Carbohydrate. Bread exchange will provide complex carbohydrate sources, and fruits contain simple sugars. Foods containing significant amounts of natural sugars should comprise approximately 15 percent of the total carbohydrate intake.

Fat. Revised lists of fat sources for the diet identify those containing saturated, monounsaturated and polyunsaturated fats to facilitate selections of foods (meat and fat exchanges) that provide a lower ratio of unsaturated fats than those used in the past. The lower cholesterol content of the unsaturated fat sources permits a lowering of the cholesterol content of the diet to 300- to 500-mg levels.

Protein. To assure a balanced amino acid content of the diet, 50 percent of protein intake should be derived from the meat exchange list. For more rigid restriction of total fat calories, meat exchanges of low fat content are used.

For diabetic patients with renal or hepatic failure, the protein ration is reduced to 30 to 40 gm daily. Restriction of potassium intake is also employed in renal insufficiency dietary programs.

Sodium restriction is required for patients with congestive heart failure, hypertension, and other fluid-retaining states.

Fiber. Nutritional studies have demonstrated that an increased fiber content in diets used in treatment of diabetes can effectively and consistently reduce the plasma glucose and lipid concentrations. An increase in fiber content from 10 to 40 gm using brans, unrefined grains, cereals, breads, fruits (not juices), vegetables, and similar components not only lowered plasma glucose but also decreased the requirements of insulin in some diabetic patients.

Artificial Sweeteners. Judicious use of saccharin as an artificial sweetener is permitted for patients with diabetes and for the obese. This is appropriate for these patients in whom sucrose and other sugars (including fructose) may rapidly elevate the plasma glucose concentrations and increase the caloric intake. Other sweeteners, such as sorbitol or mannitol, are permitted in modest quantities, since gastrointestinal absorption of these substances is low and no significant rise in plasma glucose concentrations is observed.

Alcohol. The caloric value of alcohol is 7 calories/gm. Two ounces of an 80-proof alcoholic beverage will provide approximately 170 calories. While the metabolic disposal of alcohol does not contribute to a rise in plasma glucose levels, it may lead to increased fat production. Limited amounts of alcohol may be permitted for social occasions; however, a high level of intake may lead to hypoglycemia if food intake is eliminated as a result of intoxication. On the other hand, alcoholic ketoacidosis, primarily beta hydroxybutyrate ketosis, may be observed under conditions of increased mobilization of fatty acids during periods of high ethanol intake.

Successful Use of Meal Planning for Diabetic Patients

Determine the food preference and eating habits by obtaining a thorough nutritional history.

TABLE 2 Insulins Available in the United States

Action	Lilly	Nordisk	Novo	Squibb
Rapid	Regular (R) Semilente (S)	Velosulin (R)	Actrapid (A) Semitard (S)	Regular Semilente
Combined		Mixtard (30% R) (70% N)		
Intermediate	NPH (N) Lente (L)	Insulatard (N)	Monotard (L) Lentard (L) Protophane (N)	NPH Lente Globin
Long-acting	Ultralente (U) PZI		Ultratard (U)	Ultralente PZI
	Purified pork Purified beef Single peak beef-pork	Purified pork	Purified pork Purified beef Purified beef-pork	Beef-pork

Note: N, NPH: Neutral Protamine Hagedorn; P, PZI: Protamine Zinc Insulin

Calculate the caloric requirements for the patient based upon ideal body weight and activity. Obesity requires caloric deprivation, which may significantly improve the diabetic state. The lean, insulin-dependent patient requires nutritional support with regulation of timing, regularity, and consistency of meals.

Determine the dietary composition, protein, fat, and carbohydrate, or consult a dietitian to partition the caloric calculation.

Arrange meal planning and food choices to accommodate the eating patterns of the patient or to correct unacceptable eating patterns.

Use the food exchange system to facilitate the education and training of the patient in meal planning.

Reinforce the educational process at every opportunity during the patient's visits or by periodic interviews with a dietitian.

Insulin in Treatment of Diabetes

The goal of insulin therapy is to regulate the metabolism of carbohydrate, fat, and protein by equalizing the supply and demand for the hormone. Insulin is required for the treatment of (1) type I diabetes; (2) type II diabetes during stress, trauma, major surgery, or periods of symptomatic hyperglycemia; (3) gestational diabetes not controlled by diet; and (4) diabetic ketoacidosis and hyperglycemic hyperosmolar state. For a list of insulins available in the United States, see Table 2.

Insulin requirements vary widely among individual patients and are significantly influenced by such factors as dietary intake, physical activity, environmental stress, and illness. Insulin regimens are coordinated with meal planning, physical activity, and life style of individual patients to achieve an effective program of metabolic regulation. Increasing use of combination insulin injection regimens has been found to improve glycemic control.

In patients with increased serum insulin binding, the peak actions may be delayed and duration of action prolonged (see Table 3). Other factors that affect the bioavailability of insulin include the following. (1) Site of injection: abdominal and arm injections produce more rapid and higher peak concentrations than thigh or buttock injections.

TABLE 3 Time Activity Course of Insulins

Onset of Action	Peak Effect (hrs)		Duration of Action (hrs)	
	Initial Rx*	Chronic Rx*	Initial Rx*	Chronic Rx*
Rapid				
Regular	2–3	5–6	6	16–17
Semilente	3–6		12	
Intermediate				
NPH	6–12	10–12	14–24	24–26
Lente	8–14	10–12	18–24	24–26
Slow				
PZI	16–24		36	
Ultralente	20–30		36	

*Initial Rx: patients receiving their first insulin injections; chronic Rx: patients receiving their insulin injections for more than two years

Exercised extremities rapidly release insulin from injection sites. (2) Destruction of insulin at subcutaneous injection sites may occur in rare instances. (3) Insulin-receptor interactions and postreceptor disturbances are areas in which insulin sensitivity may be significantly altered.

Treatment Programs with Insulin

The order of increasing difficulty in management entails the following schedules of insulin administration:

1. Single prebreakfast dose of intermediate insulin (NPH or Lente).
2. Split dose intermediate insulin: two-thirds prebreakfast, one-third predinner.
3. Multidose insulin combinations:
   a. Split doses of intermediate and rapid insulins. These mixtures provide two-thirds NPH or Lente and one-third regular in each injection. Of the total daily dosage, two-thirds is given prebreakfast and one-third before supper. Individual components of each dose are adjusted depending on blood glucose (home-monitored) or on urine glucose determinations.
   b. Regular insulin before each meal and intermediate insulin at bedtime.
   c. Ultralente and regular at breakfast, regular at lunch and dinner.

Each of these schedules is designed to provide a basal level of insulin overnight and between meals and to maintain heightened insulin activity during feedings. Multidose schedules, especially 3a, as described in above, have approximated glycemic control achieved with insulin pump using self-monitoring of blood glucose level for insulin adjustment.

Educating the Patient

A clear understanding is needed of the integrated roles of meal planning, exercise, and insulin activity: (1) Uniformity of meals is necessary; (2) inappropriate food ingestion is a leading cause of hyperglycemia; and (3) exercise potentiates the action of insulin.

Train the patient in methods of urine glucose and ketone determination.

Home-monitoring of blood glucose concentration using Glucometer or Chemstrip bG has become the most helpful adjunct in self-care of diabetes.

Techniques for Self-injection of Insulin

Disposable syringes are advocated, and each syringe, if properly handled, is used three times. Rotation of injection sites daily is essential, using abdomen, upper arms, buttocks, and thighs. Sterile techniques are demonstrated. For mixtures of insulin in syringe, add air to each vial equal to insulin dose, and withdraw each insulin in same sequence into syringe in correct dosages.

Ambulatory Treatment

Initial treatment on an outpatient basis is preferred for psychologic and economic reasons if (1) the patient is a nonpregnant adult, (2) there are no acute or chronic complications; and (3) educational facilities are available.

1. Single dose regimen
   a. Initial dose ranges from 10 to 20 units of NPH or Lente.
   b. Check the second voided urine glucose concentration before meals and bedtime. Home-monitored blood glucose determinations are also used (see below).
   c. Increase dose by 4 units every other day until urine is negative or trace (usually afternoon test).
   d. Reassess response in one week by checking blood glucose determinations—fasting and at 4:00 P.M.—body weight, and medical status; inspect urine records. Adjust insulin dose appropriately.
2. Split dose, intermediate insulin (NPH or Lente)
   a. Used when single dose lowers afternoon blood sugar level but fails to prevent fasting hyperglycemia.
   b. Give two-thirds before breakfast and one-third before dinner.
   c. The effect of any insulin dose is related to the blood glucose concentration at the time of its administration.
   d. A decrease in the morning dose is needed if the fasting blood sugar level is lowered by the P.M. dose.
3. Combined intermediate-regular insulin regimens

a. These are used for postbreakfast hyperglycemia, 11:00 A.M. >150 mg/dl, with regular insulin added to A.M. NPH or Lente; (2) and regular is added to P.M. NPH or Lente when postsupper hyperglycemia persists.

b. Add 4 to 10 units of regular to breakfast and supper doses of intermediate insulin.

c. A reduction of 4 to 6 units of intermediate insulin may be required when regular insulin is added.

d. In general, the higher the patient's insulin requirement, the greater the amount of regular insulin relative to intermediate insulin in the mixture.

4. Regular insulin before meals and intermediate at bedtime
   a. Used for patients with unstable diabetes unresponsive to combination insulin regimens.
   b. Total daily insulin requirement may be given in the following schedule: Breakfast, three-sevenths; lunch, one-seventh; supper, two-sevenths; bedtime, one-seventh.
   c. Each dose is adjusted to control blood glucose concentration during the intermeal and overnight intervals; home-monitoring is used.

5. Ultralente with regular in A.M., regular at lunch and dinner
   a. Ultralente dose, 10–15 units, is adjusted to control fasting blood sugar level.
   b. Regular mixed with Ultralente to control postbreakfast blood sugar level.
   c. Regular insulin given at lunch and dinner to regulate post-cibal blood glucose.
   d. Ultralente may be added to supper dose also if needed for overnight control of blood sugar level.

Self-monitoring Blood Glucose (Glucometer-Dextrostix, Chemstrip bG)

For combined insulin regimens, as well as for single dose intermediate insulin programs, home glucose self-monitoring provides an excellent method for determining dosage adjustments.

If blood sugar level is over 140 mg/dl, add 2 units of regular insulin.

If blood sugar level is over 200 mg/dl, add 4 units of regular insulin.

If fasting hyperglycemia persists, increase second dose of intermediate insulin, or increase Ultralente insulin, to maintain overnight control.

For "sick days," home glucose monitoring permits the adjustment of insulin doses depending on response to illness. Dose is reduced if the patient is anorexic and blood sugar level is low. Supplementary regular insulin, 4–8 units, is given at 2- to 4-hour intervals if blood sugar level is high. Mild DKA may be treated at home with regular insulin, 6–10 units hourly, if the patient is able to retain fluids. The physician is contacted for advice.

Insulin treatment in a hospital setting is necessary for the following conditions: (1) diabetes and pregnancy; (2) children with type I diabetes; (3) acute complications, including infection and stress; (4) cardiovascular disturbances or complications of diabetes; (5) and for education and training not available otherwise. Regular insulin is used initially before meals and at bedtime, depending upon serial blood glucose responses. In most instances, combination insulin regimens are used following a response to initial regular insulin.

Complications of Insulin Therapy

Insulin therapy is the most common cause of hypoglycemia, usually related to insulin overdosage, omission of meals, or increased physical activity. Hypoglycemia is treated, if possible, by the ingestion of concentrated sugars. The patient may carry instant glucose preparations in a plastic tube; family and friends should know how to administer glucagon injection in the event of hypoglycemic coma. Hypoglycemia may be prevented by careful evaluation and re-education; in addition, self-monitoring of blood glucose levels will detect suspected hypoglycemia and lead to its prevention. Patients should be urged to carry diabetes identification cards, wear I.D. bracelets, or both.

Insulin Allergy. Local reactions, once common, now are infrequent with purified insulin. Systemic allergy, now rare, is related to IgE insulin antibody. Rapid desensitization treatment (Lilly Desensitization Kit) is effective.

Insulin Immunoresistance. Intermittent insulin therapy, allergy, and obesity are often found in the patient's history; however, obesity may cause nonimmune resistance, as will infection and certain endocrinopathies. Immunoresistance is caused by IgG insulin-binding antibody in the serum. It may resolve spontaneously and usually responds to a change to pork insulin. For severe cases, treatment with glucocorticoids is useful.

Lipodystrophy. *Lipohypertrophy*—fibrofatty mass occurring in sites of predilection for insulin injection—will regress when affected areas are avoided. The cause of *lipoatrophy*—disappearance of subcutaneous fat—is unknown, but it may be immunogenic. Atrophic areas improve slowly if the patient's treatment is changed to purified pork preparations injected into the perimeter of the affected area.

Insulin Edema. Poorly controlled patients whose blood sugar levels are rapidly and effectively regulated frequently exhibit fluid retention and edema. Insulin edema is due to an antinatturetic effect of insulin that is readily controlled by diuretics or salt restriction. The condition clears within a few days or weeks.

Insulin Presbyopia. Sudden blurring of vision may occur with effective treatment or prolonged hyperglycemia. It is related to changes in hydration of the lens and spontaneously recedes during treatment of diabetes. Refraction should not be performed for four or six weeks after glycemic control is established.

Rebound Hyperglycemia (Somogyi Effect). Insulin-induced hypoglycemia raises the blood sugar level by (1) release of counter-regulatory hormones, and (2) hunger that stimulates food ingestion.

Hypoglycemia	Epinephrine → Glucagon Cortisol	→ Glycogenolysis Gluconeogenesis	→ ↑ Blood sugar

Treatment involves readjustment of insulin dosage or change to split dose regimen.

Purified Insulins

Chromatographic methods now used in the processing of insulin have produced a highly purified product with lower immunogenic potential. The proinsulin content is used as a standard to monitor insulin purity. The FDA standard for purified insulin is proinsulin content less than 10 ppm.

Special indications for the use of purified pork insulin include insulin allergy, immunoresistance, and lipoatrophy. It is also recommended for patients receiving short-term insulin treatment, such as gestational diabetics or type II patients during surgery or stress. Some authorities recommend purified insulin for all type I patients.

Biosynthetic human insulin (BHI) has been prepared by recombinant DNA technology in which bacterial strains containing genes for the A and B chains of insulin, synthesize the peptide moieties which, on purification, are combined to form the intact insulin molecule. The biosynthetic hormone possesses characteristics indistinguishable from porcine insulin in blood glucose lowering effects and has been subjected to extensive clinical trials in preparation for its commercial availability.

Exercise Programs for Diabetic Patients

An increase in insulin sensitivity, reduction in plasma glucose and lipid concentrations, improved muscle tone, and a sense of well-being are among the benefits derived from regular physical exercise. Preprogram stress testing is used for overweight adults; pulse-rated graduated exercise programs are recommended.

Diabetic patients react differently to exercise, depending upon the state of metabolic control. Those with adequate amounts of insulin who engage regularly in exercise will experience improvement in glucose tolerance and diminution in insulin requirements. Type I patients receiving inadequate amounts of exogenous insulin develop increasing hyperglycemia and ketonemia during exercise. Intense exercise by the patient who has not decreased his insulin nor taken extra carbohydrate (20 gm/hour) may result in profound hypoglycemia.

On the day that strenuous exercise is anticipated, the patient should decrease his insulin dose by 20 to 25 percent of the usual dose. If the patient has injected his usual insulin dose and then anticipates intense physical activity, he should examine his urine for glycosuria or perform blood glucose testing. Unless he has 1 to 2 percent urine glucose reactivity or is hyperglycemic, 20 to 40 gm of carbohydrate in the form of a beverage or candy should be ingested before commencing intense exercise and repeated hourly for sustained activity. More carbohydrate may be needed during the post-exercise period if subsequent urinary specimens are nonreactive for glucose or if lowering of blood glucose level is noted. Again, his previous experiences with similar exercise periods should aid the patient in arriving at the amount of carbohydrate to eat.

Treatment of Type II Diabetes

Non–insulin-dependent diabetes mellitus (NIDDM) occurs at any age, but the majority of patients are over 40 years of age and two-thirds of these are obese. Nonobese type II diabetes can usually be distinguished by the absence of ketonuria and the lack of a history of significant weight loss; however, the distinction between the nonobese NIDDM and type I diabetes is not always clear. In some type II patients, insulin therapy is needed to control hyperglycemia.

Office management is recommended for these patients unless there are compelling reasons for hospitalizaton. Dietary management is effective for 40 percent of these patients regardless of the initial blood glucose concentration. The meal plan is devised to achieve and maintain ideal body weight and work capacity. Daily physical activities consistent with the capabilities and health status of the patient are outlined. Instructions are provided for urine glucose testing and maintenance of the diabetic diary.

Meal planning strategies are of primary importance. A high carbohydrate, high fiber diet with restriction of saturated fats and cholesterol is advocated, as described in the section on diet. Often the blood sugar level will decrease rapidly before significant loss of weight is observed when there is dietary compliance. A reduction in plasma lipid concentrations, elevated in the untreated patient, follows the blood glucose response.

Sulfonylurea Therapy

Oral antidiabetic therapy is used for the type II diabetic patient in whom hyperglycemia persists after four to six weeks of treatment with diet and exercise. The oral agents currently available and the second generation sulfonylureas prepared for marketing in the United States are shown in Table 4.

The choice of drug depends upon the physician's experience, since all have been demonstrated to be effective. Most widely used at present are chlorpropamide and tolazamide; the former has a long half-life and thus enjoys the advantage of administration as a single daily dose.

Initial dosage is prescribed at or below the usual maintenance dosage and is increased at

TABLE 4   Sulfonylureas

Generic and Trade Names	Tablet Size (mg)	Dosage (mg) Usual	Dosage (mg) Range	Daily Dose	Duration of Action (hrs)
Tolbutamide Orinase	500	1500	500–2000	2–3	6–10
Inactivated by liver through oxidation to carboxytolbutamide, excreted by kidney and may give false positive test for proteinuria.					
Chlorpropamide Diabinese	250 100	250	50–500	1	36–60
Metabolized to several compounds; excreted by kidney.					
Acetohexamide Dymelor	250 500	750	250–1500	1–2	10–20
Metabolites formed by hydroxylation in liver; L-hydroxyhexamide is most active component.					
Tolazamide Tolinase	100 250 500	500	100–1000	1–2	12–24
Metabolized by liver to six compounds, three of which have hypoglycemic activity and are excreted by the kidney.					
Not marketed in the U.S.					
Glyburide Diabeta Micronase	2.5 5 10	20	2.5–30	1–2	12–24
Glipizide Glucotrol	5 10	30	2.5–40	1–2	12–24

three- to six-day intervals until the fasting and two-hour postcibal blood glucose decrease concentrations to acceptable ranges. An optimal response may require several weeks but usually occurs within ten days.

Criteria for Therapeutic Effectiveness

FBS: 80–130 mg/dl; postprandial BS: 120–180 mg/dl

HbA_{1c}: 8 percent or lower

If the blood glucose remains at or below these concentrations, the dosage of sulfonylurea is reduced slowly to the lowest effective levels. A continued favorable response to the minimal dosage of sulfonylurea is an indication to discontinue the drug for a trial of diet alone. The need for dietary adherence is stressed at each visit. A rise in blood sugar level accompanied by an increase of 1 or 2 pounds in body weight signals a lapse in dietary regulation. If body weight is unchanged and the blood glucose level increases, sulfonylurea therapy is resumed and the dosage adjusted to achieve a favorable response.

For the type II patient receiving insulin, conversion to sulfonylurea is easily achieved by administering the agent in appropriate dosage and discontinuing insulin if the dose is less than 40 units. Those receiving larger doses of insulin are instructed to reduce the dose by 50 percent while taking the drug. If urine glucose tests remain negative or home blood glucose tests remain normal, the insulin dose is discontinued. If the urine glucose test becomes positive, the dose of sulfonylurea is increased and insulin continued until aglycosuria and reduction in blood glucose level permits the discontinuance of insulin. By cautious monitoring of urine glucose and ketone levels, the conversion from insulin to sulfonylurea can be effected safely.

Insulinogenic Resurrection in Type II Diabetes

Patients who are clearly type II diabetics may fail to respond initially to sulfonylurea and diet. Hyperglycemia of long duration or associated with stress or infection depletes insulin reserves. For those with glucose concentrations above 300 mg/dl, exogenous insulin treatment is initiated, using regular or NPH insulins as highly purified pork preparations to avoid sensitizing the patient to insulin. Initial doses of 5–10 units twice daily are given with gradual adjustments to decrease the blood sugar level to concentrations below 180 mg/dl. Lowering the blood sugar level in this manner permits regranulation of beta cells and enhances their capacity to respond to oral antidiabetic agents. When this occurs, insulin is withdrawn and the patient is maintained on oral medication. Then, if blood glucose concentrations hold below 130 mg/dl, it is useful to try discontinuing the medication to see if diet alone is effective. This sequence has been observed in numerous patients recovering from hyperosmolar nonketotic coma, an extreme example of insulinogenic resurrection.

Sulfonylurea Failure

Primary failure is defined as an inadequate response during the first month of treatment with maximum dosage. Secondary failures are recognized by the resurgence of hyperglycemia, after an initial satisfactory response, in which infection, stress, or dietary noncompliance cannot be incriminated. In some instances failure of sulfonylurea therapy may be due to incorrect diagnosis, with the patient actually having type I diabetes. In other cases a period of exogenous insulin treatment may restore responsiveness to sulfonylurea. The average rate of secondary failure is 3 to 10 percent annually for which no explanation is apparent other than beta cell failure. Dietary noncompliance and increasing obesity are obvious causes of sulfonylurea failure.

Side Effects of Sulfonylurea Therapy

Adverse reactions are exceedingly rare; hematologic, hepatic, gastrointestinal, dermatologic, metabolic, or systemic side effects occur in an incidence of 1 percent. Hypoglycemia is prevented by careful dosage regulation and by avoidance of drug interactions that increase free sulfonylurea levels in the blood. Among the drugs involved are salicylates, phenylbutazone, sulfonamides, Coumadin, diphenylhydantoin and clofibrate. Severe hypoglycemia necessitates hospitalization for intravenous glucose administration until the blood glucose level remains normal with cessation of the infusion. Hyponatremia may occur in rare instances, usually when diuretic agents are used simultaneously with an agent such as chlorpropamide. This complication disappears on stopping the diuretic or changing to a different sulfonylurea. Another side effect is the Antabuse reaction seen in 7 to 10 percent of patients upon ingesting alcohol. If the reaction discourages the use of alcohol, it may be beneficial.

During glucosteroid therapy in lower dosages, graded increments of sulfonylurea will maintain control of blood glucose levels. With larger dosages of steroids, as in the case of stress or surgery, the use of exogenous insulin is required. Diuretic therapy does not often affect diabetic control in the stabilized patient if hypokalemia is avoided.

The Diabetic Patient During Surgery

Control of blood glucose levels is achieved by the addition of regular insulin to each liter of 5 percent dextrose solution used throughout the operation and postoperative period. Between 8 and 16 units of regular insulin are usually adequate, depending upon glycemic responses and the degree of severity of the operation. Serial monitoring of blood sugar levels three or four times daily is required; urine glucose coverage with insulin is discouraged. If the blood glucose level rises above 220 mg/dl, the patient is given 6 units of regular insulin subcutaneously and the dose of insulin is increased in the dextrose infusion. Adherence of insulin to the infusion equipment is not a problem in the application of this method. During recovery when the patient resumes oral feedings, the normal preoperative treatment for the diabetic state is usually effective. If stressful conditions persist, patients who previously responded to sulfonylurea will require continuation of treatment with insulin.

Elderly Diabetic Patients

The older diabetic patient is not treated as aggressively as those in middle age. However, asymptomatic hyperglycemia is not without hazard. Many respond with improved vitality and energy when plasma glucose level is brought into the 140 to 200 mg/dl range by low dose insulin or sulfonylurea therapy. "Renal threshold" for glucose is high in these patients and cannot be used to assess control. Low dose sulfonylurea or single intermediate insulin dose is used in these patients with persistent hyperglycemia, neuropathic disorders, infection, and other diabetic manifestations. Care is taken to avoid reductions of blood glucose levels to below 130 mg/dl. Further reduction puts the patient at risk of inadvertent hypoglycemia, a serious hazard for the elderly.

The successful use of oral antidiabetic agents requires attention to proper selection of patients and careful scrutiny of their effectiveness and safety, with particular reference to dosage adjustments and side effects. The UGDP study has raised important issues related to the treatment of diabetes. These issues remain unresolved, including the purported risk of cardiovascular mortality because of the question raised concerning the methodologies employed and the lack of confirmatory data from other studies. These reservations were echoed in the recent policy statement of the American Diabetes Association in which it was noted that decisions concerning therapeutic regimens should remain the prerogative of the informed physician.

DIABETIC PREGNANCY

JOHN W. HARE, M.D

PRINCIPLES OF TREATMENT

There is general agreement that normal or near normal glucose levels are necessary in the treatment of diabetes during pregnancy. Recent data have suggested that the best efforts at control must be applied very soon after conception. Unfortunately, the time of conception is not always known. If the pregnancy is planned, it is worthwhile for the physician to counsel the patient to make a particular effort at control as soon as pregnancy is contemplated. Previously, attempts to control diabetes once the pregnancy was discovered (which was usually a month or two after conception) were aimed at reducing perinatal morbidity and mortality rates. The current effort to control diabetes before conception and very early in the pregnancy stem from data suggesting that this may prevent congenital anomalies. The perinatal mortality rate in diabetic pregnancies is about twice that in nondiabetic pregnancies. A third to a half of the deaths are caused by congenital anomalies.

If efforts at control were successful in reducing these anomalies the perinatal mortality rate would approach that of nondiabetic women. Morbidity would remain a concern, but hopefully would be decreased by continued vigilant efforts.

In contrast to that of the fetus, maternal risk is minimal during diabetic pregnancies. There is some concern, however, when retinopathy or nephropathy is present; these conditions are discussed below.

In the last few years home glucose monitoring has become the cornerstone of management. This may be done with a reflectance meter which utilizes glucose oxidase-impregnated strips to measure capillary blood. A meter is not an absolute necessity, however, because sufficient accuracy can be obtained by the use of strips that are read by visual estimation.

Currently, ideal control for women with insulin dependent diabetes requires daily fasting capillary glucose levels to be 100 mg/dl or less and postprandial capillary glucose levels to be 140 mg/dl or less. In addition, a monthly hemoglobin A_{1c} level should be less than 7 percent (normal is 4 to 6 percent). It is not possible to achieve this degree of control in all women with type I diabetes. In some the disease is so unstable that an attempt at stringent management will result in incapacitating insulin reactions. Most women, however, are able to achieve glucose control if they and their physicians are well motivated.

Patients are examined weekly from the discovery of pregnancy. Once ideal control is achieved they may be seen every two weeks. We have a nurse knowledgeable about diabetic pregnancy instruct patients in home glucose monitoring, urine results, glucagon administration, diet, and general management of diabetes.

Most diabetic women are aware of concerns for their health and their baby's health. Often these fears are greater than need be, and if this is the case pregnancy can be a period of psychologic stress for both parents. In addition to the medical issues, there are social stresses that are increased by frequent visits to the doctor, which in turn tend to disrupt home and work patterns. It may be necessary for some women to have skilled professional help beyond the physician's capabilities. We refer them to a clinical social worker specializing in high-risk pregnancy.

In addition to the internist, the team includes an obstetrician knowledgeable in the management of diabetic pregnancy. After delivery a pediatrician must be immediately available to treat any of the several neonatal complications that may occur.

TABLE 1 Methods of Insulin Administration

Conventional use of regular and intermediate insulin once or twice a day
Premeal regular insulin plus one or two small doses of intermediate insulin
Open-loop insulin infusion pump

INSULIN USE

Insulin may be administered by one of several methods (Table 1). First, regular and intermediate insulin may be used in a conventional fashion. It is helpful to think of insulin regimens as patterns and to remember that pregnancy may require that the patient use a more complex pattern than before (Table 2). Pattern I is intermediate insulin given once a day before breakfast, pattern II a mixture of regular and intermediate insulin before breakfast, pattern III the addition of intermediate insulin in the afternoon or evening, and pattern IV a mixture of regular and intermediate insulin given both before breakfast and before supper. If the patient was taking no insulin before pregnancy, this may be considered a Pattern 0. Not all patients will progress from whatever pattern they had been on before pregnancy to a more complicated one during pregnancy in an orderly fashion, but if the information in Table 2 is kept in mind, it can help the physician decide how to arrange the insulin dosage. The action curve of regular and intermediate insulin should be kept in mind; each should be added or adjusted in such a manner as to regulate blood sugar at its peak time of action.

Less common patterns of insulin dosage may also be used, such as premeal regular insulin and small doses of intermediate insulin at night and/or in the morning to provide an approximation of basal secretion. This method has the appeal of

TABLE 2 Insulin Patterns

	A.M.*		P.M.†	
	Regu-lar	Inter-mediate	Regu-lar	Inter-mediate
Pattern 0	0	0	0	0
Pattern I	0	+	0	0
Pattern II	+	+	0	0
Pattern III	+	+	0	+
Pattern IV	+	+	+	+

*A.M. insulin is given before breakfast.
†P.M. insulin is given before supper if regular is used, and either before supper or at bedtime if only intermediate is used.

being more physiologic but has the disadvantage of often requiring more injections a day than are necessary to achieve the desired effect.

Open-loop infusion pump systems can be used at any time during pregnancy with safety and efficacy. In general, control is improved when pumps are used, but they are not an absolute essential for treatment. Careful attention to the control of diabetes will often achieve desired goals when a pump is not available, not desired, or the patient is thought not to be an appropriate candidate for it.

DIET

The diet used is similar to that for the treatment of diabetes in general, with the exception that a larger number of calories and a more generous portion of carbohydrate will be required. The extra calories provide adequate nutrition for the developing fetus and the slightly higher carbohydrate apportionment is intended to minimize maternal ketogenesis. The calorie prescriptions may be calculated in two ways. The simplest is to give 35 calories per kg of ideal body weight throughout pregnancy. Some women may have difficulty eating this much if they are nauseated in the first trimester or experience early satiety in the third trimester because of elevation of the uterine fundus into the upper abdomen. An alternative method is to give 30 calories per kg in the first trimester and recalculate the diet in the second and third trimesters so that an additional 30 calories are provided for each kg of weight gain. Either method is satisfactory.

The carbohydrate prescription should be about 45 percent of the total calories; the protein should be 1½ to 2 gm per kg of body weight, and the fat as needed to complete the total caloric prescription. Some practitioners prefer to instruct the patients to use no added salt; this concept is not universally agreed upon.

GESTATIONAL DIABETES

Gestational diabetes is a condition considered separately from insulin dependent diabetes. Gestational diabetes should first be treated by diet alone, as described above. If this fails to maintain fasting *blood* glucose levels below 90 mg percent and 2-hour postprandial glucose levels below 110 mg percent, insulin therapy is recommended. Because of the strictness of these standards, many women with gestational diabetes will not be suc-

cessfully treated with diet alone and will require insulin in the morning. If this is ineffective the pattern should be advanced as indicated by the periods of the day when hyperglycemia occurs.

Gestational diabetes is usually discovered late in the second or early in the third trimester when the diabetogenic effect of the pregnancy is maximal. Gestational diabetes is suspected when glycosuria is present, a postprandial glucose level is elevated, or if there is a history of previous gestational diabetes, diabetes in the family, stillbirth, or macrosomia. It is more common in women who are obese or of advanced age. The diagnosis is made by a glucose tolerance test with a 100-gm challenge (Table 3).

The discovery of diabetes in the first trimester suggests that the woman had unrecognized diabetes prior to pregnancy. In the absence of data to confirm this impression, she may be considered to have gestational diabetes and treated accordingly, with the understanding that its nongestational nature may be discovered after delivery when diabetes persists.

If insulin therapy is necessary in women with gestational diabetes, a highly purified preparation should be used. This is done because the women will no longer be hyperglycemic after delivery, but will be at increased risk for the development of diabetes later in life. Should insulin therapy again be required some years hence, she will be less likely to have developed antibodies to it and less likely to be allergic or resistant.

SPECIAL CONDITIONS

Retinopathy

There is a tendency for retinopathy to progress during pregnancy, whether it be background or proliferative. It usually regresses post partum, so no long-term threat is posed to the mother's eyes unless she has rapidly progressive proliferative retinopathy that causes irreversible damage during the pregnancy. The one exception to this

TABLE 3   Glucose Tolerance Test in Pregnancy*

Time	Whole Blood	Plasma
Fasting	90	105
1 hr	165	190
2 hr	145	165
3 hr	125	145

*Upper limits of normal mg/dl

is neovascularization on the disk. This condition in and of itself has a poor prognosis for vision, and some ophthalmologists consider it an indication for termination of pregnancy if it is discovered in the first trimester.

Laser photocoagulation can be used with safety in pregnancy. Women who have had previous laser coagulation successfully applied or have sustained remission of their proliferative retinopathy can anticipate going through the pregnancy without a reactivation of it.

When a woman is first seen, if there is any question about her ophthalmologic status she should be examined by an ophthalmologist. Routine examinations can then be performed in each trimester, and of course more frequently if her condition dictates.

Nephropathy

A special risk exists for the fetus in a mother who has nephropathy with over 500 mg/day proteinuria. Perinatal survival rate is somewhat less than 90 percent. Moderate azotemia with a serum creatinine level of over 3 mg/dl is usually incompatible with fetal life. Hypertension and diminished creatinine clearance are frequently associated with intrauterine growth retardation and its nonspecifically poor prognosis.

Maternal proteinuria often increases dramatically in the third trimester to levels of 5–10 gm per 24 hours. Women with this much proteinuria also are frequently hypertensive and may require therapy for this. The development of hypertension, proteinuria, and edema, which usually begin in the second trimester, may necessitate periods of bed rest beginning with 2 hours in the morning and 2 hours in the afternoon. If bed rest at home is insufficient to control edema and hypertension, hospitalization may be required, often for weeks. Women with nephropathy should be advised of this as soon as possible, because it may seriously interfere with their care of other children or their ability to work. The creatinine clearance tends not to rise during pregnancy in women with nephropathy as it does in women with normal kidneys. The presence of proteinuria, hypertension, and edema makes a diagnosis of preeclampsia a difficult one. It can often be surmised only if there is a rapid rise in the blood pressure and protein excretion. Even this is not always easy to ascertain because of the dramatic rise in proteinuria that occurs in the third trimester.

Once the woman has delivered, her renal function tends to return to prepregnancy levels. Thus pregnancy has no long-term deleterious effect on maternal renal function.

INSULIN REQUIREMENTS IN PREGNANCY
(Table 4)

First Trimester

Type I diabetes is less stable during the first trimester and reactions may be troublesome. If the woman was well controlled prior to pregnancy a slight reduction in insulin dosage may be necessary. A reduction in dosage may also be necessary if she did not adhere strictly to her diet prior to pregnancy and suddenly does so. Women who have a particularly difficult time with reactions may require glucagon. It is helpful to instruct another household member in the use of glucagon if the patient has unstable diabetes. Even though reactions may be troublesome, it may not be possible to reduce the insulin dosage in all patients. It is helpful to reassure the patient and point out the transient nature of this instability in the diabetes.

Second Trimester

In the second trimester most women experience a gradual rise in their insulin requirements. This is approximately coincident with a rise in placental peptide and steroid hormones. By the end of the second trimester, the total insulin dosage may have doubled.

Third Trimester

The insulin dosage continues to rise gradually in the third trimester. The diabetes becomes much more stable and reactions less troublesome. Furthermore, if rebound hyperglycemia has been a problem it tends to diminish, and excellent control can be achieved with surprising ease.

TABLE 4   Insulin Dosage by Trimesters

First:	Same or even decreases; more reactions; less stable diabetes
Second:	Progressive increase; more complicated pattern often needed; more stable diabetes
Third:	Continued progression until late in trimester; may then decline; stable diabetes

It is also helpful to point out that there may be a decline in the insulin dosage in the last four to six weeks of pregnancy. This does not always occur but may be striking, resulting in as much as a 20 to 30 percent decrease in the dosage. This presumably results from the fetal-placental siphonage of glucose and amino acids from the maternal compartment. Before the advent of more sophisticated tests for assessment of fetal health, a falling insulin requirement sometimes indicated fetal distress. The physician no longer needs to worry when the insulin requirement falls, because other methods that are far more sensitive and far more reliable are available to assess fetal health.

SPECIAL TESTS

Alpha Fetoprotein

Neural tube anomalies are relatively common in infants of diabetic mothers. The measurement of alpha fetoprotein in maternal serum at 16 weeks gestation detects a high proportion of these anomalies if the defect is not closed. It should be noted that in diabetic women the serum level of alpha fetoprotein lags about two weeks behind that of nondiabetic women. Therefore the presence of a high normal value or a modestly elevated value may be significant if levels are compared with standards derived from nondiabetic women. The test suffers from some disadvantage because of its lack of sensitivity, but it does have a high specificity.

Ultrasound

Ultrasonography during pregnancy is helpful in several fashions. The first one should be performed 16 weeks after the last menstrual period to confirm the accuracy of the dates. It has the added benefit at this point of detecting gross fetal anomalies and in particular will invariably detect anencephaly. A second ultrasound should be performed 10 to 12 weeks later (week 26 to 28) to reconfirm the dates and to assess fetal growth. If 12 calendar weeks have elapsed the fetus should have a corresponding increase in size. The presence of macrosomia or hydramnios may also be detected at this time.

A third or even fourth ultrasound should be performed in late pregnancy. Macrosomia as well as polyhydramnios is much easier to detect at 32 to 34 weeks. It should be remembered that the growth curve of biparietal diameter which is used in dating the pregnancy begins to level at about this time. Therefore an ultrasound done beyond 32 weeks is not particularly reliable in dating the pregnancy. If an earlier one is not available, a great deal of confidence cannot be placed in the ultrasonographic interpretation of the length of gestation.

When amniocentesis is performed (see below) after 36 weeks it is usually done with ultrasonographic guidance, and the same information may be obtained as in one done at 32 to 34 weeks. Some may prefer to delay a third ultrasound to the time of amniocentesis and not do a fourth one.

Nonstress and Contraction Stress Test

The nonstress test examines the fetal heart rate in relation to fetal movement; a normal rate and presence of beat-to-beat variability indicate fetal health with a high degree of confidence. Fetal demise within one week after a normal nonstress test occurs only about 0.5 percent of the time. If a nonstress test is equivocal or nonreactive a contraction stress test should be performed. It is done by infusing a small amount of Pitocin and causing the uterus to contract 3 times within 10 minutes. These contractions subject the fetus to anoxia because of decreased ureteroplacental blood flow, and they normally cause no change in heart rate. The presence of a deceleration in heart rate following the contraction is an indicator of fetal distress and usually prompts Cesarean section. We perform the contraction stress test only if the nonstress test is abnormal.

Nonstress tests are begun on a weekly basis at 32 weeks of gestation. After admission to the hospital they are performed twice weekly.

Estriol

Estriol is a compound that may be measured in either maternal serum or urine. It is derived from a fetal adrenal precursor that is aromatized in the placenta, conjugated in maternal liver, and excreted in the urine. The measurement of either urinary or serum levels is satisfactory. In our institution we begin urinary collections at week 30 of pregnancy to provide an indication of the level of excretion. Some women may be "low excretors," or evidence of growth retardation may be indicated. The measurements are continued weekly until admission and then daily. The laboratory must report the result on the same day that the specimen is submitted, because a fall suggests fetal distress. The estriol in urine may be compared with the creatinine (estriol: creatinine ratio) so that variances in urine collection are corrected. A fall in estriol of more than 40 percent from the mean of the previous three days' excretion requires that an immediate nonstress or contraction stress test be done. If this result is normal, delivery does not have to be effected; if not, the obstetrician has little choice but to terminate the pregnancy.

Amniocentesis

An amniocentesis may be performed early in the second trimester for chromosomal analysis or confirmation of borderline elevation of maternal serum alpha fetoprotein. Amniotic fluid alpha fetoprotein is an even more sensitive detector of neural tube defect, but this is not routinely determined unless there is a high degree of suspicion of a neural tube defect that cannot be confirmed by ultrasound. If the level of alpha fetoprotein in amniotic fluid is equivocal, an acetylcholine esterase level may be determined.

Amniocentesis is routinely performed late in gestation to assess fetal lung maturity. Since the amniotic fluid is in direct contact with the fetal lung, several compounds may be measured. The most common compounds measured are lecithin and sphingomyelin. This ratio, called the L:S ratio, is generally thought to indicate maturity when it is greater than 2:1. However, there is some discrepancy in diabetic women between the actual development of lung maturity and the L:S ratio. A ratio of 3.5:1 gives an added degree of safety; no respiratory distress or only a very mild degree occurs when this value is achieved.

It is also possible to measure the disaturated phosphatidylcholine. Pulmonary maturity is indicated when this compound exceeds 500 mg/dl. There is little point in doing amniocentesis to determine lung maturity before 36 weeks, and it is often better to delay this procedure until the thirty-seventh or thirty-eighth week if fetal health is adequate.

DELIVERY

It is preferable to continue pregnancy to as near term as possible. If control of diabetes in the mother has not been ideal, as outlined earlier in this chapter, she should be admitted between the thirty-sixth and thirty-seventh week. If she has been able to achieve ideal control it is safe to allow her to remain out of the hospital until the thirty-eighth week. With each additional gestational week, it becomes easier and easier to induce labor, which is preferable to Cesarean section. If the cervix is not inducible and the thirty-ninth week has been reached, most obstetricians will opt for delivery at this point.

There are marked changes in insulin requirements on the day of delivery. On that day and on the first day thereafter, the maternal insulin requirement may be one-quarter to one-half that required before pregnancy. Since the insulin requirement may have risen substantially during the pregnancy, this will be a far smaller dose than she was taking on her last fully pregnant day. On the day of delivery (whether this results from induced labor, spontaneous labor, or a Cesarean section) the insulin may be given in either of two fashions. The simplest method is to use a small dose of intermediate insulin in the morning, again only one-quarter to one-half of the prepregnancy dose. If glucose monitoring is available on an hourly basis, an intravenous infusion of insulin may be used. This should be started at 1–2 units per hour and maintained at a sufficient rate to provide euglycemia.

During labor, whether spontaneous or induced, the insulin requirement is quite low and the use of subcutaneous intermediate insulin or intravenous crystalline insulin will result in excellent control of the blood sugar level. Five percent dextrose in water may be needed to prevent hypoglycemia. If a Cesarean section is to be performed, it is best to schedule it in the morning.

Once the patient reaches the recovery room another glucose measurement should be determined. It may be elevated because of the stress of the procedure, or because the anesthesiologist has infused large amounts of dextrose and water, or both. If epidural or spinal anesthesia is to be used, it is helpful to request the anesthesiologist not to use dextrose and water, but instead to use normal saline for volume expansion. A moderately elevated glucose level should not be vigorously treated in the recovery room because it will spontaneously decline over the next several hours. Most patients are especially sensitive to crystalline insulin. At the beginning of the first postpartum day, a small insulin dose similar to that given the day of delivery may be administered. Over the next several days and usually within a week, there will be an increase in the insulin dosage to the prepregnancy requirement or a bit below it. This can be adjusted on a daily basis by determining blood glucose levels.

If the patient is nursing, the pregancy diet should be continued when she is able to eat. This will provide additional calories to support lactation, but somewhat less than the total calorie requirement of the mother and infant. Since there is a physiologic accumulation of maternal fat during pregnancy, this slightly hypocaloric diet will allow the mother to lose weight gradually over the next month or two without compromising the nature of breast milk.

DIABETIC KETOACIDOSIS

ELLIOT J. RAYFIELD, M.D.
and EDMUND W. GIEGERICH, M.D.

Diabetic ketoacidosis accounts for 14 percent of all diabetic hospital admissions in the United States. The high morbidity and mortality rates that still exist despite recent advances in therapy make diabetic ketoacidosis a medical emergency necessitating prompt diagnosis and treatment. Prevention of the development of ketoacidosis requires both patient education and physician awareness of potential problems facing the diabetic patient. This discussion outlines the evaluation and treatment of the patient with diabetic ketoacidosis. Preventive measures that can be taken in both ambulatory and hospital settings are also addressed.

EVALUATION OF THE PATIENT

The onset of diabetes mellitus may be heralded by ketoacidosis in a patient in whom insulin deficiency is severe and unrecognized. The main precipitating factors in a patient with known diabetes are infection, inappropriate insulin therapy by patient or physician, trauma, myocardial infarction, and emotional stress. The evaluation of the patient is incomplete if these factors are not actively sought. Despite a thorough evaluation, up to 20 percent of patients may have no obvious cause. With the widespread use of home monitoring of blood glucose during the diabetic pregnancy, the occurrence of ketoacidosis is unusual. The high risk of fetal loss during ketoacidosis makes early diagnosis and therapy imperative, and fetal monitoring is recommended during therapy. Otherwise, the treatment for pregnant women is the same as presented in this chapter.

The initial diagnosis of ketoacidosis can usually be made by a combination of history, clinical examination, and simple diagnostic testing. Treatment should be instituted rapidly without waiting for extensive laboratory assessment. The hallmarks of diabetic ketoacidosis are dehydration in the presence of hyperglycemia and metabolic acidosis due to ketone bodies. The use of glucose oxidase reagent strips—Chemstrip bG (Bio-Dynamics, Inc.) by visual inspection, or Dextrostix (Ames) with a dextrometer—will give a close approximation of blood glucose concentrations in minutes. A semiquantitative estimation of plasma and urine ketone bodies can be made by using reagent tablets. The presence of dehydration, hyperglycemia, and ketonemia or large ketonuria will be sufficient indication for the initiation of therapy. The initial laboratory assessment in a patient thought to have diabetic ketoacidosis should include arterial blood gas measurements (pH, pO_2, pCO_2), a complete blood count, urinalysis, and serum determinations of glucose, ketones, electrolytes, urea nitrogen, creatinine, calcium, and phosphorus concentrations. Microbial cultures should be obtained when there is no obvious cause for ketoacidosis, especially in patients who are hypotensive, severely ill, or elderly. An electrocardiogram and chest x-ray are also recommended.

TREATMENT OF DIABETIC KETOACIDOSIS

The consequences of insulin deficiency are hyperglycemia, metabolic acidosis, and osmotic diuresis with concomitant fluid and electrolyte depletion. The objective of treatment is to correct these abnormalities simultaneously by providing insulin and appropriate fluid and electrolyte therapy, as well as to evaluate and treat the precipitating cause. Although therapy should be initiated promptly, treatment should be controlled to prevent iatrogenic complications related to too rapid replacement of insulin, fluids, or electrolytes. (Refer to Table 1 for an outline of treatment.)

TABLE 1 Management of Diabetic Ketoacidosis

1. Rapid clinical examination with special attention to (a) mental status, (b) cardiovascular status, (c) state of hydration, (d) source of infection
2. Confirm diagnosis rapidly using blood glucose reagent strips (Chemstrip bG or Dextrostix) and blood/urine screen for acetone. STAT laboratory assessment: glucose, pH and arterial blood gases, serum electrolytes, BUN, creatinine, calcium, phosphorus, CBC, and urinalysis. Microbial cultures, EKG, and chest x-ray as indicated
3. Diagnosis DKA confirmed; initiate therapy as follows:
   A. Insulin
      1) Intravenous regimen: Priming bolus of 6 units i.v. followed by a continuous i.v. infusion of 6 units/hour (pediatric age group 0.1 U/kg/hr). 12 units/hour recommended for patients with infection. Dose adjusted on basis of hourly blood glucose determinations. When blood glucose level reaches 250 mg/dl, insulin infusion should be decreased to 1–2 units/hour to maintain blood glucose at 150–200 mg/dl.
      2) Intramuscular regimen: Loading dose of 10–20 units i.m. with subsequent doses of 6 units i.m. per hour. Monitoring as for i.v. regimen. If no change in 2 hours, switch to i.v. regimen.
   B. Fluids and Electrolytes
      1) Fluids: Isotonic saline (0.9 percent NaCl) is the fluid of choice to restore blood volume. Initial rate 1 L/hr and subsequent fluid therapy 100–500 ml/hr based on clinical response. If serum Na rises > 145 mEq/L switch to 0.45 percent NaCl. When blood glucose reaches 250 mg/dl, add 5 percent dextrose to i.v. fluid at a rate of 100 ml/hr.
      2) Potassium: Withhold therapy until K^+ level is known. Initial rate of 20–30 mEq/hr adjusted to serial serum measurements; if $K^+ < 3.5$ mEq/L infuse K^+ at 40 mEq/M and $K^+ > 5.5$ mEq/L no potassium. Potassium in the form of chloride salt and 10 mM/hour as phosphate salt (if renal failure present, omit phosphate).
      3) Serial glucose and electrolyte measurements hourly until glucose level reaches 250 mg/dl, then every 2 to 4 hours.
      4) Bicarbonate is given for pH ≤ 7.0–7.1 in the form of an infusion of 44 mEq $NaHCO_3$ added to 1 liter of 0.45 percent NaCl with 20 mEq/L KCl over 1 hour. Goal of therapy is to raise pH to 7.2.
4. Ancillary measures: Antibiotics, O_2 for $pO_2 < 80$ mmHg, volume expanders for persistent hypotension, and central venous monitoring for patients with cardiovascular and renal disease.

Insulin

The aim of insulin therapy is to correct the metabolic abnormalities with minimal risk to the patient. The major change in the treatment of ketoacidosis in the last decade has been the trend toward administering insulin in lower doses either by continuous intravenous infusion or intermittent intramuscular injection. The high-dose insulin regimen used widely before the early 1970s required large doses of regular insulin given intravenously and subcutaneously, resulting in wide fluctuations of plasma insulin levels. The problems with this form of therapy include a higher incidence of late hypoglycemia and hypokalemia. Also, of concern is the possibility of osmotic disequilibrium syndrome caused by too rapid shift in blood glucose concentration. Insulin given subcutaneously in this setting will have an unpredictable absorption when the patient is initially hypovolemic, resulting in a potential depot for later absorption of insulin with fluid administration.

The favored route of administration at present is continuous "low-dose" insulin infusion. When insulin is administered as an intravenous bolus it has a circulating half-life of approximately 5 minutes. By contrast, intravenous insulin given as a continuous infusion has the advantage of achieving a relatively constant concentration after steady state is reached by 30 minutes. In steady state studies of intravenous insulin administration, for each unit of insulin infused per hour there is an increase of plasma insulin concentration of approximately 20 μU/ml. The question of how much insulin is necessary to treat diabetic ketoacidosis is controversial. Although a priming bolus of insulin is not necessary, it does provide an immediate therapeutic level; the recommended dose is the same as for the initial infusion rate. The insulin should be administered by continuous intravenous infusion at a rate of 6 units/hour for adults or 0.1 units/kg/hr for children. Two points are relevant to the issue of how much insulin needs to be administered continuously per hour. First, it has been demonstrated in several insulin-sensitive tissues, including isolated adipocytes, that maximum stimulation of glucose transport from the periphery into the cell requires only 10 percent of the insulin receptors to be occupied. A greater increase in insulin levels will not result in a further enhancement of biologic response because the rate limiting step(s) are distal to membrane receptors. Second, there are relative sensitivities of the effects of insulin on different cellular functions. For example, lipolysis, glycogenolysis, and gluconeogenesis can be inhibited by insulin levels of 10–20 μU/ml. Insulin levels of 100 μU/ml are necessary to inhibit hepatic ketogenesis, while concentrations of up to 200 μU/ml are required for maximal stimulation of peripheral glucose uptake. Thus the rate of insulin infusion suggested here (6 units/hour) achieves an average plasma insulin level of 120 μU/ml, which is sufficient to inhibit lipolysis, ketone body formation, and hepatic glucose production. For any patient with evidence of infection at the time of presentation, an infusion rate of 12 units/hour is suggested because of the resistance to insulin action which accompanies infections.

Although insulin adsorbs to plastic and glass, it is unnecessary to add albumin to the infusion. However, flushing the solution through the intravenous lines to saturate adsorption sites is recommended. Insulin can be administered by an infusion pump inserted into a separate vein or "piggybacked" onto the i.v. line delivering rehydration fluids. Insulin should not be added to the fluid used for rehydration. One has more control over the treatment regimen when the rates of insulin and fluid delivery can be monitored independently of each other. Insulin infusion should continue until both hyperglycemia and metabolic acidosis are corrected. The progress of therapy is assessed initially by serum glucose, ketone, and electrolyte determinations done hourly until the blood glucose reaches a level of 250 mg/dl, and then every 2 to 4 hours until the patient is restarted on his daily insulin dose. A glucose reflectance meter or glucose oxidase reagent strip should be used to avoid unnecessary delay in laboratory reporting and to facilitate therapeutic decisions. Assuming adequate rehydration, blood glucose levels usually fall at a rate of 75–100 mg/dl/hr. If no change in glucose level has occurred in two hours of therapy, the rate of insulin infusion should be doubled. At this point, the patient's rehydration status as well as the possibility of an occult infection should be reconsidered. Since hyperglycemia typically resolves prior to the acidosis, insulin therapy must be continued without inducing hypoglycemia. If acidosis or ketone bodies are present when the glucose level has fallen to 250 mg/dl, a glucose infusion (5 percent) should be administered at 100 cc/hr. The insulin infusion rate should be decreased to 1–2 units/hour to maintain blood sugar in the 150–200 mg/dl range until the patient is ready to eat. The insulin infusion should be continued for 2 hours after the patient's intermediate strength (NPH, Lente, Monotard, Lentard) insulin is restarted to prevent a rebound elevation of the blood glucose level. The intermediate insulin is generally restarted at the patient's usual dose. There is no particular advantage to using subcutaneous regular insulin on a four times daily schedule after the episode is corrected unless the patient is not able to eat and continuous intravenous insulin therapy cannot be safely monitored.

A simple alternative to continuous intravenous infusion therapy is to administer insulin as intermittent intramuscular injections. The advantages and therapeutic responses are similar to those noted with continuous intravenous infusion. The simplicity and safety of intramuscular insulin injection make it advantageous in a hospital without available house staff or nurse clinicians. This modality is not recommended for the hypotensive or inadequately hydrated patient. A loading dose of 10–20 units given intramuscularly is required, and subsequent doses of 6 units/hour i.m. are given. Monitoring is the same as for intravenous therapy and lack of response in the presence of adequate hydration should prompt a change to an intravenous infusion.

Some patients with ketoacidosis may manifest insulin resistance as a consequence of concurrent infection or high titers of IgG anti-insulin antibodies. Such patients may require 20 or more units of insulin per hour by continuous infusion to decrease blood glucose levels at an acceptable rate (75–100 mg/dl/hour) and the physician should empirically double the insulin infusion rate every 2 hours until an appropriate fall in blood glucose level is observed. This patient should also be treated with a single component, highly purified pork regular insulin (for example, Novo or Nordisk). The use of corticosteroids (as may sometimes be employed in treating insulin resistance due to IgG anti-insulin antibodies in the absence of ketoacidosis) is not recommended. For more details on the treatment of insulin resistance refer to Chapter 44.

Other patients with ketoacidosis may have a current history of systemic insulin allergy, that is, diffuse urticaria usually within a half-hour of insulin administration. In this type of patient fluid and electrolyte replacement as well as treatment of the acidosis with bicarbonate (if pH<7.2) should be carried out concomitantly with skin tests using both beef and pork insulin at a dilution of 1:1,000,000 (Lilly test kit). Since beef insulin is more allergenic than pork insulin, if the patient has a positive skin test to both beef and pork or beef insulin alone, he should be rapidly desensitized to pork insulin by the administration of serial dilutions of insulin (first intracutaneously, and then subcutaneously) every 20 minutes as tolerated. If the allergy is to pork insulin, the patient should be treated with beef insulin. Desensitization can be accomplished with either the Lilly test kit or the physician's own serial dilutions of a highly purified single component pork insulin (Novo or Nordisk) in an isotonic saline vehicle. The usual precautions for anaphylactic shock should be taken, including having a tracheotomy set at the bedside, as well as epinephrine, glucocorticoids, and anti-histamines. Once desensitization is accomplished, the ketoacidosis should be treated in the manner outlined above, but the patient should receive a highly purified single component pork insulin (Novo or Nordisk). For more details on the treatment of insulin allergy refer to Chapter 44.

Fluid and Electrolyte Therapy of Diabetic Ketoacidosis

The osmotic diuresis that occurs in diabetic ketoacidosis results in profound deficits in total body water and electrolytes. Estimates from balance studies indicate average deficits: water, 5–10 liters; sodium, 500 mM; potassium, 300–1000 mM; phosphorus, 67 mM; and magnesium, 37 mM. The marked dehydration is a result of a loss of water in excess of sodium. Attention must be paid to true hyponatremia on admission, since such patients may be at risk for the development of cerebral edema. The serum sodium level may be decreased 1.6 mEq/L for every 100 mg/dl elevation in blood glucose level, and this should be accounted for in assessing the laboratory data. Pseudohyponatremia may also result from hypertriglyceridemia. Isotonic saline (0.9 percent or 154 mM NaCl) is the fluid of choice because it restores circulating blood volume and tissue perfusion and prevents a rapid reversal of osmotic gradients as blood glucose levels fall with treatment. Volume expansion should be at an initial rate of 1 L/hr and a patient in shock should be given saline and volume expanders at an even more rapid rate. Saline infusion should be slowed as volume is restored and changed to 0.45% sodium chloride (77 mM) if serum sodium level rises above 145 mEq/L. The use of isotonic saline may be associated with the development of hyperchloremic metabolic acidosis following successful therapy of diabetic ketoacidosis. The bicarbonate deficit is of no consequence to the patient when there is no primary renal defect. The renal excretion of ammonium chloride during the next 24 to 48 hours will correct the bicarbonate deficit.

In the case of hypernatremia on presentation, the fluid of choice is 0.45 percent sodium chloride after circulating blood volume has been normalized. The patient with mild dehydration may be treated with 0.45 percent sodium chloride. Right- or left-sided heart venous pressure should be monitored closely in patients with conditions that are susceptible to volume overload (cardiac disease and chronic renal failure). A recent report has noted that volume loading with large amounts of crystalloid solution (0.45 percent sodium chloride) during the treatment of diabetic ketoacidosis may produce an acute hypo-oncotic state resulting in subclinical pulmonary and cerebral edema in otherwise healthy diabetic patients. This observation underscores the need for careful monitoring of the clinical course of patients with complicating medical illness for cardiovascular and central nervous system abnormalities that may result from treatment.

The total body deficits of potassium are large despite normal or high potassium levels on admission. With treatment of diabetic ketoacidosis, rehydration and insulin therapy cause a marked lowering of plasma potassium levels, which may result in life-threatening hypokalemia. Low-dose insulin therapy is associated with less precipitous declines in potassium levels. Since the total body potassium deficit is great and, owing to urinary losses only 50 percent of administered potassium in 24 hours is retained, total body replacement will take days to achieve. The major concern, therefore, is the prevention of hypokalemia. Potassium therapy is withheld until the serum level is known, and in most cases replacement therapy is begun when the concentration is at the upper half of the normal range. The patient who presents with a low serum potassium level should have vigorous replacement from the start of therapy and electrocardiographic monitoring until the potassium levels reach the normal range. Potassium therapy in all patients should be assessed on the basis of serum levels. An initial rate of 20–30 mEq/hr of potassium can be adjusted based on subsequent serum measurements. Potassium infusion at a rate greater than 40 mEq/hr is rarely indicated and should be done with caution. The predominant form should be potassium chloride salt and the remainder as potassium phosphate (see below). Care must be taken in oliguric patients or those with renal failure, who may need potassium replacement if serum levels fall. Since the usual urinary losses of administered potassium (approximately 50 percent) are not present, replacement should be in the form of potassium chloride at a reduced rate.

Total body phosphorus depletion has long been known to be a component of diabetic ketoacidosis, and there has been recent interest in adding phosphorus replacement to the treatment regimen. Phosphorus depletion theoretically may limit oxygen delivery to tissues by virtue of decreased 2-3DPG levels (which increase hemoglobin oxygen affinity) in addition to limiting phosphorus availability for high energy phosphate bonds. Severe hypophosphatemia may result in hemolysis, rhabdomyolysis, and cardiorespiratory and central nervous system dysfunction. In all series reported to date in which phosphorus repletion has been compared with standard therapy, there have been no changes in morbidity or mortality rates. In most patients, phosphorus levels are normal or high on presentation and fall with insulin and fluid therapy in a manner similar to potassium, since phosphorus is an intracellular anion. The patient with hypophosphatemia on presentation is at greatest risk for developing consequences of phosphorus deficiency. Current recommendations are to provide approximately 10 mM of phosphate per hour as a potassium solution (K 4.4 mEq/L, PO_4 3.0 mM/ml, Abbott) with careful monitoring of phosphorus, and calcium every 4 to 6 hours, since hyperphosphatemia may cause hypocalcemia with tetany. Phosphorus therapy is contraindicated in patients with renal insufficiency.

The use of bicarbonate therapy in cases of diabetic ketoacidosis is controversial. The rationale for bicarbonate therapy is simply to counteract the deleterious effects of acidosis in the short term, since appropriate insulin therapy will increase ketone body utilization and decrease ketone body production. However, the administration of bicarbonate may cause a paradoxic fall of cerebrospinal fluid pH which could alter the patient's mental status. Also, bicarbonate therapy may reverse acidosis relatively quickly with the occurrence of hypokalemia. The circumstances under which bicarbonate therapy should be considered are severe acidosis (pH$\leq$7.0–7.1), the presence of shock unresponsive to volume expansion, and concomitant lactic acidosis. Bicarbonate therapy should never be given in the form of an intravenous bolus, but 1 ampule of sodium bicarbonate (44 mEq/Na and 44 mEq/HCO_3) should be added to 1 liter 0.45 percent NaCl with 20 m Eq/L of potassium chloride and infused over a 1-hour period. The goal of therapy is to raise pH to 7.2 or the serum bicarbonate level to 12 mEq/L. Care should be taken to avoid fluid overload, which may occur with the administration of large amounts of sodium ion with the bicarbonate.

PREVENTION OF KETOACIDOSIS

The prevention of diabetic ketoacidosis requires prompt treatment of the precipitating cause as well as intensive therapy for the patient who suddenly begins to develop poor glucose control. Patients should be instructed to maintain fluid intake and, if the normal diet cannot be taken, nutrients should be in the form of carbohydrate containing fluids (juice or nondiet beverages). The patient should continue insulin therapy even though dietary intake is decreased to offset factors that will worsen control. Urine testing and fingerstick blood glucose determinations with glucose oxidase strips every 4 to 6 hours should guide supplemental insulin therapy. The physician should keep in close contact with such a patient as well as provide the patient with a sliding scale of how much additional rapid acting insulin (regular, Actrapid) should be given. An example of such a sliding scale based on home glucose monitoring in a patient taking a total of 40 units of insulin daily would be as follows: blood glucose 150–200 mg/dl; 5 units regular insulin; 200–300 mg/dl; 10 units regular insulin; 300–400 mg/dl; 15 units regular insulin. If vomiting and dehydration exist, the patient should be advised to seek early admission to the hospital.

The diabetic who presents for surgery, obstetric delivery, or in whom oral intake is contraindicated may be at risk for developing ketoacidosis. In this group of patients, continuous intravenous administration of insulin and glucose will prevent metabolic decompensation. On the day of surgery, we recommend holding all subcutaneous insulin and placing an intravenous line to deliver 5 percent glucose at a rate of 125 cc/hr. The insulin infusion rate is started at 1–2 units/hour with the insulin added to the glucose solution. The rate of insulin administration is regulated based on frequent glucose levels determined intraoperatively and postoperatively to establish a blood glucose level of 100–180 mg/dl. Potassium levels should be monitored and replacement given as necessary. Supplemental fluids should be given as required, but separately from the insulin infusion. During labor and delivery the maintenance of normoglycemia is crucial for the diabetic mother and infant. The goal is to maintain maternal blood glucose levels between 70 and 90 mg/dl with infusion of glucose and intravenous insulin monitored by hourly blood glucose measurements by fingerstick reagent strips. During active labor and the postpartum period insulin requirements drop precipitously and careful monitoring and adjustment of the infusion is required. In the diabetic patient who requires hyperalimentation, insulin is added to dextrose or parenteral nutrition solutions and the rates of insulin administration are guided by frequent glucose monitoring. Care must be taken in all patients that infusion is not discontinued without the addition of supplemental regular or intermediate acting insulin, as subsequent metabolic decompensation will result.

HYPEROSMOLAR COMA AND LACTIC ACIDOSIS

HUGH D. TILDESLEY, M.D.,
and ANTHONY D. MORRISON, M.D.

HYPEROSMOLAR COMA

Diagnosis

The syndrome of hyperosmolar, hyperglycemic, nonketotic coma has also been described as the hyperglycemic dehydration syndrome. It most often afflicts patients in middle or old age who were not previously known to be diabetic or who are non–insulin-requiring type II diabetics. Males and females are equally affected and patients usually have a family history of diabetes mellitus. The condition is frequently associated with a severe underlying illness, such as sepsis, congestive heart failure, or cerebral vascular accident. There is generally underlying renal insufficiency that is usually the result of senile nephrosclerosis. The syndrome has also been associated with medications—notably glucocorticoids, phenytoin, and thiazide diuretics—and with endocrine dysfunction, such as acromegaly, thyrotoxicosis, and Cushing's syndrome. Patients with burns, or

those who are undergoing major surgery in which hypothermia is used, are at particular risk of developing hyperosmolar coma. The syndrome can be iatrogenically precipitated by treating severely ill patients with hyperalimentation or with hypertonic glucose solutions for nutritional support. Similarly, uremic patients undergoing peritoneal dialysis with hypertonic glucose solutions are at increased risk.

Patients usually develop the classic hyperglycemic symptoms of polyuria, polydipsia, and weight loss, which increase in intensity in association with weakness and progressive change in mental status. These symptoms persist for several days to weeks, with an average duration of 12 days, before patients seek, or are brought to, medical attention.

Treatment

The patient with hyperosmolar coma has a medical emergency. The physician should evaluate the need for intubation and respiratory assistance and institute them if necessary. An intravenous site should be established, fluid replacement started, and baseline data, such as chest x-ray, electrocardiogram, and arterial blood gases obtained. External cardiac monitoring should be continued until the patient is stable. Patients in whom large volume replacement may be hazardous require a central line to record central venous or wedge pressures. Hourly recording of pulse, blood pressure, urinary output, electrolytes and glucose levels are important during the initial phase of management. An intensive care unit is the optimal environment for the early care of the patient.

Although there is a great temptation to treat primarily the abnormal laboratory values in these patients, it is mandatory that the physician aggressively pursue and treat any underlying condition.

The problems that must be addressed in a rational fashion are: (1) free water deficit; (2) sodium depletion; (3) potassium depletion; and (4) hyperglycemia (Table 1).

A decrease in total body water will be primarily reflected in the intracellular fluid space, which will bear two-thirds of the pure water deficit. The extracellular fluid space tends to be protected by the increased oncotic pressure of the plasma proteins. Therefore, true hypovolemic shock is a very late sign of pure water loss and almost always implies an associated sodium deficit. The usual symptoms and signs of water depletion are those of hypertonic depletion of the intra-

TABLE 1   Treatment Protocol for Hyperosmolar Coma

	Immediate	*Subsequent*
Fluids	1. 0.9% NaCl at 1 L/hour 2. Replace Na deficit 4–6 hours (500 mEq). 3. Monitor electrolytes hourly.	1. When blood pressure stable, urine output adequate, change to 0.45% NaCl 250–500 ml/hour. 2. When serum glucose 250 mg/dl, add 5% glucose to i.v. fluids. 3. Replace H_2O deficit over 12–24 hours (5–10 L).
Potassium	1. If serum K^+ high, begin KCl at 20 mEq/hour after urine output established 2. If serum K^+ normal or low, begin KCl at 20 mEq/hour immediately; reduce rate by 50% if patient is oliguric. 3. Measure K^+ hourly.	1. Adjust dose of KCl by serial serum K^+ measurements.
Insulin	1. Regular insulin 0.05–0.1 U/kg/hour i.v. Monitor glucose hourly.	1. Decrease infusion rate to 1–3 U/hour. When eating, switch to s.c. insulin. 2. Monitor glucose and electrolytes every 4 hours.

cellular and interstitial fluid spaces (that is, thirst, poor skin turgor, dry mucous membranes, fever, somnolence, and coma).

A total body deficiency of sodium will be reflected primarily in the extracellular fluid spaces. There is a very significant plasma volume depletion and the signs associated with this are tachycardia, hypotension, and oliguria. As total body sodium level decreases, there is a compensatory increase in the renin-angiotensin system with secondary hyperaldosteronism. This stimulates sodium reabsorption at the expense of increased potassium excretion. Therefore, patients with hyperosmolar coma not only have a 5–10 mEq/kg sodium deficit, but also at least a 5 mEq/kg potassium deficit.

The osmotically active glucose present with hyperglycemia will expand only the extracellular fluid space and actually decrease the water content of the intracellular fluid space. This is very important in understanding a rational basis for therapy. If a patient has a low plasma sodium, it may be only the very significant hyperglycemia that is keeping the intravascular space perfused. Therefore, in an elderly patient with significant arteriosclerotic vascular disease, one should be certain that the extracellular fluid space is re-expanded first before one loses the "beneficial" effect of the hyperglycemia.

Based on these problems, rational fluid therapy in hyperosmolar coma should take place in two stages: (1) rapid replacement of marked sodium deficit, and (2) rapid but incomplete replacement of water deficit.

Since hypovolemic shock is the most immediate threat of life, we feel that it is mandatory to initiate fluid therapy with normal saline. The reflex reaction to start therapy with hypotonic saline should be avoided, as the first concern must be to maintain extracellular volume. If one were to start therapy with one-quarter normal saline, only 90 ml out of each liter would actually remain in the intravascular fluid space, and more than 90 percent would be lost to intracellular or interstitial fluid spaces. Normal saline is more appropriate than plasma or albumin for initiating therapy, because these patients usually have a high plasma oncotic pressure and hyperviscosity. Normal saline should be given rapidly, at an initial rate of approximately 1 L/hour, through a large-bore catheter until the vital signs, including blood pressure and pulse rate, are stable and urine volume has increased.

By definition these patients are not acidotic, and therefore they will not have this stimulus to elevate the serum potassium level. However, hyperosmolality per se can draw potassium out of intracellular spaces, and patients will frequently present with high or high/normal potassium levels. As noted above, there is a total body potassium deficiency and serum electrolytes must be monitored at frequent intervals. Once a good urine output has been established, and potassium levels have come down to the range of 4 mEq/L, potassium should be added to the infusate. The patient should receive 20–40 mEq/L, and, since such an individual is also deficient in both chloride and phosphate, it is best to alternate potassium chloride with buffered potassium phosphate. Once the patient's vital signs have stabilized, fluid therapy can be changed to half-normal saline, if desired. It should be noted that potassium will usually have been added to the infusate by this time, thus increasing its osmolality.

If the patient is in shock when first seen by a physician, or if the serum sodium is low initially, it is best to start therapy just with normal saline and not initiate insulin treatment until the vital signs are stable. Under normal circumstances, however, one will also start insulin therapy because of the marked hyperglycemia present. Insulin should be given intravenously at the rate of 0.05–0.1 units/kg body weight/hour. As in diabetic ketoacidosis, this rate of insulin infusion usually brings blood glucose values down close to the normal range 6 to 12 hours after initiating therapy. However, a few patients will not respond to this low rate of insulin infusion; these patients have usually suffered some severe form of stress, such as myocardial infarction, cerebrovascular accident, or a severe burn. Therefore, in addition to electrolytes, blood glucose levels should be checked at frequent intervals, approximately every 1 to 2 hours. Allowing for fluid dilution, if there has not been a significant reduction in plasma glucose level within 4 hours after initiating therapy, the amount of insulin infused should be doubled. Once the serum glucose level falls below 200–250 mg/dl, a 5 percent dextrose solution should be added to the intravenous fluids.

When the patient is rehydrated, conscious, and eating on a regular basis, a regimen of short and intermediate-acting insulin can be given subcutaneously to replace the intravenous insulin drip. Many patients will be discharged without insulin therapy, with only a diabetic maintenance diet and possibly an oral hypoglycemic agent.

The syndrome has been associated with a number of complications, including convulsions, infection, shock, renal failure, deep vein thrombophlebitis, pulmonary embolism, and pancreatitis. These should be looked for and treated appropriately. In the literature, the overall mortality rate has varied between 15 and 50 percent. We feel that, with appropriate insulin and fluid therapy as outlined above, this mortality rate can be decreased very significantly below 50 percent. The cause of death is rarely attributed to hyperosmolar coma, but rather to the associated acute underlying illness or ensuing complications.

One must always keep in mind that these patients may have a combination of two or more types of metabolic coma and may therefore have a mixed clinical picture.

LACTIC ACIDOSIS

Diagnosis

Lactic acidosis is the most common cause of increased anion gap metabolic acidosis seen in medicine today. William Huckabee's description and classification proposed in 1961 are still valid. Type A lactic acidosis is seen secondary to tissue hypoperfusion, tissue hypoxia, or both. In this syndrome, an elevated blood lactate level is caused by increased production, decreased clearance of lactate, or frequently a combination of both these factors. These patients show clinical signs that give a clue as to the etiologic agent in their acidemic state. Evidence of peripheral cyanosis implies poor tissue perfusion, whereas central cyanosis indicates poor oxygenation. For the severely hypoxic patient, who is usually in shock, it is obvious that treatment, over and above all other considerations, must be directed toward relieving the cause of the hypoperfusion or tissue hypoxia.

Huckabee's type B lactic acidosis is not associated with a clearly demonstrable cause of tissue hypoxia producing the increased anion gap in the plasma electrolyte pattern and decreased systemic pH. There is usually a history of an accompanying and precipitating illness. The latter syndrome is seen most commonly in diabetics and in alcohol-induced hypoglycemia, uremia, various hereditary enzyme defects in gluconeogenesis, glycogen breakdown, or glycolysis, and occasionally in septicemia. Patients with type B lactic acidosis have a normal blood pressure, a warm periphery, and hyperventilation.

Treatment

Lactic acidosis has a poor prognosis—the mortality rate is in the range of 50 to 80 percent. It is thus obligatory that all patients with a significant lactic acidosis and arterial pH below 7.2 be admitted to an intensive care unit if available, where they can be monitored closely with respect to pulmonary and hemodynamic functions. An adequate history must be obtained and a complete physical examination performed in an effort to determine and correct the underlying cause of either type A or B lactic acidosis.

Digitalis, diuretic, or possibly vasodilator therapy for severe acute congestive heart failure should be instituted early and the pulmonary diastolic wedge pressure monitored to detect unsuspected hypovolemia. The lactic acidosis may be corrected merely with volume replacement using colloid or normal saline. In addition, oxygen therapy is usually required, as hypoxia is generally present. Sepsis not infrequently complicates the picture, and therefore antibiotics should be administered after obtaining appropriate cultures.

The insertion of an arterial line will facilitate monitoring of arterial H^+ ion concentration, PO_2, PCO_2, and bicarbonate. Blood gases, serum electrolytes, and blood glucose levels should be obtained hourly until these values stabilize. Chest x-rays and electrocardiograms should be performed initially and repeated as clinically indicated.

In addition to the mandatory correction of underlying causes, it is usually necessary to attempt to combat the acidosis directly with the use of intravenous sodium bicarbonate. One should not attempt to bring the pH back to 7.4, because rebound alkalosis can occur, contributing to even higher blood lactate levels. Instead, the serum bicarbonate should be kept above 9–10 mEq/L, which would equal a pH of approximately 7.2. For ease of calculation, it can be assumed that bicarbonate is distributed in approximately 50 percent of the body space, and therefore, if a 70 kg person has a serum bicarbonate level of 6 mEq/L, one should administer $(10 - 6) \times (0.5 \times 70)$, or 140 mEq of bicarbonate. Each 50 ml ampule of 7.5 percent sodium bicarbonate contains 44.6 mEq. The bicarbonate also can be given as a 5 percent or 600 mEq/L infusion. We feel that a continuous infusion of bicarbonate is preferable to repeated bolus infusions. Therefore, to replace 140 mEq of bicarbonate, one would require a little more than 230 ml of a 5 percent sodium bicarbonate infusion. The physician must keep in mind that a very significant amount of sodium is also being infused, and thus it is most important to continue monitoring the hemodynamic state of the patient. If necessary, diuretics can be employed and the urine electrolytes followed to avoid fluid overload. In addition, it is most important to recognize that one is not dealing merely with an acid-base formula, but with a live patient whose status is constantly changing. Frequent monitoring of blood gases and serum electrolytes is therefore necessary to adjust the therapy.

Because lactic acidosis is a true medical emergency, it is important to use all therapeutic modalities that might potentially be beneficial (Table 2). Thus efforts to direct pyruvate metabolism away from lactate and into mitochondrial pathways are essential. In addition to stopping new lactate formation, these provide the only rational means of directing the cytosolic and mitochondrial redox

TABLE 2   Therapy for Lactic Acidosis

Most important: Relieve or correct underlying cause of type A or type B lactic acidosis (hypoxia, hypovolemia, congestive heart failure, infection, diabetes, alcoholism, and so on).
Fluid, electrolyte and drug therapy
  1. Sodium bicarbonate (5% i.v. solution) to maintain arterial levels $\geq$ 10 mEq/L or pH $\geq$ 7.2
  2. Colloid if hypoperfusion secondary to hypovolemia exists
  3. Insulin drip at 2–3 U/hour in 5–10 percent dextrose or normal saline
  4. Thiamine 300 mg
Monitoring and laboratory
  1. Admit to intensive care unit, place Swan-Ganz catheter and monitor pressures to judge volume load.
  2. Hourly blood gases, glucose, electrolytes
Employ vasodilators or dialysis if indicated.

states toward their more oxidized ratios. The key regulatory step that largely controls the flow of pyruvate is the pyruvate dehydrogenase reaction. This enzyme requires insulin for full activation and it is also inhibited by elevated fatty acid levels. Therefore, in an effort to combat any inhibition of the pyruvate dehydrogenase enzyme which might be present, we routinely utilize intravenous insulin in therapy. For the hyperglycemic diabetic patient, insulin is infused at 2–3 units/hour in a normal saline solution. Patients with normal blood glucose levels can safely receive intravenous insulin when it is given in a 5 to 10 percent dextrose solution. Frequent blood glucose measurements will safeguard against hypoglycemia. Pyruvate dehydrogenase has an obligatory cofactor requirement for thiamine, and 300 mg of this vitamin are also administered.

Finally, in patients who develop severe sodium or volume overload or both associated with lactic acidosis and its therapy, or who have severe uremia, the use of hemo- or peritoneal dialysis should be considered. The use of dialysate containing bicarbonate in place of lactate will prevent rebound alkalosis that is frequently associated with treatment. It will also remove some of the circulating lactate, although dialysis per se does not correct the acidosis.

In summary, in the therapy of lactic acidosis it is first and foremost necessary to remove the underlying cause of the increased lactate production and/or its decreased utilization. It is important to monitor the pulmonary and hemodynamic indices continuously by frequent measurements of pulmonary wedge pressure, cardiac output and arterial blood gases. The response to therapy should be followed with serial determinations of serum electrolytes, bicarbonate, and blood sugar levels.

The use of aggresive therapy with bicarbonate and insulin has improved the success in treatment of lactic acidosis over the past few years.

DIABETIC NEUROPATHY

MAX ELLENBERG, M.D.

The most important fact to emphasize in the treatment of diabetic neuropathy is that there is no such entity as diabetic neuropathy; rather there are *diabetic neuropathies* with varying etiologic factors, pathogenesis, pathology, and clinical expression. It follows therefore that this heterogeneous group cannot be treated similarly and each syndrome must be considered separately. The corollary of this is that many generalizations that have been made in the description of and in the therapeutic recommendations for the diabetic neuropathies have little or limited validity.

The diabetic neuropathic complications that tend to clear do so spontaneously, aided perhaps by medication that at best facilitates the restoration to a normal state. These include peripheral neuropathy, mononeuropathy, diabetic amyotrophy, diabetic neuropathic cachexia, diabetic diarrhea, and orthostatic hypotension. When it is part of an acute diabetic neuropathy, orthostatic hypotension will disappear along with the other reversible manifestations. At times it may tend to disappear even when it is part of the slow ongoing autonomic neuropathy.

These observations suggest that the metabolic aspect, although playing a role, is not necessarily a definitive determinant in these types of neuropathy. In fact, any of these forms of neuropathy may become clinically apparent unrelated to the degree of control. Thus they may occur during good control, as the initial clinical presenting manifestation of diabetes without overt carbohydrate metabolic derangement, or after stress situations. It would be helpful to know what determines this

reversibility and how such knowledge can be applied to other forms that are not yet reversible. Solutions to these problems may offer an insight into the nature of the diabetic neuropathies.

From the clinical point of view diabetic neuropathies are best divided into two broad categories, namely, peripheral neuropathy and visceral (autonomic) neuropathy. Each will be discussed separately.

PERIPHERAL NEUROPATHY

This is the most common form of neuropathy in the diabetic. It is bilateral, symmetric, and most often occurs in the lower extremities. It may be asymptomatic with mild paresthesias, loss of ankle jerks, and impaired vibratory sensation, or it may be an extremely painful syndrome. The subclinical or mild forms probably result from the metabolic abnormalities and may be prevented by good control. However, the very painful forms are not necessarily related to control and frequently occur after the institution of good control, or after some stressful event, such as surgery, acute myocardial infarction, severe infection, and so on. The onset of neuropathy under such circumstances is not immediate but always follows a latent period of about two to four weeks, with an average of three weeks. The onset may be abrupt or it may be an acute exacerbation of an already existing neuropathy. These are among the most painful of all the diabetic peripheral neuropathies and, paradoxically, the more painful, the better the prognosis. In the older literature the precipitation of neuropathy following the institution of insulin therapy for control was referred to as "insulin neuritis." However, this concept has been completely discredited, because continuing treatment with insulin will not impede the disappearance of neuropathy and insulin should be continued under those conditions. In addition this form of neuropathy has been observed with every other form of hypoglycemic therapeutic modality, including stringent diet and each of the available oral hypoglycemic agents. This type of neuropathy is related to an acute change in the metabolic state and not to the therapeutic agent.

Although the more painful the neuropathy the better the prognosis, many of these patients are exposed to narcotic drugs for control of the pain. It is not unusual to see patients who have recovered from their neuropathy remain narcotic addicts. Therefore all efforts must be made to minimize or eliminate the use of narcotics. To do this, various drugs have been tried and some success has been acheived with phenytoin and the related drug carbamazepine. The rationale for their use is based on neurophysiologic experiments to find a drug that would control epileptiform seizures without producing marked soporific effects as with, for example, phenobarbital. In addition to the observation that phenytoin diminished the focus of cerebral excitation that leads to convulsions, additional experiments indicated that there is a definite effect on peripheral nerves. On the supposition that pain of peripheral nerve origin could be related to repetitive discharge, the drug was tried in cases of tic douloureux and met with considerable success. On the assumption that the symptoms of diabetic neuropathy might have a similar background, a therapeutic trial was undertaken. In the usual analeptic dose of 100 mg t.i.d., it has proved to be beneficial in about 60 to 85 percent of the cases. Since its maximum therapeutic blood level is obtained in 72 to 96 hours, the drug should be discontinued if there is no response in about 10 days. Because of its similarity in action to phenytoin, carbamazepine has been introduced. It has been equally successful, though accompanied by more frequent toxic effects. The initial dose of carbamazepine is 200 mg daily, which is gradually increased to 800 mg daily. These drugs are not the definitive answer to the treatment of diabetic neuropathy and certainly not a panacea, but they offer sufficient benefit to a sufficient number of patients to justify a trial.

Anorexia and depression are associated with the severe pain. It is my impression that these symptoms are part of the syndrome and actually may clear prior to the disappearance of the pain, hence the use of antidepressive drugs is indicated. There is no antidepressive drug that has any specific or superior benefit; therefore the simplest and safest should be prescribed initially. Much attention should be paid to the psyche of the patient and much encouragement is indicated. Warm baths and massage are helpful and exercise as tolerated must be encouraged. For treatment of pain, aspirin and propoxyphene along with the antidepressant drugs help considerably.

Upper Extremities

Neuropathy in diabetes also occurs in the upper extremities. One of the significant features is that most diabetics who are blind because of diabetic retinopathy have at least some degree of impairment of the sensitivities of the tufts of the fingers because of concomitant diabetic neuropathy. This impairs their ability to learn Braille and is in keeping with the experience that diabetics are poor students of this skill. Teachers of Braille must be informed of this and urged to devote extra attention to the special problem of diabetics.

Neuropathic Arthropathy

The Charcot joint is one of the extraordinary complications in diabetes. A Charcot joint can occur only if the sensory part of the nerve is impaired whereas the motor part of the nerve is intact. In the older literature it was reported that most of these patients eventually required amputations because of development of ulceration, infection, and gangrene. That is no longer the case, and indeed hardly occurs today. The treatment is to put the joint at rest, for which a multitude of orthopedic appliances are available. In our experience the most successful method is to use a walking cast for a period of about three to four months, during which time, although bony ankylosis does not occur, sufficient fibrous ankylosis takes place, permitting the patient to get around with a remarkable degree of agility.

Neuropathic Ulcer

A neuropathic ulcer can occur only in the foot insensitive to pain and at a site of pressure. In diabetes the neuropathic ulcer is highly characteristic. It is punched out, surrounded by heaped-up callous tissue with healthy looking granulation tissue at the base indicating that this is not a vascular phenomenon, and is always at a site of pressure. Since there is no way of treating the nerve pathology, all therapy must be directed toward relieving the pressure. This can be readily accomplished by putting the patient to bed, and healing of the ulcer will then ensue. However, when the patient gets out of bed the ulcer will recur. Therefore recourse has been made to many orthopedic appliances, such as metatarsal bars, wedges, inner soles, and so on. One of the best available treatments is to have a good podiatrist make an innerspace plastic sole shaped to the patient's foot. This relieves the pressure and leads to healing. Infection in these ulcers is not uncommon. When it does occur, aggressive use of antibiotics is indicated and incision and drainage may have to be undertaken. In particularly stubborn cases it is sometimes necessary to remove the cause of the pressure, specifically the head of the metatarsal involved. Surgery of this type is feasible even in the diabetic, because this is a neuropathic complication and not related to peripheral vascular insufficiency.

The Asymmetric Neuropathies

Mononeuropathy and Mononeuropathy Multiplex

These syndromes are unilateral, accompanied by pain that may be severe and distributed along the anatomic pathway of the affected nerve and is characterized by nocturnal exacerbation. Sensitivity of the skin is limited to the involved dermatome and the prognosis is usually good. The nerves of the extremities, including the femoral, peroneal, brachial, ulnar, radial, and median, are known to be affected. Involvement of the spinal nerves of the trunk recently has been thoroughly documented. Here awareness is essential for proper differential diagnosis, since so many other diseases may be simulated, such as angina, myocardial infarction, acute cholecystitis, renal colic, acute appendicitis and intra-abdominal surgical disease. Diagnosis, which is based on the anatomic distribution of the pain, its nocturnal exacerbation and localized skin sensitivity, helps prevent unnecessary treatment, including surgery. The prognosis is good and most cases tend to clear in about three months, though some may take longer. Although they seem to be helped by phenytoin or carbamazepine, the spontaneous reversal and self-limited course make this difficult to assess.

External Ocular Motor Paralysis

This is the most common of the mononeuropathies. The paralysis is preceded by ipsilateral pain in the distribution of the ophthalmic division of the trigeminal nerve and involves the sixth, third, and fourth nerves in order of frequency. This syndrome has the best prognosis of any diabetic neuropathic complication. It almost invariably clears in about three months. Since it is spontaneously reversible, no therapy is necessary. Many therapies have been touted as being of value, but their apparent benefit is purely coincidental. Another important point to recognize is that in the older literature the association of ipsilateral facial pain and external ocular muscle paralysis always evoked the specter of internal carotid artery aneurysm. Therefore all these patients formerly were subjected to cerebral arteriography. However, if this is recognized as a self-limited, spontaneously resolving syndrome, the patient may be spared this procedure.

Diabetic Amyotrophy

The essential differences from other peripheral diabetic neuropathic manifestations are the asymmetry, the minimal to absent sensory impairment, and involvement of proximal musculature. The chief clinical features are severe pain and marked weakness of the involved lower extremity. It is far more frequent in the older diabetic, and males are more susceptible than females. The prognosis is good and there is usually a spontaneous reversion of the syndrome. The therapy used for peripheral diabetic neuropathy, namely phenytoin and carbamazepine, antidepressants, and mild pain medication, appears to be beneficial.

Diabetic Neuropathic Cachexia

This clinical picture—which has been observed only in male patients, usually in the sixth decade of life—includes profound weight loss up to 100 pounds and representing up to 60 percent of the total body weight (the picture of advanced cachexia), severe pain, the presence of bilateral symmetric peripheral neuropathy, depression and anorexia, impotence, diabetes of a very mild degree, simultaneous onset of the neuropathy with the clinical diagnosis of diabetes and an excellent prognosis with uniformly satisfactory recovery in about one year. A remarkable feature is the absence of microangiopathy, in spite of the severe neuropathic involvement. Although there is no known specific therapy available, all these patients spontaneously improve to the point of complete recovery with restoration of previous weight levels and virtual elimination of neuritic symptoms; occasionally there may be persistence of some paresthesias.

It is important to recognize this syndrome and thus minimize the usual extensive diagnostic attempts to find the nonexistent occult neoplasm, as well as to appreciate the excellent prognosis.

VISCERAL (AUTONOMIC) NEUROPATHY

Gastroparesis Diabeticorum

Gastric involvement in diabetic neuropathy results from decreased peristalsis leading to delayed emptying and marked retention. It is associated with a patulous pylorus and increase in gastric secretions. The gastric dysfunction may lead to poor control of the diabetes, since absorption becomes irregular and unpredictable. In fact, when one encounters a diabetic difficult to control and the usual reasons for this are not evident, the possibility of underlying diabetic gastropathy must be suspected. In addition, there frequently is an ulcerlike syndrome, or nausea and vomiting. Therapy until recently has been challenging. A drug that is in many respects specific for the treatment of this condition, namely metoclopramide is now available. It is a dopamine antagonist and is cholinergic, increasing the amount of acetylcholine. Given in doses of 10 mg t.i.d. either orally or, if need be, parenterally, it has been effective in controlling this condition, especially during periods of exacerbation.

Diabetic Enteropathy

This syndrome, more usually referred to as diabetic diarrhea, is quite common. It must be emphasized that any and all causes of diarrhea may attack the diabetic and an appropriate differential diagnosis is essential. The clinical picture is characterized by spontaneous remissions and exacerbations. At least half of these patients respond satisfactorily to a broad-spectrum antibiotic. Usually the drug will lead to a progressive diminution of stools and disappearance of the syndrome. The patient then learns that at the slightest suggestion of recurrence he takes the antibiotic immediately and thus either avoids or sharply minimizes an episode. With passage of time the syndrome tends to disappear.

Genitourinary Tract

Neurogenic Vesical Dysfunction

Clinically the outstanding feature is the insidious nature of onset and progression of the bladder paralysis with urinary retention. The diagnosis is almost always incorrect and the patient is admitted to the hospital because of the markedly distended abdomen. When infection supervenes, frequency, dysuria, and urgency dominate the picture. Diabetic control may be difficult because of nonrepresentative fractional urine specimens and infection. In this situation blood glucose monitoring is of considerable aid. If untreated, upper urinary tract infection occurs because of ascending hydropyeloureteronephritis.

Treatment. Once the condition is diagnosed, immediate urinary diversion is essential. At first it may be necessary to resort to catheterization or suprapubic cystotomy. Antibiotics determined by culture and sensitivity, and parasympathetic agents are indicated. After about 14 days the catheter is removed and the patient encouraged to void every 3 to 4 hours; this is reinforced by manual (Credé) pressure plus parasympathetic drugs. Occasionally partial or, if the condition is not too far advanced, even complete reversion of the signs and symptoms may occur, as happens in about 40 percent of the patients. If residual urine still persists, one must resort to surgery. In these cases, resection of the internal sphincter (the bladder neck) is definitely indicated. The operation is readily performed and in properly selected cases the results are excellent.

The rationale of the operation is based on the fact that the propulsive power of the bladder cannot overcome the resistance of the vesical outlet (internal sphincter). What is needed, therefore, is a means to restore the "balance of power." Since there is no way yet to increase the contractility of the paralyzed detrusor, surgery corrects the imbalance by weakening the vesical neck sufficiently to enable the impaired muscle to expel the bladder contents completely. The procedure does not cause urinary incontinence, which is controlled by the external sphincter, because this muscle is anatomically separate from the bladder, is innervated by the pudendal nerve which is under voluntary control, and is not involved in the surgery. Thus the operation closely approximates the ultimate goal of elimination of incontinence, residual urine, and infection. One of the side effects of the procedure may be retrograde ejaculation.

In the incipient asymptomatic neurogenic bladder, treatment is comparable to that of the nonsurgical treatment of the paralytic bladder. It involves scheduled voidings, double and triple voiding techniques, and the Credé maneuver. Scheduled voidings every 3 hours will compensate for the patient's lack of desire to void or help diminish the amount of residual urine. The patient also may be instructed to void again shortly after the initial voiding to help compensate for detrusor contraction.

Bethanechol has long been successfully utilized in diabetic cystopathy. Many patients appear to benefit from the administration of 25 to 100 mg of this substance every 6 to 8 hours. This group consists of those with a residual urine ranging from 100 to 500 cc. In more severe cases subcutaneous bethanechol, 2.5 to 10 mg, is administered every

6 to 8 hours. This is occasionally used in conjunction with intermittent catheterization. It is continued until the residual urine is lowered to approximately 100 cc of less, at which time the patient is converted to oral therapy. Phenoxybenzamine, an alpha-adrenergic blocking agent, may also be added in some cases to help decrease the outflow resistance generated by the bladder neck and external urethral sphincter. Dosages of 10 to 20 mg daily are usually effective in these instances.

SEXUAL PROBLEMS IN THE DIABETIC

In the diabetic male there are two important sexual problems: retrograde ejaculation and impotence.

Retrograde Ejaculation

Retrograde ejaculation in the diabetic is a neuropathic phenomenon resulting form involvement of the sympathetic components of the autonomic nervous system. This component regulates the closure of the internal sphincter at the time of emission and ejaculation. When it is not functioning, the sphincter does not close and the ejaculate, instead of being propelled antegrade, takes the path of least resistance and travels retrograde into the bladder. It is important to remember that this can be a cause of sterility in the diabetic male. It should also be borne in mind that progressive and as yet incomplete forms of retrograde ejaculation can lead to infertility. Hence in the investigation of sterility or infertility in diabetes one must always consider the possibility of retrograde ejaculation. In the early stages sympathomimetic drugs, such as antihistamines, have been reported to prevent retrograde ejaculation. In the presence of complete retrograde ejaculation successful attempts at impregnation have been accomplished by catheterizing the bladder immediately after masturbation or intercourse. The sperm are isolated and used for artificial insemination.

Impotence

It is important to appreciate the fact that any and all causes of impotence may affect the diabetic male. Therefore the differential diagnosis becomes especially significant. If it results from psychogenic factors, the approach must be along psychiatric lines. If vascular involvement is the cause, vascular reconstructive surgery is indicated. If due to any underlying endocrine basis, the appropriate endocrine replacement therapy is indicated, including the use of bromocriptine for hyperprolactinemia. When impotence results from poorly controlled diabetes it is a reflection of the associated malnutrition and weakness and not the diabetes per se. In such cases proper management of the metabolic aspect of the disease leading to the restoration of health and vigor will restore potency. If drugs are the cause, their withdrawal is usually followed by the return of potency; the antihypertensive drugs that often act via the autonomic nervous system have become a very important and relatively common factor in this type of impotence.

In most cases however, the cause is neurogenic and unfortunately there is no specific therapy. Hence, the prognosis in these cases is poor. However, mechanical devices have been suggested and have been found to be beneficial. The implantation of a silicone prosthesis (Small-Carrion) is a static approach that results in a permanent semi-erection that affords sufficient rigidity to permit vaginal penetration. A more complex and dynamic prosthesis consisting of a fluid storage reservoir surgically implanted in the abdomen, inflatable cylinders in the penis, and a pump in the testicular area produces an actual erection that is under control of the patient. The relative simplicity and safety of the silicone prosthesis as well as greater familiarity with its surgical and clinical aspects have made this our choice.

There are several important clinical implications. Inasmuch as patients do not readily volunteer information about sexual problems, they must be tactfully queried. The frequency of impotence is directly related to the manner in which the patient is approached. Most patients are relieved to learn that impotence is organic and hence not a reflection on their virility or manhood, a source of great insecurity and marked destruction of self-image. Further, it is important to remember that all these men had at one time been potent; with the onset of impotence they are often accused of infidelity. This can precipitate intense marital friction and distress, sometimes leading to separation and even divorce. Discussion with both partners and presentation of the facts will often allay anxiety and lead to a satisfactory emotional adjustment.

ORTHOSTATIC HYPOTENSION

This is probably the most incapacitating feature of chronic autonomic failure. Mild cases require little if any therapy but the more severe may even develop convulsions. Many modalities have been tried, but the best available and most dependable one is the use of 9A-fluorohydrocortisone. This is given in incremental dosage of 0.05 mg until the therapeutic goal is reached. One of the problems is the tendency of this drug to induce salt retention superimposed upon impaired renal function. Another approach is to use an Air Force antigravity suit, which has proven successful. Recently a beta-adrenoceptor antagonist, pindolol, has been used on the premise that those patients have low concentrations of circulating noradrenalin and have a supersensitivity to catecholamines. This suggests that beta-adrenoceptor blocking drugs with intense sympathomimetic activity might have therapeutic benefits. In a preliminary report involving three bedridden patients, the drug produced marked clinical improvement. The patients were free of all orthostatic symptoms; they could walk and standing blood pressure was maintained at above 90/50 mm hg; further studies are necessary.

POSSIBLE NEW THERAPEUTIC APPROACHES

Aldose Reductase Inhibitors

The demonstration of the existence of the sorbitol pathway and the involvement of the Schwann cell in this pathway have created interest along these lines. The accumulation of sorbitol in the Schwann cells in diabetic animals is associated with impaired nerve conduction velocity, which is restored to normal by control of the diabetes. The key feature in the sorbitol pathway is intracellular accumulation of the sorbitol resulting from the presence of unlimited amounts of aldose reductase, the enzyme which converts glucose to sorbitol. It would appear theoretically that an aldose reductase inhibitor could stop this, thereby preventing cellular damage and hopefully the subsequent development of neuropathy. One such inhibitor, CP 54634, has been used to treat diabetics with neuropathy. Although some promising results have been suggested, details are not yet available as to the clinical improvement of the diabetic neuropathic symptoms or toxic manifestations. In different study, Alrestatin, another aldose reductase inhibitor, was used for four months in nine patients with diabetic peripheral neuropathy. Most of the patients had subjective benefits but the study failed to show any objective benefits. In addition substantial toxicity was evident, including photosensitive skin rashes, nausea that limited the tolerated

dose, and hepatitis. Four of the nine patients were unable to complete the trial because of toxicity.

It would seem that although there is sufficient justification to pursue further study of this type of therapy, one must be careful about toxic effects and establish appropriate parameters to determine benefits before it is ready for general use.

Myoinositol

Myoinositol has an extraordinarily high concentration in nerve tissue. In diabetes the metabolism of myoinositol is profoundly altered in both man and experimental animal. For example, soon after the induction of experimental diabetes in the rat there is a sharp decrease in the sciatic nerve content of free myoinositol accompanied by an equally sharp decrease in the motor conduction velocity as well as a decrease in the total nerve protein content. These abnormalities can be prevented by rigid control of the blood sugar with insulin. Feeding of streptozotocin diabetic rats with a diet high in myoinositol tends to normalize the nerve content as well as the impaired motor nerve conduction velocity. Although evidence for a role of myoinositol in human diabetic neuropathy is very scant, some success has been recorded with an increase in the depressed motor nerve conduction velocity and symptomatic improvement. I have not observed this. It is tempting to speculate that any metabolic interference with the handling of myoinositol could result in both functional and structural abnormalities. However, although the depletion of myoinositol may be a factor, it is also possible that this depletion is a reflection of the metabolic deterioration that ensues with the onset of neuropathic changes.

DIABETIC RETINOPATHY

J. WALLACE McMEEL, M.D.

As the incidence of blindness due to diabetic retinopathy has increased over the past decade, there has been a commensurate development of treatments for this problem. Some treatments have been of demonstrable value, whereas others remain speculative; some are medical and others surgical; and some are prophylactic rather than reparative. Although the three aspects noted above pertain to all treatments, for this chapter the framework for presentation will be by method of treatment, which is determined by the character of the retinopathy.

The two major categories of retinopathy, nonproliferative and proliferative diabetic retinopathy, require significantly different treatment. Treatment for nonproliferative retinopathy has been primarily by photocoagulation or medical therapy, whereas proliferative retinopathy is treated not only by photocoagulation, but also by various surgical techniques.

PATHOGENESIS

A brief resumé of the pathogenesis and natural history affords an insight into the rationale of the various treatments. A relative hypoxia of the retina probably initiates the changes of nonproliferative diabetic retinopathy (NPDR). Factors suspected of being related to the production of the relative hypoxia in diabetic retinopathy are (1) impaired oxygen release from oxyhemoglobin; (2) altered rheologic characteristics of blood; and (3) altered permeability of the retinal capillaries. The above phenomena may contribute to the development of retinal edema, hard exudates, and intraretinal hemorrhages, as well as capillary closure, which in turn may accelerate their appearance. Venous dilatation, segmentation, and tortuosity may also be sequelae that contribute further to the vicious cycle producing tissue hypoxia.

These intraretinal changes warrant treatment when macular vision is threatened, or when neovascularization develops in response to some vasoformative factor related to the relative hypoxia. This neovascularization may be either flat or elevated. The tufts of new vessels away from the disk are often at the edge of an area of capillary closure, but new vessels at the disk have no such apparent relationship. Although the new vessels appear initially naked, fibrotic tissue usually develops about them, ultimately becoming more prominent than the neovascularization.

The changes in the vitreous gel itself probably are significant in the development of proliferative retinopathy. Patients with juvenile onset diabetes develop proliferative retinopathy of a significant degree much more frequently than the adult onset

diabetic whose disease does not appear until after the age of 40. One demonstrable difference between these two groups is the state of the vitreous. In the adolescent and young adult the vitreous gel is still in contact with the retina at a time when neovascularization is developing. This theoretically allows the formation of strong adhesions between these new vessels and the posterior hyaloid face. Therefore, when the hyaloid face begins to shrink, it exerts traction on these abnormal vessels. Thus not only is a potential scaffolding afforded to these vessels, but a physical factor, the mild constant traction on the abnormal vessels, may possibly enhance their growth into the vitreous cavity. Vitreous studies among diabetics show that the initial areas of vitreous detachment are in the periphery. The second most frequent area to become detached is the posterior pole itself. The last areas from which the vitreous detaches are over the disk itself and the arcade of temporal vessels. These are the areas in which the abnormal vessels associated with proliferative diabetic retinopathy are most frequently seen.

These fibrovascular proliferations often protrude into the vitreous cavity, growing along the posterior hyaloid face surface of the vitreous body along the arcades of the superior and inferior temporal vessels, or as a central mass overlying the disk. Vitreous contraction may further complicate the picture, particularly if adhesions have developed, as the centripetal traction may produce vitreous hemorrhage or various traction phenomena, such as traction detachment of the retina, traction schisis, isolated retinal holes without detachment, or rhegmatogenous detachment of the retina. Each requires a special type of therapy.

TREATMENT

The three general categories of treatment will be presented in the following order: (1) thermal destruction of tissue; (2) surgical intervention; and (3) medical treatment; this order reflects the relative degree of frequency of use and certainty of effects of these modalities.

Thermal Destruction of Tissue

Photocoagulation

The most widespread and demonstrably effective treatment for diabetic retinopathy at present is photocoagulation, introduced by Meyer-

Schwicherath over 20 years ago. The xenon arc (white light) photocoagulation of the 1960s has been largely superseded by the argon laser in the past decade. The blue-green light of the argon laser is avidly absorbed by the red hemoglobin in the blood vessels and by the melanin containing tissues (pigment epithelium and choroid). Recently, red light from the krypton laser has also been found useful in certain instances.

Conditions necessary for optimal photocoagulation are (1) maximum heat absorption at the target tissue with minimal absorption elsewhere; and (2) proper visualization of the tissue being treated. These require media that are clear or nearly so, and a pupil 5 mm or more in diameter. These conditions are less often fulfilled in diabetics who may have premature lens opacity, a hazy vitreous from protein transudation of hemorrhage from abnormal new vessels, or a poorly dilating pupil.

Instrumentation. The argon laser, which produces a continuous wave, is used with a slit lamp delivery system in all its commercially available models. The beam is prefocused to be parfocal with the plane of the slit lamp observation system, requiring a contact lens with a flat anterior surface. As the beam is prefocused, the energy in the beam is constant, with the energy density of the spot focused on the retina being inversely proportional to the spot size. Thus a small spot will receive a stronger burn than a large one with the same power setting. This requires the reduction of power when shifting to a smaller spot size. Otherwise a mini-explosion may occur in the retina. The duration of application is usually 0.1 or 0.2 sec and the spot size varies from 50 to 1000 μ. Thus the discomfort associated with the burn is slight enough so one can avoid retrobulbar anesthesia in all but a few instances.

The power delivered is sufficient to treat most problems requiring photocoagulation. These include all peripheral lesions, microaneurysms, intraretinal hemorrhages, localized areas of capillary closure, capillary dilatation, fluorescein leakage, retinal edema, and flat or elevated neovascularization, whether in a directed pattern to each specific lesion or by panretinal photocoagulation (to be described later). Perimuscular lesions and new vessels at the disk are more discretely and safely treated by small diameter burns (50–250 μ).

The commercial krypton-red lasers have the same delivery system as the argon laser. The krypton laser's main advantage is in treating through hazy media, either lens or vitreous. The red wavelength is the optimal one to penetrate the lens xanthophyll pigment in the elderly person with diffuse haze in the lens. Also, the vitreous cavity of an eye with a mild vitreous hemorrhage is penetrated more easily with the red krypton beam than with the green or blue wavelengths of the argon, which would be more absorbed by the intravitreous hemoglobin. Therefore, its greatest use is in treatment of eyes whose media are too hazy to permit treatment by the blue or green wavelengths of the argon laser. However, absence of absorption of the red wavelength by hemoglobin greatly limits its usefulness in direct treatment of abnormal new vessels.

As nonproliferative and proliferative diabetic retinopathy differ with regard to indications for treatment, technique, and results, photocoagulation of each will be discussed separately.

Nonproliferative Diabetic Retinopathy (NPDR). The rationale for treatment of the nonproliferative changes (edema, circinate exudates, intraretinal hemorrhages, capillary closure or shunt formation, and venous dilatation or tortuosity) relates to the destruction of retinal tissue in which a relative hypoxia exists. Theoretically, this destruction may reduce the relative hypoxia by lessening the nutritional needs of the retinal tissue, allowing the available nutrients to supply the remaining tissue more adequately. In support of this suggested mechanism is the observation that, by destroying areas of the external retinal layers by photocoagulation burns, the portions of the retina with the highest O_2 requirement are scarred, leaving more O_2 for the less well oxygenated inner layers. Also, a vasoproliferative factor associated with a relative hypoxia may likewise be eliminated.

Indications for treatment of NPDR are not rigid, but certain guidelines help delineate appropriate eyes for photocoagulation. In addition to the anatomic changes noted below, the visual acuity should be 20/40 or less, unless there has been good evidence of deterioration to 20/30 from 20/20. A fluorescein angiogram is most effective in uncovering microaneurysms, sites of fluorescein leakage, and capillary closure—important landmarks for placement of treatment. In the absence of these, photocoagulation is probably not indicated. Ophthalmoscopic evidence of retinal edema, circinate hard exudates, intraretinal hemorrhage, and venous changes in variable combinations may indicate a need for photocoagulation. If there is only a mild to moderate scattering of intraretinal hemorrhage, with a good visual acuity and minimal or no macular involvement by exudates or edema or fluorescein leakage, periodic observation may be preferable to photocoagulation.

Photocoagulation of NPDR is usually for maculopathy, although peripheral changes, when present, are also treated. Photocoagulation to extensive areas of capillary closure in the near periphery is occasionally indicated even though the macula appears normal and the acuity is good.

In photocoagulation of maculopathy, localized areas of disease, such as clusters of microaneurysms, fluorescein leakage, and islands of capillary closure, are prime targets, with circinate hard exudates often delimiting these areas. Less discrete are the zones where edema, intraretinal hemorrhage, and capillary dilatation merge with normal retina. Except for infrequent instances, in which only well-demarcated discrete areas are photocoagulated, treatment requires at least a perimacular barrage, and often panretinal photocoagulation (PRP) as well. The rationale for their use has been described above.

Extensive diffuse photocoagulation away from the macula evolved initially from the photocoagulation of lesions of hemorrhage, exudates, and areas of edema of NPDR as well as new vessels. Successes with this prompted experimentation with patterns of a more formalized nature, such as placement of burns along arteries or veins. The random scatter without direct photocoagulation to vascular lesions by ruby laser, as used by Beetham and Aiello, showed a beneficial effect on eyes with nonproliferative retinopathy or minimal neovascularization. The culmination of these observations resulted in the inclusion of the PRP as part of the protocol of the Diabetic Retinopathy Study (DRS), sponsored by the National Eye Institute.

The efficacy of PRP in earlier stages of nonproliferative diabetic retinopathy is now being tested in the Early Treatment Diabetic Retinopathy Study (ETDRS). This latter group represents a significantly earlier stage of the disease when the changes are primarily those of nonproliferative diabetic retinopathy.

Technique for Treatment of Focal Lesions. The technique for focal and perimacular treatment will be described first, followed by the adaptations for PRP.

Optimal treatment of focal lesions, particularly those about the macula, requires careful pretreatment documentation by fundus photography and fluorescein angiography, with referral to them intermittently during the treatment session. Several

such schemata have developed. The argon laser with the Goldmann contact lens is the best way to treat this area. The mass of the Goldmann three-mirror contact lens plus slight pressure as it is held help immobilize the eye. A magnification of $10 \times$ in the observation system affords a good compromise between adequate magnification and sufficient field. I use a burn of 250 μ applied to lesions in the perimacular region and 500 μ to those more peripheral. A gray burn that appears immediately is usually sufficient to produce the desired lesion. The initial test burn is made at the edge further from the macula, with a power setting of 100 mW. Power is increased at intervals of 50 mW until the proper intensity is obtained. More central areas of focal lesions may be more edematous and require more power to produce equivalent burns. Burns may be almost confluent if the lesions are clustered. The scatter pattern within the edematous center of a circinate rim of hard exudates is made so the treated and untreated areas are approximately equal. When there are insufficient localizing lesions, an arc of several rows of application is made, leaving only the maculopapillary bundle untreated. If there are retinopathic changes elsewhere, they may be either by focal scatter treatment directly to the lesions or a PRP.

In PRP, the burns are placed at regular intervals throughout the fundus. The intensity of the burn is similar to that in the perimacular barrage; the immediate appearance is that of gray spot. The space between burns may vary but usually approximates the diameter of the burn itself, making the treated and untreated areas approximately equal. The number of applications depends on spot size, fewer being necessary with larger burns. When using 500 μ burns, 1000 to 2000 applications are made. The total tissue destruction is approximately 20 percent of the retinal tissue. As the purpose is to destroy tissue, direct treatment of specific lesions is not necessary, except new vessels.

The posterior limit of photocoagulation is one to two disk diameters from the optic nerve, except between the arcs made by the upper and lower temporal vessels about the macula. In this area, the most posterior applications are made just within the arc of vessels and join three or four disk diameters temporal to the macula. Anterior limits vary, but approximate the level of the vortex veins.

Specifics of techniques vary little among the photocoagulation therapists.

I find the 500 μ spot size and burn duration of 0.2 sec a good compromise in obtaining adequate tissue destruction with minimal discomfort to the patient. Smaller burns (200 μ) may be given within the posterior pole. An initial power setting of 100 mW with increments of 50 mW allows one to arrive at an appropriate power level rapidly and safely. To lessen discomfort, one may reduce spot size and duration while increasing power.

PRP has been applied in both single and multiple sessions. In the latter, variables include the time interval between sessions (two days to two months), the number of sessions (two to five), and sequence of applications (quadrantic, posterior pole first, periphery first).

When treating a progressive angiopathic retinopathy in a young individual, it is preferable to treat aggressively by making the burns more closely spaced, by slightly increasing the intensity of the burns, and by making the time interval shorter between treatment episodes. The older patient may be treated in a more leisurely, deliberate fashion.

Proliferative Diabetic Retinopathy. The treatment of PDR is limited to abnormal new vessels, as the response of fibrotic tissue to photocoagulation is either nil or deleterious. The purpose of photocoagulation of new vessels is to destroy sources of potential bleeding or obliterate potential sites of development of fibrotic tissue. Certain characteristics of the lesions allow optimal energy absorption by the vessel being treated, with a minimal threat to visual loss. The features that enhance prospects for successful treatment of the new vessels are as follows: Such vessels are flat, peripheral, discrete, and devoid of fibrosis. These features may act as guidelines regarding indications for photocoagulation. Conversely, new vessels that are elevated, at the disk diffuse, or interspersed with fibrosis are less apt to respond favorably to photocoagulation. The end point one seeks in the photocoagulation of new vessels is stagnation or fragmentation of the blood column. This may be achieved at a single sitting with peripheral lesions, but constraints on strength and duration of application near the disk or macula require multiple sessions to obliterate those new vessels. The follow-up session might be from a few hours to a few days later.

Three sequences of photocoagulation may be used: (1) closing feeder arterioles before applying a barrage to the entire area of new vessels; (2) treating the periphery of the vascular network first and then working toward the base; and (3) crossing the area of new vessels in a barrage.

Closing the feeders is preferable if rapid sequence angiography in the early phases of the transit discloses the afferent arterioles. If they cannot be found, treating the most peripheral area first and working toward the area of the suspected afferent arterioles minimizes the chances of producing hemorrhage. Closing efferent venules first may dam blood in the new vessels, increasing the possibility of their rupture.

If no specific area of inflow or outflow is suggested, a barrage may be performed. The initial applications over the area should blanch the retina and constrict the vessel minimally. A barrage of stronger application is then made to immobilize or fragment the blood column. One or two rows of photocoagulation are placed around the area of neovascularization to minimize the chance of new vessels extending into the adjacent retina. It may be safer to apply photocoagulation to new vessels at a lower level three or four times during a treatment episode than to treat an area only once, but with high energy levels. Also, a slightly longer duration of application, such as 0.2 or 0.3 sec at lower intensity, is probably less apt to produce iatrogenic hemorrhage than shorter applications (0.05 to 0.1 sec) at higher power levels.

Technique for Treatment of Proliferative Retinopathy. Although the fibrotic component of PDR is important from a prognostic point of view, its presence or absence does not greatly alter the specifics of the treatment to the new vessels. The krypton-red laser is contraindicated in the direct treatment of abnormal new vessels because no significant heating of the blood column or vessels occurs owing to the minimal absorption of this wavelength by hemoglobin.

Peripheral, Flat: These lesions are the easiest to treat; there is good heat absorption and strong applications can be made without undue encroachment on the visual field or threat of thermal optic neuritis. Large, strong applications of relatively long duration can be applied until the desired vessel changes have been produced.

Peripheral, Elevated: The elevated vessels themselves usually do not contain sufficient hemoglobin to absorb enough energy to affect the vessel. Thus one must treat the feeding arteriole flat on the surface of the retina before it becomes elevated. The arteriole treatment may be part of the normal vascular arborization of the retina. The burn must be of sufficient diameter to straddle the arteriole. The initial burns should be sufficient to make the retina gray. The applications are placed five or six disk diameters posterior to the point where the elevated vessels leave the retina, and thence from "upstream to downstream" to the take-off point. The power is increased in increments of 50 mW and the process repeated. This sequence can be repeated until the vessel shows crimping. Fragmentation and stagnation are difficult to achieve and potentially dangerous to produce. In clear media, 400 mW is about the maximum power I use. Retreatment is usually indicated, preferably before the edema of the first treatment has cleared. Only infrequently are the elevated vessels sufficiently engorged with blood to absorb sufficient energy to show the effects of photocoagulation.

Disc, Flat: As many disk vessels atrophy after PRP, direct treatment of new vessels at the disk should probably be postponed until two to three months after aggressive PRP, unless the new vessel size approaches that of the major branches of normal arborization. If discovered, feeder arterioles should be treated by repeat runs of applications directly over the vessel, starting at the disk and going peripherally, in the manner described above. Direct applications to the peripheral portions of the neovascular network are followed by more centripetal burns. In the area about the disk, aggressive treatment is preferable on the initial session of treatment, as the swollen white retina protects the nerve fiber layer from the heat absorbed at the level of the pigment epithelium. The repeat episodes in the initial session can be given with relative safety. Later, when the nerve fiber layer lies in contact with the pigment epithelium, even a minimal burn may produce a large field defect. There is less danger of iatrogenic hemorrhage if more applications at lower power level are used to reach the end point of stagnation or fragmentation.

Disc, Elevated: This carries the most guarded prognosis of the four groups of new vessels. The caveats mentioned above pertain to this group as well. It is important to be aware of the danger of thermal optic neuritis if there is only partial absorption of the laser energy by an insufficient amount of hemoglobin in the vessels, particularly if the cone of laser light is focused so the spot size is smaller at the level of the disk than at the plane of the treated vessel.

The most comprehensive evaluation of the effect of photocoagulation on diabetic retinopathy is by the DRS, sponsored by the National Eye Institute. For a person to be selected for treatment by photocoagulation, his NPDR had to be moderately advanced, with at least three of the following being present: extensive retinal hemorrhages cotton-wool patches venous beading; or intraretinal microvascular abnormalities (IRMA). Selec-

tion of neovascular proliferation was over a wide spectrum of severity, limited primarily by the presence of vitreous hemorrhage, traction detachment, and extensive fibrosis. Eyes with macular ischemia or edema having a reduction in acuity to less than 20/100 were also excluded. Thus DRS conclusions may not apply to such eyes. The study design required that both eyes of each patient enrolled be suitable for photocoagulation. One eye was treated and the other observed, the selection being made by statistical randomization. The treatment by xenon arc and argon laser photocoagulation was given according to a standard protocol that required a panretinal photocoagulation in all instances and direct treatment of vessels away from the disk.

Results of Photocoagulation. The DRS showed that photocoagulation as carried out in the Study resulted in a significant reduction in severe visual loss and decreased progression to more severe stages of proliferative retinopathy in the treated eyes, as compared with the fellow eyes which had indefinite deferral of treatment. For example, although the treated eyes did not fare significantly better as regards visual loss of one or two lines, the loss of five lines of vision or more was more than twice as great in the nontreated group as in the treated group after two years.

Eyes having vitreous hemorrhage and new vessels away from the disk and new vessels at the disk all did significantly better when in the treated group as compared with the untreated group. The value of photocoagulation in early NPDR is being evaluated in a subsequent study, the ETDRS. The value of photocoagulation in extensive proliferative diabetic retinopathy with significant fibrosis, vitreous hemorrhage, or traction sequelae remains questionable.

Complications of Photocoagulation. With care, the incidence of complications following photocoagulation for diabetic retinopathy should be low, probably less than 5 percent. One should have clear media, a well-dilated pupil, a stable eye, a knowledge of the anatomy to be treated, and an awareness of the potential hazards.

Anterior segment complications of photocoagulation are associated primarily with overheating the tissues. They include paresis of miosis, pupil irregularity, iris atrophy, posterior synechiae, corneal edema, aqueous flare, and cataract formation. These risks are greater when the spot size is more than 500 μ.

When treating new vessels in the posterior segment, vitreous hemorrhage is infrequent if a longer burn is used rather than a short burn of particularly high power density. Similarly, selection of a burn of longer duration rather than high power density can minimize the risk of rupturing Brunch's membrane and allowing development of choriovitreous anastomoses. Exudative detachment and acute angle closure glaucoma may follow extensive PRP treatment. This may be associated with edema about the vortex veins and with an impediment to the venous outflow from that quadrant of the eye. Burns to the optic nerve may also occur, but are rare. If applications are placed on the macula, loss of central acuity may be expected.

Other Thermal Therapy

The use of trans-scleral diathermy temporal to the macula to treat exudative retinopathy has been supplanted by photocoagulation. Cryopexy has been used to destroy peripheral retina as in PRP in eyes with media too hazy to perform panretinal photocoagulation with either the argon or krypton lasers.

Ocular Surgery

The indications for ocular surgery are primarily complications of PDR and vitreous contraction: vitreous hemorrhage, traction detachment of the retina, and rhegmatogenous retinal detachment. Vitreous hemorrhage may occur either alone or in conjunction with one of the types of retinal detachment. As each combination of factors differs, selection of the optimal surgical procedure requires careful preoperative evaluation.

Vitreous hemorrhage requiring closed vitrectomy should be sufficiently dense to decrease vision to 10/200 or less and have been present for two or three months without clearing. The typical case of vitreous hemorrhage for which closed vitrectomy is indicated has no area of the fundus visible posterior to the equator. A red reflex indicates less density to the hemorrhage than a gray reflex. Preoperative ultrasonography of the globe will reveal if there is an underlying traction detachment or vitreous membrane formation. A combined electroretinogram (ERG) and visual evoked response (VER) will give more information regarding retinal and optic pathway function than a subjective testing of vision, particularly in a person with very low acuity.

Distinction between traction detachment and rhegmatogenous detachment is paramount because the management and prognosis differ significantly. A traction detachment usually has a taut, shiny, smooth surface that slopes from the area of vitreoretinal adhesion to the plane of the retina. Rarely does it extend anterior to the vortex veins. Arcuate demarcation lines, often seen, indicate the stepwise progression of the traction detachment. Full thickness retinal holes are not present. When a full thickness hole occurs, rhegmatogenous detachment ensues. It has a wrinkled, dull gray, convex surface that may shimmer or undulate, depending on the splinting effect of the vitreoretinal membranes. The detachment usually extends to the ora serrata. Proper diagnosis can usually be made.

The visual prognosis for untreated traction detachments is much better than for rhegmatogenous detachment. Over half of 136 traction detachments followed an average of 4.6 years maintained vision of 20/200 or better, whereas all untreated rhegmatogenous detachments lose useful vision within several months.

Judgment regarding the selection of operation and whether or not operation should be performed depends not only on the factors enumerated above, but also on the angiopathic activity within the eye at the time of surgery. The viability of the retina is also a frequently overlooked factor in judging whether or not an eye may be benefited by surgery.

Closed Vitrectomy

The most common surgery for the sequelae of diabetic retinopathy is closed vitrectomy. In this procedure, the probelike instrument is inserted into the vitreous cavity via a sclerotomy in the pars plana ciliaris. The instrument has an aspiration port near its tip that opens into a hollow tube that is connected to a suction apparatus. A blade within the tube periodically cuts across the aspiration port to excise any formed material that has been sucked into the tube. By this repetitive action, fluid, gel, and tissue are removed.

Instrumentation. There are several instrument systems available. All give intraocular illumination by a fiberoptic bundle, cut by either a rotary or guillotine mechanism, and have aspiration and infusion capabilities. Optional instruments include vitreous scissors, picks, and forceps, plus endocoagulation devices, and are used as part of a bimanual technique.

Technique. The technical requirements for optimal closed vitrectomy are good visualization, appropriate instrumentation, and the maintenance of a stable intraocular environment. Maximum preoperative mydriasis is important. An operating microscope and a contact lens with a flat anterior surface allow a view through the depths of the eye with good magnification. The fiberoptic bundle gives good illumination within the eye. In most instances it is in a sleeve about the vitrectomy instrument.

A sclerotomy for introduction of the instrument should be opposite the portion of the vitreous needing the surgery. If there is no specific area that needs maximum maneuverability of the instrument, a temporal incision is preferable, just above the horizontal meridian at 4.5 to 5.0 mm posterior to the limbus. If two instruments are used, the sclerotomies are usually at the 10 and 2 o'clock meridians.

Insertion of the vitrectomy instrument is made with a firm, constant pressure combined with a twisting motion. Once it is near the center of the visual axis, the tip should be inspected to see if pars plana has been pushed ahead of the instrument. In the two instrument technique, both incisions are prepared before the first entry is made.

The initial tissue is removed in the central axis just behind the lens to form a lacuna. Once this is formed, excursions are made into the areas of debris-filled tissue or to the membranes. This allows clearing of the aspiration port. Technique varies according to the material being removed. If there is old, dense blood, and intermittent return of the aspiration port to the enlarging central lacuna prevents the system from being clogged with debris.

The membranes in traction detachment or rhegmatogenous detachment that require excision differ. Those producing traction detachment extend anteriorly to the region of the vitreous base in a taut funnel, and are often quite dense. If occurring with dense vitreous hemorrhage, the membrane may be thicker than if no blood is present. If a membrane edge is seen, the cutting port is placed there. The aspiration usually pulls a bit of tissue into the cutting port, so one can work along this edge. Occasionally, when no free edge is available, referral to the data of the preoperative ultrasound may be valuable. Also, turning the cutting edge partially away from such a membrane minimizes the danger of aspirating and cutting an underlying detached retina.Once a hole is produced in the membrane, one can again cut into the membrane edge and extend the excision, trying to separate the elevated tissue from its anterior connections. Circumcision of this funnel-like membrane and a close cropping of the tissues posteriorly usually give significant visual improvement if the retina is functioning. In addition to atrophy of the stub of tissue, the fluorescein leakage from remaining new vessels decreases.

With the gossamer-thin tissues and rhegmatogenous detachment, it is particularly important to keep the cutting port on the side away from the mobile, elevated retina. A very slow rate of aspiration allows for greater control. Once the membranes are removed, the scleral buckling procedure is done.

With the two instrument technique, the second instrument may be used to pick up membranes too close to the retina to cut safely. Also, with dense tissues the second instrument may help to hold tissue at the cutting port, facilitating its removal.

In most instances, removal of blood and elevated membranes can be performed without undue risk. Excision of flat membranes represents a greater technical challenge and surgical risk. Removing the last 10 percent of tissue may entail 90 percent of the risk. One should cease just before, not just after.

In closing, intraocular tension should be reduced just prior to the removal of the instrument to minimize expulsion of vitreous contents from the sclerotomy site. The scleral sutures should be tightened immediately after its removal. Then the posterior fundus should be inspected for retinal tears and the sclerotomy site for incarceration or detachment of the retina.

Results of closed vitrectomy vary with the surgery being performed. Preoperative judgment in case selection for closed vitrectomy is as important as the technique itself. Most eyes undergoing closed vitrectomy have vision between 20/200 and light perception with good projection.

Surgery is to be avoided in eyes with light perception but no projection, especially if electrophysical tests show no response. If vision is better than 20/100, the risk of loss of vision must be weighed against the benefit of stabilizing vision at that desirable level. One must avoid operating on eyes with active angiopathy, as manifested by blot hemorrhages, retinal edema, beaded or dilated veins, or extensive neovascularization containing little or no fibrotic tissue. Other eyes that do poorly on a functional basis are those with atrophic retinas, as manifested by large areas of capillary closure, obliteration of arterioles so they give a silver wire appearance, or a virtual absence of intraretinal hemorrhage.

The best prognosis is with the vitreous hemorrhage with no transvitreous membranes of traction detachments. Approximately 80 percent of these cases do well. Eyes with transvitreous membranes and traction detachments have a lower success rate, particularly if the membranes for cutting lie close to the retina. In these cases, iatrogenic retinal holes become factors to be reckoned with, in addition to rubeosis iridis, glaucoma, rebleeding, cataract development, and corneal problems. Approximately one-fifth of the eyes having closed vitrectomy have these severe complications.

Other Ocular Surgery

Except for endodiathermy, operations other than closed vitrectomy are primarily to reduce traction on the retina or the rhegmatogenous detachment associated with proliferative diabetic retinopathy. Tnese include the transection of isolated dense transvitreous membranes with vitreous scissors, and operations to reduce intraocular diameter by circumferential band or scleral buckling. All may be performed in conjunction with closed vitrectomy.

Vitreous Scissors. When used alone, without internal fiberoptic illumination, visualization with indirect ophthalmoscopy affords a broad field, stereopsis, and depth of focus not available with the operating microscope. An infusion port in the shaft permits maintenance of intraocular pressure, either by injection or gravity flow. Tough membranes traversing the vitreous cavity are the prime indication for the use of scissors alone. The blades should be perpendicular to the membrane being cut. When used in conjunction with a vitreous nibbler, the membranes are more likely to be close to the retinal surface.

Endocoagulation. This is the method by which new vessels within the vitreous cavity are cauterized. Indications for endodiathermy are primarily those which prevent successful photocoagulation of new vessels, such as hazy media, location over the optic nerve or macula, or elevated vessels that are particularly large or small. In most eyes treated, vitreous hemorrhage has already occurred.

Optimal conditions for surgery include wide pupillary dialation, reasonable clarity of the media, and elevation of the vessels to be treated. Endodiathermy is now often used in conjunction with closed vitrectomy. Bimanual cautery uses the two instruments within the eye as the electrodes, with the tissue to be cauterized bridging the gap as the current is applied. Unipolar endodiathermy uses a high frequency electromagnetic wave. When using the unipolar instrument, episcleral vessels in a wet field are cauterized to test the current, a sclerotomy of proper length is made, and the instrument is inserted toward the vessels to be treated. The vessels are almost touched and the current is activated for 2 to 4 sec. If the end point, whitening with closure of the vessels, is not achieved, the power is increased and the procedure repeated. In a large fan of new vessels, closure of the edges followed by centripetal applications going to the base is the most effective way of obliterating new vessels with a minimal risk of hemorrhage.

Scleral Resection. Although most surgery for traction detachment associated with proliferative diabetic retinopathy involves closed vitrectomy, a small percentage (less than 3 percent) are probably still treated as effectively and more safely with a scleral resection procedure that shortens the anteroposterior diameter of the globe. These eyes have taut membranes extending anteriorly to the anterior vitreous base. The macula is uninvolved with proliferative tissue, but is either elevated or threatened by traction detachment. These and other findings contraindicate closed vitrectomy. The other findings may include an active angiopathy that would heighten the risk of postoperative rubeosis and glaucoma, or broad, dense adhesions between the shrunken vitreous and retina that might be difficult to remove.

The scleral resection procedure shortens the globe and primarily reduces the intraocular anteroposterior diameter. The resection, mathematically determined, covers 180 to 270° of the circumference of the globe. It is 3 mm wide, deep enough so the underlying choroid gives a bluish color to the resection bed, and lies at the equator. This procedure has been successful in either allowing the macula to settle or preventing the development of detachment in two-thirds of the 65 eyes treated. Complications, in less than 10 percent of cases, have been limited to vitreous loss, vitreous hemorrhage, and postoperative glaucoma.

Scleral Buckling. Rhegmatogenous detachment associated with proliferative diabetic retinopathy requires surgery to save vision. Discovery of breaks may be difficult because of opacities in the lens and vitreous, poor pupillary dilatation, retinal folds and the presence of fibrous tissue obscuring portions of the retina, and the possible confusion with small intraretinal hemorrhage.

Surgical modifications are often necessary, as holes lie posterior to the vortex veins in most eyes.

If a single break is present, a localized high buckle is made with a strong thermal reaction. Drainage of subretinal fluid is necessary. Closed vitrectomy is frequently used in conjunction with the scleral buckle and is performed during the same procedure, just before the buckling. Surgery has been successful in reattaching the retina in about three-fourths of treated eyes in one series. Despite the complexities in these cases, surgery can frequently be successful.

Pituitary Ablation

Although photocoagulation has become the treatment of choice in most instances of progressive retinal neovascularization, pituitary ablation remains the treatment of choice for a very limited group of patients. These include patients with eyes having large networks of new vessels over the disk which are interspersed with fibrotic tissue or are elevated, or eyes that have extensive elevated new vessels in the periphery. In addition to the above criteria, vision should be 20/100 or better in at least one eye, with the macula not being threatened by proliferative diabetic retinopathy. The general physical state should allow the patient not only to survive surgery but to have a postoperative life expectancy of at least five years. The personality must be able to cope with a perennial program of hormone replacement as demanded by the hypopituitary state. Patients over the age of 40 rarely are selected for pituitary ablation.

The surgery now used most frequently is transsphenoidal diathermy, via a probe positioned by x-ray stereotaxis. No operative or postoperative deaths have occurred in the 65 cases of our present series, which began in 1970. The usual systemic postoperative response is a decrease in insulin requirement, but with more difficulty in regulating the blood sugar level. Hydrocortisone supplement is always necessary, but thyroid hormone is necessary only if hypothyroidism ensues. The loss of menses occurs in women.

The ocular response can be measured visually and by anatomic and physiologic changes within the eye. Angiopathic changes are those most affected and are manifested by (1) a decrease in retinal hemorrhages and edema; (2) reduction in the caliber of abnormally dilated capillaries; (3) atrophy or shrinkage of new vessels; (4) reduction in the engorgement and segmentation of veins; and (5) less leakage from new vessels seen with fluorescein angiography. Fibrotic proliferation remains

unchanged after pituitary ablation. The greatest sources of visual failure postoperatively are the sequelae of fibrotic change, primarily traction detachment. In our series since 1970, two-thirds of the patients have maintained their preoperative vision, the average follow-up being more than four years. Only a few have required focal photocoagulation. Pituitary ablation remains an effective means of maintaining vision for a limited number of patients for whom photocoagulation and ocular surgery are either potentially ineffective or contraindicated.

Medical Treatment

Medical treatment of diabetic retinopathy has less apparent cause and effect relationships than either photocoagulation or the surgical procedures. The various treatments constitute attempts to rectify changes related to the production of the retinal hypoxia, impaired oxygen release from oxyhemoglobin and reduced blood flow in the retinal capillaries, or deposit of fatty exudates in the macula. These are of prime value in early nonproliferative retinopathy.

Control of Blood Glucose Level

Impaired release of O_2 from oxyhemoglobin occurs in poorly controlled diabetics, as the glycosilated hemoglobin, Hgb A_{1c}, which binds O_2 more firmly than Hgb A itself, is two or three times as high in this group as in normal persons. The concentration of Hgb A_{1c} in an erythrocyte is apparently related directly to the glucose level in the serum while the red cell is being formed. As the Hgb A_{1c} has a reduced capacity to divest itself of O_2, good control, which reduces the level of Hgb A_{1c}, may result in better oxygen release to the tissues and help to ameliorate relative tissue hypoxia. As red cells circulate approximately two months, this reading gives an assessment of control for that period, allowing a much better measurement of control than previously available.

Salicylate Therapy

Field and Powell introduced the relationship between salicylate therapy and a more favorable course for diabetic retinopathy when they noted that patients with diabetes and rheumatoid arthritis had a lower than expected incidence of retinopathy. This probably is related to two observations.

The first is that platelets in the diabetic are abnormal, having an increased sensitivity to aggregation that can be correlated with the ongoing process of their retinopathy. The second is that aspirin inhibits one of the pathways to platelet aggregation. In addition, aspirin has been found to be clinically helpful in the prophylaxis in microcirculatory thrombosis. Thus, in view of the above clinical suggestions and theoretic considerations, prophylactic ingestions of aspirin would seem to be a reasonable course for diabetic patients prior to the development of neovascularization. Two 300-mg tablets each morning is an effective dose for the above purpose and carries minimal risk of side effects.

The Medical Management

Diabetic patients with elevated serum lipids are more apt to develop retinal exudates. When circinate, exudative lesions, which have a fatty component, begin to develop in the macula in these patients, progression may be arrested if the blood level of fats is lowered. Once macular function has been lost, it does not return, even though the exudates may be particularly reabsorbed. Both a strict low fat diet or clofibrate, 250 mg 4 times daily, have been noted to reduce retinal exudates.

In the European literature, calcium dobisilate has been reported to have a beneficial effect on diabetic retinopathy, but a carefully controlled randomized study in the United States showed no difference between the progression of retinopathy in the eyes as they underwent treatment or served as controls.

Carboxyhemoglobin, which is 200 times more stable than oxyhemoglobin, may have a concentration in blood several times greater than normal in smokers of more than one pack of cigarettes a day. One might postulate, therefore, that cessation or limitation of heavy smoking could result in more O_2 being available to the retinal tissue.

In proliferative diabetic retinopathy, particularly if vitreous hemorrhage has occurred, avoidance of sudden exertion, the Valsalva maneuver, or lowering the head to the level of the waist may reduce the chances to vitreous hemorrhages. Also, once new vessels are present, aspirin is contraindicated, as its effect on platelet aggregation might allow a vitreous hemorrhage to persist a bit longer.

Other potential treatments are still in various stages of speculation, experimentation, and development. They include:

1. improved control of blood glucose levels by the use of multiple doses of regular insulin;
2. a portable pump that injects insulin according to a preset schedule or in response to blood glucose levels;
3. reduction of blood glucose levels by somatostatin—but its extremely short duration of action remains a major drawback;
4. pancreatic islet cell transplantation, which has yet to be successfully accomplished in humans; and
5. in a recent animal study, adenovirus infection destroyed beta cells in genetically susceptible animals, but the immunologic implications remain to be assessed.

FOLLOW-UP CARE

The cases that do not require treatment following the initial examination must have periodic follow-up. The time interval varies greatly. For some conditions, such as a small to moderate vitreous hemorrhage with a partially obscured fundus, a return visit in one week is indicated. In advancing active proliferative disease in which photocoagulation or surgery is contemplated, a re-examination in three or four weeks is reasonable. A two-to three-month interval is indicated in cases of extensive vitreous hemorrhage that is clearing and in cases with less active proliferative change. A two-to three-month interval is also appropriate in cases with nonproliferative diabetic retinopathy which do not yet meet the criteria for treatment, but which have visual deterioration or anatomic changes that suggest that photocoagulation will be necessary in the near future. A four- to six-month span suffices when the proliferative retinopathy appears stable or if the nonproliferative retinopathy does not have a borderline visual acuity and the signs suggesting progression (fluorescein leakage, retinal edema, blot hemorrhages) are minimal. A yearly follow-up is reserved for those with fibrotic, "burned-out" proliferative diabetic retinopathy or a similarly atrophic nonproliferative diabetic retinopathy. The other group of patients requiring yearly follow-up are those with indolent retinopathy, who have only a few microaneurysms, small round hemorrhages, or scattered hard exudates, with no fluorescein leakage and inconsequential capillary closure on fluorescein angiography.

The above discussion has dealt with eyes alone, and not with the apprehensive soul worrying and wondering about the visual future. Our charge as physicians is not only to treat patients as best we can, but also to support their psyche. One should be as optimistic as the truth allows. Utilization of low vision aids for patients with vision from 20/40 to 20/200 often allows them to read once again, a great psychologic boon. Also, informing patients of the services available to the partially handicapped as well as to those with profound vision loss is a frequently overlooked service.

The relationship that builds over the years between the concerned physician and a patient with a chronic problem can exert a strong influence on the attitude of that patient toward the disease itself and life in general. It should be made as positive as possible.

DIABETIC NEPHROPATHY

ELI A. FRIEDMAN, M.D.

Uremia resulting from microvascular degenerative disease complicating diabetes mellitus accounts for approximately 25 percent of patients starting dialytic therapy or given a kidney transplant. Only a decade ago, the prognosis for extension of useful life in diabetics with failed kidneys was so poor that their treatment was usually not advised. In 1983, it may be anticipated that the majority of treated uremic diabetics will live for at least three years; a substantial fraction will be able to return to their preuremia activity status.

In no other disease is coordinated planning of therapy more necessary than for the diabetic whose renal function is declining. Azotemic diabetics are sicker than nondiabetics with the same amount of residual renal function. The explanation for the diabetic's greater morbidity lies in the usual presence of coincident disease in multiple organs, most clinically evident in the eyes, heart, nervous system, and extremities. Success in management requires collaborative planning by all specialists sharing in the patient's care. Whereas a pediatrician or general internist may have guided decision-

making for most of the diabetic's hyperglycemic life, once nephropathy emerges as the dominant problem, a nephrologist ought to be involved in every aspect of subsequent planning.

DEVISING A TREATMENT STRATEGY

Answering five questions which arise in the assessment of every new diabetic with a renal disorder has proven helpful to construction of a treatment strategy. These are: Is the patient truly diabetic? Is the renal syndrome caused by diabetes? What is the present renal status? Which uremia therapy is appropriate for this patient? Has a life plan been formulated?

Is the Patient Diabetic?

Documentation of the diagnosis of diabetes mellitus is an initial requirement for treatment. Differentiation from renal glycosuria, carbohydrate intolerance induced by hepatic failure, and thyrotoxicosis can prevent the rare but sad mislabeling of a nondiabetic as diabetic. Renal insufficiency is a cause of significant carbohydrate intolerance; at the point when renal function declines below 5 percent of predicted normal performance, 85 percent of nondiabetic patients exhibit a diabetic response to an oral glucose load. Despite these opportunities for confusion, the diagnosis of diabetes mellitus is usually easily established by the combination of fasting hyperglycemia test, typical history, and characteristic extrarenal complications. Retinal photography aided by fluorescein angiography provides definitive proof of diabetes in at least 97 out of 100 patients in whom uremia is caused by diabetic glomerulopathy. Distinction between insulin-dependent (type I), and adult onset (type II) diabetes is important to projection of an accurate prognosis. Little is known of the natural history of type II renal disease, while a clear picture of the evolution of type I nephropathy is available.

Is Diabetes the Cause of Renal Disease?

Estimates of the number of diabetics in the United States range between five and ten million. By chance, diabetics are as likely as nondiabetics to have any kidney disease. When evaluating a diabetic with renal disease, it is therefore necessary to ascertain whether or not the kidney disorder is a consequence of diabetes. Listed in Table 1 are

TABLE 1   Diabetes-induced Renal Disorders

Infectious
    Bacteriuria
    Pyelonephritis
    Renal carbuncle

Toxic
    Contrast media-induced nephropathy

Neurogenic
    Bladder atony (hydronephrosis)

Vascular
    Nephrosclerosis
    Atherosclerosis
    Atheromatous embolic disease

Degenerative (Idiopathic)
    Diffuse intracapillary glomerulosclerosis
    Nodular intracapillary glomerulosclerosis

the renal syndromes directly associated with diabetes mellitus.

The term diabetic nephropathy has become synonymous with nodular and diffuse glomerulosclerosis. Percutaneous renal biopsy to establish the diagnosis of glomerulosclerosis is rarely indicated. A nephrotic, azotemic, type I patient evaluated in the eighteenth year of insulin dependence may safely be assumed to have glomerulosclerosis. Nephrosis in the fifth year after onset, however, is atypical and calls for a full study that may result in renal biopsy.

What Is the Present Renal Status?

To plan appropriate therapy, it is essential to determine where the patient stands in the course of progressive glomerulopathy. Measurement of serum creatinine, albumin, and phosphorus concentrations, hematocrit, and 24-hour urinary protein and creatinine excretion affords sufficient information for this assessment. Once renal insufficiency is discovered, an x-ray of the hand, and measurement of serum calcium, phosphorus, alkaline phosphatase, and parathyroid hormone levels will clarify the degree of secondary hyperparathyroidism which may be present.

TREATMENT OF RENAL DISEASE IN THE NONAZOTEMIC DIABETIC

Urinary Tract Infections.   Urinary tact infections representing a minor threat in nondiabetics may rapidly escalate to either papillary necrosis or a renal carbuncle in a diabetic. Discovery of asymptomatic bacteriuria ($>$ 100,000 organisms/ml of urine) in a diabetic is an indication for treatment using the same antimicrobial drugs as for nondiabetics. For initial management of a urinary tract infection, when renal function is not reduced significantly (creatinine clearance [CCr] $>$60 ml/min), either a sulfa drug (sulfamethoxazole) or ampicillin is an appropriate first-line drug for a seven-day course. Drugs can be changed if a clinical response is not apparent in 48 hours, or if bacteriuria persists. Should the patient improve, no change is needed even though in vitro sensitivity testing indicates that the pathogen is drug resistant. Recurrent and persistent urinary infections may be suppressed for months to years by daily administration of a single tablet containing trimethoprim (80 mg) and sulfamethoxazole (400 mg). For both acute and chronic urinary infections, a high urine flow rate is beneficial; ingestion of 2 or more L of liquid daily is to be encouraged. Incomplete bladder emptying due to a neurogenic bladder predisposes the patient to repetitive episodes of cystitis with the risk of pyelonephritis. Urologic consultation should be obtained to measure residual urine volume after voiding and to perform a cystometric study to quantify the severity of neurologic deficit. Treatment consists of a trial of Urecholine plus voiding every 2 hours, including throughout the night. Should this therapy fail, a permanent bladder catheter may be required to end the series of infections.

Treatment of Nonazotemic, Proteinuric Diabetics

This consists of reduction of hypertensive blood pressures to normal and the best attainable glucose regulation. It has been estimated that correction of hypertension in proteinuric type I diabetics slows renal deterioration by as much as 9 ml of glomerular filtration rate (GFR) per year. Within weeks of regulating blood pressure, a decrease in proteinuria is observed in the majority of type I patients. That similar benefit is obtained in the type II patient can reasonably be concluded, but this is not supported by actual trials. Nephropathic diabetics are hypertensive because of intravascular volume overload superimposed on a diseased vasular system. Therefore, a reduction in fluid retention by administration of potent diuretics is central to the treatment of hypertension. Furosemide, starting at 40 mg daily with progressive increases to as much as 180 mg twice daily, is an effective regimen for achieving a "dry weight." When the GFR is < 25 ml/min, adding metolazone, 5–20 mg daily, often sustains a diuresis when furosemide alone is inadequate. Potassium supplementation is usually required during brisk diuresis, especially for patients who are also receiving digoxin for congestive heart failure.

Reduction of blood pressure in azotemic diabetics usually necessitates prescription of a vasodilator in conjunction with diuretics. Clonidine, methyldopa, and prazosin are approximately equivalent in effectiveness and side effects and may be given in incremental doses until either the blood pressure falls or an adverse effect (most often somnolence and weakness) precludes larger doses. Resistant hypertension is an indication for use of minoxidil, a potent vasodilator that requires simultaneous administration of a beta blocker (propranolol) to modulate tachycardia. Visceral neuropathy manifested by orthostatic hypotension in a hypertensive patient may be difficult to correct. Elastic stockings, gradual shifts in position, and tolerance of intermittent dizziness usually become everyday realities for the patient.

When the creatinine clearance falls below about 25 ml/min, the azotemic diabetic risks all of the uremic complications known to occur in nondiabetics. A projection of the approximate date by which the creatinine clearance will fall to less than 10 ml/min (serum creatinine above 5 mg/dl) can be made graphically by plotting the reciprocal of the serum creatinine concentration (1/serum creatinine in mg/dl) against time (months). Variation in the rate of deterioration in type I diabetics is considerable. Elapsed time for the creatinine concentration to increase from a baseline of 2 mg/dl to 10 mg/dl ranges from 6 to 80 months, with a mean of about 27 months. The course of each patient is remarkably constant, however, permitting reasonably precise estimation of the date when uremia therapy will be required.

During the months to years of so-called conservative therapy, the basic strategy is to delay or avoid completely those complications whose pathogenesis suggests treatability. For example, uremic bone disease is a complication of renal insufficiency in which both bone matrix and mineral content become depleted, predisposing the patient to pathologic fractures and bone pain. Secondary hyperparathyroidism contributes substantially to the attack on bone integrity in uremia. In this disorder, dissolution of bone by osteoclasts under control of parathyroid hormone (PTH) is the result

of hypocalcemia in uremia; a low plasma calcium level provokes PTH release. Hypocalcemia is the consequence of diminished intestinal absorption of calcium due to impaired synthesis of active vitamin D_3 by the kidney, and retained phosphorus due to its reduced renal excretion. Hyperphosphatemic patients should be given a phosphate binding gel (either aluminum carbonate or hydroxide) prior to each meal. Hypocalcemic patients with a raised PTH level usually respond to treatment with active vitamin D (1,25 diOHD^3, 0.25 to 1.0 mcg/day) to enhance intestinal calcium absorption, plus supplemental dietary calcium, 1–2 gm per day. Repetitive measurements of the serum calcium level must be obtained, initially at weekly intervals, to protect against hypercalcemia, which is the major complication of synthetic vitamin D use.

Dietary restriction of protein to 40 gm per day and salt to 2 gm per day protects against muscle catabolism while minimizing the excretory burden of nitrogen and sodium excretion. There is no conflict between the American Diabetes Association's recommended diet (15 to 20 percent protein, 40 to 50 percent carbohydrate, 35 to 40 percent fat) and a renal failure diet. Severe azotemic acidosis (bicarbonate < 15 mEq/L) is reason to add small amounts (600–2400 mg sodium bicarbonate daily) to the diet.

TREATMENT OF THE UREMIC DIABETIC PATIENT

Selecting Appropriate Uremic Therapy

Before Scribner's epic demonstration in 1960 that chronic uremia was treatable by maintenance hemodialysis, the only option open to prolong life in patients with renal insufficiency was the slow starvation of a nearly no-protein diet. Since 1960, at least six clearly different choices for prolonging life in patients with uremia have been shown to be workable (Table 2). Depending on each patient's severity of illness; occupational, family, and home status; and emotional maturity and outlook, selection of the "correct" uremia therapy is a matter of judgment that should be made in an atmosphere devoid of crisis. Toward this end, patient and physician ought to analyze the pros and cons of what may be best under the patient's circumstances. Meetings with patients who have been treated by dialysis and renal transplantation can be particu-

TABLE 2   Selecting Optimal Therapy for Diabetics with Uremia

	Advantages	Disadvantages
Renal transplantation	Cures uremia for duration of graft function Stabilizes retinopathy Permits long intervals (months) away from treatment facility Reverses neuropathy Best rehabilitation Long-term survival	Steroids complicate glucose control Risk of infectious complication High mortality rate in cadaveric graft recipients Risk of developing diabetes in familial donors Not applicable to elderly or patients with cardiovascular instability Glomerulosclerosis can recur
Peritoneal dialysis	Avoids major surgery Minimizes burden on cardiovascular system Facilitates glucose regulation when insulin is added to dialysate Adaptable to home (intermittent PD or CAPD) in selected patients	High mortality rate Retinopathy progresses Limited long-term success
Hemodialysis	Avoids major surgery Permits care by experienced staff Available in most countries	Poor rehabilitation Retinopathy may progress Mortality rate equivalent to that for cadaveric graft recipients Inexorable "failure to thrive" syndrome in about 25 percent of patients

larly helpful to the often dazed, depressed, and frightened uremic patient.

Options in Uremic Therapy. An initial decision to be made by the uremic diabetic patient is whether or not to be treated for renal failure. A blind, hemiparetic, double amputee suffering multiple daily bouts of angina might, after discussion with his family, decline the chance for a few additional months or years of life on the grounds that there is little likelihood of achieving enjoyable, pain-free life even with the best imagined result. Informed uremic diabetics who do opt for aggressive treatment can be offered several therapies, each of which can extend life under some circumstances.

Maintenance hemodialysis is the most frequently used technique for treating uremia in type I diabetics. Several current texts paint a grim picture for survival on hemodialysis, based on the early trials at the beginning of the 1970s. At that time, the annual mortality rate of dialyzed diabetics exceeded 60 percent, and 50 percent of the surviving patients became blind. Subsequent recognition of the importance of control of hypertension and intravascular volume overload has substantially improved the lot of dialyzed patients, half of whom now live for at least three years. A typical hemodialysis prescription calls for three weekly treatments, each lasting from 4 to 6 hours. When performed at home by the patient, hemodialysis is more readily incorporated into everyday living. Disturbingly, only one in four hemodialyzed diabetics is sufficiently rehabilitated to return to gainful employment or to preillness school or home responsibilities. Death in hemodialyzed diabetics usually is caused by cardiovascular disease (30 to 70 percent of deaths), followed by cerebrovascular accidents, sepsis, or withdrawal from dialysis, each accounting for about 15 percent of deaths.

Peritoneal dialysis has re-emerged as a successful treatment for uremia which may have special value for the type I diabetic. When performed as an intermittent, thrice weekly therapy, peritoneal dialysis has had a limited one-year survival rate of only 22 to 50 percent. These poor results reflect the extreme hyperglycemia induced by dialysate glucose concentrations of 1500 to 4500 mg/dl. More recently, the application of continuous ambulatory dialysis (CAPD) with insulin added to the dialysate has increased the one-year survival rate to more than 80 percent. In CAPD, 2 L of dialysate are instilled into the peritoneal cavity via a permanently implanted silicone elastic catheter. After an equilibration period (dwell time) of 6 hours, the dialysate containing nitrogenous wastes is drained by gravity into a plastic bag, and a fresh 2 L of dialysate are infused by gravity. No machine is used. Patients dialyze themselves, performing four exchanges daily around the clock, seven days a week. By placing insulin directly into the dialysate, a form of "artificial pancreas" is created, and plasma glucose levels can be maintained very closely within a 100 to 200 mg/dl range. Advantages of CAPD over hemodialysis include rapid training (under one week), no need for a machine, minimal cardiac stress, and superior blood glucose regulation. Trials now in progress will ascertain whether these advantages outweigh the difficulties that stem from recurrent peritonitis, and the enervation related to the labor and time demanded by a seven-day-a-week therapeutic regimen.

Kidney transplantation is the best solution to the myriad problems of the uremic diabetic. A functioning renal allograft permits a degree of rehabilitation unobtainable by even the best hemodialysis. Employing an immunosuppressive regimen consisting of azathioprine, prednisone, and antithymocyte globulin, recipients of living related donor kidneys have about an 80 percent chance of retaining graft function for at least two years, while about 50 percent of cadaveric graft recipients will have a functioning graft at two years. Selected series of diabetics have had markedly better results using donor preconditioning techniques. Najarian, for example, prepares recipients with a splenectomy, and in his most recent experience, 85 percent of cadaveric graft recupients survived for two years. Conditioning recipients with donor recipient blood transfusions, Salvatierra was able to induce 83 percent of diabetic recipients of living related kidneys to hold their grafts for at least three years. Newer immunosuppressive regimens relying on Cyclosporin A and monoclonal antibodies against specific populations of T lymphocytes hold the promise of effective immunosuppression with little or no requirement for corticosteroid drugs. Diabetics, whose glucose regulation deteriorates badly during steroid therapy, stand to benefit greatly from a steroid-free immunosuppressive drug combination.

The available treatments for uremia in diabetics are summarized in Table 3. There is but scant experience in renal transplantation in type II diabetics because of their older age, often past 55 years, at the time they develop uremia. Very few diabetics have been treated for more than two years with CAPD, precluding a judgment of its worth

TABLE 3 Suggested Therapy in Uremic Diabetic Patients

Age Range (Years)	Renal Transplant	Peritoneal Dialysis	Hemo-dialysis
18–44	+ +	?	+
45–65	Selected patients	+	+
Over 65 (or presence of intractable heart failure)	—	+	+

Note: + + means strongly recommended, especially if family donor available, + means recommended, — means not recommended

and general applicability. As a generalization, it may be predicted that in the hands of a team familiar with both uremia and diabetes, the life expectancy of uremic type I diabetics now exceeds 50 percent for the majority who receive a kidney transplant or begin maintenance hemodialysis.

RETENTION OF SIGHT

One of the major advances of the past five years in uremia therapy for diabetics is the preservation of at least ambulatory vision for at least 75 percent of patients after three years of treatment. Collaboration with an ophthalmologist familiar with the natural history of diabetic retinopathy is essential to any hope for long-term rehabilitation. Employing panretinal photocoagulation for proliferative retinopathy, lensectomy for cataracts, and vitrectomy to extract intraocular clots and fibrous bands, the aggressive ophthalmologist is able to retard what was previously thought to be inevitable blindness.

MANAGEMENT OF HYPERGLYCEMIA

Induction of euglycemia throughout the day is a vital part of management of the nephropathic diabetic. First, the patient feels better when his blood glucose level is near normal. Second, a growing body of evidence suggests that it is hyperglycemia per se that is responsible for glomerular injury in diabetes. Stated as a working hypothesis to guide therapy, "Diabetic nephropathy is a hyperglycemic glomerulopathy." In the diabetic rat, correction of hyperglycemia by either insulin or islet of Langerhans transplants reverses established glomerulopathy. Furthermore, in human diabetics who receive a kidney transplant from a nondiabetic donor, tight glucose control prevents recurrent glomerulosclerosis, while restoration of euglycemia by a pancreatic transplant reverses recurrent glomerulopathy. These observations translate into a rationale for striving for the strictest attainable glucose regulation in both type I and type II diabetics before and after onset of renal insufficiency. One could hypothesize that an explanation for reduced survival rates in diabetics compared with nondiabetics treated by hemodialysis and kidney transplantation is poor glucose control achieved by conventional control protocols. To test this thesis, type I diabetic transplant recipients in an alternate case study are practicing blood glucose self-monitoring to guide daily fractional insulin doses in comparison with standard once or twice daily insulin administration regulated by urine glucose testing. It is reassuring to those about to embark on trials of tight control of blood glucose that careful glucose regulation after kidney transplantation does not seem to impose any negative consequences.

FORMULATION OF A LIFE PLAN

Throughout his life, the diabetic has been forced into decisions by the occurrence of unforeseen crises in which his feeling of well-being, sexual potency, vision, cardiac function, and kidney function have been threatened and then lost. Because uremia is predictable in a diabetic with declining kidney function, the need for dialysis or a kidney transplant should not be presented to the patient as a surprise after referral to a nephrologist. Preparatory discussions, provision of literature, and introduction to a nephrologist and transplant surgeon months to years before renal failure develops allows the patient to retain at least partial control of his destiny. The need for an arteriovenous fistula to facilitate hemodialysis, for example, should be made known to every nephrotic diabetic who becomes azotemic. Those teams having a "trust the patient" philosophy are rewarded in return by fewer depressions and more rapid adaptation to uremia therapy by diabetic patients facing a seemingly endless number of barriers to rehabilitation.

DIABETIC PERIPHERAL VASCULAR DISEASE: ULCER

FRANK C. WHEELOCK, JR., M.D.

Approximately 25 percent of the 5 to 10 million diabetics in the United States will, in the course of their lives, consult doctors with problems involving the leg or foot. In some it will be pain, weakness, or simply the inability to walk far enough to carry out essential activities. Pain at rest will develop in others with more advanced disease, occurring first in the toes and feet. The majority of people seeking professional help will have an ulcer or abscess in the foot, usually at a point where pressure or friction is great. In the latter two groups, the viability of the limb is often threatened and an amputation is a real possibility.

Proper management demands an understanding of the pathologic factors involved, both to help prevent serious problems and to treat them when they arise. Surgery is often required, and the decision as to what to do and when to do it can be very difficult. In the balance is the salvage or loss of a leg.

PATHOPHYSIOLOGY

Claudication

Pain, weakness, fatigue, or numbness of the foot, lower leg, thigh, or buttock muscles which occurs not immediately on standing but after walking some distance is almost invariably due to one or more narrowed or occluded arteries proximal to the symptomatic area. The constriction is caused by thick intimal plaques most often located at bifurcations and in the posterior wall of the arteries. The diabetic tends to develop calcification in the media of the arteries also, which may not narrow the lumen at all but does make them stiff and incompressible. An additional significant factor is the inability of these patients to develop good collateral circulation. Thus a diabetic's arteriogram

205

of a femoral artery occlusion may show 4 collateral vessels with a maximum diameter of 1.2 mm, while a nondiabetic's arteriogram of a similar block may reveal 6 or more collaterals with diameters of 2 to 2.2 mm.

The arteries involved may include one or combinations of the aorta, iliacs, femorals, popliteals, and tibioperoneals. Obviously combinations of blocks produce very severe symptoms and greatly tax the body's ability to accommodate the problem. Another peculiarity of the diabetic is the frequency of occlusions in the arteries of the lower leg and foot, locations that are usually relatively clear in the nondiabetic.

Rest Pain

In the diabetic, pain in the foot or leg may be due to diabetic neuritis or ischemia. In the former, the pain is apt to be burning in character, unaccompanied by claudication and unrelated to position. Ischemic pain is usually worse at night, is accompanied by a history of claudication, and is relieved somewhat by hanging the foot over the side of the bed.

Of course, a diabetic may have neuritis in the foot and then develop some occluded arteries and ischemia as well. If the neuritis has passed the painful stage (or never went through one) and if the foot has become numb, there may be little or no pain even with very severe ischemia.

Ulcers and Other Lesions

There are three causes of foot lesions in the diabetic: infection, neuropathia, and ischemia. Combinations of these are common.

Infection. Infection is poorly handled by diabetics, perhaps because of defects in the white blood cells. This makes it essential that we do all we can to control the problem promptly. Spread must be stopped by vigorous antibiotic treatment plus bed rest. Any activity massages the foot and helps the bacteria spread through the tissues. Heat is never used lest a burn result if the foot is numb, or tissue be destroyed if the foot is ischemic. Diabetic infections often burrow under the adjacent tissue for considerable distances and smolder there. Attention should thus be given to operative drainage of any such areas with the incision extended however far the trouble goes.

Neuropathia. Neuropathia causes a large percentage of open lesions. The sequence is most commonly (1) development of a bony deformity, such as hammer toe, hallux rigidus, "dropped" metatarsal head, bunion deformity, and so on, (2) callus formation over the prominent deformed bone or joint, (3) blister under the callus, (4) infection and ulceration. Obviously the ideal is to discover the problem at stage one or two and either correct the bony deformity or protect the area being traumatized with podiatric appliances.

Ischemia. Ischemia is the most common cause of an open diabetic foot lesion. The lack of blood may be due to proximal major arterial blocks or to more local thrombosis, or to a combination of the two. Usually the lesion develops in such a foot as the result of trauma from a tight shoe or minor injury from a shoe, socks, foreign object, nail clippers, heat, and so on. Then a vicious circle is set up of trauma, local thrombosis, necrosis, infection, more thrombosis, and on and on. Again, rest, antibiotics, and drainage are in order. Heat is never used lest it produce burns or increase metabolic demand that cannot be met.

I never use the word "gangrene." All it means, actually, is something that is dead. A small area of gangrene may in fact be healed by the body itself or successfully remedied by a conservative operation. To the patient, it means an amputation above the knee. So it's best to call these problem areas "lesions," "ulcers," or "abscesses."

DIAGNOSIS AND TREATMENT

Claudication

The diagnosis of the cause of the symptoms of claudication is usually easy, since the other common causes are diabetic neuritis and orthopedic problems. The latter two are not related to the effort of walking but are apt to occur at rest or on simply standing. Claudication due to arterial disease is usually accompanied by loss of palpable pulses.

The first step in treatment should be for the patient to stop smoking. At times this will result in significant improvement. Obese patients may increase their walking tolerance by weight loss, and graduated exercise programs within the limits imposed by pain will help any patient.

Operation is indicated often, but certainly not routinely. I advise surgery only if the symptoms interfere significantly with the patient's work or activities. Surgery is not appropriate for poor risk patients or for those with minimal symptoms. It should never be forced on the patient with the threat of limb loss if the operation is not done. The expectancy of future leg amputation in a patient with claudication as the only symptom is about 15 percent. Since there is a small mortality risk (1 to 2 percent) and an appreciable risk of eventual (five-year) arterial graft failure (5 to 8 percent for aortofemoral reconstruction and 30 percent for femoral reconstruction), this surgery should be carried out only on the basis of present need. If surgery is withheld now, it can usually be done later if increasing symptoms warrant intervention.

If a decision to operate has been reached, an aortogram or, if the femoral pulse is strong, a femoral arteriogram, is carried out. These are generally safe procedures if the renal function is normal.

If occlusions are found, surgery and balloon dilatation are the available treatments. Vasodilating medications or lumbar sympathectomy have not been found to be helpful. In general, I have referred patients for balloon dilatation if only a short segment of artery was involved, preferably in the iliac area. For claudication alone, it is usually appropriate to consider aortoiliac, aortofemoral, ileofemoral, femorofemoral, or femoropopliteal grafts. For the latter, a saphenous or cephalic vein, when of adequate size, makes a much longer lasting graft than any substitute. The success rate must be high and the risks low before these operations are offered to patients whose only complaint is claudication. The initial success rate in our hospital is 95 percent or higher, and the five-year follow-up shows 5 percent of the aortic reconstructions have occluded one limb and 20 percent of the femoral grafts have thrombosed. The result of late failure is usually only a return to the preoperative status.

Since the success rate is lower and a failure may increase the severity of the problem when the surgeon is forced to go to the tibial or peroneal arteries, this operation is seldom indicated when claudication is the only symptom.

Rest Pain

Neuropathy. Diabetic neuropathy may produce pain in the foot and lower leg at rest. Pulses may be present or absent. The pain is usually burning and not relieved by lowering the feet over the side of the bed. If pulses are absent, ischemia can still be ruled out as the cause by clinical evaluation of the circulation and by the vascular laboratory tests.

There is no specific treatment for this condition. I favor the use of Sparine and Darvon and avoid narcotics. Fortunately, the duration of the painful siege of neuritis is self-limited.

Ischemia. Pain at rest is often due to ischemia and is a very ominous symptom forecasting limb loss. It is most severe at night because of several factors (lower cardiac output and blood pressure plus loss of gravity help when the patient is horizontal). Physical examination will always show loss of pulses in the foot. Other signs to look for indicative of poor circulation are loss of hair on the dorsum of the foot; thin atrophic skin and subcutaneous tissue; thick, crumbly nails; dependent rubor; and a slow venous filling time. (To measure this the limbs are elevated until the veins on the dorsum of the foot are empty, then the patient sits and the time until any vein protrudes above the skin is measured. Normally this is about 10 seconds. If it is longer than 20 seconds, a serious ischemia is present.)

Once the diagnosis of ischemia with pain at rest is established, arterial reconstruction is clearly indicated if x-rays show it can be accomplished. Since the need is pressing here, the surgeon is justified in accepting less favorable anatomic situations for grafting, including limited runoffs and the use of the tibial or peroneal arteries for the lower anastomosis.

Since the diabetic has usually destroyed his sympathetic ganglia, sympathectomy offers little help. If artery grafting cannot be done, the patient may be lucky enough to improve by eliminating the use of tobacco, propping up the legs of the bed at the head so gravity helps the circulation, good diabetic control, weight loss (if patient is overweight), and a graduated exercise program. If these fail, a major amputation may be required.

Neuropathic Ulcers

These are ulcers in a foot with good collateral circulation (palpable pulses). Since the ulcer usually forms in areas of excess pressure caused by bony deformity and enhanced by the absence of warning pain or discomfort, prevention is a definite possibility. One can see the oddly shaped bone or identify the stiff joint or callus. If something like this exists, the patient can usually be kept out of trouble with the help of a podiatrist, by using special shoes (often broader and higher in the toe area), special inner soles built up where appropriate, or by corrective foot surgery.

If an ulcer has formed, treatment will depend on its size and the extent of surrounding infection. Small ulcers are treated on an outpatient basis with oral antibiotics, one-quarter strength Betadine dressings, and avoidance of weight bearing (by means of bed rest, crutches, and so on). Foot soaking or heat in any form is never used. The former does not do any good and introduces bacteria. The latter can cause burns in a numb limb.

More extensive ulcers, or smaller ones that have failed to heal, require hospitalization. Management will now include intravenous antibiotics, or operative drainage, or digital amputation if indicated.

Often the metatarsophalangeal joint proves to be involved, in which case that joint and the attached toe must be removed.

Since the circulation is often excellent in these patients, large skin defects may be covered with partial-thickness skin grafts. In other circumstances, defects may be closed by shortening the foot (transmetatarsal amputation).

Ischemic Ulcerations

Patients with poor circulation who develop ulcerations by the mechanisms previously described present more difficult problems. The key factors are the amount of pain involved, the location of the lesion, the degree of ischemia, and the presence or extent of infection. Depending on these factors, the treatment may vary from a Band-Aid to a series of major operations to save the foot or a major leg amputation.

Small Ulcers. Small ulcers with little cellulitis in patients with only moderate ischemia may be treated on an ambulatory basis, using crutches only if the area is weight bearing. The lesions that can be treated with this program are often on the back of the heel or the tip of a toe. The causative factors must be eliminated (poorly fitting shoes, and so on), oral antibiotics are used, any indicated drainage is instituted, and a dressing, usually of one-quarter strength Betadine, is applied once or twice a day. If ambulation is to be permitted, a sandal or shoe with the appropriate area cut out is satisfactory. Healing will be slow and the patient must be closely followed lest the condition deteriorate.

If the circulation is found to be severely impaired on physical examination, consideration must be given to arterial reconstruction, even in this group of patients with small ulcers. This is particularly true if ischemic pain at rest is present, as it signifies severe ischemia. Appropriate arteriography is obtained and arterial surgery scheduled if it is possible. In this group, the surgeon should be much more aggressive than when considering patients who suffer only from claudication. Often combinations of aortofemoral plus femoropopliteal grafts may be indicated and are carried out by two teams working simultaneously. In other instances grafts to the tibial artery are required, sometimes sequentially, that is, femoral-popliteal-tibial. If at all possible, saphenous or cephalic veins are used for at least the portion of the operation below the knee. Initial success rates above 90 percent are obtained, with only modest numbers of late occlusions.

Once adequate circulation is established, small areas of necrosis will heal. It may be necessary to remove larger areas of necrosis by conservative amputations in the foot.

Larger Areas. Larger areas of necrosis require in-hospital treatment with intravenous antibiotics if spreading sepsis is present, careful evaluation of the circulation, and arterial reconstruction if appropriate. Often some form of amputation will be needed, these will be discussed starting most distally.

Toe Amputations. Here I refer to a single digit transphalangeal procedure. The indication would usually be necrosis somewhere in the distal third or perhaps half of the toe, too large or ischemic to heal or involving the bone (except the terminal tuft of the phalanx). In the ischemic foot the skin must be closed primarily if healing is to occur, so sepsis must be confined to the ulcer prior to operation. The collateral circulation must be adequate, which practically means that the skin at the incision site must be intact and healthy in appearance, the venous filling time less than 20 to 25 seconds, and that no dependent rubor be present at the incision site. With attention to these criteria and with meticulous operating techniques, healing is to be expected 95 percent of the time.

Toe and Single Metatarsal Head. Since this operation of necessity leaves a large "dead," or open, space, it is seldom indicated in an ischemic foot. We use it frequently in the neuropathic foot with penetrating ulcers and at least fair circulation. Usually the distal 80 percent of the incision is closed and the proximal end left open for drainage.

Transmetatarsal Amputation. The transmetatarsal amputation (all toes and metatarsal heads) has the advantage of getting farther away from the diseased area and into tissue with better blood supply. It is indicated for areas of necrosis on or between the toes or over a metatarsal head. When the ulcer is beneath one of the middle metatarsal heads, a "V" of skin is removed from the plantar flap and the incision closed in a "T." Since the dorsal skin has poor circulation, the incision is straight across the top of the foot and closure is made with a plantar flap. The collateral circulation must be adequate and closure must be obtained primarily if this is to heal in an ischemic foot. Postoperatively, prolonged bed rest (three weeks) is required, followed by slow progression from wheelchair to weight bearing. When the procedure is performed for ischemia, my initial success rate is greater than 80 percent and the follow-up indicates a five-year success rate of 50 percent. Once the foot has healed, the patient can walk without a limp.

The Below Knee Amputation. The below knee amputation is employed when a foot cannot be salvaged. Rarely, it is done an inch or so above the ankle as a "guillotine" amputation (no flaps and no closure) for uncontrolled foot sepsis. A higher closed procedure is carried out a week or so later. More commonly, a closed below knee amputation is carried out, with any foot sepsis controlled by antibiotics.

Most patients requiring a major amputation can have it at this level, as opposed to an operation above the knee. It is important to operate below the knee if at all possible, because walking with a prosthesis is then relatively easy, while it is nearly impossible for many older diabetics when the leg is lost at a higher level. In general terms, a below knee amputation should heal regardless of the level at which pulses can be felt if there is no area of gangrene or of skin temperature change above the ankle.

The Above Knee Amputation. The above knee amputation, which is seldom employed at my hospital, is reserved for those patients requiring removal of a foot whose circulation would not permit a lower operation, or for those who for other health reasons could never use even a below knee prosthesis.

NECROBIOSIS LIPOIDICA DIABETICORUM

This entity should be mentioned in any surgical review of diabetic leg problems. Pathologically, it consists of subcutaneous or intracutaneous deposits of fat and cholesterol. The skin becomes discolored to a reddish-purple and eventually ulcerates. Usually the circulation is at least fairly good, so that excision and skin grafting can succeed. The important thing is not to diagnose "gangrene" and suggest leg amputation, an error that I have seen.

DIABETIC OSTEOARTHROPATHY

Diabetic osteoarthropathy is another condition peculiar to the diabetic foot. It is similar to the Charcot joint described in cases of syphilis in years past. In the diabetic neuropathic foot the tarsal and/or metatarsal bones may disintegrate. When the process is active, the foot may be unusually warm, even red in color, becomes swollen, and, as the bones deteriorate, an odd rocker shape develops. It is important not to misdiagnose this as osteomyelitis and advise surgery, which may even lead to an unnecessary amputation. The proper treatment is to avoid any weight bearing at all until the active destruction stops, as shown by loss of heat and a stable appearance demonstrated by several x-rays. This may take many weeks but must be done if a useful foot is to be salvaged. When all is quiet, a special shoe with a rocker sole may be needed.

SUMMARY

The diabetic foot can be afflicted with a variety of problems not seen in other patients. Precise diagnosis, well-thought-out treatment programs, and gentle, meticulous surgery can save these patients much misery. I hope that these comments will encourage physicians to seek out interested and informed surgeons who will care for these unfortunate patients.

INSULIN RESISTANCE AND ALLERGY

JEFFREY S. FLIER, M.D.

INSULIN RESISTANCE

Broadly defined, insulin resistance is a state in which a given concentration of insulin evokes less than the normal biologic response. When it is defined in this manner, patients with this condition span a broad clinical spectrum. At one end of the spectrum are patients in whom tissue resistance to insulin is overcome by endogenous hypersection of insulin, resulting in normal or nearly normal glucose tolerance. Examples are most patients with obesity, infection, pregnancy, and glucocorticoid or growth hormone excess, as well as certain patients with genetic syndromes of target cell resistance to insulin action. When it is available, appropriate treatment of these entities (for example, diet therapy for obesity, antibiotics for infection) leads to enhanced insulin sensitivity. However, since glucose homeostasis is, by definition, normal in this group, and compensated insulin resistance per se has no proven adverse effects, there is no clinical indication either to investigate or to treat the insulin resistance in this setting.

At the other end of the spectrum is the clinical problem of the insulin treated diabetic who does not respond to conventional doses of exogenous insulin. At what dose of insulin should we consider such a patient resistant to insulin? A commonly employed definition holds a patient to be insulin resistant when more than 200 units of insulin are required each day. However, it is now known that the normal pancreas secretes 20–50 units of insulin in the course of a day. Thus the arbitrary use of the 200-unit figure seems too restrictive. On the other hand, minor or transient increases in insulin requirements have a different significance and are best discussed separately. For these reasons, I have described an approach to patients who respond poorly to a daily dosage of more than 100 units of insulin, or to patients who display a sustained (more than two weeks' duration) and major (more than twofold) increase in a previously stable baseline insulin requirement.

Approach to Treatment of the Insulin Resistant Patient

First assess patient compliance.

This has two components, the first of which involves an assessment of the insulin injection technique. Patients should be questioned about the details of the method by which they draw up and inject insulin, and if at all possible, the patient should be observed on at least one occasion. Discovery of a faulty measurement or injection technique may obviate the need for an extended workup. Dietary history must also be assessed. Markedly increased caloric intake, especially in the obese adult diabetic, may account for poor response to a rising insulin dosage.

Second, consider the easily diagnosed and common conditions that characteristically impair insulin sensitivity, as listed below.

1. Sustained and severe emotional stress may increase insulin requirements, but rarely does this alone cause insulin needs to rise above 100 units per day.

2. Insulin resistance is a regular feature of both bacterial and viral infections, and infected patients occasionally will have uncontrolled hyperglycemia on an insulin dosage in excess of 100–200 units per day. Resolution of infection typically leads to prompt dosage reduction. Although most infections that cause major insulin resistance are clinically evident, insulin resistance may occasionally result from relatively inapparent infectious foci, such as periodontal and sinus sources, and these should always be considered. In diabetics with refractory bacterial or fungal infections, treatment of hyperglycemia with insulin should be aggressively pursued, since poor diabetic control may hamper successful control of the infection.

3. Excess production of counter-insulin hormones underlies the insulin resistance of Cushing's syndrome, acromegaly, pregnancy, and less commonly, pheochromocytoma. Development of thyrotoxicosis in a diabetic may cause increased insulin requirements as well. The insulin resistance in these cases is usually modest, and the diagnoses are usually evident once the conditions are considered.

Third, a number of uncommon syndromes associated with marked tissue resistance may be readily suspected on clinical grounds, implying the need for further evaluation and treatment. Foremost among these are a variety of syndromes in which the skin lesion acanthosis nigricans is seen. In one syndrome that affects young women (type A), an additional feature is polycystic ovaries. Resistance to administered insulin in type A patients ranges from moderately severe to extremely marked. For this reason, once the condition is diagnosed insulin doses should be escalated briskly. Individual patients have failed to respond to as many as 48,000 units daily. In those instances in which insulin therapy appears ineffective despite maximum dosages, it may be reasonable to discontinue insulin entirely. In the type B syndrome of insulin resistance with acanthosis nigricans, a variety of autoimmune features accompany the anti-insulin receptor antibodies that cause the insulin resistance of the syndrome. As in the type A syndrome, ketoacidosis is rare and huge insulin doses may be ineffective in controlling blood glucose levels. Perhaps a quarter of known patients with antireceptor antibodies had a spontaneous remission of diabetes over two to three years of observation. Individual patients have responded to trials of high-dose prednisone (60–80 mg per day) or antimetabolite drugs (Cytoxan, 1 mg/kg per day). An equal number has failed to respond, and given the fact that spontaneous remissions do occur, the overall efficacy of such therapy is unknown. In a patient with antireceptor antibodies and markedly symptomatic hyperglycemia unresponsive to any deliverable dose of insulin, I would attempt therapy with 60–80 mg of prednisone per day. I would allow up to a month for a beneficial effect to become evident, monitoring insulin effect on blood glucose level as well as antireceptor antibody titer if at all possible. It should be remembered that glucocorticoids, if unable to suppress antireceptor antibody titer, would be expected to worsen the hyperglycemia. When all else fails and treatment is required, repeated exchange transfusions have been attempted, but because there are limited data on the effectiveness of this modality, it is not recommended.

The syndromes of total or partial lipoatrophy may also be associated with marked insulin resistance, and these conditions should be readily diagnosed on physical examination. High-dose insulin therapy is the only available treatment for symptomatic hyperglycemia.

Occasionally, resistance to subcutaneously administered insulin is severe, but there is normal sensitivity to intravenously injected insulin. This syndrome can be easily diagnosed by a trial of low-dose intravenous insulin. Thus patients unresponsive to as many as 5000 units per day by the subcutaneous route have responded to 3–5 units of insulin per hour when given intravenously. The syndrome appears to be acquired and is thought to be caused by excessive protease activity in the subcutaneous tissue. Although the severity of the insulin resistance may fluctuate over time, and periods of frank hypoglycemia up to ten days in duration while the patient is off insulin have also been observed, the resistance to subcutaneously administered insulin may be sufficiently severe and prolonged to require an attempt at therapy. A number of patients have required percutaneous placement of a Silastic cannula into the superior vena cava, with constant infusion of insulin using a portable open-loop pump. Phlebitis, thrombosis,

and bacteremia have been common sequelae of this approach, and it should be avoided if at all possible. Recent reports have suggested that these patients may respond to subcutaneous insulin when it is mixed with aprotinin (Trasylol), a protease inhibitor known to inactivate certain tissue proteases in vitro. When used at a final dilution of 4–160 kallidogenase inactivating units (KIU) per unit of insulin, rapid restoration of metabolic response to conventional doses of insulin has been observed in a number of patients. Adverse effects have been limited to transient redness and itching at the injection site. The effectiveness of aprotinin may diminish after six to nine months, with restoration of the effect if the drug is withheld and insulin given intravenously for a period of weeks. Allergic sensitivity and anaphylaxis have been rare complications of intravenous aprotinin employed in the treatment of pancreatitis. Although aprotinin may be the therapy of choice in patients with subcutaneous insulin degradation, it has not been approved for this condition, and the therapy should therefore be viewed as experimental.

Fourth, the majority of patients treated with insulin who develop a sustained and marked increase in insulin requirement (> 100 and especially > 200 units per day) will not prove to have any of the conditions yet discussed. Rather, they will be suffering from the consequences of a high titer of IgG anti-insulin antibodies. Features that increase the likelihood of this diagnosis in a given patient are a history of intermittent insulin therapy, use of less purified insulins or those containing beef insulin, or a history of allergic response to insulin. In many cases, none of these features will be present.

My first step in the treatment of a patient who might have high titer anti-insulin antibodies would be to switch, if this has not already been done, to a highly purified pork insulin. This has both diagnostic and therapeutic utility. Many patients will have a modest improvement in glycemic control on the same or even lower doses of pork insulin, evident within the first few days of therapy. This is a result of lower affinity of pork versus beef insulin for binding to pre-existing antibodies. An additional improvement may often occur over the next few weeks to months, as the antibody titer falls in response to the less immunogenic challenge. In some patients, the switch to pork insulin will be sufficient therapy. If it is not, and symptomatic diabetes continues despite large doses of purified pork insulin, it is worth remembering that most patients with anti-insulin antibodies as the cause of their insulin resistance will spontaneously remit over the course of 6 to 12 months. Thus it is possible to continue pork insulin therapy at whatever high dosage is necessary to avoid metabolic decompensation. If the dosage of insulin itself becomes a problem because of the large volume administered, it may be helpful to obtain U-500 insulin. This concentrated insulin is crystalline zinc insulin (regular), but it has a time course of action that lies between that of rapid- and intermediate-acting insulins. Two doses per day are usually prescribed. In some patients resistant to large doses of U-100 NPH or lente, improved response to lower doses of U-500 has been observed, suggesting that the switch from high-dose U-100 to U-500 insulin should initially be associated with a modest dose reduction (about 30 percent), followed by a brisk increase in the administered dose (about 10–20 units at a time) if the response is poor.

If high-dose pork, U-100, or U-500 insulin has failed to control hyperglycemia over a period of weeks, I will usually measure an anti-insulin antibody titer. In those cases in which anti-insulin antibodies are responsible for the insulin resistance, the titer is substantially higher than that routinely found in the plasma of insulin treated patients. A low antibody titer suggests another etiologic agent for the insulin resistance. If the titer is high, and poorly controlled, symptomatic diabetes has persisted for weeks to several months, I will consider two other therapeutic maneuvers.

The first maneuver to be considered is the administration of glucocorticoids. The decision to employ glucocorticoids must be carefully weighed, since these medications of themselves increase tissue resistance to insulin and worsen hyperglycemia, and they have numerous other well-known complications. For these reasons, I will not employ these drugs unless (1) the presence of immunologic insulin resistance is confirmed by reliable antibody titers, and (2) the severity of the uncontrolled diabetes can no longer be tolerated. If these conditions are met, 60–80 mg of prednisone are administered in divided doses. When effective (in 20 to 50 percent of cases), the response is sometimes surprisingly rapid: within several days to two weeks. Glycemic control must be carefully monitored to avoid hypoglycemica from the increasingly effective high doses of insulin, as well as hyperglycemia from the additive effects of the glucocorticoids themselves. Most patients would benefit from hospitalization in the initial phases of this therapy.

If insulin sensitivity is restored, tapering of prednisone should be rapid (over two to three weeks), with due concern for the usual issues regarding glucocorticoid withdrawal. If at all possible, prednisone should be completely discontinued when insulin sensitivity is restored. If a major beneficial effect has not been seen after three weeks of prednisone treatment, the therapy should be discontinued.

Occasional patients with severely uncontrolled diabetes clearly due to anti-insulin antibodies will fail to respond to these therapies. It may then be necessary to obtain sulfated insulin, which is usually rapidly effective but is unfortunately not generally available in this country. Sulfated insulin, a beef or pork insulin that has been chemically modified by treatment with sulfuric acid, retains about half of its original activity on a weight basis, but possesses markedly less affinity for anti-insulin antibodies. Thus, when switching to sulfated insulin, patients require an average of 15 percent of their previous insulin dosage, and this is usually evident from the first dose administered. The dosage requirement often falls further as antibody titers decline over ensuing weeks with the diminished antigenic stimulation. Sulfated insulin is currently available in Canada and in the United States as an investigational drug. Although currently unavailable, fish insulin would be expected to have a similar mode of action and efficacy.

A final and poorly recorded syndrome of insulin resistance is that of the adult, typically obese patient whose insulin resistance cannot be explained by any of the above considerations. Insulin resistance persists despite (1) supervised diet, (2) ruling out of all relevant stresses and unusual syndromes, (3) a negative trial of intravenously administered insulin, and (4) a trial of pork insulin plus demonstration of unimpressive anti-insulin antibody titer. Some patients of this description have an excellent response to a sulfonylurea, either alone or when added to a lower dose of insulin. These patients are presumed to have developed an unusually marked degree of tissue resistance to insulin, and the sulfonylurea is presumed to have acted by increasing the tissue response to insulin. It would be prudent to admit such a patient to the hospital for close monitoring of blood glucose levels, unless the patient is both reliable and adept at glucose self-monitoring techniques. Along with addition of the sulfonylurea, such as 500 mg of

Tolinase, the insulin dosage should be reduced by at least 50 percent. Response is often rapid—within days—and may persist indefinitely. Some patients may not require further insulin therapy. Because the efficacy of this treatment is unpredictable, close follow-up of glycemic control is mandatory.

INSULIN ALLERGY

The insulin currently available for the treatment of diabetes is obtained by extraction of animal (beef and/or pork) pancreas. Because the insulins of these species are not identical to human insulin (pork differs by one and beef by three amino acid residues), and because of hormonal and other impurities that are not removed during industrial preparation, allergic responses to administered insulin are well-known complications of insulin therapy. These reactions, which are becomming much less common now that the level of impurities has been markedly reduced in standard insulin preparations, may be transient and local or, less commonly, systemic and severe. The occurrence of severe reactions may be as much a function of genetic susceptibility as of the nature of the insulin preparation.

Preferred Approach to Treatment of Insulin Allergy

Prevention. There are several therapeutic practices that can reduce the prevalence of allergic reactions to insulin. The first involves avoidance of intermittent insulin therapy wherever possible, since intermittence appears to increase greatly the prevalence of future allergic responses.

Now that all commercially available insulin has lower levels of contaminants as compared with insulin available only two or three years ago, the major therapeutic decision that remains relates to the choice of insulin species (that is, mixed species versus pure beef or pork). When insulin therapy is acutely needed, but the need is likely to be transient (for example, with gestational diabetes, extreme stress, and so on), highly purified pork insulin is clearly indicated, since the patients have a high risk of insulin allergy and pork insulin is less immunogenic than pure beef or beef/pork mixtures in the majority of patients. Although there is no proof that, at the current high level of purity, monospecies pork has a clinical advantage over

beef-containing preparations in the routine treatment of diabetes, I am currently prescribing monospecies pork insulin to all new insulin treated patients, since supplies appear to be adequate, price differentials are relatively small, and a small number of patients would be expected to benefit.

Treatment of Local Insulin Allergy. Insulin injection technique should be assessed and viewed by the physician or nurse if at all possible, since occasional patients induce local swelling by faulty injection technique. If this is not the case, I will switch the patient to monospecies pork insulin if he is not already using it. Many patients appear to respond to this maneuver, either because of the lower immunogenicity of pork versus beef insulin, or because most local reactions are typically transient, regardless of changes in therapy. When troubling local reactions persist despite one week of pork insulin therapy, or earlier if reactions are severe, antihistaminic therapy may be helpful. Systemic therapy (50 mg of Benadryl) may be tried, but this is not often effective. Benadryl is more effective when mixed in the insulin syringe and directly administered with insulin. A dose of 1 mg of Benadryl with each 10 units of insulin produces improvement of many local reactions. For particularly severe local reactions unresponsive to Benadryl, addition of 2–5 mg of hydrocortisone to the insulin syringe is worth an attempt for 2 to 3 days. Throughout this period, the patient can be assured that such reactions are typically self limited.

Treatment of Systemic Insulin Allergy. Systemic insulin allergy may be manifested as serum sickness, purpura, angioedema that may progress to respiratory failure and shock, or an Arthus-like reaction with LE cells, eosinophilia, and hypergammaglobulinemia. Concurrent local reactions are often but not always present. When systemic reactions occur, it is reasonable to switch to monospecies pork insulin, but this is not very helpful in most cases.

Desensitization is the most effective therapy for systemic insulin allergy, and over 90 percent of patients can be successfully desensitized using the regimen presented here. The patient must first be hospitalized. It is important to diminish the circulating levels of insulin prior to desensitization. Thus insulin injections should be discontinued for as long a period as possible given the metabolic state of the patient. It is my practice to change to a regimen of regular pork insulin given every 6 hours, and then to stop all insulin for at least 24 hours if possible. Intravenous saline, KCl, and

HCO_3 are administered as needed. The desensitization is most easily carried out with a kit made available by the Eli Lilly Company. The kits employ monospecies beef or pork insulin, serially diluted with human serum albumin to prevent sticking.

Prior to desensitization, it is prudent to advise the patient that severe allergic reactions may occur. All anti-inflammatory drugs that might obscure a reaction are discontinued. The procedure should be initiated by intradermal testing with 0.1 ml volumes of saline followed by beef and pork insulin, the latter at 1/1000 unit. Unless the reaction is clearly greater with pork insulin, as rarely occurs, desensitization should be carried out with pork insulin, according to the scheme in Table 1. Because of the danger of life-threatening anaphylactic reactions, epinephrine, Benadryl, and intubation equipment must be available, and a physician should be present or easily available. Once desensitization has been successfully carried out, the desensitized state should be maintained by insulin injections once or twice daily for an indefinite period. Occasionally, patients have required multiple desensitizations despite apparently continuous insulin therapy.

In the unusual circumstances in which desensitization is ineffective, the available therapeutic alternatives are few, and these have little data to support their use. They include glucocorticoid therapy and use of sulfated insulin (see above, in the section on treatment of insulin resistance).

TABLE 1 Schedule for Rapid Insulin Desensitization

Time (hours)	Dose (units)	Route
0	1/1000 (may need less)	intradermal
½	1/500	intradermal
1	1/250	subcutaneous
1½	1/100	subcutaneous
2	1/50	subcutaneous
2½	1/25	subcutaneous
3	1/10	subcutaneous
3½	1/5	subcutaneous
4	1/2	subcutaneous
4½	1	subcutaneous
5	2	subcutaneous
5½	4	subcutaneous
6	8	subcutaneous

Note: If a reaction occurs, drop back two dilutions and continue.

After last dose (8 units), give 2–10 units every 4 to 6 hours for the next 24 to 36 hours before switching to intermediate-acting insulin.

HYPOGLYCEMIA

POSTPRANDIAL HYPOGLYCEMIA

JOHN W. ENSINCK, M.D.

THE DILEMMA IN DIFFERENTIAL DIAGNOSIS

In recent years, there has been much heated debate concerning the prevalence of postprandial (reactive or rebound) hypoglycemia in Western societies and about the options for its treatment. This controversy stems in part from the confusion in the minds of physicians as to how to establish its diagnosis definitively, as well as from misconceptions among lay people who have been led to believe that hypoglycemia is a common disorder. The diagnosis has become a popular explanation for the symptoms emanating from the substantial stresses of everyday living in our complex society. Unfortunately, this preoccupation by hypochondriacal patients with the idea that their complaints are due to hypoglycemia has been exploited by some medical practitioners for their financial gain. Moreover, a number of ethical physicians have perpetuated this notion unwittingly because of their dependence upon diagnostic criteria that, although held to be gospel, are inadequate and misleading. Therefore it is not difficult for both patient and physician to become convinced that the cluster of symptoms occurring within a few hours of food intake is due to hypoglycemia. Owing to the lack of a precise means of diagnosis, the frequency of this disorder in the population cannot be validly assessed. How then have we arrived at this dilemma?

Hypoglycemia is operationally defined as an abnormality of fuel homeostasis reflected by a fall in blood glucose level below 45 mg/dl. This definition has been arbitrarily arrived at from observations that the majority of normal persons will have blood glucose levels that are higher than this during fasting or after food intake. The clinical manifestations of hypoglycemia are the result of responses of the central nervous system to counteract the decline in its major source of energy. Depending upon the rate of fall of the blood glucose level, its nadir, and maintenance at a given level, distinctive clinical patterns accompany the activation of the adrenergic nervous system and perturbation in cortical and subcortical functions. In general, an abrupt increase in sympathetic nervous system activity is likely to be triggered during a rapid fall of circulating glucose, but it also may be further stimulated when the blood glucose level falls below a threshold between 40 and 50 mg/dl. Activation of the adrenergic nervous system accounts for the symptoms of restlessness, anxiety, hunger, sweating, palpitations, and malaise. Deranged cortical and subcortical cerebral function is usually preceded by heightened sympathetic activity and is rarely encountered when blood glucose levels are greater than 40 mg/dl. It is obvious that the neuroglucopenic syndrome that is the consequence of decreased availability of glucose may simulate a wide array of psychiatric and neurologic disorders.

Oral Glucose Tolerance Test

Postprandial hypoglycemia occurs during the transition between the fed and fasting phases, and virtually all the symptoms relate to activation of the adrenergic nervous system caused by the rapid descent of circulating glucose levels. Based upon a number of recent studies, it is abundantly clear that the oral glucose tolerance test (OGTT), the time-honored test for postprandial hypoglycemia, should be abandoned and replaced by responses of blood sugar levels within 6 hours after the ingestion of a regular meal. This recommendation to discard the hallowed OGTT is based on considerable data accumulated in the past decade, which indicate that up to 20 percent of normal individuals may have blood glucose levels below 45 mg/dl and yet are asymptomatic. Since intraduodenal instillation of glucose into normal subjects results in rapid glucose absorption with augmented insulin release proportional to the glycemic stimulus with frequent hypoglycemia, it is not surprising that the ingestion of hypertonic solutions of glucose may lead to variable rates of glucose absorption, depending upon gastric transit time. The OGTT is prone to wider excursions in the glycemic level than are encountered with food of mixed nutrient composition, which tends to retard rates of monosaccharide absorption. The OGTT is thus an unsuitable model to replicate the perturbations in glucose levels following food intake and has no validity in establishing a diagnosis of postprandial hypoglycemia. Unfortunately, the OGTT is still widely used by physicians, and its interpretation has led to the conviction that postprandial hypoglycemia is a widespread disorder.

Food Tolerance Test

A number of authorities now recommend a standardized breakfast tolerance test as a substitute for the OGTT. A meal of specified calories and composition has not as yet been widely evaluated; however, it seems reasonable to recommend a food tolerance test that involves the ingestion of food containing a third of the patient's typical daily caloric intake, with 50 percent complex carbohydrates, 30 percent fat, and 20 percent protein. Since many of the patients may already be undergoing treatment for their alleged hypoglycemic symptoms by restriction of dietary carbohydrate, which has been shown to accentuate the hypoglycemic responses to the OGTT, it is advisable to request that patients rearrange their food patterns to increase the portion of complex carbohydrates to approximately 50 percent of total calories seven days before undertaking the test. Although it is clear that the OGTT has led to the diagnosis of an excessive number of false positive cases of reactive hypoglycemia, experience with the diagnostic sensitivity of the meal tolerance test is not extensive. In a recent study comparing the glucose responses to an OGTT with those to a mixed meal in patients with apparent idiopathic postabsorptive hypoglycemia, 78 percent had identical groups of symptoms regardless of the oral challenge. Nonetheless, glucose levels after food ingestion never achieved hypoglycemic levels. In 118 patients with suspected reactive hypoglycemia, Lev-Ran and Anderson found that only 16 had glucopenia after an OGTT, whereas 5 of the 16 had symptomatic hypoglycemia after ingestion of a meal. Therefore, although postprandial hypoglycemia may be far less common than heretofore thought, it is not to say that symptomatic hypoglycemia related to food ingestion does not exist. Previous classifications of reactive hypoglycemia probably still hold true in terms of etiologic agents and pathogenesis. Thus, those patients with bona fide hypoglycemia have in common a relationship between food ingestion and the rates of delivery of nutrients to the bloodstream, and the response of the B cells in releasing insulin to the particular substrate, notably glucose.

CLASSIFICATION OF HYPOGLYCEMIAS

Postprandial Hypoglycemia

Based on the OGTT, three groups of patients are most likely to experience symptomatic hypoglycemia in the postprandial phase.

In patients who have undergone gastrointestinal surgery (including partial or total gastrectomy, gastrojejunostomy, or pyloroplasty) symptomatic hypoglycemia is not uncommon after food ingestion. It is attributed to the rapid transit of nutrients into the lumen of the small intestine, leading to rapid absorption and triggering excessive insulin secretion coincident with the rapid ascent of high levels of circulating glucose.

Whether or not reactive hypoglycemia is found in patients with non–insulin-dependent diabetes mellitus early in its development is uncertain, but it is now thought to be a rare occurrence. Based on profiles obtained with the OGTT, the alleged hypoglycemia is preceded by hyperglycemia and the nadir and blood sugar "lags" 4 to 5 hours after eating. This phenomenon has been ascribed to dysfunctional B cells that are inappropriately responsive to glucose and other physiologic signals.

Despite the inappropriateness of labeling hypoglycemia as the cause of stress-related symptoms in the vast majority of patients, it is nonetheless likely that there is a small but distinct group of patients who develop glucopenia after eating. Since no systematic evaluation of meal tolerance test results has been undertaken to search for an abnormality in either intestinal absorption or in pancreatic endocrine responses, it seems reasonable to continue to designate them as idiopathic.

Pseudohypoglycemia

In contrast, the designation "pseudohypoglycemia" has been given to the hordes of patients whose symptoms mimic those of legitimate reactive hypoglycemia but who do not have documented glucopenia. Because of the overlap between the two groups of patients and the quandary in which I have frequently been placed in attempting to treat them, I describe in the following sections therapeutic approaches that might apply to both.

STRATEGIES FOR TREATMENT OF PATIENTS WITH POSTPRANDIAL HYPOGLYCEMIA AND "PSEUDOHYPOGLYCEMIA"

I have attempted to place in perspective my opinion that symptomatic hypoglycemia occurring in the postprandial state is indeed an uncommon, if not rare, benign disorder in the adult. However, in those patients in whom the diagnosis has been established by a meal tolerance test, as well as in a number of individuals who have adrenergic manifestations following food intake without hypoglycemia, it is appropriate to consider the options for treatment that might alleviate their symptoms. It is obvious that, if there is substantial uncertainty as to whether a patient's complaints are due to hypoglycemia, it is unlikely that a specific treatment will definitely be successful. This may account for the many nostrums that became fashionable but were eventually discarded by the patients who did not benefit from their use. Unfortunately, some of these are not innocuous; for example, the use of adrenal cortical extracts has led to clinical manifestations of glucocorticoid excess or, when withdrawn, to chronic adrenal suppression. Similarly, the belief in the salutary effects of a variety of vitamins in large doses has no foundation other than perhaps a psychologic one. It is hoped that, when studies have been undertaken to identify the subset of patients who have symptomatic hypoglycemia related to their meals (idiopathic), and an underlying cause for the pathogenesis has been identified, a coherent, rational treatment targeted to rectify the specific defect will be forthcoming. In the meantime, time-honored approaches are still available to the physician treating patients who have legitimate hypoglycemia as well as those with "pseudohypoglycemia." Since many of the latter share symptoms that may be attributable to adrenergic hyperactivity, the methods described below may be successful in alleviating the symptom complex.

Counseling

In view of the overlap of symptoms in patients with bona fide idiopathic reactive hypoglycemia and those who have been labeled as having "pseudohypoglycemia," it is relevant for the physician to attempt to distinguish between the two groups. Since patients with hypoglycemia may share with the pseudohypoglycemia patients personality descriptions such as intense, driving, conscientious, tense, emotionally labile, nervous, and apprehensive, it is not unreasonable to infer that a rapid fall in blood glucose levels postprandially may contribute to symptoms in such patients, and they may thus benefit from efforts to identify and mitigate obvious causes of stress. In addition, the patients should be encouraged to "ventilate" to their physician or surrogate. If the psychologic disturbances are more deep-seated and beyond the scope of the physician's skills, professional psychiatric care may be indicated. Patients with pseudohypoglycemia should be informed that hypoglycemia is not the cause of their symptoms. It is a disservice to them to maintain the illusion that a metabolic disorder is at the root of their complaints. Of course, the decision as to when to break this news to the patient must be individualized and tact must be used in bringing the patient to the realization that he or she may have substituted a fashionable disease for less acceptable alternatives, such as depression or anxiety. Since the idea of hypoglycemia may be firmly entrenched in some patients' minds; the sensitive issue of a psychologic cause for their problems must be approached with care. In some instances, it may be that the patients' symptoms are partly explained by sympathetic nervous system activation during the postprandial phase without glucopenia, and they may therefore benefit from dietary measures that are also recommended for patients with idiopathic reactive hypoglycemia (see below). Nevertheless, the physician is not advised to use this to perpetuate the belief that the patient may have a metabolic abnormality. The prescription of appropriate psychotropic drugs (Table 1) may be beneficial. On the other hand, if such benign measures fail, it may be necessary to refer the patient to the care of a psychiatrist.

The physician should also be aware of the possibility that, in those patients in whom the symptom complex can be convincingly linked to biochemical glucopenia, treatment with diet, drugs, or surgery may not reverse the symptoms. Based upon evaluation of patients with symptoms of rebound hypoglycemia during OGTT who have undergone the Minnesota Multiphasic Personality Inventory, those who experience reactive hypoglycemia were more likely to have psychologic disturbances, including depression and hysteria. Nonetheless, because the diagnosis was based upon the OGTT, the prevalence of true hypoglycemia in these patients has not been definitely established. Whether or not there is an increased association of neurosis in the patients with idiopathic reactive hypoglycemia remains to be ascertained.

Diet

Because patients with true hypoglycemia as well as those who have pseudohypoglycemia experience symptoms within a few hours of eating, the composition of the meal, its size, and when it is eaten are major factors in the attempts to relieve patients' symptoms. Numerous studies have shown that the composition and physical properties of food are critical determinants in the speed of absorption of the dietary components. Thus the rates at which nutrients are delivered to the absorptive segments of the small intestine are governed not only by the propulsive force through the stomach, but also by the relationship between the proportions of proteins, fats, and carbohydrates and their physical states. Therefore, it is not surprising that persons most prone to experiencing a rapid absorption of glucose are those who have increased gastric transit times of food, in particular, of mono- and disaccharides, which comprise refined carbohydrates. This principle underlies the likelihood that patients who have had surgical resection of various portions of the stomach will have accelerated absorption of glucose, accounting for the early hyperglycemia and consequent hyperinsulinemia resulting in rebound hypoglycemia. It is also conceivable that the food of patients with idiopathic reactive hypoglycemia is more rapidly passed into the intestinal lumen, thereby leading to increased glucose absorption and insulin release—although this may be less dramatic than in patients who have had gastric surgery. Hence, efforts to match the physiologic processes of digestion and absorption form the basis of the modification of the dietary regimen in an attempt to mitigate exaggerated rates of monosaccharide absorption and concomitant inordinate insulin release.

Due to the varied food preferences among various populations, no universally accepted dietary prescription can be applied to all patients, and the kinds of foods and the frequency of intake must be tailored within the context of ethnic dietary habits. Since the efficacy of any specific diet has not been rigorously proven, the physician, with the aid of the dietitian, may have to improvise meal plans to attempt to alleviate the individual patient's symptoms. Because of the nature of the neuroglucopenic symptoms experienced by patients with both "pseudo-" and "true" hypoglycemia, it is mandatory to avoid stringent constraints on food selection, since they may further "cripple" patients who already have underlying personality disorders. Therefore, to optimize potential benefits from dietary manipulation and to assure the compliance of the patient the following are needed: (1) a sympathetic physician with insights into mechanisms underlying the patient's symptoms; (2) a dietitian skilled in imaginatively coping with the patient's individual dietary idiosyncrasies and constructing a flexible diet geared to palatability and minimizing monotony; and (3) continuing follow-up and revision of the diet to ensure its efficacy.

The traditional modification of meals for treatment of patients with reactive hypoglycemia entails rearrangement of the elements in the average western diet, in which carbohydrate comprises approximately 50 percent. This widely accepted dietary prescription is derived from studies performed in the 1930s and 1940s by Conn and others, who advised substitution of protein for carbohydrate to minimize the glucose-mediated excursions in insulin secretion. To meet these objectives the rearrangement of dietary composition also necessitates inclusion of foods high in animal fat. In addition, it has become standard practice to recommend that the amount of food taken at each meal be diminished and the number of feedings increased; the meals are interspersed throughout the day both to remove the dietary load and to ensure the continuous absorption of nutrients, thereby decreasing the chance of glucopenic episodes.

A weight-maintaining diet consisting of approximately 30 percent protein, 50 percent fat, and 20 percent carbohydrate is generally recommended. Throughout the years patients have asserted that their symptoms have abated with rigid adherence to this dietary formula. Nevertheless, several practical problems arise with these diets: (1) restricted food options that make the diet monotonous, (2) expense of protein-containing foods, and (3) concern about the possibility of increased atherogenesis due to inclusion of foods high in animal fat. Moreover, studies by Permutt have indicated that diets high in fat and protein are likely to predispose one to hypoglycemia if refined carbohydrate is ingested, as might occur in patients who do not adhere to the "hypoglycemia" diet. There is also considerable evidence that diets that are restricted to less that 100 g of carbohydrate per day lead to ketosis and decreased ability to dispose of amino acids. Therefore, total carbohydrate elimination should not be advised. Unfortunately, because of problems in determining which patients have idiopathic reactive hypoglycemia, no systematic controlled evaluation of dietary therapy has been undertaken. In a few patients studied by Anderson, diets high in protein (51 percent) and low in carbohydrate (26 percent), compared with those high in carbohydrate (54 percent) and low in protein (13 percent), failed to show any differences in terms of rebound hypoglycemia based on the OGTT. Furthermore, those patients consuming the high-protein diet for five to seven days felt worse. Only one patient with a total gastrectomy experienced a dramatic improvement in symptoms.

Recently there has been increasing enthusiasm for the inclusion in foods of undigested carbohydrate, which has been shown to ameliorate glucose intolerance in diabetics. Monier and colleagues have reported that, in patients with reactive hypoglycemia who have had chemical diabetes, the inclusion of pectin—a dietary fiber that forms gels and is resistant to digestion and absorption—attenuated the late rebound hypoglycemia, as measured by the OGTT. Jenkins and colleagues have also noted a blunting of the glucose profile after an OGTT in nine patients with postprandial hypoglycemia associated with gastric surgery, with remission of "hypoglycemic symptoms" in two; the diarrhea associated with the "dumping" syndrome also improved in seven of the affected subjects. Dietary fiber comprises a complex group of substances and it is uncertain precisely how they modify carbohydrate tolerance. One of the possibilities is that fiber alters intestinal motility, thereby diminishing not only the rates of hydrolysis of complex carbohydrate but the rates of delivery of mono- and disaccharides to the absorptive cells. It is appealing, therefore, to consider that patients with reactive hypoglycemia and

selected individuals with pseudohypoglycemia may benefit from food that is more liberal in carbohydrates in the form of complex starches and dietary fiber.

Although no controlled studies documenting the efficacy of such a regimen are available, within the past two years I have recommended for the nonobese patient a weight-maintaining diet in which protein comprises 15 to 20 percent, total fats 30 percent and the remaining 50 to 55 percent of the energy requirements in the form of carbohydrate, three-quarters of which is in the form of complex carbohydrate with fiber content of 30–40 gm per 2000 k/cal. I have also endorsed artificial sweeteners, such as saccharin, which are not likely to precipitate glycopenia. Similarly fructose, unlike sucrose, glucose, and lactose, does not stimulate insulin secretion nor provoke reactive hypoglycemia, and it may be substituted, if need be, for refined sugar as a sweetener. Although ethanol attenuates glucose-stimulated insulin secretion under certain circumstances, it has not been established that, when ingested in moderation with meals, it contributes to reactive hypoglycemia. In a practical setting, modest alcohol intake should not be proscribed, but rather its effects on hypoglycemia symptoms should be individually assessed.

The cardinal principle of this dietary approach is its flexibility in the content of meals and in the frequency and size of the portions to be eaten, depending upon individual preference and remission of symptoms. The overall goal is to ensure a graduated absorption of nutrients so that there are no extreme gradients of ambient blood glucose levels that trigger excessive insulin secretion, leading to rapid glucose disposal and hypoglycemia with its attendant activation of the adrenergic nervous system. It must be stressed that the frequency of the meals and the size of the portions may be modified depending upon the patient's caloric needs, sense of satiety, and symptoms. Thus meals normally taken 3 times daily may be adjusted to divert more calories to snacks every 2 to 3 hours. Adherence to a dietary plan that entails frequent small portions of food is particularly helpful to the patient with gastric outlet surgery who may also have symptoms associated with "dumping." It is also wise to counsel the obese patient to restrict total calorie intake within the framework of the above-mentioned dietary regimen to attempt to achieve an acceptable body weight. In those patients who may fall into the category of having reactive hypoglycemia associated with mild diabetes mellitus—

TABLE 1   Drugs That *May* Be Useful in Treatment of Reactive Hypoglycemia

Class	Representative Drug	Major Action	Average Dose	Major Adverse Effects
Beta-adrenergic receptor antagonists	Propranolol	Blockade of catecholamine action	10–20 mg p.o. t.i.d.	Bradycardia, hypotension, CNS depression, bronchospasm
Cholinergic antagonists	Propantheline	Inhibition of gastric motility	15–30 mg p.o. t.i.d.	Dry mouth, blurred vision, urine retention, CNS disturbances
Sulfonylureas	Acetohexamide	Potentiation of insulin release and action	250–500 mg p.o. q.i.d.	Hypoglycemia
Antidepressants	Amitriptyline	Increased central catecholamine uptake	25–50 mg p.o. t.i.d.	CNS disturbance, GI upset
Anxiolytics	Diazepam	Inhibition of limbic system	2–10 mg p.o. t.i.d.	CNS depression
Insulin-secretion inhibitor	Diazoxide	Blockade of insulin release Stimulation of hepatic glycogenolysis	50–100 mg p.o. t.i.d.	Hyperglycemia, fluid retention

and who are frequently obese—modest weight reduction coupled with the high-carbohydrate, high-fiber diet makes the most sense in attempting to mitigate the symptom complex and improve carbohydrate tolerance.

Drugs

In some patients in whom counseling and dietary maneuvers may not relieve symptoms related to hypoglycemia, various drugs have been advocated. A list of these agents, their actions, doses, and side effects are given in Table 1. It must be strongly emphasized that none of these agents has been systematically evaluated over the long term in patients with meal-related reactive hypoglycemia. Their benefits and, conversely, their lack of efficacy appear in scattered case reports or are anecdotal. Therefore the following discussion represents my opinion of those drugs that may have some role in the management of these patients.

Neupharmacologic Agents

Beta-adrenergic receptor antagonists exemplified by propranolol, have been reported by Permutt and colleagues to be effective in abating symptoms in patients with postgastrectomy hypoglycemia. It has been suggested that benefits that may accrue from their use are a result of actions suppressing glucose-mediated insulin release as well as a reversible blockade of the beta receptor-mediated symptoms associated with catecholamine discharge. Thus, in theory, use of beta-adrenergic receptor antagonists might be considered useful in treating patients with reactive hypoglycemia, as well as those with "pseudohypoglycemia" in whom symptoms are attributable to adrenergic hyperactivity. Although concern has been expressed that beta-adrenergic antagonists may block hepatic adrenergic receptors, leading to diminished glycogenolysis, and thereby prevent sugar rebound after glucopenia, this is not likely to be a serious problem in patients with idiopathic reactive hypoglycemia, because their glucagon responses to glucopenia are normal, allowing physiologic counterregulation of hepatic glucose output. I believe that in those patients whose symptoms are refractory to dietary modification, a trial with a beta-adrenergic blocker is justified—specifically in subjects with idiopathic reactive hypoglycemia and "pseudohypoglycemia."

Anticholinergic drugs have also been examined by Permutt and colleagues in six patients in whom the diagnosis of idiopathic reactive hypoglycemia was made by OGTT. They noted a dramatic flattening of the plasma glucose response and absence of glucopenia when these patients were given propantheline prior to a repeat OGTT. It seems plausible that the effects of the cholinergic blockade on the OGTT were attributable to a delay in the rate of glucose transit and absorption, since both glucose and insulin levels in these patients were lower. Whether or not the long-term use of oral anticholinergics, such as propantheline, before each meal abolishes symptomatic hypoglycemia has not been proven, and the side effects may be so disturbing as to outweight any potential benefit. Nevertheless, I favor the trial of this drug in selected patients should they be unresponsive to other measures.

Since anxiety and a depressive syndrome may accompany or underlie the symptoms attributable to hypoglycemia in those patients with genuine glucopenic syndromes or those with "pseudohypoglycemia," it may be essential to use specific medications to relieve the patient's symptoms. Drugs such as *amitriptyline* are often useful in alleviating the symptoms in patients with underlying depression. *Benzodiazepines* are generally considered the mainstay of antianxiety pharmacotherapy, and compared with barbiturates and other hypnotic agents, they are more selective and anxiolytic, with less sedation, and lower morbidity and mortality rates on overdose withdrawal. They allegedly relieve anxiety by reason of their affinity for certain neuroreceptors in the limbic system. Antipsychotic drugs, such as *phenothiazines,* are usually best avoided for most anxious patients, but in low doses they may occasionally prove salutary during periods of emotional turmoil with anxiety and agitation. I prescribe them judiciously.

Sulfonylureas have been prescribed for patients with early onset diabetes and reactive hypoglycemia. This approach stems from the notion that the "lag" in insulin secretion may be restored in such patients by improving the sensitivity of the B cell in responding to glucose and other physiologic signals, thereby "normalizing" glucose tolerance. Since the validity of reactive hypoglycemia as part of the spectrum of diabetes is disputed, it is not clear that the few case reports attesting to its benefits justify its use. However, in patients with diabetes mellitus, the physician may wish to use a sulfonylurea as treatment for the hypoglycemia, and if the symptoms attributable to glucopenia diminish, it makes sense to continue to recommend it as a treatment option.

Diazoxide, a drug that has been shown to suppress the secretion of insulin, has been given to patients with reactive hypoglycemia due to gastric outlet surgery with equivocal improvement in their symptoms. Intuitively, one would not wish to use this agent without documented proof of its benefit. Furthermore, it is contraindicated in patients with diabetes who already have impaired insulin secretion. It has been claimed that *phenytoin* alleviates symptoms in a very few patients with idiopathic reactive hypoglycemia diagnosed by OGTT. It has been proposed that this drug interferes with insulin release; therefore, for the same reasons that apply to the use of diazoxide, and because of the possibility of toxic reaction associated with this agent, its protracted use does not appear warranted. I have never used it.

Biguanides, which interfere with glucose absorption from the intestinal tract, have been reported to block symptoms in patients with reactive hypoglycemia after OGTT. Again, no systematic evaluation of such agents has been undertaken, and, although they are still prescribed in Europe for treatment of diabetes, they are no longer available in the United States because of the unacceptable risk of lactic acidosis.

Surgery

In some patients who experience postprandial hypoglycemia as a consequence of gastric resection or vagotomy and drainage for duodenal ulcer disease, symptoms may be disabling despite frequent small portions of food and trials with beta-adrenergic agents and anticholinergic drugs. In such instances, the possibility of an operation to revise the distorted anatomy of the GI tract should be considered. In 11 such patients, Fink and colleagues have reversed 10-cm segments of the jejunum either immediately distal to the gastric outlet or beyond the ligament of Treitz and have claimed that all patients have sustained improvement in the symptoms of rebound hypoglycemia, one as long as three years afterward. Since not all patients who undergo surgical manipulations of the upper gastrointestinal tract have symptoms associated with glucopenia, experience with the jejunal reversal procedure is extremely limited. Nonetheless, it should be considered an option in the event that the patient would otherwise be crippled by the deranged fuel homeostasis as a consequence of inappropriate nutrient absorption.

SUMMARY

There is increasing evidence that postprandial hypoglycemia in adults is an uncommon disorder and that previous high estimates of prevalance have been arrived at erroneously through interpretations derived from the unphysiologic oral glucose tolerance test. The majority of patients with adrenergic-mediated symptoms after eating do not have low blood glucose levels and have been designated as having "pseudohypoglycemia." Nevertheless, there are patients who have legitimate hypoglycemia after food intake. For the most part they have had gastric outlet surgery, and there is also an undetermined number of individuals with "idiopathic" causes. Treatment strategies are aimed at ameliorating the symptoms in these patients as well as in a number of those with pseudohypoglycemia. They involve modification of eating patterns and the composition of meals, emphasizing those that lead to delay in the absorption of monosaccharides. In selected patients treatment also involves drugs that attenuate the rates of carbohydrate absorption or directly inhibit the symptoms caused by adrenergic activation.

INSULINOMA AND NON-ISLET TUMORS PRODUCING HYPOGLYCEMIA

C. RONALD KAHN, M.D.

Fasting hypoglycemia may occur for a variety of reasons, but it almost always signifies an important underlying organic disease. After drug-related causes of hypoglycemia (patients taking insulin, oral hypoglycemic agents, or experiencing alcoholic hypoglycemia), the most common causes are tumors—either islet cell tumors producing insulin (insulinoma) or non-islet cell tumors. The hypoglycemia produced by these two types of tumors is indistinguishable, but the two disorders can usually be readily differentiated by laboratory and clinical tests, and this should be done prior to treatment, since the approach to these two problems may be quite different.

INSULINOMA

Diagnosis of insulinoma should be based upon strict biochemical criteria, in particular the demonstration of fasting hypoglycemia with inappropriately elevated insulin levels. In up to 75 percent of patients with insulinoma, symptomatic hypoglycemia occurs within 24 hours of fasting and almost all patients are hypoglycemic by 72 hours. Inappropriate secretion of insulin is observed after fasting and after provocative stimuli, such as tolbutamide, glucagon, leucine, or calcium infusion. C-peptide levels are also elevated. In 50 percent of patients with benign insulinoma and in almost all patients with malignant insulinoma, the percentage of immunoreactive insulin in plasma in the form of proinsulin is elevated.

About 80% of insulinomas are benign, single lesions, and the majority are less than 3 cm in diameter. Ten percent of patients have malignant tumors, defined by metastases present at the time of diagnosis (not histology). The remainder of patients may have multiple adenomas (MEN) or islet cell hyperplasia (rare in the adult) with or without other lesions. Multiple adenomas occur most often in patients with multiple endocrine neoplasia (MEN) type I.

Assuming the biochemical diagnosis of insulinoma is secure, the first factor in making an appropriate therapeutic decision is the attempt to localize the tumor and determine if it is benign or malignant. Selective arteriography is the most useful test in localizing insulinomas and is positive in about 60 to 70 percent of cases. Insulinomas may be detected by computerized tomography in up to 30 percent of cases and with ultrasound somewhat less frequently. Pancreatic venous sampling may help with rough localization of the tumors, but it should be done only in specialized centers because of the difficulty and morbidity associated with the procedure. A malignant tumor may often show radiographic evidence of frank metastatic disease and should also be suspected if the tumor is greater than 3 cm in diameter or if there are symptoms or signs related to tumor mass. Elevated plasma levels of HCG or its alpha-subunit are also observed in about 50 percent of patients with malignant tumors, but not in patients with benign disease. In patients with MEN type I suspect multiple adenomas, even if they cannot be visualized.

Therapy for insulin secreting islet cell tumors, like that for other functioning endocrine tumors, can be divided into antihormonal therapy, that is, attempts to block hormonal secretion or its effects, and antitumor therapy, that is, attempts to remove or ablate the tumor. For the patients with benign adenomas, antihormonal therapy is necessary only as a temporary measure to control the hypoglycemia prior to definite surgery; in those patients with malignant tumors or tumors that cannot be found at surgical exploration, the antihormal therapy may be needed on a prolonged basis.

Antihormonal Therapy (Table 1)

As with other forms of hypoglycemia, the primary form of therapy for the hypoglycemic symptoms associated with insulinoma is dietary. Frequent feeding between meals, at bedtime, and even throughout the night can often ameliorate attacks of hypoglycemia during the early stage of disease. The composition of the diet may be important. Islet cell tumors often respond more dramatically to amino acids than to glucose and thus a reactive hypoglycemia-type diet (high protein, low carbohydrate) may actually exacerbate symptoms rather than relieve them.

A major advance in the antihormonal therapy of insulinomas has been the introduction of diazoxide (7-chloro-3-methyl-2H-1, 2,4-benzothiadiazine 1,1-dioxide or Proglycem). This benzothiadiazine has potent hyperglycemic properties when given orally. Its mechanism of action is twofold. The primary effect of diazoxide is to inhibit insulin's secretion directly. This has been demonstrated in isolated perfused preparations of the pancreas, as well as in intact animals; since the drug has no effect on the synthesis of insulin, there is an accumulation of the hormone within the beta cell. Diazoxide may also have extrapancreatic effects, including stimulation of hepatic glycogenesis and inhibition of the peripheral utilization of glucose.

The usual dosage for diazoxide in adults is 3–8 mg/kg/per day, divided into 2 or 3 equal doses. The most frequent and serious adverse reaction is retention of sodium and fluid. This may be corrected by thiazide diuretics, which also act to potentiate the hyperglycemic effect of diazox-

TABLE 1   Antihormonal Management of Insulinoma

First Line (Most effective, least toxic)
  Frequent feeding
  Glucose infusions
  Diazoxide

Second Line (Occasionally effective, moderate toxicity)
  Phenytoin
  Glucocorticoids

Third Line (Variable or uncertain efficacy, significant toxicity)
  Mithramycin
  L-asparaginase

Fourth Line (Use limited to research institutions)
  Somatostatin
  Growth hormone

ide. Additional adverse reactions include gastrointestinal irritation, thrombocytopenia, neutropenia, postural hypotension, hyperuricemia, and hirsutism (particularly in children). Ketoacidosis and nonketotic hyperosmolar coma have been reported in patients treated with diazoxide, usually during an intercurrent illness. If possible, the patient is best initially treated with suboptimal doses (50 mg b.i.d. orally), which minimizes the gastrointestinal side effects. Since the half-life of the drug is long (approximately 30 hours), the patient should be carefully followed for at least 3 or 4 days at each dosage level before evaluating whether the therapy is satisfactory and increasing the dosage.

Experience with other agents that inhibit release or synthesis of insulin is limited. Phenytoin (Dilantin) blunts secretion of insulin, presumably by an effect that decreases intracellular concentrations of sodium. Phenytoin in high doses (300 to 600 mg per day) diminished the response of insulin to provocative stimuli in patients with benign insulinomas; however, it does not appear to be as potent as diazoxide in this action. In patients with seizures due to unsuspected hypoglycemia, phenytoin may partially mask the diagnostic clinical and chemical features of an insulinoma. L-asparaginase, an antileukemic drug that depresses the synthesis of a number of proteins, and mithramycin may also palliate the hypoglycemia caused by an insulinoma by decreasing the synthesis of insulin, without any direct tumoricidal action.

A logical drug with potential in the antihormonal therapy of insulinoma is somatostatin, which inhibits the release of insulin in normal humans and has been shown to be effective in some patients with beta-cell tumors. This drug, however, has numerous effects, including inhibition of the secretion of glucagon and other hormones, diminution of absorption of glucose from the intestine, and alteration of splanchnic blood flow. Thus its net effect is often to decrease rather than to increase the concentration of glucose in blood. Also owing to its very short half-life, therapy would require continuous intravenous administration or development of some long-acting, absorbable form of the drug.

In addition to these agents hormones that counteract insulin's effects on target tissues may be of some benefit. Glucocorticoids, growth hormone, epinephrine, and long-acting preparations of glucagon have all been used with some success, but in most cases the effects of these agents are only temporary, and thus I rarely find them of use. Glucagon is also a potent stimulus to insulin's secretion for some insulinomas, and in these cases glucagon may produce a paradoxic exacerbation of hypoglycemic symptoms. Unfortunately, at present no true competitive antagonists of the action of insulin are known.

Surgical Therapy

Eventual cure of the hypoglycemia due to islet cell tumors requires effective surgery or antitumor therapy. Approximately 80 percent of insulinomas are benign and single and therefore are amenable to simple surgical excision.

Prior to surgery, tumor localization by selective arteriography should be attempted in all patients. If arteriography is negative, then I proceed to a therapeutic trial of diazoxide. In those patients who respond appropriately, the latter not only provides additional confirmation of the diagnosis but also allows one to postpone surgery and repeat the arteriogram at some later time, perhaps six months, in hopes of having a more clearly defined tumor at the time of operation. If the arteriogram is positive or if there is no response to diazoxide, I proceed immediately with surgery.

Beta-cell adenomas occur with almost equal frequency in the head, body and tail of the pancreas. It is thus, frequently necessary to mobilize the pancreas to facilitate detection of small tumors by palpation. If no palpable lesion is found, surgical management is controversial. Assuming a nonlocalizing arteriogram and a poor response to diazoxide, a blind distal pancreatectomy in hopes of resecting the lesion is reasonable. The morbidity rate with distal resection is similar to that with pancreatic mobilization, and the morbidity rate with a second exploration is considerably higher. The major disadvantage of this approach is that if the lesion is not found in the resected specimen (which is the case 40 to 60 percent of the time, depending on the extent of resection), a second operation usually means a total pancreatectomy and all of the morbidity and fatalities associated with that procedure. On the other hand, if the patient has had a preoperative trial of diazoxide and is known to respond, one could argue that the blind distal resection can be avoided and, in fact, that surgery should be done only if the arteriogram is localizing. In the patients with malignancy or hyperplasia, palliative surgery may alleviate symptoms by decreasing the mass of tissue that is secreting insulin. With malignant insulinoma the hypoglycemia will eventually recur and chemotherapy is indicated.

Antitumor Chemotherapy (Table 2)

Chemotherapy has been shown to be effective only in patients with malignant tumors. Patients with benign tumors, even those that cannot be found at surgery, or with hyperplasia should not be treated with any of the chemotherapeutic agents discussed below, since none has been shown to be effective in such cases. It is important to have as many biochemical (and anatomic) measures of disease as possible in all patients with malignant tumors in whom chemotherapy is undertaken, since all forms of therapy are potentially quite toxic. We have found evidence in some patients after treatment, of persistent disease based on only one test, for example, elevated proinsulin levels, even when other test results have returned to normal. Also, if possible, patients with rare and highly malignant tumors such as these should be transferred to referral centers with special interest and expertise in their therapy.

At present the drug of choice in the management of malignant insulinoma is streptozotocin (glucopyranose-2-deoxy-2 [3-methyl-3-nitrosoureido-D]). This antitumor antibiotic was isolated from fermentation cultures of Streptomyces acro-

TABLE 2 Antitumor Agents Used in Patients with Insulinoma*

Drug	Dosage	Toxicity	Comments
Streptozotocin	1.5 g/m^2 rapid i.v. or i.a. q week 500 mg/m^2 per day rapid i.v. or i.a. for 5 days q 6 weeks	Nausea, vomiting Renal tubular damage Liver function abnormalities Myelosuppression (high dose)	Give antiemetic before Give saline infusion before and after to induce diuresis Reduce dose or without if proteinuria develops
5-fluorouracil	12 mg/kg i.v. q week 400 mg/m^2 per day i.v. for 5 days q 4–6 weeks	Myelosuppression	Reduce dose by 25% for low WBC or platelets May be given in combination with streptozotocin
Adriamycin (Doxorubicin)	50–75 mg/m^2 i.v. q 3 weeks (up to total of 500 mg/m^2)	Cardiac Myelosuppression	May be given with streptozotocin and/or 5-FU
Tubercidin (7-Deazaadenosine)	1500 μg/kg days 1 and 8, then 750 μg/kg monthly	Proteinuria, azotemia Nausea, vomiting Leukopenia, thrombocytopenia Liver function abnormalities	Very toxic Incubate drug with 500 ml RBC for 1 hr at 37°, then reinfuse RBC
Alloxan	50–100 mg/kg i.v.	Renal Nausea, vomiting	Too toxic to use

*Given in order of perference

mogenes and was found to be selectively betacy-totoxic in animals. The acute diabetogenic activity of streptozotocin has been related to the compound's ability to inhibit the synthesis of pyridine nucleotides. In man the drug may be administered intravenously or intrarterially. The latter route results in about a twofold increase in concentration in the blood that reaches the tumor; however, it is not clear if this maneuver results in any increase in therapeutic efficacy. The usual schedule of administration is 1–1.5 gm/m^2 as a single dose per week, or 500 mg/m^2 per day for 5 consecutive days. I prefer the single dose regimen, since the patients have nausea and vomiting for only the one day of therapy. Theoretically, the effect of the drug is also related to peak blood level. The median time to response has been approximately three weeks. The most encouraging report on the use of this drug has been that of the National Cancer Institute, which has claimed that 62% of patients with malignant insulinoma have less severe hypoglycemia, and in 26 percent of patients the concentrations of insulin and glucose in blood return to normal. Other experience has been much less encouraging, with only about 20 percent of patients showing a clear-cut remission of disease. The median duration of remission is about 16 months.

Renal tubular damage is the most serious and common toxicity. This may be the result of methylation of tubular proteins, since about 10 to 20 percent is excreted in the urine with the N-nitroso group intact. The earliest manifestation is proteinuria, which usually is reversible. With continued treatment, extensive proximal tubular damage, with aminoaciduria, phosphaturia, uricosuria, glycosuria, and renal tubular acidosis, may result. I also usually administer at least 500 ml of normal saline intravenously before and after giving the drug to produce a diuresis in hopes of minimizing renal damage. Serious renal toxicity can be avoided by careful monitoring of renal function, as well as by keeping doses below 1.5 mg/m^2. Attempts have also been made to minimize renal damage by infusing nicotinamide into the renal artery during streptozotocin therapy. Other side effects include nausea and vomiting, transient elevations in serum transaminase levels, and, rarely, myelosuppression.

Chlorozotocin, a chloroethylnitrosourea, exhibits less renal toxicity than streptozotocin and is currently under study for therapy of islet cell tumors. The efficacy of this drug appears to be similar to that of streptozotocin and the major complication is delayed bone marrow toxicity. At present, the drug is available under research protocols only.

Experience with other antitumor agents is limited. 5-fluorouracil (5-FU) and adriamycin have both been shown to be effective as single agents in patients with malignant insulinoma, but the percentage of good responders is clearly lower than with streptozotocin. Combinations of streptozotocin and 5-FU have been suggested to be more effective than either drug alone. Theoretically, three-drug therapy (streptozotocin, 5-FU, and adriamycin) might be used, since the toxicities are different; however, at present there are insufficient data on this combination to determine if it is more effective.

Historically, alloxan was the first drug with proven diabetogenic action. However, it has rarely been used in patients with islet cell carcinoma because of its marked toxicity. Tubercidin (7-deazaadenosine) has also been successfully used in chemotherapy of insulinoma, but it is both highly toxic and difficult to administer. Dosage regimens for all of these agents are given in Table 2.

Other

In general, islet cell tumors are not radiosensitive and thus radiotherapy is not useful. The tumors may be vascular, however, and a few difficult patients have been treated by attempts to infarct the tumor by embolization through arterial catheters or ligation of the hepatic artery. These may produce temporary remissions but should be used only in cases in which a single large vessel feeding the tumor can be identified and when other more conventional approaches have failed.

HYPOGLYCEMIA DUE TO NON-ISLET CELL TUMORS

Fasting hypoglycemia may occur in association with tumors of non-islet cell origin. In these patients insulin levels are invariably low. The tumors may be of many histologic types (Table 3) and are almost always large and easily detectable on physical examination or x-ray. The origin of the hypoglycemia is probably multifactorial. Because of the large size of these tumors (characteristically 0.5 to 10 kg) and their inefficient utilization of glucose, it has been suggested that the hypoglycemia may be due to excessive utilization of glucose by the tumor itself. However, in about

TABLE 3 **Non-Islet Cell Tumors Associated with Hypoglycemia**

Tumor	Percentage
Mesenchymal	45
Hemangiopericytoma	
Mesothelioma	
Fibrosarcoma	
Leiomyosarcoma	
Hepatoma	20
Adrenocortical carcinoma	10
Gastrointestinal tumors	10
Lymphoma and leukemias	6
Other	8

40 percent of cases, plasma levels of insulinlike growth factors are elevated by radioreceptor assay. This is a peptide with insulinlike biologic activity but no reactivity toward anti-insulin antibodies. In some patients with hepatoma, an acquired form of glycogen storage disease may be responsible.

Therapy for these tumors and the associated hypoglycemia has been difficult. Antihormonal measures are at best palliative, and oral diazoxide in our experience is rarely beneficial. Appropriate chemotherapy or radiotherapy remains the next best alternative. In one patient with a high level of insulinlike growth factors and a hemangiopericytoma, we have produced separate long remissions by both radiotherapy and chemotherapy with adriamycin. Unfortunately, in many cases neither of these therapies is very effective. Some of these tumors are benign or very slow growing malignant tumors, and for these, aggressive surgical resection may be very beneficial.

OBESITY

OBESITY

LESTER B. SALANS, M.D.

Most experienced clinicians and researchers consider obesity to be a heterogeneous group of related disorders of different underlying etiologic factors but sharing the common clinical manifestation of increased adiposity. Thus it is now common to refer to "the obesities" of man as a means of underscoring the heterogeneity of this condition and emphasizing the need for individual and specific therapies.

Unfortunately in the overwhelming majority of obese persons an underlying cause of obesity cannot be determined and a specific treatment cannot be initiated. Under these circumstances therapy is directed toward achieving weight loss through a combination of caloric restriction and exercise.

At the simplest level, obesity is the result of a positive energy balance: calories are ingested in excess of caloric expenditure and the excess calories are stored as triglyceride in an expanding adipose tissue. Most obesity is probably due to overeating, that is, the ingestion of excess calories relative to the energy requirements of a sedentary existence. However, some obese individuals do not appear to overeat yet they gain weight, suggesting that positive caloric balance and weight gain may be the result either of enhanced caloric efficiency (extracting more utilizable calories from ingested nutrients) or diminished caloric expenditure in physical activity. Although it is quite likely that both of these caloric expenditure factors contribute to the perpetuation of established obesity, there is considerable controversy over whether differences in caloric efficiency or physical activity are directly responsible for the development of any or a significant number of human obesities. While an answer to this question is of great importance, the reality of the moment is that currently available therapies for the obesities of unknown cause can only be directed toward controlling food intake or physical activity.

A variety of weight reduction programs combining caloric restriction and exercise have been advanced for the treatment of obesity. Unfortunately, none has had much success when examined over time. While initial weight loss may be impressive, recidivism is too often the rule. Since the significant health benefits of the treatment of obesity come from the long-term effects of weight reduction, the goal of treatment of obesity is not merely to lose weight but to keep it off. It is the latter objective that is only rarely achieved through current medical management of obesity. Yet medical management remains the primary therapeutic approach to obesity at this time.

At the same time, it is clear that traditional medical therapeutic approaches employed by most physicians, namely, diet prescription and a return visit in three to six months, are inadequate. Attention must be directed not only to developing effective measures for inducing weight loss but also to maintaining weight loss. New approaches based more broadly than on the narrow confines of traditional medical settings are required. The approach described here is based on the concept that while the diagnosis of obesity and formulation of a medical treatment plan are the responsibility of the physician, a successful outcome over the long term requires the physician and patient to identify, mobilize, and utilize various other resources in the community to provide an environment conducive to the development of more healthy life styles with respect to eating and physical activity.

The following discussion focuses on the treatment of patients with obesity of unknown origin. Even in these patients, classification of obesity may be of practical importance, since it may afford some indication of prognosis and thus better define the objectives of treatment and the therapeutic approach to be taken. On the basis of clinical experience the medical management of the massively hypercellular obese patient must be viewed with pessimism, at least in terms of weight reduction. Hypercellularity of the adipose tissue, especially when its onset is early in life, appears to be irreversible, a phenomenon paralleled by the frustrating clinical observation that weight reduction in these patients is difficult at best and almost inevitably followed by regain of weight and restoration of the original obesity. This observation has focused attention on prevention of obesity, as will be discussed later in this chapter. In the meantime, the evidence currently available indicates that once massive hypercellular obesity is established it cannot be readily reversed by diet, exercise, drugs, behavior modification, or psychotherapy. Treatment of morbid obesity by these methods has been uniformly unsuccessful. Furthermore, prolonged unsuccessful attempts at dietary management for this type of obesity may be potentially harmful; the cycle of weight loss and regain of weight with associated cyclic fasting and refeeding may enhance atherogenic risk factors such as hyperlipidemia as well as generate enormous frustration and cost.

Failure of the medical approach to this type of obesity has led to the introduction of more dramatic surgical interventions, including intestinal and gastric bypass. While these have been effective in achieving weight loss and may be justified in selected massively obese patients faced with life-threatening medical problems or severe psychosocial limitations, they are somewhat hazardous and remain experimental.

In view of this author a more acceptable approach to the hypercellular massively obese patient is one in which an intensive effort is made to implement the treatment plan described below. If unsuccessful, the therapeutic regimen is altered to one that is primarily supportive. In this approach less emphasis is placed on weight reduction and more on minimization of additional weight gain and management of the associated medical, emotional, functional, and socioeconomic problems of the individual.

Most frequently, obesity is of the hypertrophic type and mild or moderate in degree. This form of obesity should be more amenable to treatment and is the type to which the approach described below can most successfully be applied.

DIET

Diet, especially caloric restriction, forms the cornerstone of obesity therapy. Weight loss depends upon caloric deficit and caloric deficit depends upon the total number, not the kind, of calories consumed relative to calories expended. The degree of caloric restriction required to achieve weight loss will vary according to the physical activity and the age, sex, general health, and life style of an individual. In most instances, drastic reduction in caloric intake and rapid weight loss are unnecessary.

A satisfactory rate of weight loss can be achieved through diets containing approximately 1000 to 1200 calories per day, with appropriate adjustments for variations in physical activity and for coexisting conditions, such as diabetes, renal disease, and so on. This degree of caloric restriction can be expected to induce a weight loss of from 1 to 2 lb per week. In those situations in which obesity is associated with severe metabolic or other abnormalities, such as marked hyperosmolarity, hyperlipidemia, and cardiorespiratory failure, a more severe degree of caloric restriction may be indicated, for example, reduction of caloric intake to less than 600 calories per day or total starvation. Since severely restricted diets are associated with severe ketosis and an increased risk of postural hypertension, cardiovascular disorders, electrolyte imbalance, hyperlipidemia, and hyperuricemia, such a vigorous approach should be instituted only under close supervision and monitoring in the hospital. Marked improvement usually occurs with only modest weight loss and treatment can then be continued on an outpatient basis. In obese diabetics with severe metabolic abnormalities, this author prefers the more conservative approach of modest caloric restriction and small amounts of insulin to the more vigorous approach of severe caloric restriction. This author does not initiate a weight reduction program during pregnancy.

Hypocaloric diets can be "balanced" to provide the conventional distribution of carbohydrate (40–50 percent), protein (15–20 percent), and fat (40 percent), or unbalanced so as to limit specifically, or to emphasize, a particular nutrient. The low carbohydrate/high fat diet and diets comprised only of protein (protein sparing modified fast) are examples of unbalanced diets that manipulate dietary composition.

This author prefers the more traditional balanced diet in the treatment of most obese persons because of the significant and potentially serious health hazards associated with unbalanced diets. Moreover, there is little or no evidence to suggest that unbalanced hypocaloric diets are more effective than are balanced hypocaloric diets in achieving the long-term goal of maintaining reduced body weight. Indeed, when viewed from the standpoint of the need to alter previous attitudes and practices and to change eating habits as a means of achieving long-term success, the use of unbalanced fad diets is probably more likely to lead to the eventual resumption of undesirable eating habits and a return to obesity. However, some individuals may prefer, and therefore may be more likely to adhere to, unbalanced hypocaloric diets for reasons of taste, socioeconomics, or culture. If taken under proper supervision and if not used in the face of contraindications, such diets may be of value to certain persons in achieving weight reduction.

The total daily allotment of calories is spread over five meals, with the largest portion of calories given at lunch and dinner. Patients are instructed to eat only in the "meal" room at home and at work, to record the type and amount of food eaten at each meal in a notebook, and to avoid eating alone whenever possible. These practices tend to enhance adherence to hypocaloric diets in many patients.

In the end, the effectiveness of any diet to achieve weight loss is directly dependent upon a reduction in total caloric intake below levels required for weight maintenance. A change or modification of the individual's beliefs, attitudes, and behavior with respect to eating and exercise, that is, life style, is essential to long-term success. Indeed, it is probable that the approach to changing life style after the weight is lost is more important than how the weight is lost.

EXERCISE

A daily exercise program, carefully planned and tailored to the patient's abilities and physical condition, is an important component of a long-term weight reduction and weight maintenance program. At the same time, while exercise can be a positive adjunct to the treatment of obesity, it is not an effective means of inducing weight loss and maintaining reduced weight unless combined with caloric restriction.

A daily program of low levels of aerobic physical activities, such as walking, swimming, or cycling, can have several potential benefits, including an enhanced rate of weight loss, an improved self-esteem, an increased feeling of well-being, and an improved effectiveness of insulin to regulate glucose metabolism in diabetic individuals.

Sudden increases in physical activity are, however, contraindicated. Exercise should be gradually incorporated into the daily schedule so that it becomes part of the patient's routine. Walking may be the best activity with which to initiate such a program. Regular exercise is not only important during the weight loss period but must be incorporated into the daily routine of the obese individual who has lost weight as part of the program to achieve the long-term goal of maintaining reduced body weight. This author has observed that in terms of persuading patients to incorporate exercise into their daily schedule, there is some advantage to having them exercise at the same time each day.

BEHAVIOR MODIFICATION

Behavioral management techniques have been increasingly applied in the treatment of the obesities. These techniques are aimed at modifying the obese patient's eating habits and physical activity. A person's attitudes, beliefs, and experiences have a profound influence on eating behavior and physical activity throughout life, and it is only through successful modification of these attitudes and practices that long-term success can be realized. As suggested earlier, it is probable that the approach to changing life style after the weight is lost is more important than how the weight is lost.

While the goal of behavior modification is permanently to alter eating behavior and physical activity so that postreduction weight maintenance is assured, the program of behavior modification should be initiated early in the course of a weight loss program, at a point when weight reduction is proceeding successfully and the patient is highly motivated.

A number of different behavior modification programs exist; since the patterns of, and attitudes toward, eating behavior and physical activity vary among obese people, the particular approach must be individualized. The most effective programs are those administered over the long term, which emphasize positive self-control rather than aversion behavior and which provide frequent positive reinforcement. There are several weight control self-help groups that may be of considerable value in the modification of individual eating behavior and physical activity patterns.

PHARMACOTHERAPY

Drugs should rarely be used in the treatment of obesity and, when administered, only as part of an overall management plan. The potential for abuse of and addiction to amphetamines is very high, and this risk is not outweighed by the potential short- or long-term benefits of these drugs; they should not be used in the treatment of obesity. Other "safer" drugs, such as phenylpropanolamine, phenmetrazine, or fenfluramine have either no effect or effects that are of short duration. If they are to be employed they are best used for short time periods (weeks) rather than for prolonged periods (months) throughout weight reduction.

Pharmacotherapy should only be used as part of a total treatment program comprising caloric restriction, exercise, and behavior modification, and should be undertaken with full recognition of the risks of addiction and abuse. Digitalis, diuretics, and thyroid hormones should be administered only for specific indications, such as congestive heart failure, edema, hypertension, stasis ulcers, or hypothyroidism. In view of the lack of efficacy and the risk of harm associated with the currently available drugs, it is this author's opinion that there is little place for pharmacotherapy in the treatment of obesity at this time.

SURGICAL TREATMENT

Failure of the traditional medical management of obesity has provided the rationale for more drastic surgical approaches. The most widespread surgical procedure currently in practice is jejunoileal bypass. This procedure is associated with significant and permanent weight loss and often is accompanied by an improvement in psychosocial function. There may also be an improvement in obesity-associated health risk factors, such as diabetes, hyperlipoproteinemia, hypertension, respiratory symptoms, and symptoms of arthritis. At the same time, however, jejunoileal bypass surgery is associated with significant and serious complications. Mortality rates following jejunoileal bypass have been reported to be as high as 11 percent. Diarrhea and malnutrition are among the most prominent postoperative complications. The development of impaired liver function has not infrequently been observed in association with this surgery, and hepatic failure has been reported in

2 to 4 percent of cases. Urinary calculi have been reported with a frequency varying between 3 and 10 percent. Other major complications include polyarthritis, peptic ulcer, acute cholecystitis, and intestional obstruction.

Newer surgical approaches, including gastric bypass and gastric stapling, have been introduced as alternative therapies. These procedures can be effective and appear to be associated with less morbidity than jejunoileal bypass. Experience with these newer surgical approaches has, however, been limited.

In the opinion of this author, surgical therapies for the obesities should be limited to selected massively obese patients faced with lif-threatening medical problems or severe psychosocial impairments. When utilized as a form of treatment in such patients, the procedure should be conducted in a setting in which short- and long-term follow-up can be provided.

MOBILIZATION OF NONPHYSICIAN COMMUNITY RESOURCES

Given the consequences of obesity for the public health (for example, diabetes, hypertension, hyperlipidemia, coronary heart disease) and the limited success of a wide spectrum of therapeutic interventions, it seems clear that renewed efforts and new approaches to the treatment of obesity are required. Involvement of community resources in the management of obesity is based on the premise that life style factors contribute to the development and perpetuation of obesity and that such influences are more likely to be affected through the broader resources of the community than through the narrower confines of traditional medical settings. The cooperation and coordination of all health and allied personnel of the community should be enlisted in this effort, not only during the period of weight loss but also during the critical postreduction period of weight maintenance. Commercial self-help organizations in the community can be of considerable value in motivating patients to adhere to hypocaloric diets and in modifying individual patterns of eating behavior and physical activity. The mass media, places of employment, schools, supermarkets, community centers, churches, and the home, in addition to the traditional health care establishments, can be important resources in the intensive effort to combat obesity.

MANAGEMENT OF ASSOCIATED PROBLEMS

Treatment of the obese diabetic is primarily dietary; reduced caloric intake and weight reduction will frequently improve the diabetic state sufficiently to eliminate symptoms and to reduce or even eliminate the requirement for insulin or oral hypoglycemic therapy. If the dietary approach is unsuccessful, and if the obese patient suffers from the clinical symptoms of hyperglycemia and glycosuria, insulin administered in doses sufficient to eliminate these symptoms is recommended. Restoration of normoglycemia is generally not sought in these individuals because obese patients are insulin resistant and extremely large doses of insulin would be required, doses that stimulate lipogenesis and appetite, thereby worsening the obesity. Insulin treatment is also indicated in the treatment of the obese diabetic with ketoacidosis; this type of diabetes improves with weight loss, and although the need for insulin may not be entirely eliminated in all patients, insulin requirements usually are markedly diminished at a lower body weight.

Weight reduction through reduced caloric intake is the primary therapeutic approach to those hyperlipidemias associated with obesity. In obese hyperlipidemic individuals who are not successful at weight reduction, manipulation of dietary composition and pharmacologic intervention are required.

Hypertension is commonly associated with obesity, and the combination of obesity and hypertension is particularly hazardous to health. Weight loss is a major tool in the control of hypertension and should be combined with pharmacologic treatment of the obese hypertensive. Reduction in total calories is sufficient without the need for further salt restriction. If hypertension is severe or is responding slowly to weight loss, antihypertensive drugs are indicated.

As discussed earlier, in a small percentage of patients an underlying cause of obesity can be identified. Hypothyroidism, hypercortisolism, hyperinsulinism of either endogenous or exogenous origin, hypopituitarism, and ingestion of certain drugs are some examples. In these instances, specific therapies can be instituted and the obesity will be cured. Thus, even though these are rarely the cause of obesity, it is important to consider them in every obese patient and to initiate appropriate treatment. These conditions may also coexist with obesity due to other causes; they should be appropriately treated but, in these cases, the obesity will not disappear. Almost any other condition may coexist with obesity, for example, congestive heart failure, severe edema, psychiatric illness, and should be treated in accordance with good medical practice.

PREVENTION OF OBESITY

Social, economic, cultural, and psychologic factors are important contributions to the development and perpetuation of many of the human obesities. A program of prevention must, therefore, direct attention to these life-style factors. Since early life can be critical in the development of obesity in adult life, efforts should be directed towards preventing obesity during infancy and childhood. This can best be accomplished by directing attention to the home, the school and the mass media. Modification of the life style of adults, specifically with respect to attitudes about eating, nutrition, exercise, and body weight, should have an impact on childhood obesity, since the eating habits of children are often a reflection of those learned from parents and other adults.

HYPERLIPIDEMIA

HYPERLIPO-PROTEINEMIA

W. VIRGIL BROWN, M.D.

Elevated plasma cholesterol or triglyceride levels are due to increases in one or more of the plasma lipoproteins. These are large, complex, dynamic particles responsible for the transport of fatty substances from the liver and intestine to most other tissues in the body. Triglycerides are a major energy source for muscle and provide for fuel storage through their uptake from the lipoproteins by adipose tissue. Transport of the cholesterol component allows for a balance of this important structural element among the cells of various tissues and assures a source of the sterol for hormone synthesis in the adrenal and gonads. The uptake of cholesterol from most organs and its transport to the liver for excretion is also an important function of lipoproteins.

THE LIPOPROTEINS

There are five major groups of lipoproteins which should be considered by the clinician.

Chylomicrons

These are large particles (100 to 1000 nM in diameter) produced by the intestine during absorption of dietary fat. They usually contain over 90 percent triglyceride and less than 5 percent cholesterol. Normally they are cleared rapidly from the plasma and should be absent within a few hours following a meal. Like cream or milk, they float to the top of plasma or serum.

Very Low Density Lipoproteins (VLDL)

These lipoproteins are continuously produced by the liver. They are 30 to 100 nM in diameter, containing 50 to 80 percent triglyceride and about 10 to 20 percent cholesterol. Triglyceride to cholesterol ratio averages about 5:1. These particles float at plasma density (p = 1.006 gm/ml) when subjected to ultracentrifugation.

Intermediate Density Lipoproteins (IDL)

Normally very little lipid is present in human plasma in the density range 1.006 to 1.019 gm/ml. This represents VLDLs that have been partially digested by lipase enzymes and that are being rapidly converted to low density lipoproteins (LDL). These particles (25 to 50 nM in diameter) contain less than 50 percent triglyceride but 20 to 30 percent cholesterol. In certain forms of hyperlipoproteinemia, the IDL may become markedly elevated.

Low Density Lipoproteins (LDL)

These are relatively uniform particles of about 20 to 25 nM in diameter (with hydrated density of 1.019 to 1.063 gm/ml). They are primarily the products of VLDL and IDL degradation, resulting from triglyceride lipase action. They contain about 40 percent cholesterol (two-thirds esterified with fatty acids), 25 percent protein, 25 percent phospholipid, and 10 percent triglyceride. In normal fasting plasma, about two-thirds of the cholesterol resides in LDL.

High Density Lipoproteins (HDL)

This is a heterogeneous group of particles ranging in density from 1.063 to 1.21 gm/ml. These small particles (8 to 18 nM) are protein rich (40 to 55 percent). Cholesterol (25 percent), phospholipid (25 percent), and triglyceride (5 percent) together make up about half the mass.

HYPERLIPOPROTEINEMIA

Elevations of the plasma lipoproteins are frequently the result of genetic metabolic disorders, only a few of which are understood at the molecular or biochemical level. In certain individuals, marked increases in lipoproteins may accompany hypothyroidism, proteinuria, diabetes mellitus, gout, and a variety of less common disorders. The intake of diets high in calories, saturated fat, and cholesterol is also an important factor in determining lipoprotein levels. The dietary effect varies tremendously among individuals. In a few, this may appear to be the major cause for the hyperlipoproteinemia, while in others, dietary change may have only a modest effect on the lipoprotein levels. The marked differences found in the "normal range" of plasma cholesterol for different population groups are usually due to differences in the intake of saturated fat.

The strong and progressive increase in risk of arteriosclerotic cardiovascular disease associated with plasma cholesterol levels in western man has been repeatedly confirmed by epidemiologic studies. Measurement of the specific lipoproteins carrying this cholesterol increases the power of this prediction, since it is the low density lipoprotein (LDL) which shows a positive relationship to vascular disease. High density lipoprotein (HDL) cholesterol provides exactly the opposite message, since the higher the level, the less the risk of heart attack and stroke. Most studies have found only a modest relationship between total triglycerides and vascular disease, and this may be due to the associated reduction in HDL and the increase in LDL seen in some subjects with triglyceride elevation. From comparative studies of many populations around the world, varying widely in their prevalence and incidence of cardiovascular disease, it has been suggested that reduction of LDL cholesterol to less than 100 mg/dl and the maintenance of HDL at 50 mg/dl or greater would be ideal with regard to eliminating risk from this source. From a public health point of view, this means preventing the rise in plasma LDL from a mean of 100 mg/dl seen in the second decade of life to the 150 mg/dl or greater levels found in the 50- or 60-year-old citizen of Europe, the United States, or Canada. Many believe that this could be accomplished by an appropriate change in diet and exercise.

The term hyperlipoproteinemia has been reserved for elevations of plasma lipids to such levels that a physician's evaluation and management are indicated. By convention, the age and sex adjusted value at the 95th percentile for the total plasma triglyceride, cholesterol, and/or LDL cholesterol is used to diagnose hyperlipoproteinemia in a given individual. Table 1 gives such values as obtained from recent population surveys in the United States by the Lipid Research Clinic Program sponsored by the National Institutes of Health. Individuals with these extreme levels are particularly likely to have inherited metabolic abnormalities, making family screening important. It is in this group that drug therapy may be appropriate.

PRINCIPLES OF THERAPY

General Approach

The following is recommended as an approach to all patients seen in a general medical practice. Measure the total plasma cholesterol and triglyceride at least every five years in all adult patients. If vascular disease has appeared in first degree relatives prior to the age of 50 years, cholesterol levels should be measured at the first opportunity in children and adults. For the child with a cholesterol level under 150 mg/dl or an adult with a level under 200 mg/dl, no specific recommendations need to be made. It should be noted that many experts feel it prudent to follow moderate dietary guidelines, such as those recommended by the American Heart Association, even for individuals in this lower range of plasma lipid levels (Table 2). If the cholesterol level exceeds the values above, or if the triglyceride exceeds the 95th percentile for age and sex (see Table 1), the values should be repeated and an HDL cholesterol value should be obtained. This allows an estimate of the LDL cholesterol by the following formula:

LDL Cholesterol = total cholesterol
— (triglyceride/5) — HDL cholesterol

This formula is applicable only if the triglycerides are under 500 mg/dl, chylomicrons are absent, and the VLDL has normal composition (that is, triglyceride to cholesterol mass ratio of five). The presence of chylomicrons is most easily and accurately determined by observing a white layer floating after allowing the plasma to stand in the refrigerator overnight. When the triglyceride level is less than 500 mg/dl and a chylomicron layer is

TABLE 1   The Lipid and Lipoprotein Levels Found for the American Population*

	Age	Male Percentiles			Female Percentiles		
		5	50	95	5	50	95
Cholesterol	20–29	124	167	223	125	167	215
	30–39	145	193	262	135	179	236
	40–49	157	207	267	147	195	260
	50–59	158	212	275	169	224	294
Triglyceride	20–29	45	83	185	40	65	120
	30–39	49	106	285	38	73	157
	40–49	56	121	229	44	85	185
	50–59	62	122	288	55	104	247
LDL Cholesterol	20–29	68	108	156	66	103	146
	30–39	80	128	187	72	113	160
	40–49	93	138	194	79	125	181
	50–59	88	144	200	92	144	213
HDL Cholesterol	20–29	30	45	63	37	-53	81
	30–39	29	44	63	36	52	79
	40–49	29	44	65	34	55	86
	50–59	28	45	67	37	58	88

*Lipid research clinic data from studies in the early 1970s

present, failure to fast for 12 hours is the usual reason. In dysbetalipoproteinemia (type III hyperlipoproteinemia), the VLDL is usually very rich in cholesterol (see below).

The proper interpretation of lipid and lipoprotein values requires that the patient be fasting for 12 hours and have a stable body weight. The physician should obtain a dietary and medical history. A family history with emphasis on early vascular disease and hyperlipoproteinemia should be recorded. In the event that either triglyceride or cholesterol is elevated, other laboratory tests should include urinalysis, T_4, fasting glucose, and liver function tests.

Specific Approaches

Hypertriglyceridemia

Chylomicronemia (Type I Hyperlipoproteinemia). The plasma triglycerides in these patients are usually 1000 mg/dl or greater (up to 25,000 mg/dl). The plasma is turbid and a fat layer floats to the top after a few hours. The cholesterol may be normal or moderately elevated. Lipemia retinalis, eruptive xanthomata, and hepatosplenomegaly are often present. The patient frequently notes abdominal pain and may develop pancreatitis. Paresthesias, organic mental syndromes, and shortness of breath may also be present with severe elevation of chylomicrons. Triglycerides above 5000 mg/dl should be considered a medical emergency, since death may result from pancreatitis.

Lipoprotein lipase deficiency and deficiency of the apolipoprotein activator (apo-CII) are two well defined genetic abnormalities leading to this syndrome. Rarely, lipoprotein lipase deficiency may appear as a transient idiopathic disorder. The most common cause is severe insulin deficiency in certain patients who may have a genetic predisposition. The first treatment for such patients is complete fat restriction. If pancreatitis or diabetic ketoacidosis is present, all oral feedings should be denied until pain disappears, acid base balance returns, or both. A diet with less than 5 gm of fat is advised until the triglycerides are less than 1000 mg/dl. Patients with lipoprotein lipase or apo-CII deficiency should be restricted to less than 10 percent of calories from fat. Supplementation with medium chain triglycerides, such as shortening for cooking, is advised and need not be counted as part of the "fat calories." Adequate insulin treatment usually resolves the problem in the diabetic.

Chylomicronemia with Elevated VLDL (Type V Hyperlipoproteinemia). The triglycerides in these patients may be in the same range (1000 to 25,000 mg/dl) as those above with type I hyperlipoproteinemia, but they differ in several respects. The cholesterol level is usually elevated from 300 to 1000 mg/dl. On standing, the plasma below the floating chylomicrons remains densely turbid and usually has a yellow color. This is due to the high levels of VLDL. The clinical signs and symptoms are identical to those noted in chylomicronemia above. This disorder may be due to a primary metabolic defect, presumably genetic, but no biochemical causes have been established. Overproduction of VLDL has been found in those studied by research techniques. This disorder usually appears in adults and is aggravated by obesity and diabetes mellitus. Estrogen treatment may induce this syndrome in certain susceptible patients.

Short-term treatment involves fat restriction as noted above. After the triglycerides are below 1000 mg/dl, the major emphasis should be on long-term improvement of those factors that aggravate the underlying and idiopathic disorders of lipoprotein metabolism. Caloric restriction and increased exercise to bring about weight loss usually result in complete clearing of chylomicrons and reduction of VLDL triglyceride levels to less than 500 mg/dl. Insulin treatment should be considered if hyperglycemia is present and discontinuation of estrogen administration is also indicated. If the triglycerides remain above 1000 mg/dl after this therapy, administration of nicotinic acid, clofibrate, or gemfibrozil might be considered (see below).

VLDL Elevation (Type IV Hyperlipoproteinemia). The great majority of subjects with elevated triglycerides have fasting levels that range between 200 and 500 mg/dl. These are usually due to primary metabolic disorders that result in overproduction of VLDL. Many of these individuals have normal or low LDL and often (but not always) have low HDL levels. Another common pattern seen in familial VLDL elevations is an associated increase in LDL. This is discussed below. Elevated VLDL is commonly seen in obese patients and those suffering from nephrosis, gout, hypothyroidism, and diabetes mellitus. Less common causes include glycogen storage diseases and other liver disorders. Alcohol and estrogens may markedly accentuate the problem.

A number of considerations are involved in treating these patients. Satisfactory reduction of VLDL usually follows appropriate management of other underlying disorders, and in this sense the triglycerides may be considered a marker of metabolic control. VLDL elevation with plasma cholesterol levels at 200 mg/dl or below may confer no increased cardiovascular risk. However, the prudent approach is to recommend a reduction in calories and an increase in exercise to trim excess body fat, as well as a reduction in dietary fat and cholesterol. Some substitution of polyunsaturated fat for saturated fat is also recommended (Diet A, Table 2). An associated low level of HDL cholesterol (less than 40 mg/dl) is often found and adds impetus to this recommendation, since it is an independent risk factor.

In those few individuals who maintain triglycerides in the 500 to 1000 mg/dl range, there is concern that pancreatitis may result from a sudden rise in these levels. Drug therapy with nicotinic acid, clofibrate, and gemfibrozil might be considered (see below).

Elevated LDL (Type II Hyperlipoproteinemia). Patients with high LDL levels have a significant increase in the incidence of vascular disease. Patients in this group—which makes up (by definition) 5 percent of the population—have many metabolic abnormalities. Approximately 4 percent of patients with elevated LDL (1:500 in the general population) have familial hypercholesterolemia. This is an important group of patients because their condition results from a defined genetic defect in specific cell surface receptors for LDL. Patients with this defect have a severe impairment in the clearance of LDL manifested as an autosomal dominant trait with virtually complete penetrance. Tendon and tuberous xanthomata as well as early xanthelasma and corneal arcus are seen in such patients. The rare (1:1,000,000) patient with homozygous familial hypercholesterolemia has all these clinical signs and usually suffers from vascular disease by the second decade of life. In most patients elevated LDL results from unexplained metabolic defects. The most common abnormality may be due to overproduction of LDL, and this is often accompanied by increased VLDL and thus hypertriglyceridemia as well. Within this group, one frequently discovers other family members with increased LDL or VLDL as well as individuals with elevations of both lipoproteins. The lipoprotein pattern may change over time in the same individual. This has been referred to as familial combined hyperlipoproteinemia and probably represents a group of biochemical abnormalities.

When triglycerides are normal, the use of the

TABLE 2 Diets Used for Reducing LDL Levels

	Proteins	Carbohydrate	Fat	P/S	Cholesterol
A	12–18%	50–50%	30–35%	0.8–1.0	300 mg
B	12–18%	55–60%	25–30%	1.0–1.5	200 mg
C	12–18%	60%	25%	2	100 mg

Diet A is the American Heart Association diet recommended for general use.
Diet B is a significant departure from the usual American diet, but still leaves a wide choice of meats, poultry, and fish.
Diet C severely restricts animal fats, eliminates eggs, and increase oils from vegetable and ocean fish.
Composition as percent of total daily calories.
P/S is the ratio of the mass of polyunsaturated to saturated fat in the diet.
Cholesterol is given as maximum allowable per day.

formula above to estimate LDL is quite satisfactory. When triglycerides are elevated, the possibility of dysbetalipoproteinemia (type III hyperlipoproteinemia) must be considered (see below). More extensive laboratory tests are then needed to be certain that the VLDL is of normal composition and that the cholesterol elevation is due to increased LDL. These tests are usually available in large commercial laboratories or major medical centers.

The treatment goal should be the reduction of the LDL cholesterol level to less than 150 mg/dl. Diet treatment of elevated LDL should begin with diet B (Table 2). When the subject demonstrates adequate acceptance and proficiency, a graduation to diet C may be undertaken, if the LDL remains above 150 mg/dl. Drugs should be considered for all those whose LDL level is above 175 mg/dl on a diet. If the HDL is below 40 mg/dl, one might consider an LDL cholesterol level of 150 mg/dl as sufficiently high for use of certain drugs, such as bile acid binding resins. For patients over 60 years old, LDL is a less powerful risk factor and the rationale for treatment is less clear.

Drugs, in order of preference, include the bile acid binding resin (colestipol and cholestyramine) nicotinic acid, neomycin sulfate, and probucol. If the VLDL is elevated, and particularly if the diagnosis of familial combined hyperlipoproteinemia can be made, gemfibrozil or clofibrate might be used initially. Many of these patients will need combination drug therapies, the most effective of which have proven to be use of colestipol (or cholestyramine) with nicotinic acid or clofibrate (or gemfibrozil).

Dysbetalipoproteinemia (Type III Hyperlipoproteinemia). Elevated cholesterol and triglyceride levels are found in subjects with this uncommon form of hyperlipoproteinemia. It is important because it leads to vascular disease and is usually responsive to treatment. Patients with this disorder have elevated VLDL and IDL, but often have low or normal LDL levels. The VLDL is particularly rich in cholesterol, and within this lipoprotein the triglyceride to cholesterol ratio may range from 3 to 1 or even lower instead of the usual 5. This disorder results in part from the presence of the homozygous state for an abnormal allele of apolipoprotein E. This apolipoprotein is normally present in VLDL and appears to facilitate the conversion of VLDL and IDL to LDL in the liver. The development of the elevated lipoprotein levels seems to require an additional metabolic abnor-

mality, such as the overproduction of VLDL. The diagnosis requires examination of the VLDL for cholesterol and triglyceride content after ultracentrifugation. Determination by isoelectric focusing of the abnormal apolipoprotein E can be done in many lipoprotein research laboratories.

Although the apolipoprotein abnormality is present from birth, the required second metabolic abnormality usually does not become fully manifest until the fourth decade, and therefore this form of hyperlipoproteinemia is a disorder seen in adults. A few patients note planar xanthomata in palms and tuberous xanthomata on the knees, elbows, and buttocks. Peripheral vascular disease is very frequently seen, as are coronary heart disease and stroke. Weight loss and the use of diet B or C (Table 2) usually reduce the lipid levels to near normal. Clofibrate, gemfibrozil, or nicotinic acid may be used if the total plasma cholesterol level remains above 250 mg/dl. Reduction to levels below 200 mg/dl is desirable.

DRUG TREATMENT

General Considerations

The balance of risk versus benefit for the patient requires good clinical judgment when drugs are considered in the treatment of hyperlipoproteinemia. In specific patients and in monkeys, where LDL has been markedly reduced by aggressive drug treatment, objective evidence of reduction in angiographically demonstrated lesions and in pathology specimens (monkeys) has been published. Only one large trial of a lipid lowering agent has been completed in patients with hyperlipoproteinemia and without pre-existing cardiovascular disease. Clofibrate in the WHO study reduced the number of new myocardial infarctions even though the total cholesterol reduction was only 9 percent. Unfortunately, the side effects of the drug eliminated any lessening of overall morbidity or mortality. In those studies in which moderate elevations of total plasma cholesterol levels were required, the specific lipoprotein elevation has not been determined and the drug treatment was not tailored to achieve a large reduction in LDL or VLDL cholesterol levels. Well-designed drug trials that should eliminate these deficiencies are currently underway. In the interval, physicians must care for these high-risk patients using diet and the prudent selection of one or more of the drugs listed below. Before beginning any drug treatment, a thorough testing of the diet effect should be undertaken, since many patients require time to learn the new daily habits required for dietary adherence. The regimen will not cure these metabolic disorders, and documentation of the effect of each therapeutic intervention (diet and drug) is therefore most important. Addition of the first drug should be followed by lipoprotein measurements at one or two month intervals for six months or longer. The impact of a second or third drug can be judged against a trustworthy baseline. The purpose is to design a safe and efficacious regimen that the patient will follow for five or more years, that is, "until something better comes along."

Drugs Reducing LDL Levels

Colestipol and Cholestyramine. These agents lower LDL cholesterol almost specifically, producing a 15 to 30 percent reduction in many subjects. Both drugs are bile acid binding resins and they are equally effective. Colestipol (Colestid) is a powder of fine plastic beads containing a positive charge. The usual dose is 15 gm taken twice each day (30 gm per day) as a suspension in water or any other beverage or food as selected by the patient. Cholestyramine is taken in a dose of 12 gm twice each day. This is formulated with an additional 15 gm of filler and flavoring (orange). On passage through the intestine and into the stool, 1 or 2 additional gm of bile acids are bound each day and the net sterol loss from the body is increased by this fraction. The liver, sensing the reduced bile acid pool, increases LDL clearance from the plasma to provide additional cholesterol for increased bile acid synthesis. Plasma triglycerides may rise as a result of increased synthesis, but this is usually transient and pretreatment levels are found after three to six months.

Constipation occurs in 10 to 20 percent of patients and thus a history of anorectal disorders should be taken before prescription. This problem usually responds to stool softeners and mild laxatives and resolves within two or three months. Gastric fullness, eructation, and even vomiting are complaints of a small minority (less than 5 percent). This is helped by beginning with small doses (4 or 5 gm) and increasing at weekly intervals to full dose. Reduction in fat-soluble vitamin levels may in part be due to reduced LDL levels. Vitamin supplements of A, D, and E are wise for long-term

treatment, even though true deficiencies have not been documented except in occasional patients who had complicating illnesses, such as chronic liver disease or malabsorption syndromes. Adherence is compromised by the expense—$60 to $70 per month—and the inconvenience of suspending the powder. It is best to prescribe other drugs, such as digoxin, thyroxine diuretics, and anticoagulants, 1 or 2 hours before or 5 or 6 hours after these resins, since some adsorption of these drugs to the resin has been reported.

These agents are particularly effective when used in combination with nicotinic acid or clofibrate (or gembrozil), as noted below.

Nicotinic Acid. The vitamin niacin, when given as nicotinic acid in doses of 3 to 7.5 gm per day, is particularly effective in lowering LDL levels. It has the added advantage of lowering VLDL and therefore triglycerides, while raising HDL cholesterol. When used alone, a 10 to 15 percent reduction in plasma cholesterol is usually seen; however, in combination with colestipol or cholestyramine, a reduction in LDL cholesterol level of 40 to 60 percent may be expected. All patients experience cutaneous flushing due to capillary vasodilation in the skin and other tissues. Drop in blood pressure and (rarely) postural dizziness may result. This can be held to a minimum if the drug is started at a small dosage level, such as 50 mg 3 times a day, and increased by doubling the dose each 3 or 4 days until 1.0 gm 3 times a day is given. An aspirin 1 hour before the dose may markedly reduce the flushing, which appears to be a prostaglandin mediated process. After evaluating the lipid reduction, increases by 0.5 gm 3 times a day (1.5 gm per day) may be made at monthly intervals until a maximum dosage of 7.5 gm per day is reached. Uric acid, plasma glucose, and liver function tests should be measured, since these may become abnormal in an occasional patient on nicotinic acid. Induction of gout is very rare and the blood glucose and liver function abnormalities return to normal after the drug is discontinued. Peptic ulcer or other inflammatory conditions of the bowel may be aggravated by this drug.

Neomycin Sulfate. This poorly absorbed antibiotic interferes with bile acid and cholesterol absorption. Used in doses of 0.5 gm 4 times a day (2 gm per day) only traces of the drug are absorbed, and when it is restricted to those with normal hepatic and renal function, significant toxic effects are rare. The marked renal and neurotoxicity (eighth nerve) observed with intravenous use or in those given 8–12 gm per day orally should caution the physician to monitor appropriate laboratory tests before and during treatment. A 15 to 20 percent reduction in LDL is often found and this may be sustained for years in some patients.

Probucol. This drug lowers serum choles-terol levels by about 10 to 15 percent in most subjects when taken at the recommended dosage of 0.5 gm twice daily. The effect is variable, with only a 5 percent reduction in some and up to 30 percent in others. The drug is poorly absorbed, with up to 90 percent appearing unaltered in the feces. A large fraction of that absorbed is stored in the adipose tissue and this may explain a continuing hypolipidemic effect for six months after discontinuing the drug. In general, it has been well tolerated and few significant side effects have been reported. However, a large reduction in HDL cholesterol level is frequently found and the consequences of this are not known. Diarrhea, nausea, and flatulence are common and eosinophilia has been observed in 10 to 30 percent of subjects. Cardiac arrhythmias in dogs and in case reports of humans are worrisome. This is particularly true because large-scale, long-term trials have not been conducted with this drug as with several of the other lipid lowering agents.

Drugs Reducing VLDL Levels

Clofibrate. Reduced VLDL (and therefore, triglyceride) levels are achieved in many patients with clofibrate (Atromid S). The usual dosage of 1.0 gm twice daily increases lipoprotein lipase and may reduce VLDL synthesis as well. The most consistent effect is seen in patients with dysbeta-lipoproteinemia (type III hyperlipoproteinemia). In other patients with elevated VLDL, the effect is less predictable, and LDL levels may actually rise in some individuals. There is an increase in hepatic cholesterol excretion with a modest reduction in bile acid output. This effect may explain one of the significant side effects, which is a two- to fourfold increase in the incidence of cholelithiasis in clinical trials. Nausea, vomiting, and a rise in muscle and liver enzymes are also well-documented side effects. Large trials have found a higher than expected incidence of sudden death and cardiac arrhythmias, and in one study a small rise in the cancer rate was found. This drug suffers from having been studied so extensively, but since it is so well known, we should be able to use it most wisely. Patients who respond dramatically, such as those with dysbetalipoproteinemia, should be treated while they continue to be observed for the known side effects. Moderate VLDL elevations with normal LDL levels do not justify its use.

Gemfibrozil. This is a relatively new drug which has many structural and clinical features that place it in the same category as clofibrate. Gemfibrozil (Lopid) is given in a dosage of 600 mg twice each day. It lowers triglycerides as effectively as clofibrate, but it also raises HDL levels. This may prove to be an advantage. It may reduce LDL by 5 to 10 percent. The effects on gallstone production and other gastrointestinal complaints may not be as frequent as with clofibrate, but this remains to be determined in clinical trials with large numbers of patients.

SURGICAL TREATMENT

Reduction of LDL levels can be achieved reproducibly by surgically bypassing the distal third of the ileum. This operation has been used in several hundred subjects with type II hyperlipoproteinemia, producing an average 40 percent reduction in cholesterol levels. It is quite safe in the hands of an expert surgical team and offers the advantage of complete patient adherence. The principal problem has been diarrhea, which is apparently due to the irritation of the colon by the excess bile acids that arrive after failing to enter the small bowel—a normal function of the distal ileum. Small doses of colestipol or cholestyramine usually treat this successfully. Vitamin B_{12} absorption is also compromised, requiring monthly parenteral replacement. In patients who fail to improve on the medical regimens, this procedure may offer significant advantages. A large scale clinical trial is currently underway in the United States.

Portocaval shunting is a second surgical procedure that has been used to lower the extremely high levels of LDL in subjects with homozygous familial hypercholesterolemia. This unusual and somewhat heroic approach to cholesterol reduction should be confined to these rare patients who face such a poor prognosis owing to impending diffuse, rapidly progressive vascular disease. The procedure was found empirically to lower LDL from the 500–900 range to 200–400 mg/dl in many such patients. This is due principally to a reduction in VLDL and LDL synthesis, perhaps secondary to bypass of substrate directly to peripheral tissues. Since these patients have no capacity to synthesize normal receptors for LDL in response to drugs such as the bile acid binding resins, they are not able to effect increased hepatic uptake. Presumably, for similar reasons, ileal bypass is also not effective in such patients.

CARCINOID SYNDROME

CARCINOID SYNDROME

KARL ENGELMAN, M.D.

DIAGNOSIS AND CLINICAL COURSE

The carcinoid syndrome is a complex group of varied signs and symptoms which result from humoral products produced by carcinoid tumors. These tumors arise from argentaffin cells in the bronchial tree and the upper gastrointestinal tract, including the stomach, common bile ducts, pancreas, and small intestine, with the majority of tumors arising from the ileum. Rarely, tumors of the ovary and medullary carcinoma of the thyroid may also result in this condition. Diarrhea, flushing, and bronchospasm are the primary symptoms of the syndrome, though structural heart disease leading to congestive heart failure also is common. Most of the elements of the syndrome have been found to result from tumor production of chemical substances, including serotonin, kinin peptides, prostaglandins, and histamine. Other features of the syndrome, such as abdominal pain and intestinal obstruction, may occur from direct involvement with tumor. Patients with carcinoid tumors almost never manifest the carcinoid syndrome until extensive metastases, largely to regional lymph nodes and liver, are present.

Thus, once patients present with the classic symptoms of the carcinoid syndrome, they are considered incurable in almost all instances. Therapy is currently confined to symptomatic and palliative measures that pharmacologically inactivate or reverse the effect of tumor products that cause the most prominent symptoms of this condition. Because the tumor is not totally resectable, surgery should be reserved for special situation, and chemotherapy has unfortunately proved not to be very effective in most patients.

An understanding of the natural history of the average patient with carcinoid syndrome is important in determining the approach to therapy. The onset of symptoms (usually flushing, diarrhea, or both) is usually insidious and may be slowly progressive over years before the proper diagnosis is made. The diagnosis of a variety of functional disorders, especially functional bowel disease, is usually made in these patients whose symptoms may wax and wane with periods of spontaneous remission. Eventually the growing frequency and severity of symptoms result in the proper diagnosis being suspected. Even when symptoms occur daily, episodes of exacerbation may be interposed by days to weeks of relative remission. The whole course from initial onset of symptoms through progression of the full-blown syndrome to eventual death may occupy a period of 5 to 10 years, and it is not uncommon for patients with the full-blown syndrome to survive for 20 years or more, indicating that many tumors, while metastatic, may be relatively slow-growing.

The most common causes of death are (1) inanition due to intractable abdominal pain, diarrhea, and malabsorption, (2) abdominal catastrophe due to mechanical obstruction or bowel infarction, and (3) severe chronic congestive heart failure due to the development of structural and valvular right-sided heart disease.

In considering the therapy of the patient with carcinoid syndrome, one must recognize that the primary antitumor approaches of surgical resection, chemotherapy, or radiation are almost universally palliative, and almost never cure the patient. Furthermore, because the tumor produces its primary symptoms through chemical mediators that it produces, the primary and most effective approach to treating these patients is pharmacologic therapy directed toward controlling the often incapacitating flushing and diarrhea.

ANTITUMOR THERAPY

On initial diagnosis of the syndrome, confirmed by symptoms and increase in urinary 5-hydroxyindoleacetic acid (5-HIAA), there seems to be a nearly universal urge for surgical exploration of the patient, resection of the primary tumor, and attempts to cure the patient by removal of metastases. This is almost always doomed to failure by the already established presence of metastatic disease deep in mesenteric or other regional lymph nodes as well as in the liver. Especially in the more common type of carcinoid syndrome associated with the presence of the primary tumor in the ileum, not only will extensive resection not benefit the patient, but it is very likely to produce eventual significant morbidity and greatly complicate control of diarrhea and maintenance of nutrition. The primary tumor is usually very small and by itself rarely causes local mechanical problems or obstruction. The latter more commonly occurs because of fixation and kinking of the bowel due to extensive metastatic disease in the mesentery. Mechanical small bowel obstruction is one of the most common serious problems confronting the patient with malignant carcinoid syndrome, and its surgical relief should be directed toward restoring continuity of intestinal flow while maintaining the maximal residual amount of small intestinal absorptive surface. If large segments of small bowel, especially ileum, are resected either to relieve obstruction or in the misguided hope that it will cure the patient with otherwise evident metastases, the common sequela is the marked worsening of the already present diarrhea.

Patients with carcinoid syndrome are thought to have diarrhea because of the effects of serotonin and histamine, both secreted by the tumor, which cause increased gastric and small bowel secretion as well as increased small bowel motility. If large quantities of ileum are resected surgically, a marked decrease in reabsorptive surface results, not only for electrolytes, nutrients, and fluid, but especially for bile salts. The entrance of these cathartic substances in large quantities into the large bowel thus causes further exacerbation of diarrhea, malabsorption, malnutrition, and incapacity. Therefore, if intestinal obstruction occurs, it should be the aim of the surgeon to preserve small bowel contents even if they are involved in metastatic disease in the mesentery. A useful approach is the creation of enteroenterostomies to bypass areas of obstruction while preserving bowel length and absorptive surface. As will be further explained below, adrenergic stimulation, whether endogenous or with most vasopressors, results in marked exacerbation of flushing. It has been found that administration of norepinephrine, epinephrine, and related sympathomimetic drugs may produce profound paradoxic hypotension. In contrast, the direct acting vasoconstrictor methoxamine (Vasoxyl) does not produce this hypotensive response and is the only generally available vasoconstrictor that may be used if hypotension occurs during surgery.

Surgical "debulking" has been attempted in some patients with carcinoid syndrome. Given the nature of widespread metastases, primarily in the liver and mesentery, this does not seem to offer a very useful approach for the patient. Another approach to this problem which has limited usefulness is transarterial embolization of the hepatic artery with nonabsorbable thrombotic material to infarct large areas of tumor metastases. While attractive and quite effective from a purely mechanical standpoint, this approach is *extremely dangerous*. The danger lies in the fact that with tumor infarction, extremely large quantities of vasoactive substances, including serotonin, prostaglandins, and kinin peptides, may be released from the tumor and cause extremely severe flushing, hypotension, and diarrhea. This approach has been used successfully only when very large doses of inhibitors of serotonin synthesis, antiserotonin drugs, and massive doses of steroids and inhibitors of proteolytic enzymes have been administered prior to and following embolization. With the benefit of this adjuvant therapy, reports of several dramatic remissions have appeared.

Chemotherapy in treatment of malignant carcinoid tumors has generally been very disappointing, and radiotherapy is generally conceded to be ineffective. Cyclophosphamide, 5-fluorouracil, methotrexate, phenylalanine mustard, and streptozotocin have been reported to produce objective remission and regression of tumor in occasional patients, though no uniform response has been observed. In administering chemotherapy to patients with carcinoid metastases, the physician must balance the expected toxicity of chemotherapeutic drugs against the generally established slow progression of the tumor.

Many patients with the more common small bowel carcinoids may present with a clinical picture suggesting obstruction. This is usually associated with abdominal pain, especially in the right upper quadrant, fever, leukocytosis, nausea and vomiting, and an x-ray picture consistent with small bowel obstruction. Experience has proved that these patients frequently suffer not from irreversible mechanical obstruction, but either from kinking of bowel in an area where the bowel wall may be fixed by mesenteric metastases or from sympathetic ileus resulting from spontaneous hemorrhagic infarction and necrosis of large liver metastases. It is frequently possible to avoid surgery in these patients by use of long tube intubation of the small bowel and conservative therapy. These exacerbations frequently remit after a period of days, and this approach saves the patient the dangers of surgery, hypotension, and bowel resection.

THERAPY OF FLUSHING

Flushing is among the earliest symptoms noted by patients with carcinoid syndrome, and while in many instances its appearance may be embarrassing or uncomfortable, it is rarely dangerous. A distinct exception occurs in patients with primary bronchial tumors in whom flushing, rather than being evanescent, may be extremely prolonged and profound and is usually associated with hypotension, oliguria, and may be fatal. As noted previously, flushing is usually precipitated by an event that induces adrenergic discharge, such as pain, anger, embarrassment, or excitement. Flushing may also occur spontaneously and is especially likely to occur after the ingestion of alcohol or spicy foods. Flushing in the carcinoid syndrome is thought to be due to the peripheral manifestations of kinin peptides, histamine, and prostaglandin release from tumor metastases.

Mild flushes may be treated with antiadrenergic drugs and those that have antikinin properties. Phenothiazines, especially prochlorperazine (Compazine), 5–10 mg, or chlorpromazine (Thorazine), 25–50 mg orally every 4 to 6 hours may be helpful, and the alpha-adrenergic blocker phenoxybenzamine (Dibenzyline) in a dose of 10–50 mg orally each day may also be helpful. Because of the antiadrenergic effect of these drugs, some hypotension may also result. Antihistamines have been reported to be very effective in treating carcinoid flushes, especially in patients with gastric carcinoid tumors in whom production of histamine is greatest. Combined use of H_1- and H_2-histamine antagonists appears to be more effective in some patients than the use of either class of drugs alone. Diphenhydramine (Benadryl), 50 mg 4 times daily, and cimetidine (Tagamet), 300 mg 4 times daily have been effective. Inhibitors of prostaglandin synthesis may be especially helpful in patients with bronchial carcinoid flushing, and indomethacin (Indocin), 25 mg 3 or 4 times daily has been shown in several instances to be useful in a patient with severe flushing due to the bronchial carcinoid syndrome. In the absence of benefit from this more conservative therapy, patients with devastating bronchial carcinoid flushes may have to be treated with large doses of oral or parenteral glucocorticoids (prednisone, 10–20 mg p.o. 2 to 4 times daily), with the attendant undesirable side effects.

Avoidance of alcohol and spicy foods and effective reduction of diarrhea and tenesmus are also useful in reducing flushing by avoiding inciting factors.

THERAPY OF DIARRHEA

Patients with carcinoid syndrome have diarrhea due to the combined pharmacologic actions of several neurohumors produced by the tumor cells. Serotonin (5-hydroxytryptamine), the amine resulting from the decarboxylation of 5-hydroxytryptophan (5-HTP) is thought to be the primary tumor product producing diarrhea. Serotonin has direct stimulatory effects on small bowel motility. Bowel active prostaglandins are also produced in large quantities by these tumors, and the stimulatory effect of histamine on gastric secretion is also thought to contribute to the development of diarrhea. Finally, a "short bowel" syndrome due to ileal resection may result in malabsorption of fats and especially of bile salts and acids which have a cathartic effect in the large bowel.

Conservative and simple approaches usually are quite effective in patients who have mild diarrhea. It is fairly typical for patients, even those with more severe diarrhea, to have a formed or semiformed stool on awakening with progressive increase in frequency, liquidity, and volume during the day. Eating usually results in marked stimulation of tenesmus and diarrhea, since these patients seem to have an exaggerated gastrocolic reflex. Rather than to follow the common procedure of administering antidiarrheal drugs after the development of diarrhea, it is much more logical and effective to prevent diarrhea by administering the drugs 30 to 60 minutes prior to eating.

Patients with mild to moderate diarrhea will usually benefit from the use of tincture of paregoric either in anticipation of meals or following one or two loose bowel movements. For patients with more severe diarrhea, Lomotil (1 or 2 tablets before meals) or loperamide (Imodium), 2–4 mg before meals, usually provides significant control, although it is often difficult, and even sometimes undesirable, to relieve the patient of diarrhea completely. Paradoxically, this sometimes causes increase in abdominal pain due to distention and tenesmus. Cimetidine (Tagamet), 300 mg before meals, may also prove a useful adjunct to the use of narcotic antidiarrheal agents, since it reduces gastric secretion and the volume of fluid content in the small bowel. In patients with prior small bowel resection, especially that of the terminal ileum, use of the bile acid binding agent cholestyramine (Questran), 4–8 gm before meals, may be especially effective as an adjunct to other agents.

In patients with even more severe diarrhea, two additional drugs with antiserotonin activity may also prove useful. Their use in this condition is relegated more to "last resort" status because of associated side effects. Cyproheptadine (Periactin), a drug with antiserotonin, antihistamine, and anticholinergic effects, may be used in doses of 4–8 mg 3 to 4 times daily. Methysergide (Sansert), an analogue of LSD with potent antiserotonin effects, may be very effective in reducing diarrhea in doses of 2–4 mg 3 to 4 times daily. Both drugs, but especially methysergide, have been reported to result in the development of extensive fibrosis of pleural, peritoneal, and retroperitoneal tissues, a complication normally already present in patients with carcinoid syndrome. In addition, methysergide used chronically may also produce endocardial fibrosis and valvular disease indistinguishable from that produced by the carcinoid syndrome, as well as significant fluid retention. These side effects and toxicity make methysergide, while effective in controlling diarrhea, a potentially dangerous drug for use in this condition.

Inhibitors of serotonin synthesis have also been shown to be useful in controlling the diarrhea of carcinoid syndrome. Parachlorophenylalanine, an experimental inhibitor of the rate limiting enzyme in serotonin synthesis, tryptophan hydroxylase, has been shown to reduce serotonin synthesis effectively by more than 50 percent and to have a favorable effect on diarrhea; in some cases the patient begins to have completely normal bowel movements. While inhibitors of decarboxylation of 5 hydroxy-tryptophan, the next step in serotonin synthesis, might be expected to result similarly in reduction of serotonin production, they have not proved to be useful in patients with the usual types of carcinoid syndrome. However, drugs inhibiting this enzyme may be uniquely useful in patients with carcinoid syndrome due to metastatic gastric tumors. The reason for this singular applicability is that, while almost all carcinoid tumors of tissue derivation other than stomach produce large quantities of serotonin, gastric carcinoids appear to be incapable of metabolizing the tryptophan derivatives beyond 5-hydroxy-tryptophan. These tumors are devoid of the aromatic-L-aminoacid decarboxylase, and they produce 5-hydroxy-tryptophan rather than serotonin. The tumor-derived 5-hydroxy-tryptophan is further metabolized to serotonin in other tissues where the decarboxylase enzyme is present. Therefore, in this condition it is possible to inhibit serotonin synthesis by inhibiting the decarboxylase enzyme. Initially, methyldopa (Aldomet) in a dose of 750–2000 mg per day proved useful in inhibiting 5-HTP conversion to serotonin and the symptoms of diarrhea. Undesirable side effects of Aldomet are sedation and reduction of blood pressure, especially in the standing position. Hydrazino-alphamethyl dopa (Carbidopa), a peripheral decarboxylase inhibitor not producing hypotension or sedation, has been used to enhance the central effects of L-dopa administration in patients with Parkinson's syndrome because it effectively reduces peripheral tissue decarboxylation of this amino acid. Similarly, Carbidopa could be used in a dosage of 25–50 mg 4 times daily in patients with gastric carcinoid syndrome, though availability of this drug singly, rather than in combination with L-dopa, is limited and use for this purpose would be considered experimental. A potential advantage of the use of Carbidopa in this situation is that it is just as effective as methyldopa in inhibiting peripheral decarboxylation but produces none of the central or hemodynamic effects of the latter agent.

GENERAL SUPPORTIVE MEASURES

Maintenance of adequate nutrition is often the major problem confronting the physician caring for a patient with a malignant carcinoid syndrome. Traditional concepts concerning foods to be avoided by patients with diarrhea do not seem to be valid in this condition. Patients should be encouraged to try a wide variety of foods and to eliminate selectively those that seem to cause some problems. The use of more frequent smaller meals may also be helpful in patients who are otherwise distended or who develop severe diarrhea after larger meals. Because the tumor acts as a metabolic parasite shunting tryptophan from the niacin pathway toward the production of 5-hydroxy-indoles, patients with large tumor masses, very high serotonin production, diarrhea, malabsorption, and poor food intake may develop niacin deficiency and pellagra. Dietary supplementation with multivitamin tablets and additional niacin, 100–200 mg daily, should prevent the development of vitamin deficiency.

With adequate nutrition, control of diarrhea, reduction of symptomatic flushing and other appropriate conservative measures, it is usually possible to sustain the patient with malignant carcinoid syndrome for years. The clinical course will be marked by periods of remission and exacerbation, often associated with prolonged bouts of pain and discomfort. Psychologic support and involvement of the patient and family in an understanding of this unique syndrome, its symptoms, and prognosis may be especially helpful in making the remaining years of the patient more tolerable and comfortable.

DISORDERS OF CALCIUM AND BONE METABOLISM

RICKETS

NORMAN H. BELL, M.D.

Rickets occurs in children and is caused by defective mineralization of the organic matrix of bone. Impairment in calcification produces the greatest abnormalities in bones where growth is most rapid. Since the rate of growth of different bones varies with age, the clinical picture of rickets is dependent on age. At birth, craniotabes is common because of the rapid growth of the skull. During infancy and early childhood, widening of bones of the forearm at the wrists and of the costochondral junctions, causing the ricketic rosary, is related to the rapid rate of growth of the arms and ribs, respectively. In later years, the bowing of the legs especially around the knees is related to the rapid rate of growth of the lower extremities. Secondary hyperparathyroidism often occurs in rickets, may produce erosion of metaphyses of long bones, and may be the most prominent form of the skeletal disease. The skeletal abnormalities thus may provide clues to the age of onset and severity of the disorder. With early and adequate treatment, skeletal deformities can be prevented.

Rickets can result from a variety of disorders: an alteration in the metabolism of vitamin D, deficiency of phosphate or calcium, or a mineralization defect (Table 1). Often there may be more than one contributing factor. In a given patient, a clear understanding of the underlying pathogenesis is essential not only for establishing the correct diagnosis and the most effective means of therapy, but in some instances for prevention of treatment that may be either harmful or unnecessary.

Hypocalcemia often occurs in association with rickets and can cause tetany, cataracts, diarrhea, laryngeal stridor, grand mal seizures, and increased intracranial pressure with papilledema. Chronic hypocalcemia in childhood may produce mental retardation, behavioral abnormalities, and psychoses. Early detection and treatment are therefore essential.

METABOLISM OF VITAMIN D

Vitamin D_2 (ergocalciferol) is absorbed from food via the intestinal lymphatic system. Absorption requires the presence of bile acids and takes place in the proximal small intestine. Vitamin D_3 (cholecalciferol) is produced in the skin by the photochemical synthesis of 7-dehydrocholesterol. Upon exposure to ultraviolet light, 7-dehydrocholesterol absorbs one photon of light energy and is converted to previtamin D_3, which is thermally labile. Previtamin D_3 then undergoes a temperature-dependent rearrangement of double bonds to form vitamin D_3, which is thermally stable. Vitamin D_3 is removed from the skin by vitamin D-binding protein, which has a high affinity for the vitamin, by way of the dermal capillaries.

Vitamin D_2 and vitamin D_3 themselves have little in the way of biologic activity. Both undergo hydroxylation in the liver to form 25-hydroxyvitamin D by action of the enzyme vitamin D-25-hydroxylase. 25-hydroxyvitamin D is the major storage form of the vitamin. The normal range in the circulation is from 8 to 60 ng/ml. 25-hydroxyvitamin D undergoes further hydroxylation to form 1,25-dihydroxyvitamin D by action of the enzyme 25-hydroxyvitamin D-1α-hydroxylase. This hydroxylation takes place primarily but not exclusively in the kidney and is tightly regulated by parathyroid hormone. Production is not as well regulated in children. The normal range of serum 1,25-dihydroxyvitamin D in adults is from 20 to 50 pg/ml. Values in infants and children are somewhat higher. In man, the metabolites of vitamin D_3 are present in higher amounts than those of vitamin D_2. The biologic activities of the metabolites of vitamin D_2 and D_3, however, are the same.

TABLE 1 Pathogenesis of Rickets

I. Alteration in vitamin D metabolism
  A. Vitamin D deficiency
    1. Dietary deficiency or lack of exposure to sunlight
    2. Malabsorption syndromes
      a. small bowel disease
      b. pancreatitic insufficiency
  B. Impaired 25-hydroxylation of vitamin D
    1. Liver disease (primary biliary cirrhosis, biliary atresia)
    2. Anticonvulsant therapy (phenobarbital, diphenylhydantoin)
    3. Neonatal rickets
  C. Impaired 1α-hydroxylation of 25-hydroxyvitamin D
    1. Hypoparathyroidism
    2. Pseudohypoparathyroidism
    3. Chronic renal failure
    4. Vitamin D-dependent rickets type I
    5. Hypophosphatemic rickets
    6. Oncogenic rickets
  D. Impaired target-organ response to 1,25-dihydroxyvitamin D
    1. Vitamin D-dependent rickets type II
    2. Anticonvulsant drugs (phenobarbital, diphenylhydantoin)
II. Phosphate deficiency
  A. Diminished intake
    1. Neonatal rickets
  B. Excessive renal loss
    1. Primary renal tubular defects
      a. Hypophosphatemic rickets
      b. Fanconi syndromes (Wilson's disease, Lowe's disease, tyrosinemia, glycogen storage disease, cystinosis)
    2. Secondary renal tubular defects
      a. Primary hyperparathyroidism
      b. Renal tubular acidosis
      c. Oncogenic rickets
III. Mineralization defect
  A. Enzyme deficiency
    1. Hypophosphatasia
  B. Circulating inhibitor of calcification
    1. Chronic renal failure
  C. Drugs and ions
    1. Diphosphonates
    2. Fluoride
    3. Aluminum
  D. Abnormal bone collagen or matrix
    1. Chronic renal failure
    2. Osteogenesis imperfecta

25-hydroxyvitamin D is converted to 24,25-dihydroxyvitamin D by action of the enzyme 25-hydroxyvitamin D-24-hydroxylase. This reaction also takes place primarily but not exclusively in the kidney. There is considerable controversy as to whether this metabolite has a physiologic role with regard to bone and mineral metabolism. Evidence on the one hand indicates that 24,25-dihydroxyvitamin D may be important in healing osteomalacia and rickets, and on the other hand that 24-hydroxylation may be of importance only as a pathway for degradation. Both 24,25-dihydroxyvitamin D and 1,25-dihydroxyvitamin D undergo further hydroxylation to form 1,24,25-trihydroxyvitamin D before cleavage of the side chain and excretion.

Vitamin D, 25-hydroxyvitamin D, 24,25-dihydroxyvitamin D, and 1,25-dihydroxyvitamin D are all transported in the circulation by the vitamin D-binding protein, an α_2 globulin that is also the group-specific component protein, or Gc protein. Patients with heavy proteinuria sometimes lose significant amounts of the metabolites in the urine and thus are at risk for developing vitamin D deficiency. Vitamin D and the metabolites listed above undergo an enterohepatic circulation and are conjugated in the liver to form sulfates and glucuronides. Vitamin D deficiency can result from disruption of the enterohepatic circulation.

Clinical and basic studies show that hydroxylation of vitamin D in both the 25 and 1α positions is necessary for optimal biologic activity. Dihydrotachysterol resembles 1α-hydroxyvitamin D_3 in structure: The A ring is rotated 180° so that the hydroxyl group in the 3 position acts as a pseudo-1-hydroxyl group. Both 1α-hydroxyvitamin D_3 (which is not clinically available in the United States) and dihydrotachysterol must undergo 25-hydroxylation by the liver for full biologic activity. Indeed, dihydrotachysterol is inactive. The rank order of biologic activity experimentally is:

$$1,25(OH)_2D_3 > 1\alpha,25\text{-}OHD_3 > 25\text{-}DHT \\ > 25\text{-}OHD_3 > D_3 > DHT$$

MECHANISM OF ACTION OF VITAMIN D

1,25-dihydroxyvitamin D_3 binds to a cytosol receptor in target tissues, predominantly the intestine and skeleton, and is transported to the nucleus where it initiates events related to translation and transcription. The major actions are to augment the intestinal transport of calcium and phosphorus and to stimulate release of these ions from the skeleton. Inhibition of secretion of parathyroid hormone is mediated indirectly through increases in the intestinal absorption of calcium. In vitamin D intoxication, serum 25-hydroxyvitamin D is markedly increased and serum 1,25-dihydroxyvitamin D is normal or only slightly increased because 25-hydroxyvitamin D 1α-hydroxylase is tightly

TABLE 2 Preparations of Vitamin D and its Derivatives

Drug	Dose Required (μg/day)	Period for Optimal Activity (weeks)	Duration of Action (weeks)	Available Preparations (μg)	Trade Name
Vitamin D$_2$ (ergocalciferol)	250–2500	4–8	6–18	250 solution* 1250 capsules	Drisdol Drisdol
25-Hydroxyvitamin D$_3$ (calcifediol)	50–200	2–4	4–12	20 capsules 50 capsules	Calderol
Dihydrotachysterol	125–1000	1–2	1–3	125 capsules 200 capsules 400 capsules	Hytakerol, dihydrotachysterol
1,25-Dihydroxyvitamin D$_3$ (calcitriol)	0.5–3	0.5–1	0.5–1	0.25 capsules 0.50 capsules	Rocaltrol

Note: 40,000 IU of vitamin D is 1,250 μg.
*250 μg per ml

regulated. At high concentrations, 25-hydroxyvitamin D is thought to occupy and activate the receptors in target organs.

DRUGS

Preparations of vitamin D and its metabolites which are available for clinical use in the United States are listed in Tables 2 and 3. The onset of optimal biologic activity, duration of effect after cessation of treatment, dosage forms available, and trade names are listed in Table 2. The pharmacologic advantages and disadvantages of the drugs are listed in Table 3.

Vitamin D$_2$ and 25-hydroxyvitamin D$_3$ have the theoretical advantage that they are the precursors of the other vitamin D metabolites, including 24,25-dihydroxyvitamin D, which may prove to be of value in treating rickets. Also, 25-hydroxyvitamin D$_3$ should be used in patients with liver disease who have decreased activity of vitamin D-25-hydroxylase. The major practical advantage of vitamin D$_2$ is that it is inexpensive and can be used in selected patients. In contrast to 25-hydroxyvitamin D$_3$, however, vitamin D$_2$ tends to be chemically unstable and to lose its activity with storage. It also tends to accumulate in fat and muscle during long-term administration so that its effects may become cumulative. With both compounds, the therapeutic dose approaches the toxic dose, a long period is required for optimal biologic effect, and activity may persist after cessation, a disadvantage in the event of intoxication. Also, the two sterols

are not consistently effective, especially when the metabolism of vitamin D is abnormal.

The advantages of dihydrotachysterol and 1,25-dihydroxyvitamin D$_3$ are that they require only a short period for optimal biologic activity and their effects last only a short period after cessation of treatment. The biologic activity of dihydrotachysterol, however, may be prolonged on occasion. Also, both are effective when 1α hydroxylation of 25-hydroxyvitamin D is defective. On the other hand, both drugs are relatively expensive, neither may be completely effective in curing rickets in patients who are deficient in some of the other metabolites, and toxicity can occur spontaneously in patients who are receiving long-term treatment. The hypercalcemia, however, is easily managed by stopping the drug and is prevented by reducing the dose. 1,25-dihydroxyvitamin D$_3$ may be highly effective in promoting normal or near normal growth and development in some children with deficiency of the metabolite. This may also be the case with optimal treatment when the other preparations of vitamin D are utilized.

TREATMENT OF RICKETS

The goals are (1) to correct hypocalcemia, alleviate related symptoms, and prevent grand mal seizures and cataracts; (2) to prevent or alleviate the skeletal deformities of rickets and excess parathyroid hormone; (3) to prevent hypercalcemia, hypercalciuria and their sequelae; and (4) to pro-

TABLE 3　Advantages and Disadvantages of Vitamin D and its Derivatives

Drug	Advantages	Disadvantages
Vitamin D_2	Inexpensive Precursor of vitamin D metabolites	Therapeutic dose approaches toxic dose Long period for onset of biologic effect Prolonged duration of effect after cessation May not be effective, particularly when vitamin D metabolism is defective Unstable, undergoes oxidation, photochemical decomposition, and loss of activity with storage
25-Hydroxyvitamin D_3	Chemically stable Precursor of vitamin D metabolites Should be useful in liver disease when 25-hydroxylation is impaired	Moderately expensive Except for stability, disadvantages are same as vitamin D_2
Dihydrotachysterol	Does not require 1α-hydroxylation; can be used when this is impaired Short period for onset of biologic effect Duration of effect after cessation usually short but may be prolonged	Therapeutic dose approaches toxic dose Moderately expensive 25-hydroxylation required for biologic effectiveness; may be ineffective in liver disease May be less effective in osteomalacia than in osteitis fibrosa cystica
1,25-Dihydroxyvitamin D_3	Short period of onset for biologic effect Short duration of effect after cessation Can be highly effective when 1α-hydroxylation is impaired and may provide normal or near normal growth	Expensive May be less effective in osteomalacia than in osteitis fibrosa cystica Toxicity may occur spontaneously

mote normal growth and development. Treatment must be individualized with regard to pathogenesis and severity of the disorder.

Administration of elemental calcium is useful. Calcium content varies with oral presentations: calcium carbonate (40 percent), calcium chloride (36 percent), calcium lactate (13 percent), and calcium gluconate (9 percent). Thus, 2.5 gm, 2.8 gm, 7.7 gm, and 11.0 gm are required, respectively, to provide 1.0 gm of elemental calcium. One preparation is calcium lactate powder, which can be obtained from health food stores. One level teaspoonful provides about 1.0 gm of elemental calcium. It can be administered in a glass of water and is well tolerated.

VITAMIN D DEFICIENCY

Regardless of age, vitamin D-deficient rickets is treated by the daily administration of 125 μg (5000 IU) of vitamin D_2 and 1.0 gm of elemental calcium for 4 to 6 weeks or until the rickets is healed. Thereafter, the dose is 10 μg (400 IU) per day. Additional calcium is required only if the dietary intake is not adequate.

ANTICONVULSANT THERAPY

Phenobarbital and Dilantin impair the target-organ response (intestine and skeleton) to 1,25-dihydroxyvitamin D_3 and may cause rickets. Anticonvulsant drugs also cause the production of more polar, biologically inactive metabolites of vitamin D. Rickets can be treated and prevented by small but pharmacologic doses of vitamin D, 125 μg (5000 IU) per day.

HYPOPARATHYROIDISM AND PSEUDOHYPOPARATHYROIDISM

Serum 1,25-dihydroxyvitamin D values are diminished in hypoparathyroidism and pseudohypoparathyroidism because of lack of parathyroid hormone and abnormal response to parathyroid hormone, respectively. Patients with rickets may respond to vitamin D_2. The dose is from 1.25 to 2.5 mg (50,000 to 100,000 IU) per day. Elemental calcium should be given in an initial dose of 1.0 gm per day. The dose can be increased to as much as 3.0 gm per day to bring the serum calcium to the lower range of normal. The serum phosphate will then often decrease to within the normal range. If hypocalcemia persists, the dose of vitamin D can be increased, but this should be done very slowly at intervals of from one to two months.

If rickets and hypocalcemia persist, vitamin D should be stopped and treatment with 1,25-dihydroxyvitamin D_3, 0.5 μg per day, should be started. The dose can be increased at about two-week intervals if required to correct hypocalcemia. Healing of the rickets may require some two months or longer.

VITAMIN D-DEPENDENT RICKETS TYPE I

Rickets in this disease is caused by impaired renal production of 1,25-dihydroxyvitamin D_3. Treatment is 1,25-dihydroxyvitamin D_3, 0.5 to 2.0 μg per day (or 0.04 μg per kg body weight per day). This results in correction of the hypocalcemia, hypophosphatemia, increased serum alkaline phosphatase, and healing of the rickets within one to two months.

VITAMIN D-DEPENDENT RICKETS TYPE II

Rickets in this disease is caused by defective target-organ response to 1,25-dihydroxyvitamin D. The disease is particularly severe in patients with associated alopecia who may be refractory to as much as 20 μg a day of 1,25-dihydroxyvitamin D_3. Some patients respond to large doses of vitamin D. Therefore, vitamin D_2 in doses of 1.25 to 2.5 mg (50,000 to 100,000 IU) or more and 3.0 gm a day of elemental calcium should be tried initially. If the response is poor, treatment with 1,25-dihydroxyvitamin D_3 may be tried with an initial dose of 1.0 to 2.0 μg per day.

HYPOPHOSPHATASIA

This is a disease of unknown cause which is characterized by rickets and low serum alkaline phosphatase. There is no known treatment.

HYPOPHOSPHATEMIC RICKETS

Hypophosphatemic rickets is caused by a defect in renal tubular transport of phosphate which results in renal phosphate wasting and hypophosphatemia. Serum 1,25-dihydroxyvitamin D is inappropriately low for the serum phosphorus, does not respond normally to exogenous parathyroid extract, and may represent a secondary impairment resulting from the abnormal renal phosphate transport.

Treatment is with elemental phosphate, 2.0 to 4.0 gm per day by mouth, and 1,25-dihydroxyvitamin D_3, 1.0 to 2.0 μg per day (or 0.04 μg per kg body weight per day). With this regimen, the serum phosphorus may be brought into the normal range, there is a decline in the serum alkaline phosphatase toward normal, and healing of the rickets occurs. Treatment is lifelong.

Corrective osteotomies should be carried out after cessation of growth. Reduction of the dose of 1,25-dihydroxyvitamin D_3 may be required during prolonged bed rest because of immobilization and the potential development of hypercalcemia.

SIDE EFFECTS AND COMPLICATIONS OF TREATMENT

Intoxication can be a major problem with vitamin D or any of its metabolites. Patients with intoxication are often asymptomatic, but they may have anorexia, nausea, vomiting, weight loss, polyuria, polydipsia, and alterations in mental status. Children and infants often show listlessness and are hypotonic. Hypercalcemia and hypercalciuria result from increased intestinal absorption of calcium and mobilization of calcium from the skeleton and may lead to impairment in renal function, nephrocalcinosis, nephrolithiasis, urinary tract infections, renal failure, and death. In patients on long-term treatment, the development of hypercalcemia and hypercalciuria is not uncommon. Unfortunately, there is no way of predicting when or in whom intoxication will occur.

Intoxication with vitamin D, 25-hydroxyvitamin D_3, and dihydrotachysterol is related to the fact that there is very little difference between toxic and therapeutic doses. On the other hand, toxicity to 1,25-dihydroxyvitamin D_3 appears to be related to an alteration in the metabolism of the drug. There are suggestions that this may be the case with regard to vitamin D, since lower doses are sometimes required after a hypercalcemic episode.

The treatment for intoxication is to stop the drug and force fluids. If intoxication is profound, a short course of steroids or salmon calcitonin may be required, usually only when hypercalcemia is produced by the longer-acting sterols. Use of lower doses of the drugs after episodes of hypercalcemia will usually prevent recurrences. Patients who are difficult to treat with vitamin D may be more easily managed with 1,25-dihydroxyvitamin D_3.

The best treatment for intoxication is prevention. Patients should be closely followed at regular intervals of four to six weeks with measurement of serum calcium and creatinine. They should be informed of the possibility of intoxication, the symptoms to be on the lookout for, and the potential harmful effects.

OSTEOMALACIA

GEOFFREY M. MAREL, M.B., B.S.,
and BOY FRAME, M.D.

The term osteomalacia covers a heterogeneous group of hereditary and acquired diseases that have in common (1) defective mineralization of newly formed preosseous matrix (osteoid) of mature lamellar bone, with impaired appositional bone formation seen on histologic studies; (2) a clinical syndrome of variable severity in adults, whose childhood counterpart is rickets and whose features are bone pain and tenderness, skeletal fracture and deformity, muscle weakness, and typical biochemical and radiologic findings; (3) a pathogenesis involving one or more of the following: phosphate depletion, deficiency of vitamin D or one of its metabolites, alterations in vitamin D metabolism, or defective bone matrix synthesis.

This chapter outlines an approach to management and the principles of pharmacologic therapy in the commonly encoutered forms of osteomalacic disorders.

PHYSIOLOGIC CONSIDERATIONS

Vitamin D_3 (cholecalciferol) is formed in the skin under the influence of ultraviolet light. It is then transferred to the circulation, bound to plasma vitamin D binding globulin, and converted to 25-hydroxy vitamin D_3 (25 OH D_3) in the liver. This conversion is partially product-inhibited by increasing plasma levels of 25 OH D_3, so that 25 OH D_3 production rises only fourfold and twentyfold in response to D_3 increments of tenfold and hundredfold respectively. The result is a weak but not insignificant feedback control against vitamin D overdosage. The principal circulating form of D vitamin is 25 OH D_3, and its levels in plasma correlate well with vitamin D body stores. The normal turnover time of 25 OH D_3 is three to four weeks. Further metabolism of 25 OH D_3 to 1,25 $(OH)_2D_3$ and to other, less potent metabolites occurs in the kidney. Normal plasma levels are listed in Table 1. The production rate of 1,25 $(OH)_2D_3$ is closely regulated by plasma concentrations of parathyroid hormone (PTH), calcium, phosphate, and 1,25 $(OH)_2D_3$ itself, as well as intracellular phosphate levels. Turnover time for 1,25 $(OH)_2D_3$ in plasma is about one day. Adequate plasma and intracellular phosphorus levels are required for normal skeletal mineralization. Nutritional phosphorus deficiency, intestinal malabsorption, or diminished renal tubular reabsorption of phosphorus is present in almost all cases of osteomalacia, though for different reasons in different etiologic groups. Since body stores of phosphorus are either intracellular in soft tissues or deposited extracellularly in mineralized bone, plasma phosphorus levels may be normal in the presence of significant phosphorus depletion. Intracellular phosphorus depletion may play an important role in the pathogenesis of muscle weakness and impaired osteoblast function in osteomalacia.

THERAPEUTIC PRINCIPLES

The clinical manifestations and diagnostic evaluation of osteomalacia are beyond the scope of this chapter. However, once the diagnosis of osteomalacia is established, generally from bone biopsy, its etiologic agent must be determined, since the choice of appropriate therapeutic agents, dosage level, and duration of treatment usually depend on the nature of the underlying disorder. Table 2 summarizes the common varieties of osteomalacia based upon an etiologic classification that forms the basis for a logical approach to therapy.

There are certain guidelines to therapy for

TABLE 1   Vitamin D Derivatives in Hypocalcemia and Osteomalacia*

	Ergocalciferol	Dihydro-tachysterol	Calcifediol	Calcitriol
Abbreviation	D_2; EC	DHT	25 OH D	$1,25(OH)_2D$
Trade name	Calciferol	DHT	Calderol	Rocaltrol
Antirachitic (physiologic) daily dosage (mcg)	2–10	20–100	1–6	0.1–0.8
Relative potency (antirachitic)	1	$^{1}/_{10}$†	2	20
Normal plasma levels	0.5–2 ng/ml (vitamin D_3)	Unmeasurable routinely	10–40 ng/ml	20–50 pg/ml
Estimated daily dosage range in Vitamin D "resistance" (pharmacologic dosage)	1–10 mg	0.1–1 mg	50–200 mcg	0.5–3 mcg
Daily dosage in hypoparathyroidism (mcg)	750–3000	250–1000	50–200	0.5–2
Relative potency in hypoparathyroidism	1	3†	15	1500
Time to reach maximal effects (lag time) (weeks)‡	4–10	2–4	4–20	½–1
Persistence of effect after cessation (weeks)	6–18§	1–3	4–12	½–1
Approximate cost per month of therapy§§ (pharmacologic doses)	$6	$25	$42	$128

*Adapted from Frame and Parfitt.

†DHT more potent than D_2 in raising plasma calcium levels (hypoparathyroidism), but less potent than D_2 for rickets and osteomalacia

‡Assumes constant daily dosage. Shorter if loading dose is used (see text)

§Up to 18 months with severe intoxication

§§Based on cost of 100 tablets/capsules in Detroit in March 1982, and daily doses of 2.5 mg D_2, 0.8 mg DHT, 100 mcg 25 OHD, 2.0 mcg $1,25(OH)_2D$

osteomalacia. The therapeutic response to appropriate measures in most subgroups of the disease is generally excellent, with resolution of symptoms within 2 or 3 months, and healing of skeletal lesions within 4 to 18 months, depending on cause and severity. Osteomalacia always requires treatment; the earlier it is commenced, the better will be the chance for complete skeletal healing. If osteopenia, or loss of total bone volume, accompanies osteomalacia (frequently the case in intestinal osteomalacia or in cases in which there has been prolonged immobilization or glucocorticoid therapy) healing will be incomplete, and the risk of fractures will remain.

The first approach to therapy should be to correct underlying abnormalities or remove obvious precipitating factors. Table 3 lists several remediable predisposing factors whose correction may be all that is required in mild or moderate cases. A search for, and correction of, such underlying conditions must be made in every case, since unnecessary and expensive treatment may be avoided. As a corollary, vitamin D requirements will diminish as an underlying disease improves, so that dosages required initially may later lead to vitamin D intoxication.

PHARMACOLOGIC CONSIDERATIONS OF VITAMIN D

The irradiated plant sterol, ergocalciferol (vitamin D_2), for all intents and purposes is as potent as natural vitamin D_3 in man and undergoes identical metabolism. Having been identified and synthesized before vitamin D_3, vitamin D_2 is the most widely used preparation in the prophylaxis and therapy of rickets and osteomalacia. Dosage of vitamin D is still commonly expressed in the traditional units of antirachitic activity in the rat—

TABLE 2   Etiologic Classification of Common Forms of Osteomalacia*

Diagnostic Category	Therapeutic Dosage Range Approximate Daily Maintenance Vitamin D_2 (mgm)	Alternative Agent	Phosphate Supplements
Nutritional deficiency	0.05–0.125	—	–
Vitamin D malabsorption			
± 25 OH D deficiency			
Gastrectomy	0.1–0.2	—	–
Small intestinal disease	1.0–10.0	Calcifediol, 20–200 mcg†	±
mucosal (gluten enteropathy)		or 250–1000 mcg	
jejunal-ileal bypass		(10,000–40,000 IU) vitamin	
scleroderma, blind loop		D_2 per week i.m.	
Hepatobiliary disease	0.25–1.0	Calcifediol, 20–100 mcg†	±
Pancreatic disease	0.25–1.0	or 2.5 mg (100,000 IU)	±
		vitamin D_2 i.m. per month	
Accelerated catabolism/excretion			
Anticonvulsant-induced	0.1–1.0	Calcifediol, 20–100 mcg†	–
Nephrotic syndrome	0.1–1.0	Calcifediol, 20–100 mcg†	–
Impaired renal 1-hydroxylation			
Vitamin D dependency (type I)	1.0–2.5	Calcitriol, 1–2 mcg‡	–
Primary (X-linked) hypophosphatemia	1.0–5.0	Calcitriol, 2–4 mcg‡	+
Tumorous hypophosphatemia	1.25–5.0	Calcitriol, 1–3 mcg‡	+
Sporadic adult-onset hypophosphatemia	1.25–2.5§	Calcitriol, 1–3 mcg‡·§	+
Hyperchloremic acidosis			
RTA	0.25–1.0		+
Ureterosigmoidostomy	0.25–1.0		+
Multiple renal tubular defects			
Fanconi syndromes	0.1–1.5		+

*Excluding renal osteodystrophy
‡Preferred choice as first-line therapy (± phosphate)
†Second-line therapy for vitamin D resistant cases, or initial choice in those with severe or extensive disease
§Cure may be possible (but not advisable) with phosphate alone (see text).

where 1 international unit (IU) equals 25 ng of chemically pure vitamin D_2, or 40,000 IU equals 1 mg. Vitamin D_2 is available in tablets or capsules containing 1.25 mg (50,000 IU) per dosage unit; in an injectable form, as 12.5 mgm (500,000 IU) per ml in sesame oil, in 1 ml ampules; and, for orally administered physiologic doses, in solution with propylene glycol, containing 6.25 mcg (250 IU) per drop, which can be administered by mixing with milk. The inconsistency of potency that characterized preparations of vitamin D in the past is less problematic with currently available commercial preparations. However, the clinician should bear in mind the possibility of irregularities in pharmaceutic formulation when an unexpected response to ergocalciferol is encountered. Vitamin D_2 in liquid form is subject to deterioration with exposure to air or light and thus should be stored in tightly stoppered amber bottles, or administered in opaque capsules. Care should be taken to avoid any preparations containing vitamin D_2 in addition to calcium salts (which promote decomposition of

ergocalciferol), or components of multivitamin preparations (which may inactivate vitamin D_2 by isomerization).

Used therapeutically, vitamin D, through its hydroxylated derivatives, (1) stimulates intestinal calcium and phosphorus absorption (mainly in the jejunum); (2) mobilizes calcium from bone and facilitates bone remodeling; (3) reverses secondary hyperparathyroidism (frequently present in osteomalacia itself or due to phosphate therapy), not only by raising plasma calcium levels, but also probably via a direct effect on parathyroid glands; and (4) moderately increases renal tubular reabsorption of phosphorus, both directly and through suppression of PTH release.

The net effect of these actions is to raise the plasma concentrations and the availability for mineralization of calcium and phosphorus ions. In addition to the effects listed above, vitamin D metabolites (but not those of tachysterol, see below) probably possess direct stimulatory effects on bone mineralization, most likely through restoring im-

TABLE 3   Potentially Remediable Underlying Causes of Osteomalacia

Diagnostic Category	Therapy
Substrate deficiency	Nutrition, sunlight
Gluten enteropathy	Gluten-free diet
Jejunal-ileal bypass	Surgical reversal
Pancreatic insufficiency	Pancreatic enzyme supplements Medium chain triglyceride oil
End-stage renal disease	Renal transplantation
Tumorous hypophosphatemic osteomalacia	Resection of mesenchymal tumors
Renal tubular acidosis Ureterosigmoidostomy	Correct acidosis with sodium bicarbonate 2 mEq HCO_3 per kg per day
Fanconi syndromes (multiple renal tubular defects)	Correct acidosis, as above Dietary exclusion in galactosemia Chelating agents for heavy metal toxicity D pencillamine in Wilson's disease Specific therapy for Sjögren's disease, multiple myeloma, paraproteinemias
Medications known to produce osteomalacia under some circumstances	Phosphate-binding antacids, laxatives, cholestyramine, anticonvulsants, diphosphonates, fluoride, glutethimide, amphotericin, acetazolamide

paired osteoblast function. Vitamin D metabolites also appear to stimulate linear bone growth in childhood and adolescence.

Physiologic and Near-Physiologic Dosages

In vitamin D depleted subjects, small "physiologic" doses (2.5 mcg, or 100 IU) of vitamin D daily will induce a positive calcium and phosphorus balance by increasing the fractional intestinal absorption of these ions, with minimal changes in their urinary excretion, and a normalization of low plasma levels and of abnormal skeletal mineralization.

With single doses of vitamin D ranging from 35 mcg (1400 IU) to 1 mg (40,000 IU), about 80 percent is normally absorbed. Vitamin D is largely inert, and its need for serial biotransformations before activity largely explains the lag time between administration and response. In vitamin D depletion, treatment with physiologic doses results in rapid conversion of hydroxylated metabolites within the first few days, and the first histologic evidence of bone healing (return of a mineraliza-

tion front) is evident by the end of the first week. Radiographic evidence of healing may not appear for several weeks, however. This reflects the normal delay between the fairly rapid renewal of bone mineralization and osteoblast function, and the effects of complex healing processes, ongoing repletion of tissue vitamin D stores, and the correction of secondary hyperparathyroidism. The duration of the delay depends on the extent and severity of the skeletal disease; it can vary from several weeks to many months in some cases.

When near-physiologic doses are required, our practice is to start with a larger dose than the anticipated maintenance (or prophylactic) dose level and to continue this until signs of healing occur. This approach is based not on the erroneous belief that a higher dose is necessary to initiate healing but on the observation that healing begins more rapidly this way. In vitamin D deficiency, for example, the duration for skeletal repair might be reduced from 6 months to 3 months by using 50–125 mcg vitamin D daily (2000–5000 IU), but 12.5–25 mcg daily (500–1000 IU) would have been equally effective over a longer time. The risk of intoxication with such an initial approach in this group (vitamin D deficient patients) is minimal.

Monitoring Response to Vitamin D (Vitamin D-depleted Subjects)

While receiving initial high-dose therapy (2 to 4 times the anticipated maintenance dosage), the following should be monitored, initially every month, then every 3 to 6 months: (1) 24-hour urinary calcium, phosphorus, and creatinine levels, and creatinine clearance; (2) plasma calcium, phosphorus, creatinine, and 25 OH D levels; and (3) appropriate radiographs. The earliest changes to be anticipated with vitamin D administration in D-depleted patients are (1) rise in plasma phosphorus level, with no change or a fall in urine phosphorus level—generally well within seven days; (2) initial fall in urine calcium level, more marked if intake is inadequate, and occasionally (espeicially in children), a fall in plasma calcium level; (3) rise in plasma alkaline phosphatase level during the first few weeks (phosphatase "healing flare"), then a progressive fall toward normal as ongoing healing occurs; and (4) normalization of 25 OH D levels.

Indications to reduce dosage to maintenance levels (usually only after vitamin D stores are replenished, which may take several months) are listed below:

1. Significant improvement in clinical, radiologic, and histologic findings

2. Rise in urine calcium excretion or plasma calcium level

3. Fall toward normal of alkaline phosphatase

4. Any evidence of incipient renal deterioration

Factors that may delay the predicted response to vitamin D include the following:

1. Inappropriate dosage selection

2. Pharmacologically substandard preparations

3. Phosphorus or calcium depletion. Dietary calcium intake should be equivalent to at least 1 gm elemental calcium per day, and up to 2 gm per day may be necessary for severe osteomalacia or hypocalcemia.

4. Intestinal malabsorption of orally administered vitamin D metabolite

5. Magnesium depletion, particularly likely with steatorrhea, which will impair both intestinal and skeletal response to vitamin D

6. Pharmacologic doses of glucocorticoids which may antagonize intestinal and skeletal effects of vitamin D metabolites.

Pharmacologic Dosage

In vitamin D-replete patients requiring pharmacologic dosage (see below), hydroxylation of metabolites occurs more slowly, and body stores of vitamin D and its derivatives require saturation to a certain level before renewal of normal mineralization and osteoblast function occurs. Once stable tissue levels are achieved (after four or so weeks of constant daily dosage with vitamin D_2), a state of vitamin D equilibrium ensues, and ongoing effects on target tissues will induce skeletal healing. If the initial dosage chosen is excessive, body stores will continue to increase and will eventually overcome the homeostatic mechanisms that normally guard against vitamin D toxicity and hypercalcemia. The time required to attain stable tissue levels varies among the different therapeutic metabolites now available. Accepted ranges are given in Table 1, which compares these and other characteristics. With pharmacologic doses, an initial high-dose regimen, such as that described above for vitamin D depletion, significantly increases the risk of intoxication. This risk is less if the bone disease is severe and widespread and if initial plasma calcium levels are low. In such cases, or in patients with severe disability due to symptomatic disease (skeletal pain and muscle weakness), we would select an initial dose that was two to four times that of the expected maintenance level. Very close observation in such circumstances in mandatory, with repeated clinical assessment and charting of 24-hour urinary calcium, creatinine clearance, plasma fasting calcium, phosphorus, alkaline phosphatase, albumin, and creatinine levels, initially at once weekly intervals. Serial plotting of these variables is the only means by which biochemical trends will be obvious before clinical toxicity supervenes. In children with rickets or adults with Looser's zones, appropriate x-rays should be repeated every four to six weeks while the high-dose regimen is continued. Reduction of dosage to maintenance levels is indicated when either incipient vitamin D intoxication or clinical, biochemical, or radiographic evidence of healing becomes evident.

If no indication exists for an initial high-dose protocol, therapy should commence at a dosage level slightly below the range of anticipated maintenance dosage for the appropriate disease category (Table 2). The dosage can then be progressively increased, in increments no greater than 25 percent of the initial dose, and at intervals of four weeks plus the appropriate lag period of the compound being used (Table 1). The same measurements should be made, and plotted serially, as in the initial high-dose regimen, but at less frequent intervals; every two to four weeks at first, and finally every three months once appropriate maintenance dosages are established.

If desired, a loading dose may be administered, followed by dosage increments, to minimize the lag period between dosage adjustment and therapeutic response. Only the increment itself is used in the calculation, not the whole dose. This principle is best illustrated by the following example: For a dosage increment from a daily dose of 2 mgm (80,000 IU) to one of 2.5 mgm (100,000 IU) of vitamin D, 4 times the increment (2 mgm per day) may be added to the daily dose for the first 2 days, then twice the increment (1 mgm per day) for the next 2 days, before commencing the new maintenance dose. The next dosage increment will then be possible in four weeks plus half the usual lag period, a total interval of six instead of eight weeks.

Vitamin D Intoxication

The toxic effects of excess vitamin D are primarily those of hypercalcuria and hypercalcemia, with or without hyperphosphatemia. The clinical manifestations are well known and include renal tubular dysfunction, acute and chronic renal impairment, nephrocalcinosis, soft tissue and vascular calcification, and neurologic dysfunction. Direct toxic effects of vitamin D metabolites on bone and renal tissue, independent of those caused by hypercalcemia, are likely. Early symptoms include constipation, lethargy, weakness, dry mouth, metallic taste, and nausea. Polyuria and polydipsia may be the first indications of renal tubular impairment.

Contributing factors to vitamin D intoxication include inappropriate dosage selection, excessively frequent dosage increment, failure to monitor urinary calcium excretion and serum calcium levels adequately, increased dietary calcium intake, concomitant thiazide administration, and any significant improvement in underlying disease states (for example, successful treatment of intestinal mucosal disease with gluten-free diet, rever-

sal of an intestinal bypass shunt, or renal transplantation).

Therapy for vitamin D intoxication is described elsewhere in this volume. Some salient points however, are that a reduction in intestinal calcium absorption (low-calcium diet with cellulose phosphate, 5 gm t.i.d.) may be sufficient in mild to moderate cases; hydrocortisone is invariably effective in vitamin D intoxication and should be given to those with moderate to severe symptomatic manifestations (200–300 mg per day); duration of intoxication depends on the level of body tissue stores of the vitamin D metabolite, not on the degree of hypercalcemia, and will vary with different metabolites (Table 1).

Currently Used Therapeutic Agents

Several metabolites and analogues of Vitamin D, other than the more familiar ergocalciferol, are efficacious in specific varieties of osteomalacia. Comparative data are presented in Table 1. Several therapeutic points are further outlined below.

Calcitriol. Calcitriol is synthetic $1,25(OH)_2D_3$, marketed as Rocaltrol by Hoffman-LaRoche Laboratories in gelatin capsules of 0.25 mcg and 0.50 mcg. It is the most potent naturally occurring metabolite of vitamin D in stimulating calcium absorption from the small intestine and in mobilizing bone calcium. Since it does not require in vivo metabolism for activity, its effects occur rapidly following oral administration. Increased intestinal calcium absorption is evident within 2 to 5 hours of a single dose of 0.5 mcg. Calcitriol is minimally protein-bound in plasma and is not stored, in contrast to its precursors, vitamin D and 25 OH D. Its plasma half-life is thus short (about 2 hours), necessitating a twice or thrice daily administration regimen, and the duration of its biologic effects is similarly brief. While cumulative toxicity is not a risk with calcitriol, hypercalcemia may occur quickly. Thus we recommend that monitoring of serum and urinary calcium levels be undertaken more frequently during the early treatment phases of dosage titration than with other vitamin D compounds.

Calcitriol is approved by the United States Food and Drug Administration for use in renal osteodystrophy. In pharmacologic doses, calcitriol is effective also in treating X-linked, vitamin D-resistant osteomalacia, and certain cases of sporadic acquired hypophosphatemic osteomalacia in adults. In slightly supraphysiologic doses, calcitriol is effective in vitamin D dependency or pseudo-vitamin D deficiency (Table 2).

Dihydrotachysterol. Crystalline dihydrotachysterol (DHT) is a chemical reduction product of tachysterol, which undergoes hepatic 25-hydroxylation to 25-hydroxy DHT, an analogue of $1,25(OH)_2D$. It is generally available in tablet form in strengths of 0.125, 0.2, and 0.4 mg. DHT is about three times as potent as D_2 in raising plasma calcium levels, but only one-tenth as potent in healing rickets and osteomalacia. It is conceivable that this difference may reflect the ability of naturally occurring vitamin D metabolites to affect mineralizing cells directly in addition to their effects in elevating plasma calcium and phosphorus levels, a function not shared by DHT.

Since DHT does not require a 1-hydroxylation step in the kidney for biologic activity, it is of particular use in renal osteodystrophy and hypoparathyroidism (in which renal 1-hydroxylation is suppressed). Its rapidity of onset and cessation is exceeded only by that of calcitriol (Table 1).

Calcifediol. Calcifediol is the generic or approved name for synthetic 25-hydroxyvitamin D (25 OHD), marketed as Calderol by Upjohn Laboratories. It is available in capsules of 20 mcg and 50 mcg. Experience with this agent is not extensive. It may be of particular use in vitamin D deficiency associated with intestinal malabsorption, hepatobiliary disorders (in which 25 OH D deficiency may result from reduced synthesis, biliary secretion, or enterohepatic circulation of this metabolite), and anticonvulsant therapy (in which accerated hepatic catabolism of vitamin D and 25 OH D occurs).

Its onset of action is more rapid than that of ergocalciferol; therapeutic levels can be directly monitored if necessary via reliable assay methods. It has a relatively long plasma half-life (12 days), and resolution of hypercalcemia may require up to 30 days. In doses of 100–500 mcg/ per day it is, somewhat surprisingly, effective in anephric and uremic subjects, for whom it appears to be a reasonable alternative to 1-hydroxylated forms of vitamin D. It is approved by the United States Food and Drug Administration for prophylaxis and treatment of renal osteodystrophy.

Alfacalcidol. Alfacalcidol is 1-alpha-hydroxy vitamin D (1α OH D), a synthetic analogue that is hydroxylated in the liver to $1,25(OH)_2D$. The obligatory 25-hydroxylation step probably accounts in large part for its slightly slower onset of action than that of calcitriol itself.

It is similar to calcitriol in clinical efficacy, appearing useful in hypoparathyroidism, hypophosphatemic rickets and osteomalacia, vitamin D dependency, and renal osteodystrophy. Hepatic conversion of alfacalcidol may be incomplete, and some degree of tissue storage is likely. The resulting higher dosage requirements than those for calcitriol (1–3 mcg/per day), and its general unavailability (it is unavailable in the United States and Australia but available in Japan, Europe, Canada, and the United Kingdom) have resulted in comparatively less clinical experience with this agent compared with other 1-hydroxylated vitamin D metabolities. It appears to offer no particular advantage over calcitriol.

On a theoretic basis, the replacement of a deficient natural metabolite appears the most logical approach to any individual case of osteomalacia. However, long-term experience with these newer agents in various forms of the disease and firm guidelines as to optimal dosage and duration to therapy are lacking. Moreover, considerations of relative metabolite potencies, bioavailability, rapidity of onset and cessation of action, and cost may well be more important determinants in the choice of therapeutic agents in individual cases (Table 1). These incompletely resolved questions of long-term efficacy and safety, especially with regard to renal function, dictate that use of these agents be confined to those situations in which a clear superiority has been demonstrated over the more familiar forms of vitamin D and in which adequate supervision and laboratory monitoring are available. Table 2 outlines appropriate forms and maintenance dosage levels of therapeutic agents in several of the more common forms of osteomalacia. Further points are discussed below.

NUTRITIONAL OSTEOMALACIA

This diagnosis is not uncommon within certain groups in our society, such as the impoverished, the elderly, and food faddists. A combined chronic deficiency of dietary intake (less than 70 IU vitamin D per day), together with inadequate cutaneous solar exposure, is almost invariably present. Prophylactic dietary vitamin D requirements are about 400 IU, or 10 mcg, daily for infants, children, and pregnant or lactating women, and 100 IU, or 2.5 mcg, daily for adults. Vitamin D requirements may be greater in those over age 60. Several factors contribute to this, including age-related malabsorption of calcium (and possibly vitamin D also), diminished sunlight exposure, age-related skin changes that may affect the efficiency with which vitamin D is synthesized from 7-dehydrocholesterol, and inadequate dietary vitamin D.

Nutritional vitamin D deficiency characteristically responds to vitamin D in doses of 500–1000 IU (12.5–25 mcg) daily, but doses on the order of 2000–5000 IU (50 mcg–125 mcg) are generally used in adults, for the reasons previously discussed.

FAT MALABSORPTION SYNDROMES

Intestinal, hepatobiliary, and chronic pancreatic diseases result in malabsorption of calcium and vitamin D and often in the loss of the 20 to 30 percent of circulating 25 OH D_3 which undergoes enterohepatic circulation. In biliary and pancreatic disease, losses correlate relatively closely with the degree of steatorrhea. This is not necessarily the case in intestinal mucosal disease and bypass or short-loop syndromes, since the mere reduction in the small intestinal luminal surface available for absorption may be sufficient to result in malabsorption. Similarly, a strict gluten-free diet leading to reversal of intestinal mucosal disease may completely cure even severe associated osteomalacia.

Chronic hepatocellular disease may further contribute to hepatobiliary malabsorption by leading to impaired 25 OH D_3 and vitamin D binding protein production. Patients should be treated with calcium supplements (calcium carbonate, 1 gm per day), and vitamin D (Table 2). We use calcifediol in cases requiring, or likely to require, large doses of vitamin D over a relatively short period (for example, those with severe gluten enteropathy or advanced biliary cirrhosis), in whom plasma 25 OH D_3 levels are 7 ng/ml or less. Before starting therapy in those with intestinal disease, we establish the adequacy of calcifediol absorption after a single oral dose, using a protocol of 10 mcg/kg body weight and monitoring plasma 25 OH D_3 levels every 8 hours for 24 hours. We favor the use of oral preparations whenever possible, assuming that, with adequate dosage, a proportion will be absorbed. Absorption of parenteral (intramuscular) preparations of vitamin D varies from patient to patient. Moreover, there are no parenteral preparations containing less than large pharmaco-

logic doses. If oral administration is impossible, even with the addition of medium chain triglyceride oil, or if compliance with oral medication is dubious, 250–1000 mcg (10,000–40,000 IU) vitamin D_2 may be administered intramuscularly every week to patients with intestinal malabsorption, and 2.5 mg (100,000 IU) vitamin D_2 intramuscularly once a month to those with hepatobiliary or pancreatic insufficiency. Doses or oral preparations are given in Table 2.

If underlying absorptive defects cannot be corrected, lifelong therapy with calcium supplements (1 gm elemental calcium daily) and vitamin D, in maintenance dosage, may be required.

ANTICONVULSANT-ASSOCIATED OSTEOMALACIA

In some series, osteomalacia has been described in up to 60 percent of subjects receiving long-term therapy with phenytoin, phenobarbital, primidone, and pheneturide. Accelerated hepatic microsomal degradation and biliary excretion of vitamin D and 25 OH D, probably in addition to direct intestinal and skeletal effects (in the case of phenytoin), underlie this association. Deficient vitamin D intake and sunlight exposure, as well as reduced physical activity, frequently in an institutional environment, also contributes in most cases. Treatment is with 0.1–1 mg (4000–40,000 IU) of vitamin D daily, generally for 6 months or more. Following adequate healing, long-term prophylaxis with 50–200 mcg (2000–8000 IU) daily should be given.

VITAMIN D DEPENDENCY OSTEOMALACIA

Vitamin D dependency (VDD), or pseudovitamin D deficiency, is an autosomal recessive condition that usually appears in infancy or early childhood with hypocalcemia, but rarely may be diagnosed in adolescence or early adulthood. Defective renal 1-hydroxylation of vitamin D underlies the disease in the overwhelming majority of cases (VDD type I), and slightly supraphysiologic dosages of calcitriol (1–2 mcg in divided doses daily) are curative. Calcium supplementation (1–2 gm calcium carbonate per day) is usually required during the early months of calcitriol therapy, if plasma calcium levels remain low and urinary calcium excretion falls. Lifelong calcitriol therapy in the same or slightly lower dosage is necessary to prevent recurrence. Plasma and urinary calcium and creatinine level monitoring at three- to six-month intervals should be continued indefinitely.

PRIMARY X-LINKED HYPOPHOSPHATEMIC OSTEOMALACIA

Primary hypophosphatemia, X-linked hypophosphatemia (XLH), and familial vitamin D resistant rickets (FVDRR) are synonyms for a hereditary disorder involving (1) a selective phosphate transport defect in the terminal brush border membrane of the renal tubular epithelium, and probably (2) a disproportionately low rate of renal 1-hydroxylation of vitamin D. In adults, XLH is present both in patients who have been diagnosed and treated since childhood, and in those who first developed symptomatic osteomalacia between ages 20 and 60. The objectives of therapy in this group differ from those in pediatric patients since symptomatic relief and skeletal healing take precedence over consideration of linear bone growth and prevention and management of growth-related skeletal deformities. If patients have received vitamin D supplementation since childhood, we advocate this be continued in a small dosage to prevent recurrence, for example, 250–500 mcg daily (10,000–20,000 IU). If the plasma phosphorus level is persistently less than 3.0 mg/dl or if the mean 24-hour urinary calcium excretion exceeds 200 mgm on a normal calcium diet, we prescribe dietary phosphorus supplementation. This should be the maximum dose tolerated by the patient, at least 1–2 gm per day of elemental phosphorus as phosphate salts, given in 6 to 8 divided doses. Gastrointestinal side effects, especially diarrhea, or else an appropriate improvement in plasma phosphorus levels should be used as end points in determining dosage. Side effects can be minimized by using powdered phosphate preparations in drinks or in cooking.

Adequate phosphorus therapy should result in a rise in plasma phosphorus levels of at least 0.5 mg/dl, an increase in 24-hour urinary phosphorus levels of 60 to 80 percent of the administered daily dose, and a substantial fall in urinary calcium excretion. In XLH, phosphorus repletion alone does not heal the skeletal lesions. Thus if osteomalacia is present on bone biopsy, vitamin D or calcitriol should be administered in addition. We believe calcitriol is preferable. Phosphate-induced hypocalcemia and hyperparathyroidism are suppressed by 1–2 mcg of calcitriol per day, which can be titrated once phosphorus requirements are stabilized over a matter of weeks. When used in a slightly higher dosage (3–4 mcg per day in divided doses) so as to achieve supraphysiologic plasma levels of $1,25(OH)_2D_3$ calcitriol in conjunction with oral phosphate supplements continued over several months appears to lead to complete cure of the osteomalacia. This is the only therapeutic approach to date which has been shown to be so effective. Frequent monitoring (once a week initially) to avoid hypercalcemia and renal dysfunction, as outlined earlier, is mandatory with such a protocol.

ADULT SPORADIC HYPOPHOSPHATEMIC OSTEOMALACIA

This generally severely disabling form of osteomalacia occurs in the absence of a childhood or family history and is often characterized by severe symptoms of bone pain and muscle weakness. In some cases the identification and removal of a benign or malignant mesenchymal tumor can result in cure or significant improvement. Severity of symptoms and disability usually justify an initial high-dose regimen of 5 mg (200,000 IU) vitamin D_2 daily, together with 1–3 gm elemental phosphorus as phosphate salts. Maintenance pharmacologic dosage is usually 1.25–2.5 mg (50,000–100,000 IU) vitamin D_2 with somewhat less phosphate than initially. Alternatively, calcitriol may be used as the agent of first choice in doses of between 1 and 3 mcg daily together with phosphate salts. Its rapidity of action probably makes calcitriol preferable in severely symptomatic cases.

Phosphate salts are more uniformly successful in this group than in XLH, and in a few cases may be effective treatment alone. However, slowness of onset, uncertainty of success, and patchiness and irregularity of skeletal mineralization in the absence of vitamin D or $1,25 (OH)_2D$ in addition, preclude the routine use of phosphate therapy alone in all but mild asymptomatic cases.

METABOLIC ACIDOSIS

Appropriate alkali therapy will, in time, heal the osteomalacia associated with most cases of renal tubular acidosis (most commonly, distal type). However, the need for prompt healing and the presence of distressing symptoms dictate the use of vitamin D together with alkali. We find 250–1000 mcg (10,000–40,000 IU) vitamin D_2, together with approximately 10–15 gm sodium bicarbonate per day, to be satisfactory in initiating healing. This regimen is generally necessary for six to eight months, together with administration of phosphate salts if phosphorus depletion is present. Correction of metabolic acidosis is monitored by serial measurement of plasma chloride and bicarbonate. Care must be taken with such high sodium loads in those with cardiac and hypertensive disease. Once osteomalacia has healed, and acidosis is corrected, alkali therapy alone should prevent recurrence of the skeletal disease. If acidosis cannot be adequately corrected, or if alkali therapy is poorly tolerated, slightly supraphysiologic dosages of vitamin D_2 may be continued.

FANCONI SYNDROME—MULTIPLE ABNORMALITIES OF TUBULAR REABSORPTION

Identification and correction of underlying primary causes should be attempted: galactose restriction in galactosemia, penicillamine administration in Wilson's disease, or chelating agents in heavy metal toxicity.

Compensatory replacement of solutes, electrolytes, and phosphate, together with correction of acidosis and modest doses of vitamin D (often around 125 mcg or 5000 IU daily) are usually required, in various combinations, according to the severity and nature of the particular syndrome phenotype.

OSTEOPOROSIS

B. LAWRENCE RIGGS, M.D.

Osteoporosis is defined as an absolute decrease in the amount of bone; the remaining bone is morphologically normal when analyzed by routine histologic techniques. The reduced bone mass leads to an increased risk of fracture, especially at sites in the axial skeleton. Back pain from vertebral fracture is usually the symptom that prompts the patient with osteoporosis to seek medical help. The goals of treatment are to relieve pain and to maintain or increase bone mass, thereby reducing the incidence of new fractures.

GENERAL MEASURES

Relief of Pain

Treatment of acute pain caused by a new vertebral fracture depends on its severity. Mild pain often responds to simple analgesics, and more severe pain may necessitate the use of codeine sulfate, often in combination with aspirin. Parenterally administered opiates rarely are needed. Severe pain may mandate bed rest for a one- to three-week period. A hard mattress or insertion of a bed board between the mattress and springs is recommended. Local administration of heat (electric pad or infrared heating lamp) and massage to diminish paraspinal spasms often is helpful. If pain persists after a reasonable period of bed rest, ambulation with a back support (usually a semirigid dorsolumbar support with shoulder straps) is prescribed. Treatment of chronic mechanical back pain due to vertebral deformity differs. The patient is instructed in posture and gait training and in regular back-extension exercises (to strengthen flabby paraspinal muscles). In selected patients a back support is prescribed. Because the pain is chronic, the use of codeine and other opiates should be avoided. Buffered aspirin may be prescribed in dosages of 0.6 to 0.9 gm 4 times daily to maintain the blood salicylate level within the analgesic range. Selected patients benefit from local injection of a glucocorticoid preparation into interspinal ligaments. Those most likely to respond are identified by point tenderness in a localized area of chronic pain.

Protection of Spine

Patients should avoid heavy lifting and, for picking up objects, bending at the knees is preferred to bending of the spine. Sports activities that involve twisting of the spine are interdicted, and precautions should be taken to avoid falls.

Other General Measures

The patient's diet should contain at least 1 gm of elemental calcium (3 glasses of milk daily or an equivalent exchange in terms of cheese or other dairy products) and be adequate in protein and calories. All patients should daily receive a multiple vitamin preparation that contains 1000 units of vitamin D. Nontraumatic exercise, such as long walks and swimming, is encouraged.

DRUG THERAPY

Calcium

The rationale underlying calcium supplementation in the treatment of osteoporosis is twofold. First, intestinal calcium absorption decreases with aging and is lower in patients with osteoporosis than in age-matched control subjects. Heaney and colleagues have shown that the daily dietary calcium requirement needed to prevent negative calcium balance is about 1.0 gm in premenopausal women and 1.5 gm in postmenopausal women. In contrast, several dietary surveys have shown that the average calcium intake of adult women in the United States is only about 0.5 mg per day. Second, administration of calcium supplements has been shown to decrease parathyroid hormone secretion and thus to reduce the level of bone resorption.

Calcium supplementation should be prescribed at a dosage of 1.0–1.5 gm of elemental calcium daily. Calcium carbonate, which is 40 percent elemental calcium, is preferred over other calcium salts, which are only 10 to 15 percent elemental calcium. Each 650-mg tablet of calcium carbonate, therefore, contains about 250 mg of elemental calcium. Calcium carbonate is generally well tolerated. Although an occasional patient will complain of gas and constipation, these symptoms usually disappear when another preparation, such as calcium phosphate or calcium gluconate, is substituted. The urinary calcium concentration may increase slightly, but unless a vitamin D preparation is administered concomitantly, hypercalcemia does not occur.

Estrogen

Research during the last 40 years has documented a central role for estrogen deficiency in the pathogenesis of postmenopausal osteoporosis and has affirmed the value of estrogen replacement therapy.

Estrogen replacement retards the rate of bone loss from the appendicular skeleton and probably has a similar effect on the axial skeleton. The mechanism of estrogen action is to decrease bone turnover; bone resorption decreases more than bone formation, and these factors lead to improved calcium balance. This effect may be mediated by decreased responsiveness of bone-resorbing cells to circulating parathyroid hormone. Estrogen may act on bone indirectly since estrogen receptors have not been demonstrated in bone cells.

The effect of estrogen—and, indeed, the effect of any active agent for osteoporosis that reduces bone resorption—has two phases. Initially, a positive calcium balance is induced by a positive uncoupling of the components involved in bone turnover (bone resorption is decreased but bone formation is unchanged). After several months of continued therapy, however, formation is gradually decreased until a new steady state is reached. Thereafter, the net therapeutic effect is to maintain existing bone mass or to slow the rate of loss.

The therapeutic dosage of estrogen in the treatment of osteoporosis is 0.625–1.25 mg daily of conjugated estrogen (Premarin, Ayerst) or its equivalent in another estrogen preparation.* Dosages of less than 0.625 mg daily are not consistently effective, and dosages of more than 1.25 mg per day are often poorly tolerated. Estrogen should be given cyclically to mimic the normal menstrual cycle. It is convenient to tell the patient to omit the dosage for the first seven calendar days of each month.

Estrogen preparations, although quite effective in the treatment of osteoporosis, have potentially severe side effects. Estrogen stimulates the breast and may lead to mastodynia. At the lower therapeutic dosage (0.625 mg per day of conjugated estrogen), only about half the women who have been postmenopausal sufficiently long (5 to 10 years) to produce endometrial atrophy will have estrogen withdrawal bleeding. Most patients who receive concurrent progestins with this dosage and those who receive the larger dosage (1.25 mg per day) will have regular menses.

Estrogen increases sodium retention and thus aggravates edema formation in susceptible patients. Moreover, because orally administered estrogen is absorbed via the portal vein, the dosage to the liver is disproportionately greater than that to other tissues. This increases hepatic synthesis of many plasma proteins, including renin substrate (which increases the risk for hypertension) and coagulation factors (which increase the risk for thrombosis).

---

*An estimate of equivalent dosages with respect to effects on bone is 0.625 mg of conjugated estrogen, 0.025 mg of ethinyl estradiol, or 1 mg of estrone sulfate.

Many case-control studies have shown that estrogen replacement therapy in postmenopausal women increases the relative risk of endometrial carcinoma eightfold; there also is some evidence of an increased risk of breast carcinoma. Recent studies, however, suggest that induction of carcinoma in estrogen-responsive tissues may result from an unopposed action of estrogen and can be offset by administering a progestational agent concomitantly. This can be accomplished by giving medroxyprogesterone acetate (Provera, Upjohn), 2.5–5 mg daily, or an equivalent dose of another progestin during the last 12 days of the cycle. Alternatively, an anticontraceptive tablet combining a progestin and a reduced amount of the estrogen component, such as Loestrin (Parke-Davis), could be prescribed. It must be recalled, however, that addition of the progestin may exacerbate sodium retaining effects of estrogen. Regardless of whether a progestin is given, all patients receiving estrogen therapy should have annual breast and pelvic examinations, and abnormal bleeding (except for that occurring with estrogen withdrawal) should be promptly investigated.

Androgens and Synthetic Anabolic Agents

Although androgens should not be used for treatment of osteoporosis in women because of their virilizing effect, synthetic analogues with equivalent anabolic activity but reduced virilizing potency provide an alternative to estrogen therapy. Although use of these agents avoids the problem of estrogenic stimulation, they also have major side effects. These agents increase the plasma cholesterol and low-density lipoprotein concentrations and, in some patients, induce liver dysfunction. Moreover, in about one-quarter of patients treated with therapeutic dosages, severe androgenicity develops. The recommended dosage is 4–6 mg daily of stanozolol (Winstrol, Winthrop) or a comparable dosage of another anabolic agent.

Vitamin D and Vitamin D Metabolites

Although vitamin D in dosages of 50,000 units once to twice weekly is commonly prescribed, my experience has been that it may induce hypercalciuria and hypercalcemia in about one-quarter of the patients on long-term treatment. Therefore, pharmacologic doses of vitamin D should mainly be used for those patients with a demonstrable impairment in intestinal calcium absorption. Although documentation of this disorder necessitates a test of radiocalcium absorption, a decrease in calcium absorption can be inferred clinically for those patients with osteoporosis who have an average amount of calcium in their diet but a urinary calcium excretion of less than 50 mg daily.

Reports that serum 1,25-dihydroxyvitamin D is decreased in some patients with osteoporosis provide the rationale for administration of this active metabolite. If this agent is to be used, the dosage should be only 0.25 µg twice daily, because higher dosages are associated with a substantial incidence of hypercalcemia or hypercalciuria, either of which may occur unpredictably. Because of the short half-life of 1,25-dihydroxyvitamin D in the circulation, however, the hypercalcemia remits promptly when use of the drug is discontinued. If either vitamin D or its metabolites is to be employed, it is mandatory to monitor levels of serum calcium, creatinine, and phosphorus and urinary calcium periodically.

Calcitonin

This antiresorptive agent recently has been approved for use in patients with osteoporosis by the United States Food and Drug Administration. A recent study showed that administration of salmon calcitonin (Calcimar, Armour), 100 MRC units daily, and calcium carbonate, 1.2 gm daily, resulted in an increase in total body calcium levels during the first 24 months but not thereafter. The expense, the need for parenteral administration, and the development of neutralizing antibodies in some patients limit the usefulness of this regimen.

Fluoride

Sodium fluoride, a potent stimulator of bone formation, increases bone mass of the axial skeleton substantially in most patients with osteoporosis. Although fluoridic bone may be structurally less sound than normal bone, a recent study at the Mayo Clinic demonstrated that responding patients had a reduced number of new fractures.

In at least one-third of patients treated with fluoride, gastric or rheumatic side effects develop. The former are due to irritation of the gastric mucosa. The rheumatic symptoms of painful joints or feet are due to a chemical synovitis or fasciitis. Both types of symptoms disappear on discontinuing treatment and usually do not recur after reinstitution at a lower dosage.

Sodium fluoride is given in divided doses of 50–75 mg daily. Elemental calcium (1.0–1.5 gm daily) is administered concomitantly to facilitate bone mineralization. Gastric side effects are minimized by administering sodium fluoride and calcium carbonate together during meals, although this may decrease fluoride absorption by 15 to 25 percent.

Unfortunately, a subset of patients with osteoporosis (25 to 40 percent) fail to respond to sodium fluoride therapy, possibly because of an intrinsic abnormality in osteoblast function. These patients do not have an increase in bone mass after long-term therapy and continue to have vertebral fractures.

Sodium fluoride has not been approved for the treatment of osteoporosis by the United States Food and Drug Administration and thus is not generally available in a high-dose form. Formal prospective trials evaluating the efficacy of sodium fluoride in reducing fractures, however, are underway. If these studies confirm published reports of antifracture efficacy, medical practitioners may be able to prescribe sodium fluoride in the near future.

ASSESSMENT OF THERAPEUTIC EFFECT

All available regimens for the treatment of osteoporosis are only partly successful and are ineffective in some patients. A simple and reliable way to assess therapeutic effect is to measure the patient's standing height serially. Untreated patients and therapeutic nonresponders commonly lose 12.7 cm (5 inches) of height or more within a 5-year interval during the early phase of their disease. Another practical method is to obtain annual roentgenograms of the lumbar and thoracic spinal column. A decrease of more than 15 percent in the height of a vertebral body from that on the roentgenogram from the preceding year indicates the presence of a new vertebral fracture. Fracture rates for various therapeutic groups obtained by using this criterion are given in Table 1. Assessment of bone mass in the appendicular skeleton by single photon absorptiometry or radiogrammetry is useful for group studies but is of little help in assessing the response of individual patients. Changes of bone mass in the axial skeleton are larger and correlate more closely with fracture risk than do those of the appendicular skeleton; these can now be assessed by dual photon absorptiometry or by quantitative computed tomography. Although currently confined to only a few research centers, these procedures should soon be widely available.

TABLE 1 Comparison of Incidence of Vertebral Fractures in Various Therapeutic Groups of Patients With Postmenopausal Osteoporosis

Treatment	Person-Years of Observation	Fracture Rate/1000 Person-Years
Placebo or none	91	834
Calcium*	74	419
Calcium and fluoride*	138	205†
Calcium and estrogen*	144	181
Calcium, fluoride, and estrogen*	113	53

*Approximately half the patients received vitamin D, 50,000 units once or twice weekly. Dosages of other components of therapy are as suggested in text.

†For data after first year of treatment

Note: All treatment groups had lower fracture rates (p < 0.001) than the untreated patients. The addition of fluoride or estrogen to the calcium regimen further decreased the fracture rate (p < 0.001). The combined use of calcium, fluoride, and estrogen was more effective (p < 0.001) than any other combination.

AN APPROACH TO TREATMENT OF THE INDIVIDUAL PATIENT

Postmenopausal Osteoporosis

Therapy should be individualized, depending on the severity of the disease (Table 2). For patients with mild disease, particularly for those older than 75 years, I prescribe only calcium supplementation. I add low-dose estrogen therapy (the equivalent of 0.625 mg daily cyclically of conjugated estrogen) for women with more extensive disease, especially when they are less than 15 years postmenopausal. The incidence of side effects (including induction of endometrial carcinoma) associated with this estrogen dosage is low, and when it is combined with calcium supplementation, it is probably as effective as high-dose therapy. If the disease progresses when this regimen is used, I increase the dosage to 1.25 mg daily cyclically of conjugated estrogen or its equivalent. Because the risk of endometrial carcinoma is substantially greater with use of this higher dosage, I concurrently administer a progestin. Women older than 75 years generally tolerate synthetic anabolic steroids better than estrogens. Patients with a past history of gastrointestinal surgery, hepatic disease, or small bowel disease should receive pharmacologic dosages of vitamin D, particularly if a low serum 25-hydroxyvitamin D level has been recorded.

TABLE 2 Recommended Treatment Regimen for Patients With Postmenopausal Osteoporosis

Use general measures for all patients
For mild disease, give 1.0–1.5 gm per day of supplementary calcium (for example, $CaCO_3$, 6 tablets daily in divided doses)
For moderate or severe disease, add *cyclic* low-dose estrogen (for example, conjugated estrogens, 0.625 mg per day, or add progestin (for example, medroxyprogesterone acetate, 2.5 mg per day) for the last 12 days of the cycle
For disease that progresses during therapy: Double the dose of estrogen and progestin. Reconsider diagnosis
Elderly women may prefer anabolic steroids to estrogen

Osteoporosis in the Young Female

This uncommon disease probably is etiologically heterogeneous. It is relatively refractory to therapy. Becauuse the women are premenopausal, there is no reason to prescribe sex steroids. Some patients with the disorder seem to have impaired calcium absorption, which can be corrected by administration of vitamin D. The mainstay of treatment, therefore, is calcium supplementation with or without pharmacologic doses of vitamin D. Calcitonin can be added in an attempt to reduce any component of increased bone resorption that may be present.

Osteoporosis in the Male

As with osteoporosis in young women, this condition in male patients usually is not associated with a deficiency of sex steroids; hence, no rationale for hormonal treatment exists. Approximately 10 to 20 percent of males with osteoporosis, however, have partial or complete hypogonadism of varying cause. Thus patients with documented low plasma testosterone levels should receive replacement therapy, such as testosterone enanthate (Delatestryl, Squibb), 200–400 mg i.m. every 4 weeks. I also prescribe calcium supplementation with or without pharmacologic doses of vitamin D.

Osteoporosis Associated with Glucocorticoid Excess

The most common cause of secondary osteoporosis is chronic use of pharmacologic dosages of glucocorticoids. The most important single treatment is to reduce the dosage or, if possible, to discontinue glucocorticoid therapy. Administering the glucocorticoids once daily or on alternate days may maintain a more favorable balance between anti-inflammatory or immunosuppressive effect and the osteopenic effect in some patients. All patients should be given calcium supplements, and postmenopausal women should be given estrogens. Although glucocorticoids inhibit calcium absorption, the use of pharmacologic dosages of vitamin D or its metabolites in this circumstance is controversial. There is increasing evidence that glucocorticoids do not induce major alterations in vitamin D metabolism.

HYPOCALCEMIA

LOUIS V. AVIOLI, M.D.

Hypocalcemia, which presents either as a serendipitous finding in routine blood screening tests or as a medical emergency, results from a variety of seemingly unrelated disorders (Table 1). Therapy is often mandatory in severe hypocalcemic states in order to prevent acute muscle spasm seizures, increased intracranial pressure, cardiac arrythmias, and in children, inspiratory stridor due to spasm of the muscles of the glottis. More chronic and less severe forms of hypocalcemia, which often result in cataract formation, intermittent paresthesias of the extremities, and intermittent losses of cognitive function, should also be treated.

HYPOPARATHYROIDISM AND CHRONIC RENAL FAILURE

The most important causes of hypocalcemia are those attending disorders of parathyroid function. Acute symptomatic hypocalcemia, which characteristically follows thyroid or parathyroid surgery, should be treated with intravenous calcium. One usually administers calcium gluconate, 15–20 mg of calcium per kg of body weight over 4 to 6 hours. It should be recognized that a 10 percent calcium gluconate solution contains 9 mg/ml of elemental calcium. In severe hypocalcemia with spasm, tetany, and stridor, 20–30 ml of a 10

TABLE 1 Pathogenesis of Hypocalcemia

Hypoparathyroidism
  Post-thyroidectomy
  Postparathyroidectomy
  Idiopathic
  Pseudohypoparathyroidism
Hypomagnesemia
Chronic renal failure
Malabsorption syndromes
Acute pancreatitis
Osteoblastic metastasis
Chemotherapy of acute leukemia
Chronic anticonvulsant therapy
Phosphate enemas or infusions
Neonatal hypocalcemia
Osteomalacia or rickets due to:
  Vitamin D deficient states
  Poor sunlight exposure
  Inadequate vitamin D intakes
Transfusion of citrated blood
Tumors producing vitamin D "antagonists"*

*Specifically tumors that produce substance(s) that interfere with the biologic activation of vitamin D

percent gluconate solution can be administered intravenously over 10 to 15 minutes. If additional intravenous therapy is required to maintain the serum calcium in the range of 8.5–10.0 mg/dl after the initial 4- to 6-hour period, continued infusion of the calcium gluconate solution in a dose of 15–20 mg of calcium per kg of body weight should be continued, with heart rate and blood pressure monitoring at frequent intervals.

Although the addition of vitamin D (or its biologically active metabolites) may ultimately prove essential to maintain a normal serum calcium level in patients with low circulating parathyroid hormone levels, this type of therapy should be reserved for those patients who do not respond to treatment with oral calcium preparations. In this regard it should be acknowledged that the function of the parathyroid glands may be deranged for seven to ten days following surgical procedures (either thyroidectomy or subtotal parathyroidectomy), and that intermittent intravenous and supplemental oral calcium therapy may be essential during this period.

In prescribing oral calcium supplements, which usually range from 1.5–2.5 gm of elemental calcium per day, the physician must also recognize that various forms of calcium differ in the content of elemental calcium. Tablets of calcium gluconate (9 percent calcium), calcium carbonate (40 percent calcium), and calcium lactate (13 percent calcium) are all appropriate as supplemental agents. Calcium chloride should not be prescribed, because

it often causes gastrointestinal irritation. When oral calcium supplementation fails to reverse the hypocalcemia, treatment with pharmacologic quantities of either vitamin D or one of its biologically active metabolites is essential.

Patients with hypoparathyroid disease or chronic renal failure usually require 50,000–100,000 IU of vitamin D per day supplemented with 1.0–2.0 gm of elemental calcium. Even with this regimen vitamin D intoxication with hypercalcemia may occur. The hypercalcemia that results from the vitamin D overdosage is treated by discontinuing the vitamin, vigorous hydration with normal saline, and glucocorticoid therapy (30–40 mg prednisone per day for 6 to 10 days). The physician should also recognize that vitamin D therapy in the pharmacologic doses required to reverse the hypocalcemia always results in hypercalciuria. In fact, during the early stages of therapy in hypocalcemic hypoparathyroid patients, hypercalciuria precedes the reversal of the hypocalcemia. Consequently, appropriate management of the hypocalcemic patient on vitamin D therapy demands occasional monitoring of 24-hour urinary calcium levels to prevent the subtle changes in renal function which result from nephrocalcinosis in an asymptomatic patient with chronic and progressive hypercalciuria. It should also be stressed that the onset of action of the administered vitamin D may be prolonged owing to a lag period essential for the hepatic and renal bioactivation of the vitamin to its active hydroxylated metabolites, and to the large storage depots that gradually release the vitamin D. For this reason, the vitamin D dosage should not be increased for at least three to four weeks if the patient is still relatively hypocalcemic following the initiation of vitamin D therapy. Dihydrotachysterol (Hytakerol) acts more rapidly than vitamin D and can also be administered to hypoparathyroid patients in dosages of 0.5–1.25 mg per day.

Two active vitamin D metabolites have recently become commercially available for the treatment of hypocalcemic disorders (Table 2). Both 25-hydroxycholecalciferol (Calderol) and 1.25-dihydroxycholecalciferol (Rocaltrol) have proven their effectiveness in reversing the hypocalcemia of hypoparathyroidism, rickets, and chronic renal insufficiency.

The onset of action of both these agents is faster than that of vitamin D, and, as noted in Table 2, the time for reversal of the toxic effects is decreased. Moreover, because blood assays for blood vitamin D metabolites are routinely available commercially, therapeutic levels are easily

TABLE 2 Vitamin D and Structurally Related Compounds used for the Therapy of Hypocalcemia

Abbreviation	Commercial Name	Effective Daily Dose	Time for Reversal of Toxic Effects (Days)
Vitamin D$_3$	Calciferol	1–10 mg	17–60
Dihydrotachysterol	Hytakerol	0.1–1 mg	3–14
25(OH)$_2$D$_3$	Calderol	0.05–0.5 mg	7–30
1,25(OH)$_2$D$_3$	Rocaltrol	0.5–1 μg	2–10

monitored. Maximal response to these agents can only be assured with concomitant oral calcium therapy in a range of 1.0–2.0 gm of elemental calcium per day.

GASTROINTESTINAL DISEASE

Chronic alcoholism and intestinal malabsorption syndromes often lead to both hypomagnesemia and hypocalcemia. In these patients the clinical symptoms are comparable to those cited above for hypocalcemia. Not infrequently, the hypocalcemia is not corrected until magnesium therapy is instituted. The hypomagnesemia can be rapidly corrected with intramuscular MgSO$_4$ in a dosage of 8–16 mEq thrice daily for 3 days; a more gradual reversal of the hypomagnesemia occurs with oral MgO capsules in a dosage of 35 mEq (10 gr) once or twice daily. Once the hypomagnesemia is reversed, the serum calcium usually returns to the normal (or low normal) range. Oral calcium therapy in dosages of 1.5–2.0 gm of elemental calcium per day is usually sufficient to maintain a normal serum calcium level. One should also recognize that some patients with chronic hepatic disease present with hypoalbuminemia and low serum calcium levels. In these particular instances the hypocalcemia need not be corrected, since it represents a decrease in the protein-bound calcium moiety and not the functional ionized or ultrafilterable calcium fractions.

RICKETS AND OSTEOMALACIA

The hypocalcemia seen in patients with either rickets or osteomalacia due to dietary deficiencies or inadequate sunlight exposure is readily reversed with vitamin D and supplemental calcium. In childhood rickets, 1000–5000 units of vitamin D and at least 0.8–1.0 gm of elemental calcium per day are usually adequate to control the hypocalcemia and the underlying bone lesions. In adult forms of simple vitamin D-deficiency osteomalacia and hypocalcemia, vitamin D, 50,000 units per day for 1 to 2 months, followed by a normal diet (400–800 units vitamin D and 1 gm calcium per day) is adequate. In each case, vitamin D and calcium therapy should be instituted to treat the hypocalcemia *and the underlying bone disease.* The osteomalacia and mild hypocalcemia in patients with increased hepatic vitamin D catabolism due to anticonvulsant drug regimens should be treated with vitamin D, 50,000 units per day, with calcium supplements of 1.0–1.5 gm per day for a 3- to 6-month interval until serum calcium and circulating 25-hydroxycholecalciferol levels are normal. At that juncture, prophylactic therapy with 800–2000 units of vitamin D and 1.0–1.5 gm of calcium per day should be instituted for the duration of the anticonvulsant therapeutic interval. Hypocalcemia that results from fat malabsorption syndrome should be approached by combining the treatment of the underlying disorder (that is, gluten-free diets, pancreatic extracts, and so on) with calcium supplementation (1.5–2.5 gm per day) and vitamin D (50,000 units 3 to 7 times weekly). In this instance careful monitoring of serum and urinary calcium levels is mandatory, since the patient may become hypercalcemic while responding to therapy of the primary disease process.

TRANSFUSION HYPOCALCEMIA

Finally, consideration should be given to the hypocalcemia that may occur during massive transfusion with citrated blood. Since citrate is metabolized by the liver via the Krebs cycle, patients with liver disease have an increased susceptibility to hypocalcemia when subjected to massive transfusion with citrated blood. Although specific guidelines for calcium replacement in transfused patients have not been established, 0.6 mg of CaCl$_2$ is usually added to each unit of citrated blood with heparin to prevent clotting. In patients without liver disease who require repeated transfusions, 10 ml of a 10 percent solution of calcium chloride should be given for every 2 units of citrated blood. Individuals with severe hepatic impairment and various blood magnesium and calcium levels should be monitored frequently and calcium infusions initiated as soon as hypocalcemia is evident.

HYPOPARATHYROIDISM

CHARLES F. SHARP, JR., M.D.
and FREDERICK R. SINGER, M.D.

Hypoparathyroidism is an endocrine problem characterized by hypocalcemia and hyperphosphatemia, and either transient or permanent impairment of secretion of parathyroid hormone. Its most common cause is previous thyroid or parathyroid surgery. Idiopathic hypoparathyroidism is far less common. Congenital aplasia, infiltrative disorders (cancer, hemochromatosis), and postradioiodine thyroid ablation are extremely rare causes. A reversible state of hypoparathyroidism is a major feature of moderate to severe magnesium deficiency and is a not uncommon problem in patients with alcoholism, intestinal malabsorption, and in patients unable to eat for prolonged periods after surgery. Transient hypoparathyroidism is also thought to occur in some patients with primary hyperparathyroidism after removal of a parathyroid adenoma. In hypoparathyroidism a variety of neuromuscular and neurologic syndromes may occur, most commonly paresthesias of the extremities, muscle cramps, and frank tetany. Urinary retention and laryngeal stridor, especially in children, are less common neuromuscular symptoms. Seizures and increased intracranial pressure with frank papilledema may occur, raising the question of intracranial pathology. Extrapyramidal signs, including Parkinsonism, chorea, and athetosis, may occur in conjunction with calcification of the basal ganglia. The electrocardiographic change in hypoparathyroidism is characteristic. Prolongation of the Q-T interval occurs, without S-T segment or QRS complex alteration. Longstanding hypocalcemia may be associated with integumentary changes, especially cutaneous *Monilia* infection, dry skin, alopecia, and ectopic ossification. Cataracts are another serious consequence of untreated hypoparathyroidism.

THERAPEUTIC ALTERNATIVES

The treatment of hypoparathyroidism primarily involves raising the serum calcium concentration into the physiologic range. This can be accomplished by administration of intravenous or oral calcium compounds (Table 1), by treating with vitamin D or a related agent (Table 2) in combination with adequate calcium intake (Table 3), or, in the case of magnesium deficiency, by administration of parenteral or oral magnesium salts.

PREFERRED APPROACH

The aims of the treatment of hypoparathyroidism are the rapid correction of symptoms arising from neuromuscular irritability, the prevention of hypocalcemic episodes, and the prevention of long-term complications of hypocalcemia. Avoiding hypercalcemia and/or hypercalciuria induced by the therapeutic regimen is also an important objective.

Pharmacologic amounts of calcium salts given intravenously provide the most rapid means of raising the extracellular calcium concentration.

TABLE 1 Oral Calcium Preparations

Salt	Trade Name(s)	Calcium Content Per Gram
Calcium carbonate	Titralac suspension, 1 gm/5 cc Tablets: 420 mg OS-CAL, 650 mg and 1.25 gm tablets Tums tablets, 500 mg	400 mg
Calcium glubionate	Neo-Calglucon syrup, 1.8 gm/5 cc	64 mg
Calcium gluconate	325 mg, 500 mg, 650 mg, and 1 gm tablets	90 mg
Calcium lactate	325 mg and 650 mg tablets	130 mg

TABLE 2 Vitamin D Preparations

	Trade Name	Dosage in Hypopara-thyroidism	Onset of Maximal Effect (Approx.)
Vitamin D$_2$	Drisdol Calciferol	50,000–200,000 IU/day	30 days
Dihydrotachy-sterol	Hytakerol	0.4–1.6 mg/dl	15 days
25(OH) vitamin D$_3$	Calderol	50 μg/day	15 days
1,25(OH)$_2$ vitamin D$_3$	Rocaltrol	0.25–2 μg/day	2–3 days

TABLE 3 Calcium-Rich Foods

Food	Amount	Elemental Calcium (mg)
Almonds (dried)	⅔ cup	254
Cheddar cheese	¾'' cube	109
Chocolate milkshake	8 oz	363
Collards (cooked)	½ cup	152
Cottage cheese (creamed)	1 tbsp	26
Ice cream (vanilla)	⅛ quart	104
Macaroni and cheese	1 cup	407
Milk (whole or skim)	8 oz	298
Sardines (canned)	8	354
Sour cream	1 oz	31
Spinach (cooked)	½ cup	93
Swiss cheese	1 oz	259
Tofu (soybean curd)	3 ½ oz	128
Yogurt	1 cup	282

Oral calcium in large doses (> 4 gm daily) can also reverse the hypocalcemic state. Vitamin D or a related agent facilitates intestinal calcium absorption and allows the intake of physiologic amounts of oral calcium to control the serum calcium concentration. At the doses of vitamin D used to maintain a normocalcemic state there is little evidence to indicate that vitamin D induces an increase in bone mineral release. In hypocalcemic magnesium deficient patients either parenteral or oral magnesium salts will increase parathyroid hormone secretion and improve target organ response to parathyroid hormone.

Rapid relief of disturbing symptoms of hypoparathyroidism is best achieved by intravenous injection of 10–20 cc of 10 percent calcium gluconate (90–180 mg Ca^{++}) over a 5- to 10-minute period. This usually produces improvement of symptoms for hours despite the observation that the serum calcium concentration quickly reverts to pretreatment levels after the injection is completed. The injection may be repeated as often as is needed to control the symptoms. In patients with magnesium deficiency intravenous calcium is not predictably effective in relieving symptoms. Magnesium sulfate solution ($MgSO_4·7H_2O$), 1 gm (8.13 mEq Mg) i.v. over 10 minutes usually will quickly relieve tetany. If significant renal failure is known or suspected the dose should be reduced by ⅓ to ½.

The chronic treatment of hypoparathyroidism almost invariably requires the administration of some form of vitamin D together with a dietary and/or supplemental calcium intake of 1 gm daily. Most of our experience is with vitamin D_2, which is administered orally in an initial dose of 50,000 to 100,000 USP units daily. The serum calcium

response to therapy is usually not maximal until 30 days after initiation of treatment because of the slow conversion of vitamin D_2 to 25-hydroxyvitamin D_2 in the liver. Dihydrotachysterol and 25-hydroxyvitamin D_3 have a more rapid onset of maximal calcemic effect but are more expensive than vitamin D_2. There is much to be gained by the use of $1,25(OH)_2$ vitamin D_3 in hypoparathyroid patients; it can be used as the sole form of vitamin D therapy or in conjunction with vitamin D_2 to achieve a rapid resolution of hypocalcemia during the initial few weeks of treatment. The maximal effect is observed in several days and the relatively short biologic half-life of this potent agent allows for much easier manipulation of the dosage. Most patients require a single dose of 0.5 μg daily, although unusual patients require several micrograms daily and a rare patient is refractory to treatment. The high cost of this agent is a limiting factor in its use.

The ingestion of approximately 1 gm of elemental calcium daily is an important component of the therapeutic regimen. This is the recommended daily intake of dietary calcium for children and most premenopausal adults. We recommend initially that the patient manipulate his diet so that it provides 1 gm of calcium daily. This is mainly achieved by ingesting an appropriate amount of dairy products, but Table 3 provides alternative sources of dietary calcium. Calcium supplements are used if the patient cannot obtain the desired amount of calcium by dietary means because of lactose intolerance or distaste for the particular foods rich in calcium. Another indication for calcium supplements is the occasional persistence of hyperphosphatemia after correction of hypocalcemia. In these patients it is necessary to reduce the intake of the phosphorus-rich dairy products. An alternative but less desirable approach is to reduce intestinal phosphorus absorption by administering frequent doses of aluminum hydroxide, a therapy sometimes used in hyperphosphatemic patients with renal failure.

Of the available oral calcium salts we have found that calcium carbonate is best tolerated by patients, although occasional complaints of a "chalky" taste or of mild constipation with higher doses are heard. Calcium glubionate has a sweet taste that is relished by some patients, but flatulence is not uncommon with this compound.

The correction of hypocalcemia secondary to magnesium deficiency is most efficiently achieved by administration of parenteral magnesium sulfate. Most patients will respond well to administration of 1 gm of $MgSO_4·7H_2O$ (8.13 mEq Mg) given every four to six hours over a five day period. $MgSO_4$ is available in either a 10 percent or 50 percent solution; the latter is preferable for intramuscular use. If the patient is on intravenous therapy the magnesium can be given throughout the day to avoid painful intramuscular injections. Restoration of normocalcemia usually requires four to five days of this regimen. If it is thought to be clinically desirable because of the severity of the illness, up to 100 mEq daily for 5 days could be safely administered to patients with normal renal function. The dose should be reduced by approximately 50 percent in patients with impaired renal function, and the serum magnesium level should be monitored daily. If the hypocalcemic magnesium deficient patient is only mildly symptomatic and able to eat a normal diet this may be sufficient to correct the hypocalcemia. Oral magnesium supplements are available in the form of sulfate, lactate, hydroxide, chloride, and glycerophosphate. Oral magnesium supplementation is essential in preventing magnesium deficiency in the rare patients who have a permanent disorder of magnesium homeostasis, such as renal magnesium wasting. Supplementation of dietary magnesium by 10–160 mEq of magnesium daily has been reported to prevent symptomatic magnesium deficiency.

A number of factors may significantly alter the dosage of vitamin D and calcium required for optimal regulation of the serum calcium concentration. These include the following:

Change in Vitamin D Preparation. This has not been a recent problem in our experience, but in the past overdosage or underdosage with vitamin D_2 in some patients has been related to a variable potency of the preparations used.

Thiazide Diuretics. Administration of any thiazide diuretic to a hypoparathyroid patient taking vitamin D may provoke a hypercalcemic response. This may occur in part because of the reduced renal calcium clearance known to be induced by thiazide diuretics. This effect has led to the suggestion by one group that thiazide therapy alone could be used to treat the hypocalcemia of hypoparathyroidism. We have not had any success with this type of therapy in the few patients we have treated in this manner.

Anticonvulsant Drugs. In patients who require anticonvulsant therapy the dose of vitamin D may have to be increased above the average. This may result from a combination of abnormal metabolism of vitamin D and a state of resistance to the peripheral actions of vitamin D.

Corticosteroid Therapy. Administration of glucocorticosteroid therapy to a vitamin D treated patient might provoke a hypocalcemic response. The antagonistic effect of glucocorticoids on the action of vitamin D has been extensively documented.

Estrogen Status. Because of the inhibitory effect of estrogens on bone resorption, the onset of the menopause in a previously stable hypoparathyroid patient may result in hypercalcemia. Correction of estrogen deficiency in a stable postmenopausal patient will produce the opposite response, a fall in serum calcium concentration.

Pregnancy and Lactation. Relief of tetany has been reported to occur during both pregnancy and lactation in hypoparathyroid women. Frank hypercalcemia may occur in vitamin D treated patients during lactation. The mechanism of the reduced need for vitamin D therapy is not known.

Intestinal Malabsorption. Diseases of the small intestine may result in impaired absorption of fat soluble vitamin D, calcium, and magnesium. Larger amounts of these nutrients may be needed to achieve adequate control in the appropriate patients. Parenteral administration of vitamin D_2 may prove necessary.

TOXICITY

The complications that may occur as a consequence of overtreatment with vitamin D and calcium include hypercalciuria, renal stones and nephrocalcinosis, hypercalcemia, and extrarenal soft tissue calcification. Hypercalciuria is the earliest detectable abnormality and will occur in the absence of frank hypercalcemia primarily because of the absence of the renal calcium conserving effect of parathyroid hormone. To avoid hypercalciuria, careful attention is paid not only to the serum calcium concentration but also to urinary calcium excretion. During the initial phases of therapy with vitamin D_2 we obtain urinary calcium excretion and serum calcium estimates every two weeks until the desired levels are achieved on two consecutive occasions. If 1,25 $(OH)_2D_3$ is used urinary and serum calcium measurements should be made daily until the desired levels are reached. Subsequently, monthly follow-up, and then evaluations at least every four months are done if the patient is stable. We ask the patients to collect 24-hour urine specimens for calcium analysis rather than fasting specimens, since the former is a better reflection of intestinal calcium absorption. Creatinine is also measured to assess the adequacy of the collection. It is our aim to keep the urinary calcium excretion below 4 mg/kg body weight per 24 hours to minimize the risk of renal stone formation and nephrocalcinosis. This usually is achieved at a serum calcium concentration of 8.5–9.0 mg/dl, levels at the lower range of normal. In our experience using these guidelines patients remain asymptomatic. In patients who develop symptomatic hypercalcemia all therapy should be immediately discontinued. Depending upon the clinical urgency intravenous saline combined with furosemide, oral glucocorticoid therapy, or salmon calcitonin could be used to control the hypercalcemia.

Hypermagnesemia may result from overzealous treatment with magnesium salts. This is much more likely to occur in patients with renal failure. Signs and symptoms of hypermagnesemia include disappearance of deep tendon reflexes, somnolence, paralysis of voluntary muscles, bradycardia, cardiac arrest, and hypocalcemia. Usually no symptoms occur at magnesium levels below 4 mEq/L. Discontinuation of the magnesium therapy is promptly followed by resolution of hypermagnesemia.

It is critical that patients with hypoparathyroidism be aware of the need for lifelong followup of their disease. In addition, they should be familiar with the symptoms of hypercalcemia which might develop, so that prompt treatment can be instituted.

PSEUDOHYPOPARA-THYROIDISM

GERALD D. AURBACH, M.D.

Pseudohypoparathyroidism (PsHP) is a state of hypoparathyroidism resistant to parathyroid hormone. Management of hypoparathyroidism in PsHP is identical to that for any other form of chronic hypoparathyroidism (such as idiopathic or postsurgical). The classic form of PsHP is associated with Albright's hereditary osteodystrophy (AHO), that is comprised of the following features: short stature, round face, obesity, certain skeletal defects, subcutaneous calcifications (actual subcutaneous bone formation), and mental retardation. Skeletal defects include bowing, shortening of the metacarpal and metatarsal bones (particularly the fourth metatarsals and metacarpals), and loss of tubulation of the long bones. Pseudohypoparathyroidism with AHO is attributable to a defect in the renal adenylate cyclase system normally responsive to parathyroid hormone. Recent studies show that in many cases the defect is due to a reduced complement of the guanine nucleotide regulatory unit (G unit), the protein coupling receptor function to adenylate cyclase activity. This defect also causes resistance to thyrotropin in over 80 percent of the cases and possibly gonadal dysfunction in some. In pseudohypoparathyroidism without AHO, G unit content of cells is normal and resistance to hormone action is limited to the renal effects of parathyroid hormone.

The pathophysiology of pseudohypoparathyroidism is complex, involving reduced PTH-dependent generation of cyclic AMP in the kidney with consequent low 25(OH) D 1-α-hydroxylase function and low renal clearance of phosphate. The resultant increase in plasma phosphate concentration also tends to suppress formation of 1,25-dihydroxyvitamin D. The low synthesis rate of 1,25-dihydroxyvitamin D leads to diminished calcium absorption from the gut and areas of osteomalacia in bone. Indeed, the bone may show mixed areas of osteomalacia and osteitis fibrosa cystica, the latter attributable to an increased rate of secretion and effect of parathyroid hormone.

PROBLEMS AND THERAPEUTIC ALTERNATIVES IN PSEUDOHYPOPARATHYROIDISM

Pseudohypoparathyroidism presents several problems with regard to therapy. The principal immediate problem facing the physician is hypocalcemia; other problems found in the syndrome include cataracts, dystonic reactions to drugs, hypothyroidism, obesity, and growth and mental retardation.

The following approaches have been advocated:

1. Increase in calcium intake utilizing dairy products and calcium salts (for example, calcium lactate tablets) by mouth. This simple approach may be effective in a small number of cases.

2. Administration of thiazide diuretics and sodium restriction. This approach offers the potential advantage of obviating hypercalciuria but has not been evaluated sufficiently for long-term therapy.

3. Administration of vitamin D or its metabolites along with an adequate oral intake of calcium.

VITAMIN D: CHEMISTRY, METABOLISM, AND ACTIONS

Vitamin D is a sterol produced exogenously (vitamin D_2) by irradiation of ergosterol, the previtamin found in plants or generated endogenously (vitamin D_3) through the natural radiation of 7-dehydrocholesterol, the precursor found in the skin. Vitamin D is fat soluble, and given exogenously it can accumulate and be stored in fat for prolonged periods up to six months or more. Vitamin D itself is not active directly but must be converted in vivo through two hydroxylation steps to 1,25-dyhydroxyvitamin D. The first hydroxylation, at the 25-position, is catalyzed by a 25-hydroxylase enzyme in the liver. 25-hydroxy D [25(OH)D] released from the liver is bound in the plasma compartment by a binding protein. 25(OH)D in the circulation reaches the kidney where a second hydroxylation takes place at the 1-α position. This 1-α hydroxylation step is controlled by parathyroid hormone. With reduced secretion or effect of parathyroid hormone (for example, in hypoparathyroidism and pseudohypoparathyroidism), the rate of conversion of 25(OH)D to 1-α-25-dihydroxyvitamin D [1,25(OH)$_2$D] in the kidney is impaired in at least two ways. Lack of parathyroid hormone or resistance to the hormone, as in pseudohypoparathyroidism, engenders a reduced production of cyclic 3',5'-AMP, one of the intracellular factors normally stimulating production of 1,25(OH)$_2$D. The 25(OH)D 1-hydroxylase step also is inhibited by high plasma concentrations of phosphate, which is another result of reduced parathyroid hormone activity on the kidney. 1,25(OH)$_2$D elaborated by the kidney reaches intestinal and skeletal cells where it regulates flow of calcium into the extracellular fluid compartment. In the intestine it stimulates synthesis of proteins mediating calcium absorption. For further discussion of vitamin D, see Chapter 50.

Pseudohypoparathyroidism can be treated with vitamin D or any of several metabolites or synthetic analogs. Vitamin D, being stored in fat, acts more slowly and, once effective, shows the most prolonged activity of any of the congeners. This is an advantage for long-term therapy wherein vitamin D is provided to the extracellular fluids at a relatively uniform rate from the fat stores. The slow equilibrium with fat storage sites is a disadvantage when rapid correction of hypocalcemia is desirable; this property of vitamin D is also disadvantageous in the event of overtreatment and production of hypercalcemia or hypercalciuria. The cost of therapy with vitamin D also is much less than with the synthetic congeners 25-hydroxyvitamin D, dihydrotachysterol (DHT),* or 1,25-dihydroxyvitamin D. DHT must be 25-hydroxylated in the liver to yield 25(OH)DHT. With either 1,25-dihydroxyvitamin D or dihydrotachysterol, the need for the parathyroid hormone-regulated 1-α-hydroxylation step in the kidney is circumvented.

Interactions with Other Drugs

Certain drugs interfere with the actions of vitamin D congeners. Corticosteroids as well as anticonvulsants, including phenytoin and barbiturates, disturb normal metabolism of vitamin D to its active forms and also may inhibit action of the metabolites. Furosemide promotes renal clearance of calcium, while thiazide diuretics decrease renal clearance of calcium. The thiazides can be therapeutically useful in raising serum calcium concentrations without causing hypercalciuria, but they can produce harmful hypercalcemia when superimposed upon already effective management. Cholestyramine can interfere with gastrointestinal absorption of vitamin D. It also should be noted that hypocalcemia in pseudohypoparathyroidism or hypoparathyroidism sensitizes subjects to dystonic reactions from the phenothiazine drugs.

GENERAL APPROACH

A high calcium intake should be assured; dietary and supplemental calcium intake equivalent to at least 1 to 2 gm of elemental calcium daily should be given in the form of dairy products and/or calcium glubionate. In a few patients this mod-

---

*1-α-hydroxyvitamin D has similar action at approximately 1/700 the dosage but is not currently approved for use in the U.S.

erately high calcium intake alone will suffice to control hypocalcemia. Most of the remaining patients will require vitamin D, 50,000–100,000 units per day (1.25 to 2.5 mg per day of crystalline vitamin D_2). Since pseudohypoparathyroidism is hereditary and existed chronically in the patient before the physician was consulted, there is usually no need for rapid correction of the problem through use of the more expensive vitamin D metabolites or analogs. In the remainder of cases, resistant to treatment with vitamin D itself or those requiring rapid control of hypocalcemia, the patients are given 1,25-dihydroxyvitamin D in divided doses totaling 0.5–1 μg per day. Parenteral administration of vitamin D or analogs will only rarely be required, for example, in patients unable to take anything by mouth. In acute hypocalcemia causing laryngeal stridor or convulsions, calcium gluconate should be given by vein, equivalent to 15 mg of elemental calcium/kg body weight per day.

The above recommended doses of vitamin D or $1,25(OH)_2D$ should be increased if necessary until tetany and marked hypocalcemia are controlled. Frequent monitoring (see Table 56–1) will be required until reasonable control is achieved without hypercalciuria or hypercalcemia. Side effects and complications of treatment with vitamin D or analogs relate solely to results of overtreatment, namely, hypercalcemia and hypercalciuria. Hypercalciuria is a potential complication, sometimes leading to nephrolithiasis or azotemia, that

may arise in treatment of any form of hypoparathyroidism with vitamin D or its analogs. Under normal physiologic conditions, parathyroid hormone acts in part to enhance reabsorption of calcium from the renal tubular lumen. In hypoparathyroid states, this control mechanism is lost. Thus restoration of normocalcemia in hypoparathyroidism with the use of vitamin D congeners can cause inordinate hypercalciuria at serum calcium concentrations that approach normal. Frank hypercalcemia due to excessive treatment with vitamin D congeners is a complication that, if sustained, could lead to irreversible renal impairment. Both hypercalcemia and hypercalciuria can be avoided by using the minimum dose of vitamin D compatible with alleviation of symptoms and maintenance of serum calcium concentration near normal.

Assessment of Response

Correction of symptoms, that is, alleviation of tetany, is the most urgent goal of therapy. Over the long term one should attempt to keep serum calcium concentration near normal with avoidance of hypercalciuria (24-hour urinary calcium excretion should be kept below 200 mg). This may require maintenance of serum calcium just below normal, which is usually possible with avoidance of symptoms of tetany. One must monitor serum calcium and urinary calcium concentration at intervals that are short at first and gradually lengthened as satisfactory control is achieved (Table 1).

TABLE 1 Treatment of Pseudohypoparathyroidism with Vitamin D and Metabolites

Drug	Dosage	Advantages	Disadvantages	Follow-up Required
Vitamin D_2	1.25–2.5 mg/d*	Economy Easier to control in chronic therapy	Slow onset of actions Prolonged half-life in vivo	Serum and urine calcium weekly initially, then biweekly, monthly, half-yearly
$1.25(OH)_2D_3$	0.5–1 μg/d	Fast acting Short half-life in vivo Circumvents renal 1-α-hydroxylase	High cost Difficult to regulate—rapid swings in serum Ca May require assays for plasma $1,25(OH)_2D$	Serum and urine calcium, every 3 days, then biweekly Switch to D_2 or DHT for chronic treatment
Dihydrotachysterol (DHT)	1–2 mg/d	Faster acting than D_2 Circumvents renal 1-α-hydroxylase Perhaps easier to control than $1,25(OH)_2D$	High cost No assay available for 25(OH)DHT	Serum and urine calcium weekly initially, then biweekly, monthly, half-yearly

*1.25 mg of crystalline vitamin D_2 is equivalent to 50,000 units of vitamin D_2.

If 1,25-dihydroxyvitamin D is used as therapy, frequent monitoring of serum and urinary calcium concentration will be necessary; with this drug rapid swings in serum calcium concentration may be evidenced. Patient compliance in pseudohypoparathyroidism can be a problem. One could monitor for plasma concentration of 25(OH)D or 1,25(OH)$_2$D, depending on whether vitamin D$_2$, 25(OH)D, 1,25(OH)D, or 1-α-(OH)D is used for treatment, but this is expensive. The defective urinary cAMP response to parathyroid hormone in pseudohypoparathyroidism is not corrected by treatment with vitamin D congeners or calcium.

Treatment of Coincident Defects in Pseudohypoparathyroidism

Coincident clinical problems in pseudohypoparathyroidism include hypothyroidism, obesity, growth deficiency, mental retardation, and cataracts. Approximately 80 to 90 percent of patients with pseudohypoparathyroidism have mild primary hypothyroidism as described in the introduction to this chapter. This is readily correctable with standard thyroid replacement, for example, thyroxine, 175–200 μg daily. Since hypothyroidism in pseudohypoparathyroidism is mild (indeed, it may be compensated for adequately by compensatory TSH secretion), there is generally no need for the usual cautious and gradual institution of thyroid treatment as in the case of frank myxedema. There is no satisfactory treatment for obesity in pseudohypoparathyroidism. Obesity may be yet another manifestation of the biochemical abnormality (reduced complement of the G unit) in pseudohypoparathyroidism. The actions of lipolytic hormones are also mediated by cyclic AMP. Intestinal bypass surgery is probably contraindicated, as consequent reduction in bowel function can further impair absorption of vitamin D and calcium. There is no known therapy or prevention for the growth and mental retardation problems. Cataracts are the result of long-term hypocalcemia. It is presumed but unproven that early recognition of the disease and early institution of treatment to correct hypocalcemia will prevent or moderate the development of cataracts.

Genetic counseling should be a part of caring for patients with pseudohypoparathyroidism. Prenatal diagnosis may be possible in the near future. In vitro culture of cells obtained by amniocentesis may provide a means to test for the guanine nucleotide regulatory unit.

HYPERCALCEMIA

JOHN P. BILEZIKIAN, M.D.

The purpose of this chapter is to summarize current approaches to the management of hypercalcemia. With the variety of therapeutic modalities available, the serum calcium level can be lowered readily in most patients. Etiologies and mechanisms responsible for hypercalcemia will not be emphasized because they are thoroughly covered in many textbooks. Nonetheless, the differential diagnosis of hypercalcemia should always be considered, along with the management of the hypercalcemic state, because selective approaches to hypercalcemia are based in part upon the underlying etiology. The causes of hypercalcemia are listed in Table 1. Despite the diverse and numerous etiologies on this list, the vast majority of hypercalcemic patients have either primary hyperparathyroidism or a malignant disorder.

Hypercalcemia itself may be a medical emergency associated with specific signs and symptoms, in which case it requires aggressive therapy. However, not every patient with hypercalcemia necessarily suffers from the direct effects of an elevated serum calcium level. The measures outlined in this chapter should be reserved for those individuals whose symptoms can be attributed directly to hypercalcemia. These symptoms, which are noted in Table 2, include dysfunction of the central nervous system (impaired concentration, altered states of consciousness), the gastrointestinal tract (anorexia, nausea, vomiting, constipation), and the kidneys (polyuria). Abnormal function of these organ systems can be due to the hypercalcemia itself, and thus be independent of specific etiologic factors. These symptoms depend both upon the rate of rise of the serum calcium level, which may be difficult to delineate with precision unless a recent serum calcium level is available, and also upon the absolute calcium level.

The reported value for the serum calcium should be assessed with attention to the serum albumin, the major circulating calcium binding protein. Under normal circumstances, the form of calcium that is physiologically relevant, namely, the ionized calcium, constitutes approximately one-

TABLE 1   The Etiologies of Hypercalcemia

Most Common
  Primary hyperparathyroidism
  Neoplasms
    Multiple myeloma
    Malignancies with evident metastases in bone
    Humoral hypercalcemia of malignancy (without
      detectable bone metastases)

Uncommon
  Hyperthyroidism
  Thiazide diuretics
  Hypervitaminosis D
  Sarcoidosis
  Lithium administration
  Immobilization (in children and in Paget's disease of bone)
  Recovery phase of acute renal failure

Rare
  Other granulomatous diseases (tuberculosis,
    histoplasmosis)
  Hypervitaminosis A
  Adrenal insufficiency
  Hypophosphatasia
  Familial hypocalciuric hypercalcemia
  Milk-alkali syndrome

TABLE 3   Signs of Hypercalcemia

Cardiovascular
  Hypertension
  Electrocardiographic changes (shortened QT interval)
  Increased sensitivity to digitalis

Renal
  Insufficiency
  Decreased concentrating ability
  Nephrocalcinosis
  Nephrolithiasis

Gastrointestinal
  Pancreatitis
  Peptic ulcer

Dehydration

Metastatic Calcification

half of the total serum calcium. Calcium bound to albumin usually comprises the other half. The calcium reported from most hospital laboratories is the total serum calcium, consisting of both the ionized and the bound calcium. If the serum albumin is reduced, as is not infrequently the case in very sick patients, the ionized calcium becomes a disproportionately greater fraction of the total calcium. The general rule is that for every gm/dl reduction in the serum albumin, the total serum calcium is lower than it should be, relative to the

TABLE 2   Symptoms of Hypercalcemia

General
  Weakness
  Polydipsia

Central Nervous System
  Impaired concentration
  Increased sleep requirement
  Altered states of consciousness (confusion, stupor, coma)

Gastrointestinal Tract
  Anorexia
  Nausea
  Vomiting
  Constipation

Renal System
  Polyuria

actual ionized calcium, by approximately 0.8 mg/dl. For example, a serum calcium level reported to be 12.0 mg/dl should be regarded as 12.8 mg/dl if the serum albumin level is below normal by 1 gm/dl. This point should always be borne in mind when assessing the degree of hypercalcemia in a given patient.

In most laboratories the normal range for the serum calcium level is 8.5–10.5 mg/dl. In general, patients whose serum calcium level is no more than 12 mg/dl will not have obvious symptoms from their hypercalcemia, although they may be very symptomatic of the disease process underlying the hypercalcemic state. For these individuals acute therapeutic intervention is not usually necessary, and their clinical condition usually is not improved when the calcium level returns to normal. If the serum calcium level is moderately elevated, between 12 and 14 mg/dl, patients may or may not have symptoms. In this range of hypercalcemia, close clinical observation is required to determine how aggressive one should be in lowering the serum calcium level. When the serum calcium level is greater than 14 mg/dl, treatment should be instituted, not only because patients are invariably symptomatic in this range, but also because they are at significant risk for developing signs of hypercalcemia with target organ damage. The signs of hypercalcemia are noted in Table 3.

GENERAL MEASURES

General principles of management of hypercalcemia are listed in Table 4.

TABLE 4   General Management of Hypercalcemia

Rehydration with intravenous fluid
Saline administration
Diuresis with furosemide
Dialysis (if necessary because of renal failure)
Mobilization

Hydration

Patients with hypercalcemia may become dehydrated because of a calcium-related defect in renal concentrating mechanisms. Polyuria develops, and because of anorexia, nausea, or vomiting that may also be present, the polydipsia that accompanies polyuria may not compensate for renal fluid losses. Fluid replacement therefore is of primary importance to the hypercalcemic patient. The intravenous route is usually necessary. The serum calcium level may decline significantly simply by virtue of rehydration and expansion of the relatively concentrated plasma volume. An additional advantage of rehydration is improved renal glomerular filtration, which in turn facilitates the clearance of calcium.

Diuresis

Saline is the most appropriate intravenous solution to employ for the purposes of rehydration. When presented with a saline challenge, the renal tubule clears, in an obligatory manner, both sodium and calcium. The degree of calciuresis is directly linked to the degree of saliuresis. To this end, saline administration is a principal therapeutic approach to hypercalcemia. The rate of saline administration should be adapted to the individual patient. Many patients with hypercalcemia are elderly, and the tolerance of their cardiovascular systems for vigorous fluid and saline challenge may be marginal. In addition, the coexistence of significant renal dysfunction, even if only temporary and reversible, may stress their hemodynamic capacity even further. In the hypercalcemic patient with a history of previous cardiac dysfunction, intravenous saline administration requires careful and regular monitoring of cardiac function to avoid the possible complication of acute congestive heart failure. A loop diuretic, such as furosemide, may prevent this complication. Furosemide also inhibits the tubular reabsorption of sodium and may therefore augment calcium clearance in these pa-

tients. Furosemide should be used only after fluids have been initiated, to avoid further dehydration and temporary worsening of hypercalcemia. Thiazide diuretics are absolutely contraindicated in this setting because they decrease the glomerular filtration rate, increase renal tubular calcium reabsorption, and may aggravate hypercalcemia. With intravenous saline (200–250 cc/hr) and furosemide (10 mg every 4 to 6 hours), urinary calcium excretion can be increased to as much as 1000 mg per day. If the serum calcium level is extremely high (that is, more than 17–18 mg/dl), one can be even more aggressive with saline (500–1000 cc/hr) and furosemide (40 mg every 4 to 6 hours) and cause even more impressive urinary calcium losses. However, such vigorous diuresis may lead to serious electrolyte disturbances, such as hypokalemia and hypomagnesemia. To prevent these complications, serum and urinary electrolytes should be monitored closely.

Dialysis

Peritoneal or hemodialysis should be considered seriously in the special circumstance of the patient whose hypercalcemia is associated with renal failure. Under these conditions, the generally useful initial therapeutic approaches of saline administration and furosemide are limited. When dialysis is performed against a calcium-free dialysate, the serum calcium level will decrease significantly within the first two days. Although emergency dialysis may not be readily available in many hospitals, this approach should be considered when other options are limited and hypercalcemia is severe. If dialysis is employed, phosphate may have to be supplemented in the dialysate fluid to prevent substantial losses from the body and worsening hypercalcemia.

Mobilization

Another general measure to be employed whenever possible in the hypercalcemic individual is mobilization. The ambulatory patient is less prone to the negative calcium balance that occurs inevitably with immobilization, a feature that may further aggravate the underlying cause of hypercalcemia. Although the patient with hypercalcemia may not be ambulatory when admitted to the hospital, every effort should be made to meet this goal as soon as possible.

TABLE 5   Specific Management of Hypercalcemia

Mithramycin
Diphosphonates
Calcitonin
Glucocorticoids
Phosphate
Prostaglandin inhibitors
Therapy of underlying etiology

SPECIFIC MEASURES

Specific principles of management of hypercalcemia are listed in Table 5.

Mithramycin

Mithramycin has become a mainstay in the therapy of severe hypercalcemia. In contrast to the general measures of rehydration, saline diuresis, and mobilization, mithramycin acts to prevent, in a specific manner, the resorption of calcium from bone. It is cytotoxic to the osteoclast, the cell in bone responsible for the mobilization of calcium. Because virtually all causes of hypercalcemia involve, at least in part, the accelerated loss of bone calcium through the mechanism of osteoclast activation, it is not surprising that mithramycin should be effective in all hypercalcemic patients. The drug is usually administered intravenously as a 4- or 8-hour infusion (15–25 μg/kg). The infusion is repeated daily for up to five days or until the serum calcium level starts to decline. The time course and duration of action vary considerably among patients. To a certain extent, this variability depends upon the intensity of ongoing bone resorption. Unfortunately, mithramycin is not without significant and potentially serious adverse effects, including thrombocytopenia, hepatic dysfunction, and nephrotoxicity. These adverse consequences are related both to the cumulative amount of drug administered as well as to its repetitive use. Single doses given less frequently than daily may minimize the development and severity of these side effects. However, the condition of severe hypercalcemia usually does not permit this theoretically more desirable approach. Despite the possibility of adverse consequences, mithramycin is a very important agent for the acute management of severe hypercalcemia. If the serum calcium level is markedly elevated and associated with life-threatening signs or symptoms, mithramycin should be used without hesitation.

Diphosphonates

The diphosphonates represent another specific approach to hypercalcemia which is directed at inhibiting bone resorption. In particular, dichloromethylene diphosphonate (Cl_2MDP) and amino-hydroxypropylidene bisphosphonate (APD) both have been shown to be effective in reducing hypercalcemia due to a wide spectrum of causes. Similar to mithramycin, the general mechanism of diphosphonate action involves the impairment of osteoclast function. However, the specific mechanisms by which mithramycin and the diphosphonates affect this cell are different. Recent experience with Cl_2MDP has been particularly encouraging with respect to its ability to lower both serum and urinary calcium levels. When Cl_2MDP is administered intravenously in daily infusions (5 mg/kg), the serum calcium level will start to decline within 2 to 3 days and, in most patients, will eventually normalize. The degree to which Cl_2MDP may lead to adequate control of the serum calcium level in the postinfusion period, with or without the institution of oral Cl_2MDP, is variable and depends partly upon the extent of ongoing osteoclast activity. Unfortunately, neither Cl_2MDP nor APD is available in the United States at this time. The only diphosphonate that is available, ethane hydroxy 1,1 diphosphonic acid (EHDP), is an oral preparation and has not been shown to be effective in the acute therapy of hypercalcemia.

Calcitonin

Calcitonin acts to decrease the skeletal release of calcium and to increase urinary calcium excretion. These properties of calcitonin should make it an ideal agent in the management of hypercalcemia. In fact, several conditions such as thyrotoxicosis and vitamin D toxicity have been reported to be responsive to the administration of calcitonin. However, the general experience with calcitonin in the more common causes of hypercalcemia, primary hyperparathyroidism and malignancy, has been less impressive. The serum calcium level will decline by no more than 1–3 mg/dl and often soon returns to pretreatment levels. Nevertheless, calcitonin may be useful as an adjunct to other approaches. In particular, the combination of calcitonin and glucocorticoids has been reported to be more effective in hypercalcemia associated with malignancy than calcitonin alone. Salmon calcitonin, the most potent form of calcitonin, can be administered by the intravenous, intramuscular, or subcutaneous routes. A dosage of 200–400 MRC units may be given daily in divided doses. Calcitonin is relatively free from adverse effects; an occasional patient may develop allergic manifestations.

Glucocorticoids

The glucocorticoids may be very effective in selected conditions associated with hypercalcemia, namely hypervitaminosis D, sarcoidosis, and certain malignant states, such as multiple myeloma, leukemia, lymphoma, and carcinoma of the breast. If any of these disorders is present, glucocorticoid therapy should be considered as an early approach to effective management. Glucocorticoids appear to have many different mechanisms of action, including inhibition of calcium absorption from the gastrointestinal tract, altered vitamin D metabolism, increased urinary calcium excretion, direct actions on bone, and in some instances, antitumor activity. In the acute setting, 100–300 mg of hydrocortisone (or its equivalent) are administered intravenously in 4 divided doses. The time course of response varies from reasonably rapid (within 12 to 18 hours) to deliberate (48 to 72 hours). Unfortunately, hypercalcemic patients with primary hyperparathyroidism or with a malignancy generally do not respond to the hypocalcemic actions of the glucocorticoids. For those disorders that are sensitive to steroid administration, chronic therapy also has a potential role in controlling the serum calcium level. The many well-known adverse effects of the glucocorticoids should be evaluated along with the potential benefits before embarking upon a course of chronic oral therapy.

Intravenous Phosphate

The use of intravenous phosphate presents a significant therapeutic dilemma. There is little doubt that intravenous phosphate administration is invariably associated with a rapid reduction in the serum calcium level. Phosphate inhibits bone resorption and promotes the deposition of calcium-phosphate salts into bone. However, calcium-phosphate salts may also be deposited into soft tissues. It is this latter effect that probably accounts for phosphate's extremely rapid onset of action in

lowering calcium levels. This same observation, however, has led to serious reservations regarding its place in the acute management of hypercalcemia. Precipitates of calcium-phosphate complexes deposited into tissues other than bone could result in serious organ damage. This potentially life-threatening complication has led most investigators to regard intravenous phosphate as a last resort in the management of hypercalcemia. It should be reserved for those rare individuals whose hypercalcemia cannot be controlled adequately by any other means. The chelating agent EDTA also forms a complex with circulating calcium; it should be reserved for only the most desperate situations because its use may be associated with renal failure and severe, acute hypocalcemia.

Oral Phosphate

The oral use of phosphate to manage hypercalcemia has no place in treatment of the acute condition, especially if the calcium level is markedly elevated. However, oral phosphate is sometimes useful in the management of disorders associated with more moderately elevated levels. Most patients can tolerate 1 gm of elemental phosphorus before diarrhea develops. Some patients will tolerate up to 3 gm. The phosphate is almost completely absorbed from the gastrointestinal tract and is incompletely cleared by the kidney. The resulting increase in the serum phosphate level predisposes for calcium-phosphate deposition into bone. The same relative contraindication to the use of intravenous phosphate—namely, the potential for soft tissue calcification—applies to its oral use as well. But the pharmacokinetics and actions of oral phosphate are much less rapid, making this consideration less worrisome than in the case of intravenous phosphate.

Prostaglandin Inhibitors

Interest in the potential usefulness of prostaglandin synthesis inhibitors, such as aspirin and indomethacin, in the therapy of hypercalcemia has developed over the past five years. The rationale for this approach is based upon the observation in some patients with malignancy and hypercalcemia that the tumor appears to be a source of prostaglandin production. In several experimental models, prostaglandin E_2 has been directly implicated as a humoral factor responsible for the resorption of bone. Despite encouraging early reports, however, neither aspirin nor indomethacin has been very effective, even in settings in which there did seem to be good evidence for the production of endogenous prostaglandins. These agents do not offer much likelihood for beneficial results in tumor-associated hypercalcemia. They should be reserved for those special clinical circumstances in which humoral hypercalcemia of malignancy appears to be present and in which other measures have failed.

Therapy of the Underlying Etiology

The final but perhaps the foremost consideration in the management of hypercalcemia is the diagnosis of the underlying cause. The most definitive approach to the hypercalcemic patient is focused specifically upon treating the etiology. As soon as the patient has been stabilized by a judicious combination of approaches discussed above, measures can be taken to treat the underlying disease itself. If the patient has primary hyperparathyroidism, a neck exploration should be considered. If the patient has a malignancy, surgical removal, chemotherapy, or irradiation all are potentially very useful. Without effective therapy of the underlying cause, management of the hypercalcemic crisis will be merely temporary. However, if aggressive diagnostic measures are associated with the initial approach to management, more definitive action may be possible as soon as the patient's condition has been stabilized. On the other hand, if the diagnosis is a malignancy that has no potential for cure or even for palliation, one's aggressive approach to the therapy of a symptom of the rampant disease process may be tempered by the realities of the situation.

SUMMARY

Symptomatic hypercalcemia can be managed successfully in most instances by a combination of general and specific measures. Rehydration and saline administration in combination with the judicious use of furosemide are generally useful in all patients, regardless of the cause of hypercalcemia. Due regard for the specific cause of the elevated serum calcium level permits, in addition, a reasoned and tailored approach to the patient. Acute management of hypercalcemia affords the time required to make a diagnosis and to embark upon a course of definitive therapy of the underlying condition.

PRIMARY HYPERPARATHYROIDISM

CLAUDE D. ARNAUD, M.D.
and ORLO H. CLARK, M.D.

The natural history of untreated primary hyperparathyroidism is unknown, because the majority of patients with this disease are subjected to neck exploration and removal of the abnormal parathyroid glands and are cured. The natural history and progress of patients with "biochemical" or minimal hyperparathyroidism (serum calcium level less than 1 mg/dl above the upper limits of the normal range) and no apparent manifestations of the disease appear to be variable.

Based on studies carried out in a group of 147 patients in Rochester, Minnesota, it appears that a relatively small proportion (10 to 30 percent) will develop complications of this disease or will progress to a more severe form of the disease within 5 years. Unfortunately, even in retrospect, there were no clinical or biochemical measurements that could predict such progression. It is currently an open question whether patients without apparent complications or progression require therapy.

It is presumed that patients with mild to moderately severe manifestations of primary hyperparathyroidism progressed from the "biochemical" form of the disease. However, it is clear that a relatively small portion of this group of patients attains some degree of disease stability, because some have been observed for as long as 10 to 15 years without apparent worsening of their disease. A very small number develop severe disease, whereas the remaining patients probably suffer slow progression with gradual deterioration of renal function and the development of bone disease. Patients with severe primary hyperparathyroidism (serum calcium > 15 mg/dl) will almost certainly die of their disease unless it is detected and appropriately treated.

Surgical resection of benign parathyroid lesions is generally curative in primary hyperparathyroidism. Recurrences are rare in patients determined at surgery to have single gland disease or multiple gland disease without familial hyperparathyroidism or multiple endocrine neoplasia. Recurrences are common in patients with multiple gland disease of a familial nature. Several short studies suggest that surgical treatment results in restoration of previously impaired renal function and improvement in hypertension, but long-term studies are required. Active nephrolithiasis generally becomes inactive unless factors other than primary hyperparathyroidism are present to perpetuate this problem. There have been anecdotal reports that severe psychiatric symptomatology has disappeared after the removal of abnormal parathyroid glands. All but the more severe forms of osteitis fibrosa cystica demonstrate improvement within months, and essentially complete resolution within a year of parathyroidectomy. It is not known if the surgical treatment of hyperparathyroidism in patients who also have postmenopausal or senile osteoporosis results in improvement of the osteopenic disease. However, this will be important to determine, because as many as 8 to 10 percent of patients with age-related osteopenia have increased circulating levels of immunoreactive parathyroid hormone and may very well suffer from some form of curable hyperparathyroidism.

TREATMENT

Medical

There is currently no satisfactory medical treatment for primary hyperparathyroidism. In general, medical treatment is used in two relatively well defined situations and directed primarily at controlling hypercalcemia. The first is in patients who cannot undergo surgery (that is, in cases of inoperable parathyroid cancer, unacceptable surgical risk) and who have chronic increases in serum calcium levels above 11.5–12.0 mg/dl. The second is in patients who present with life-threatening hypercalcemia (serum calcium > 15.0 mg/dl) when acute lowering of the serum calcium level might reverse or prevent severe symptoms, signs or conditions that can be associated with hypercalcemia (for example, somnolence, coma, or pancreatitis).

Chronic Hypercalcemia. The therapy for chronic hypercalcemia is difficult and will tax the therapeutic innovativeness of the physician. Pharmacologically, attempts are made to increase the urinary excretion of calcium (accepting the risk or worsening or inducing active nephrolithiasis), increase bone accretion, or decrease bone resorption.

Sometimes increasing the urinary excretion of calcium by the combined administration of increased water (3–4 l per day), sodium chloride (400–600 mEq per day), and furosemide (40–160 mg per day) will suffice. The major problems associated with this approach include annoying polyuria, electrolyte disturbances, aggravation of heart failure, and, if water intake is not adequate, renal stone diathesis and dehydration. Thus patients receiving such a regimen require close monitoring of serum Na, K, Cl, Ca, Mg, and PO_4, and must be watched for signs of worsening heart failure and diminished urine output.

Oral phosphate may be used as an antihypercalcemic agent, provided patients are not taking glucocorticoids. Some clinicians have found that the combination of oral phosphate and glucocorticoids occasionally induces nephrolithiasis, although the cause of this phenomenon is not known. Either neutral phosphate or potassium phosphate may be given in doses as high as 2–4 gm per day in divided doses. Initial doses should be relatively low (1–2 gm per day in divided doses every 6 hours) because of gastrointestinal side effects, which disappear with time. The mechanisms by which phosphate lowers serum calcium levels are poorly understood. They are not renal, because phosphate therapy lowers urinary calcium. Evidence suggests that phosphate increases the accretion of calcium in the skeleton as well as in soft tissues. Therapy with phosphate should be monitored by measuring serum calcium and creatinine levels to give assurance of the desired effect and to detect the possible development of renal functional impairment. In general, decreases in the serum calcium level during phosphate therapy are not observed unless serum phosphate concentrations increase. However, increases in serum phosphorus above 5.0 mg/dl should be avoided at all costs because of the danger of inducing extraskeletal calcifications. Such therapy with phosphate can be used as a temporizing measure during a period in which diagnostic studies are being pursued and the definitive diagnosis made. Phosphate may also be given along with hydration, furosemide, and salt loading. Phosphate therapy may cause hypokalemia, requiring the administration of potassium supplements.

The use of the hormone calcitonin (which inhibits bone resorption) in the treatment of chronic hypercalcemia has been disappointing. Recently, however, there have been occasional reports of good therapeutic responses to high-dose therapy

(500–1000 units of salmon calcitonin per day). Such treatment requires daily self-administered injections.

Mithramycin, a toxic antibiotic that inhibits bone resorption as one of its cellulicidal effects, should be used only in cases of severe hypercalcemia or inoperable parathyroid cancer, because it can cause severe thrombocytopenia. It is generally effective in doses of 25 μg/kg given as an i.v. push every 2 to 3 weeks, provided platelet counts have not been dangerously suppressed and the patient has not had a bleeding diathesis.

Recently reports have appeared that several investigational diphosphonate compounds are effective in the treatment of hypercalcemia by inhibiting bone resorption.

Acute Hypercalcemia. The medical therapy of acute severe hypercalcemia (serum calcium > 15 mg/dl) is quite different from the treatment of chronic, moderate hypercalcemia (12–14 mg/dl). Immediate treatment of severe hypercalcemia is important because the condition is life-threatening. First, dietary calcium restriction should be instituted and all drugs that might cause hypercalcemia discontinued (for example, thiazide diuretics, vitamin D). Serum electrolytes and renal function tests should be determined. If the patient is digitalized, consideration should be given to reducing the dose of the digitalis preparation being administered because the hypercalcemic patients may be more sensitive to the toxic effects of digitalis. Ideally, the patient should be admitted to an intensive care unit where electrocardiographic monitoring can be done while antihypercalcemic measures are being applied. If possible, the patient should not be permitted to remain in bed. The mainstay of therapy is a regimen consisting of hydration, saline administration, and furosemide or ethacrynic acid. The overall objective is to increase the urinary excretion of calcium rapidly, thus decreasing the exchangeable calcium pool and the serum calcium concentration. Saline is given to increase the sodium excretion because sodium clearance and calcium clearance parallel one another during water or osmotic diuresis, independent of any changes in urinary ionic strength or acidity. Furosemide inhibits the tubular reabsorption of calcium and helps to maintain diuresis. Practically, as long as the kidneys are functional, approximately 4–8 l of isotonic saline should be given daily, along with furosemide in doses up to 100 mg every 1 to 2 hours or ethacrynic acid in doses up to 50 mg every 1 to 2 hours. Such a regimen should increase the urinary calcium level to 500–1000 mg per day and lower the serum calcium level by 2–6 mg/dl after 24 hours. With such a regimen, potassium and magnesium depletion must be anticipated and appropriate replacement therapy instituted early. Thus it is important to monitor serum calcium, magnesium, sodium, and potassium levels on a regular 2 to 4 hour basis. In patients who are in danger of developing heart failure, central venous pressure should be monitored so that appropriate cardiotonic measures can be taken if significant and consistent increases in this index are observed. After the serum calcium level has decreased into a reasonably safe range (< 13 mg/dl), a chronic regimen may be instituted. This should consist of furosemide (40–160 mg per day) or ethacrynic acid (50–200 mg per day), sodium chloride tablets (400–600 mEq per day) and at least 3 l of fluid per day. Serum calcium, magnesium, and potassium levels are monitored daily initially and weekly when the serum calcium level has stabilized. Magnesium and potassium should be replaced when necessary.

Finally, mithramycin may be given in doses of 25 μg per kg of body weight intravenously per day for 3 to 4 days early in the course of the treatment of acute hypercalcemia. In most situations it is not necessary to give mithramycin to individuals suspected of having primary hyperparathyroidism, because the above treatment is generally effective and because such patients are likely to require surgery and mithramycin can cause marked thrombocytopenia. Patients receiving mithramycin should be followed carefully with platelet counts and serum creatinine and liver function tests because of the liver, kidney, and marrow toxicity potential of the drug.

Surgical

Preoperative Localization of Abnormal Parathyroid Tissue. It is important to recognize that the abnormal parathyroid tissue causing primary hyperparathyroidism will be discovered and excised in more than 90 percent of patients at initial neck exploration by a competent parathyroid surgeon. Thus there is no need for preoperative localization (using invasive techniques) except under very unusual circumstances (see below).

Generally, localization procedures are reserved for those patients whose first neck exploration was unsuccessful or who suffer from recurrent disease. There are both noninvasive and invasive localization procedures. The noninvasive procedures include esophagography, ultrasonography, and computerized axial tomography. The invasive procedures include differential (selective) venous catheterization of the neck and mediastinum with measurement of immunoreactive PTH (iPTH) in the serum samples obtained; arteriography; and, rarely, fine-needle aspiration (23 gauge) with cytologic confirmation of the tumor localized by ultrasonography.

Esophagography may occasionally identify a relatively large parathyroid gland, deep in the tracheal esophageal groove, which was inadvertently missed on first exploration because of its aberrant shape and posterior position. However, the procedure is mostly unrewarding, as false positive and negative results occur. Ultrasound technology has improved so rapidly in recent years that it is now possible to identify parathyroid lesions in the neck as small as a centimeter in diameter. Further technologic development in this area is expected, and because of the simplicity of the procedure, ultrasound evaluation prior to initial neck exploration may become feasible and advisable.

Whereas ultrasonography is not useful in identifying mediastinal lesions, computerized axial tomography is and should be routinely employed with ultrasonography and esophagography in the patient harboring a missed or recurrent parathyroid lesion(s). These noninvasive procedures designed for localization are especially helpful diagnostically in the severely hypercalcemic patient who has not undergone previous neck exploration, because treatment is urgent and most of these patients have large parathyroid tumors that are more likely to be identified.

Differential catheterization of the neck and mediastinal veins for the purpose of obtaining serum for iPTH analysis is helpful because localization of the tumor depends on its secretory ability and not on the size of the parathyroid tumor. The procedure is safer than arteriography and is especially helpful if the results from this study correspond to those of the noninvasive studies. The principle of these tests is that there is ipsilateral venous drainage of the parathyroid secretory products. In general, all of the small veins in the neck should be entered and blood samples obtained for iPTH determination. It is frequently difficult to obtain blood from small veins because of obstruction of the lumen by the catheter tip. However, it is critical that the operator not yield to the temptation to withdraw the catheter into the mainstream of a larger vein where blood is easy to aspirate. Blood flow is so great in such larger veins that step-up increases in serum iPTH can be obliterated even if the catheter tip is near a small vein draining a parathyroid tumor.

It is important that a radioimmunoassay of PTH which recognizes only intact PTH (aminoregion or intact specific) be used in measurements of iPTH in sera obtained during differential venous catheterization procedures. Step-up differences in iPTH concentrations between peripheral sera and sera from veins draining parathyroid lesions are greater when such assays are used because of the relatively low concentrations of intact PTH in the peripheral circulation. By contrast, carboxyl-region-specific assays measure the high concentrations of carboxyl-region fragments in the peripheral circulation and are excellent for screening hypercalcemic patients for hyperparathyroidism. Interpretation of the results obtained by differential catheterization should be cautious. Because of the distortion in venous anatomy produced by previous surgery and extensive individual variation and venous anastomoses, the best that can be obtained is usually lateralization rather than localization of a parathyroid lesion. In general, less than two-fold step-up changes should be ignored unless all other values for iPTH are almost identical. It is also difficult to interpret differential catheterization PTH results when the highest levels are in the innominate vein. This can reflect a cervical parathyroid gland draining in a caudal direction or a mediastinal parathyroid gland draining in a cephalad direction. Significant step-up increases in iPTH have also been recorded in sera draining normal parathyroid glands, obviating the need for differential venous sampling in the diagnosis of hyperparathyroidism.

Of the invasive procedures, thyroid arteriography is most useful to the surgeon because it demonstrates the site of the tumor, not just the general area. However, because of the risk of serious sequelae, arteriography is only occasionally used and only in patients who have undergone unsuccessful parathyroid operations by an experienced surgeon. Neurologic complications, such as transient occipital blindness and hemiplegia, and also deaths have been recorded, and it is the authors' practice to avoid the procedure in patients who are at risk for neurovascular disease. The risk of such complications can be minimized if the following precautions are taken: hydrate the patient adequately; use low quantities of radiopaque contrast materials; avoid injecting the small costovertebral trunk and wedging the catheter; and secure the services of an experienced arteriographer.

Surgery for the Removal of Abnormal Parathyroid Tissue. Neck exploration should be considered in all patients in whom the diagnosis of primary hyperparathyroidism has been established. There is some evidence to suggest that even patients with biochemical hyperparathyroidism benefit metabolically from parathyroidectomy. This, as well as the fact that the majority of patients with hyperparathyroidism have histologic evidence of osseous hyperparathyroidism, should be kept in mind before a long-term medical follow-up program is embarked upon, especially in older women who may have already suffered considerable bone loss as a result of age-related factors. In this regard, it is the authors' opinion that age, per se, should not be a contraindication to neck exploration. A parathyroid exploration is a minimal operation when performed by an experienced surgeon, and most patients are discharged from the hospital within 48 hours of the operation. In general, it is better to perform elective parathyroidectomy in an older person than to find it necessary to deal with hypercalcemia as a complication of another age-related serious illness (for example, myocardial infarction).

In the long-term follow-up study of biochemical hyperparathyroidism commented upon earlier, one of the authors (CDA) and his colleagues at the Mayo Clinic developed a group of arbitrary indications for neck exploration. They include (1) x-ray evidence of metabolic bone disease, (2) demonstration of decreasing renal function, (3) active nephrolithiasis, (4) serum calcium concentrations greater than 11.0 mg/dl, and (5) the development of one or more "complications" of hyperparathyroidism, such as serious psychiatric disease, peptic ulcer resistant to treatment, pancreatitis, and severe hypertension. In any patient proposed for long-term follow-up, certain systematically applied follow-up studies should be done. At a minimum, these should include yearly history and physical examinations, serum calcium and creatinine clearance determinations, x-rays of the hand on fine-grain industrial film to detect subperiosteal bone resorption, and a plain film of the abdomen to check for renal calcifications. If inactive nephrolithiasis has been detected on initial examina-

tion, nephrotomograms should be done to determine if new stones or stone enlargement occurred. By definition, either of the latter would be interpreted as the recrudescence of active stone disease, which would in turn be an indication for surgery. Patients should also be warned that if they develop diarrhea or vomiting they should seek medical attention because dehydration could produce profound hypercalcemia.

The most critical consideration in the surgical treatment of patients with primary hyperparathyroidism is the selection of the parathyroid surgeon. He or she should not only have extensive experience in parathyroid surgery, and be able to distinguish between an abnormal and a normal parathyroid gland, but should also know the ectopic places where parathyroid tumors may be situated.

There are two common approaches to the actual surgery. The first, and most widely accepted, involves the identification of all 4 parathyroid glands (using biopsy if absolutely necessary), the removal of a single enlarged parathyroid gland or the removal of 3½ parathyroid glands if it is determined that multiple gland disease exists. In patients prone to recurrence, all remaining parathyroid glands or remnants should be marked with individual sutures or clips so as to make future identification of the parathyroid tissue easy if repeat surgery is necessary. The other, less commonly used, approach is first to explore only one side of the neck and remove any single enlarged parathyroid gland. The nature of this tissue should be confirmed by microscopic examination and oil-red-O staining. If the second parathyroid gland on the same side is normal by gross and microscopic examinations, exploration of the other side of the neck is not performed. If the second parathyroid gland is abnormal, the other side of the neck is explored and all abnormal parathyroid tissue removed except for one-half of the smallest gland or the gland most distantly situated from the recurrent laryngeal nerve. The second approach has the advantage of leaving the unoperated side without scar tissue and easier to explore at a future time for recurrent hyperparathyroidism. Persistent hyperparathyroidism, however, is more common because of failure to remove all the abnormal hypersecreting parathyroid glands. No matter which approach is taken, it is important for the surgeon to make meticulous and absolutely accurate records of the number and location of glands identified and removed. This information, along with histologic confirmation of the removed parathyroid glands, is essential in assessing the possible locations of missed parathyroid lesions in patients with persistent or less frequently recurrent hyperparathyroidism.

Parathyroid autotransplantation to the muscles of the forearm is a recognized procedure of considerable value in special circumstances. This is particularly true of the situation in which the last known parathyroid gland is removed because of recurrent or persistent primary hyperparathyroidism. The chances are reasonably good that such patients will be rendered hypoparathyroid or aparathyroid without successful transplantation. The functioning of such transplants can be easily assessed by measuring serum parathyroid hormone in venous blood from both forearms. A step-up in the concentration of serum iPTH from the nontransplanted to transplanted forearms is indicative of a functioning graft. Cryopreservation of the abnormal parathyroid tissue is also a very helpful procedure in these patients, because if the patient does not develop hypoparathyroidism, transplantation of this abnormal parathyroid tissue is not necessary.

Approximately 20 percent of abnormal parathyroid glands are present in the mediastinum. However, 95 percent of these are in the superior part of the cavity attached to the thymus or mediastinal fat pad. These abnormal glands are readily identified and removed during routine neck exploration by mobilizing and removing the thymus and perithymic tissues as well as tissues from the posterior mediastinum. Since the blood supply is from the neck, there is little danger of hemorrhage. The remaining 5 percent of all abnormal parathyroid tissue is located elsewhere in the mediastinum and can be approached for excision only by a sternal splitting procedure. Median sternotomy is not recommended at the intial operation unless the patient has profound hypercalcemia (calcium > 14.0 mg/dl). Before the advent of localization procedures (see above), the success rate in removing mediastinal abnormal parathyroid tissue was only 50 percent. The decision to carry out mediastinal exploration depends to a great extent on the accuracy and completeness of the information obtained during initial neck exploration. If the previous exploration was inadequate or the records are incomplete, repeat neck surgery is almost always indicated. The only exception is when four normal parathyroids are identified in the neck. An elusive parathyroid gland is then usually in the mediastinum. Virtually all studies of patients with persistent or recurrent hyperparathyroidism reveal that repeat neck exploration is successful in 80 percent of cases.

Postoperatively, serum calcium concentrations decrease to within the normal range or below within 24 to 48 hours. It is possible to determine if all of the abnormal parathyroid tissue has been removed by measuring decreased urinary phosphate or cyclic AMP within 2 hours of parathyroidectomy. Patients who have significant bony demineralization with osteitis fibrosa cystica and elevated blood alkaline phosphatase levels may develop rather severe degrees of hypocalcemia postoperatively. This is presumably caused by the avidity of demineralized bone for extracellular fluid calcium. It is called the "hungry bone syndrome," and it can be distinguished from the development of hypoparathyroidism by the absence of hyperphosphatemia and the presence of increased concentrations of serum iPTH. Treatment of this problem may be difficult and requires very large quantities of intravenous calcium given continuously by infusion (as much as 5–10 gm elemental per day) and administration of calcium carbonate by mouth in doses of 1–5 gm per day depending upon the serum calcium response. Administration of the biologically active metabolite of vitamin D, $1,25\text{-}(OH)_2\text{-}D_3$ (Calcitriol, 0.25 µg once or twice daily) may provide an additional effective therapeutic agent.

Most patients who develop hypocalcemia and mild hyperphosphatemia have temporary hypoparathyroidism as evidenced by low normal serum iPTH. A very small percentage (<1.0 percent) of these patients will develop permanent hypoparathyroidism requiring treatment.

Other complications that may occur in the postoperative period include worsening of renal function (either temporary or permanent), metabolic acidosis, hypomagnesemia, pancreatitis, and gout or pseudogout. The problem of deterioration in renal function should be anticipated in patients who have abnormal renal function preoperatively, and preoperative hydration or prophylactic mannitol infusions given early in the postoperative period to initiate an osmotic diuresis are helpful. Likewise, a flaring of gout or pseudogout should be anticipated in patients with intra-articular calcification or a history of prior arthritic attacks.

Primary hyperparathyroidism is a common, often subtle, endocrine disease that is frequently discovered by routine determinations of serum calcium concentrations. Although surgery is an effective treatment for this disease, more studies are needed for us to learn how to select patients who will benefit most from parathyroidectomy.

RENAL OSTEODYSTROPHY

SHAUL G. MASSRY, M.D.
and ELAINE M. KAPTEIN, M.D.

Disturbances in divalent ion metabolism are common in patients with renal failure. The major features of these abnormalities are listed in Table 1. The processes causing disordered divalent ion metabolism and osteodystrophy begin in the early stages of renal insufficiency, continue throughout the life of the patient, and may be influenced beneficially or adversely by various therapeutic approaches employed.

The goals of the therapy of these disorders are (1) to maintain the blood concentrations of calcium and phosphorus as near normal as possible; (2) to prevent the development of secondary hyperparathyroidism, and, if the latter already exists, to suppress the activity of the parathyroid glands; (3) to prevent and reverse soft tissue calcification; and (4) to ameliorate or reverse the proximal myopathy, bone pain, pruritus, and soft tissue necrosis.

Despite our increased knowledge of the pathogenesis of the deranged divalent ion metabolism in patients with renal failure, there is still no unified approach to optimal therapy. The various therapeutic modalities currently in use are neither completely effective nor without hazards. The overall management includes the use of one or more of the following therapeutic approaches: (1) control of phosphate retention and hyperphosphatemia, (2) supplementation of calcium, (3) treatment with vitamin D or one or more of its metabolites, (4) parathyroidectomy, and (5) appropriate dialysate composition in the dialysis patients.

CONTROL OF PHOSPHATE RETENTION AND HYPERPHOSPHATEMIA

Phosphate retention and hyperphosphatemia play an important role in the pathogenesis of the disorders of divalent ion metabolism of renal failure. The prevention of phosphate retention in patients with mild or moderate renal insufficiency

TABLE 1 Major Features of Disordered Divalent Ion Metabolism in Renal Failure

Hyperphosphatemia
Hypocalcemia
Elevated serum levels of alkaline phosphatase
Secondary hyperparathyroidism
Defective intestinal absorption of calcium and phosphate
Altered vitamin D metabolism resulting in relative or absolute deficiency of 1,25 dihydroxyvitamin D
Bone disease
  Enhanced bone resorption
  Increased endosteal fibrosis
  Defective mineralization (rickets or osteomalacia)
Soft tissue calcification
  Vascular
  Visceral
  Periarticular
  Cutaneous
  Ocular
Alterations in renal handling of phosphate (increased fractional excretion), calcium (hypocalciuria), and magnesium (increased fractional excretion)
Pruritus
Proximal myopathy
Skin ulcerations and soft tissue necrosis

and the control of hyperphosphatemia in those with advanced renal failure are major factors in the management of these patients. The hyperphosphatemia of uremia may be reduced by dietary restriction of phosphate, the use of phosphate binding antacids, increased frequency of hemodialysis, and by the inhibition of parathormone (PTH)-mediated bone resorption.

The dietary intake of phosphate is a function of the meat and dairy products ingested by the patient. The usual phosphate intake by a normal adult in the United States ranges between 1.0 and 1.8 gm per day. One can reduce dietary intake of phosphate by 40 percent (600–900 gm per day) by the elimination of dairy products and the restriction of protein intake. Further reduction may be difficult to achieve without jeopardizing adequate protein intake or compromising the palatability of the food. Thus restriction of dietary phosphate intake in proportion to the decrease in glomerular filtration rate (GFR) as the sole measure for the prevention of phosphate retention is feasible only in patients with moderate renal failure (GFR 60–30 ml/min). Indeed, this approach has been successful in reversing many of the abnormalities in divalent ion metabolism in such patients.

In patients with advanced renal failure, dietary phosphate restriction alone is not adequate to control the hyperphosphatemia. In a group of patients with creatinine clearances of 2 to 10 ml/min who were treated with rigid protein restriction

TABLE 2   Partial List of Available Phosphate Binding Compounds

Generic Name	Proprietary Name	Manufacturer	Form Available
Aluminum hydroxide gel	Amphogel	Wyeth	Tablets (0.3 and 0.6 gm)
Aluminum hydroxide gel	Alu-Cap	Ricker	Capsules (0.6 gm)
Aluminum carbonate	Basaljel	Wyeth	Solution (3.6 gm/30 ml) Tablets (0.5 gm) Capsules (0.5 gm)
Aluminum hydroxide and magnesium hydroxide	Aludrox	Wyeth	Tablets
Aluminum hydroxide and magnesium hydroxide	Maalox	Rorer	Tablets
Aluminum hydroxide, magnesium hydroxide, and simethicone	Gelusil	Parke-Davis	Tablets
Aluminum hydroxide, magnesium hydroxide, and simethicone	Mylanta	Stuart	Tablets

(20 or 40 gm per day) for 30 to 60 days, serum phosphorus levels remained elevated, with mean levels of 7.2 ± 0.86 and 7.3 ± 0.72 mg/dl respectively, despite continued negative phosphorus balance in some of the patients. It is evident that in patients with advanced renal failure other measures are needed to maintain serum phosphorus levels within the normal range. This could be achieved with the use of phosphate binding antacids, which would render the ingested phosphate and the phosphate contained in the saliva (12 mmol/l), bile (5 mmol/l), and intestinal juices (1 mmol/l) unabsorbable.

Several compounds that bind phosphate in the intestinal tract are available in liquid, tablet, and capsule forms (Table 2). The capsules are less effective than liquid gels in binding phosphate, but patient compliance is easier to achieve with capsules than with either the liquid or the tablets. The most frequently used compounds are Alucaps, Amphogel, and Basaljel concentrate. The latter is tasteless and only a small volume is necessary per dose; hence the patients more readily follow the prescribed regimen. The goal of treatment is to reduce the level of serum phosphorus to near normal. Care should be exercised to avoid both a fall in serum phosphorus to a very low level and phosphate depletion with these agents. Phosphate depletion per se may aggravate bone disease and even cause osteomalacia. Therapy may be started with 2 to 3 tablets of Amphogel or capsules of Alucaps, or 5 to 10 ml of Basaljel with each meal. The levels of serum phosphorus should be monitored at least twice per month and the dosage of the phosphate binders adjusted accordingly. Continued coaxing and emphasis on the importance of this treatment are essential to obtain adherence to this therapy by the patients. These compounds are ineffective in controlling the concentration of serum phosphorus if phosphate intake exceeds 2.0 gm per day.

The fall in serum phosphorus concentration during therapy with dietary phosphate restriction and the use of phosphate binding antacids is usually associated with a rise in the level of serum calcium; if the magnitude of the latter is adequate, a fall in the blood levels of PTH may occur, and this in turn will contribute to the maintenance of the concentration of serum phosphorus at lower levels.

The aluminum in the phosphate binding antacids is absorbed by the intestine and may accumulate in various tissues of the body, such as brain and bone. Increased aluminum burden of the brain has been incriminated in the pathogenesis of dialysis encephalopathy, and accumulation of aluminum in bone may be responsible for the low turnover osteomalacia that is refractory to therapy. Despite these potential hazards, these compounds are still recommended to control hyperphosphatemia in patients with advanced renal failure and in dialysis patients. The use of magnesium containing compounds should be avoided because of the risks of hypermagnesemia.

CALCIUM SUPPLEMENTATION

The low dietary intake of calcium and the defect in intestinal calcium absorption which is more evident at low intake put the patients with renal failure in double jeopardy regarding their calcium metabolism. Evidence exists indicating that normal amounts of calcium could be absorbed by the gut of these patients when their calcium intake is high. Indeed, long-term calcium supplementation has been associated with beneficial effects, such as a rise in the concentration of serum calcium, a fall in the serum levels of alkaline phosphatase and PTH, and a reduction in bone resorption and the number and incidence of fractures; such therapy, however, did not result in normal mineralization of osteoid. Thus there is a good rationale for calcium supplementation, but the time in the course of renal insufficiency at which such therapy should be initiated is not clear. It is reasonable to suggest that patients with GFRs between 40 and 10 ml/min should receive 1.2–1.5 gm of elemental calcium per day. Calcium supplements may be given to these patients to bring their total daily intake to this level. Patients with advanced renal failure (GFR<10 ml/min) may need a supplement of 1.0–2.0 gm of calcium per day.

Treatment with calcium salts is not without hazards. It is dangerous to administer large quantities of oral calcium compounds in the face of marked hyperphosphatemia because of the danger of an elevation in calcium-phosphorus product, which predisposes to soft tissue calcification. It is thus imperative that hyperphosphatemia be controlled and the level of serum phosphorus be less than 5.5 mg/dl prior to treatment with calcium salts. Hypercalcemia may also appear during therapy with large doses of oral calcium, especially in patients with advanced renal failure; this is particularly true when there has been a concomitant reduction in the levels of serum phosphorus to less than 2.0 mg/dl. A variety of symptoms may accompany even mild hypercalcemia in uremic patients. Nausea, vomiting, mental confusion, lethargy, pruritus, dysesthesias, and severe hypertension have been encountered. Therefore, weekly or bimonthly monitoring of the concentration of serum calcium and phosphorus is advisable. If the serum concentration of calcium exceeds 10.5 mg/dl, calcium supplements may be cut in half or may even be discontinued temporarily.

Elemental calcium constitutes 40 percent of calcium carbonate, 12 percent of calcium lactate, and 8 percent of calcium gluconate. Calcium chloride should be avoided in uremic patients because of its acidifying properties. Calcium carbonate is inexpensive, tasteless, and relatively well tolerated. Calcium carbonate is available in several proprietary preparations, such as Titralac, Tums, or Oscal. Titralac provides 0.42 gm of calcium carbonate and 0.18 gm of glycine per tablet (160 mg of elemental calcium per tablet). Neo-Calglucon syrup is another preparation well accepted by patients, but it is costly; each 4 ml contains 92 mg of calcium ion. To maximize calcium absorption, the amount prescribed should be ingested in several small doses divided throughout the day rather than in one or two large doses.

USE OF VITAMIN D COMPOUNDS

Since many of the features of abnormal calcium metabolism in uremia resemble those of vitamin D deficiency, this compound and its related steroids have been used in the management of renal osteodystrophy. The forms of vitamin D metabolites currently available for clinical use in the United States are vitamin D_2 (ergocalciferol); vitamin D_3 (cholecalciferol), which is the naturally occurring form of the steroid in mammals; dihydrotachysterol (DHT); $25OHD_3$; and $1,25(OH)_2D_3$. Another vitamin D analogue, $1\alpha OHD_3$, is available for clinical use outside the United States.

Because of its low cost, vitamin D_2, a steroid obtained from plant sources, has been most widely used in medicine. Vitamin D_3 can now be prepared inexpensively but it does not enjoy widespread use. Moreover, there is little evidence to indicate that vitamin D_2 differs in activity from vitamin D_3 in man.

Vitamin D_2 and D_3

The amount of vitamin D required by patients with advanced renal failure varies greatly. Doses as high as 50,000–200,000 IU per day (1.25–5.0 mg) may be needed to achieve beneficial effects. Long-term therapy with large doses of vitamin D causes a rise in serum calcium level and may be followed by a fall in serum levels of alkaline phosphatase and PTH, reduced bone resorption, and amelioration or healing of rickets in uremic children or of osteomalacia in uremic adults. Because of the need for large doses of vitamin D, hypercalcemia is a real and frequent hazard. *Such hypercalcemia may persist for weeks* after the discontinuation of therapy. In addition to the clinical side effects of hypercalcemia, the elevation in the serum levels of calcium in a hyperphosphatemic patient would cause a marked rise in calcium-phosphorus product, predisposing to soft tissue calcification. Therapy with vitamin D should not be started prior to the normalization of the serum levels of phosphorus. Frequent monitoring of the levels of serum calcium and phosphorus during such therapy is advisable.

25 Hydroxyvitamin D_3

Despite the block in the conversion of 25OHD to $1,25(OH)_2D$, therapy with 50–100 μg of 25OHD$_3$ per day has been shown to be beneficial. Treatment with this metabolite was associated with amelioration of bone pain and proximal myopathy, a rise in serum calcium concentration, and a fall in serum levels of alkaline phosphatase and PTH. A decrease in the degree of osteitis fibrosa and even improvement in bone mineralization have been noted.

1,25 Dihydroxyvitamin D_3

A relative deficiency of this active metabolite exists in patients with mild and moderate renal failure, and absolute deficiency exists in those with advanced renal failure. Furthermore, the kidney is required to convert the parent vitamin D to this active metabolite. Therefore, it is rational to treat renal failure patients with this metabolite to correct the vitamin D deficient state. Indeed, such therapy has proven beneficial. It is important to emphasize at this point that some or most of the beneficial effects of $1,25(OH)_2D_3$ in the management of renal osteodystrophy could be produced by other vitamin D compounds. The smaller dose of $1,25(OH)_2D_3$ that is needed to achieve beneficial effects and its shorter half-life make it a better and safer agent than other vitamin D compounds. On the other hand, the high biologic potency of $1,25(OH)_2D_3$ is mandatory.

Dosage Schedule. The suggested initial dose is 0.5 μg per day, although it may be safer to begin therapy with 0.25 μg per day. Although the limited data suggest that 0.5 μg per day of $1,25(OH)_2D_3$ is beneficial and safe in patients with GFRs of 30–50 ml/min and normophosphatemia, it is possible that smaller or larger dosages may be required by patients with higher or lower GFRs, respectively. Caution should be exercised in the use of $1,25(OH)_2D_3$ in patients with GFRs less than 25 ml/min. These patients may be hyperphosphatemic, and a rise in blood calcium concentration in the presence of elevated blood phosphorus concentration would result in an increase in the calcium-phosphorus product to a hazardous level. In such an eventuality, calcium deposition

may occur in various tissues, including the renal parenchyma. The latter effect could be associated with deterioration in renal function.

The changes in the concentrations of serum calcium provide the best clinical guide for modification of the dosage. Failure of the level of serum calcium to rise by at least 0.5 mg/dl with any particular dosage given for 4 to 6 weeks justifies increasing the dose by 0.25 to 0.5 μg per day. Such an approach may be used until serum calcium level reaches the upper normal range (10.0–10.5 mg/dl). When this is achieved, frequent monitoring of serum calcium is needed, and if the latter approaches hypercalcemic range, a reduction of the dosage or temporary discontinuation of therapy should be considered. It is our experience and that of others that the requirement of and the tolerance for $1,25(OH)_2D_3$ may decrease progressively during treatment in many patients; therefore, reduction of the maintenance dosage after a prolonged period of therapy may be needed.

Effect on Serum Calcium. The most consistent effect of $1,25(OH)_2D_3$ in uremic and dialysis patients is the elevation in the serum concentration of calcium. Although it is reasonable to assume that the higher the dosage of the metabolite the greater the rise in serum calcium concentration, many variables in addition to the dosage may modify the calcemic response to therapy with $1,25(OH)_2D_3$. These may include duration of treatment, dietary calcium intake, changes in intestinal absorption of calcium, type of bone disease and its response to treatment, and the severity of the state of secondary hyperparathyroidism. Occasionally, serum calcium concentration may fall during the first one to two weeks of therapy, probably owing to rapid remineralization of the skeleton.

Hypercalcemia is a frequent complication of treatment with $1,25(OH)_2D_3$. It has been reported that 30 to 67 percent of the patients treated with this metabolite developed one or more hypercalcemic episodes during the course of their therapy. The overall incidence of one episode was 42 percent. Hypercalcemia occurred with a dosage of 0.5–3.0 μg per day of $1,25(OH)_2D_3$ and was more frequent with a dosage of 1.0–30 μg/day. Certain patients are more prone to develop hypercalcemia: (1) patients with osteitis fibrosa and pretreatment serum calcium concentration greater than 10.5 mg per day, and (2) patients with low turnover osteomalacia, low serum concentration of PTH, and absent bone marrow fibrosis. Hypercalcemia may appear at any time during therapy with $1,25(OH)_2D_3$. It usually occurs after 2 to 3 months of therapy but has been encountered as early as 5 days and as late as 6 to 18 months after treatment. A high starting dose may be the cause for the early appearance of hypercalcemia. In patients with severe osteitis fibrosa and pretreatment serum calcium concentration of 10.5 mg/dl, early hypercalcemia within one to four weeks of therapy may also occur. Extreme caution should be exercised in the management of such patients with $1,25(OH)_2D_3$. It has been noted that the incidence of hypercalcemia increases as serum alkaline phosphatase activity returns to normal, and it is recommended that the dose of $1,25(OH)_2D_3$ be reduced when serum levels of alkaline phosphatase normalize. The hypercalcemia is usually mild and asymptomatic, but serum calcium concentrations greater than 13.0 mg/dl and occasionally even higher than 15.0 mg/dl have been encountered during therapy with $1,25(OH)_2D_3$. The elevated levels of serum calcium usually return to normal shortly after reduction of the dose or discontinuation of therapy. The hypercalcemia may occasionally persist for several weeks. It is advisable to stop treatment completely rather than reduce the dose when hypercalcemia appears and reinstitute therapy with a small dose as serum calcium concentrations return to normal.

Effect on Serum Phosphorus. The effect of $1,25(OH)_2D_3$ treatment on the concentration of serum phosphorus in uremic or dialysis patients is not consistent. Increases, decreases, and no change have been reported. This variability among patient populations may be related to differences in dietary intake of phosphate and/or the ingestion of phosphate binding antacids, the dosage of $1,25(OH)_2D_3$, the effect of the metabolite on intestinal absorption of phosphate, the degree of suppression of the parathyroid gland activity, and the status of the remineralization of bone. Monitoring of serum phosphorus concentrations during therapy with $1,25(OH)_2D_3$ is mandatory because the development of hyperphosphatemia, especially in the face of rising serum calcium concentration, would result in elevation of calcium-phosphorus product and augment the hazards of soft tissue calcification. If hyperphosphatemia occurs and calcium-phosphorus product approaches 55, every effort should be made to control the levels of serum phosphorus with phosphate binding antacids. If this procedure is not successful, the dose of $1,25(OH)_2D_3$ should be reduced or temporary cessation of therapy should be considered. Under no circumstances should the calcium-phosphorus product be allowed to exceed 55.

Effect on Alkaline Phosphatase, PTH, and Calcium Absorption. Serum alkaline phosphatase activity usually decreases during therapy with $1,25(OH)_2D_3$, but several months may elapse before levels return to normal. Occasionally, serum alkaline phosphatase may rise during the critical phase of therapy. Monitoring the serum alkaline phosphatase could provide an additional guide for the adjustment of the dosage of $1,25(OH)_2D_3$ for two reasons. First, normalization of serum levels of alkaline phosphatase reflects improvement in bone disease, and second, the occurrence of hypercalcemia increases as serum alkaline phosphatase returns to normal.

Long-term therapy with $1,25(OH)_2D_3$ may be associated with a marked fall in or even normalization of the serum levels of PTH. No change, or even an increase in serum levels of the hormone has also been encountered during therapy with this metabolite. The reduction in the serum levels of PTH during therapy with $1,25(OH)_2D_3$ is probably due to the rise in the concentration of serum calcium. We have found an inverse correlation between the percentage change in serum calcium concentrations and PTH levels.

Intestinal absorption of calcium is usually increased in uremic patients during therapy with $1,25(OH)_2D_3$. The increment in calcium absorption is most evident during the first 2 hours after calcium ingestion, which suggests that the metabolite exerts its effect in the duodenum and proximal part of the small intestine. This metabolite may also affect calcium absorption in the jejunum, since this segment of the intestine has receptors for $1,25(OH)_2D_3$. There is a dose-response relationship between $1,25(OH)_2D_3$ and intestinal absorption of calcium. Finally, the quantity of the sterol required to elicit an increase in intestinal calcium absorption in the uremic patients is greater than in normal subjects, which indicates that uremia, per se, may interfere with the action of the sterol on the gut. $1,25(OH)_2D_3$ also augments intestinal absorption of phosphate. The metabolite may produce a modest rise in urinary calcium in uremic patients.

Clinical Response. Among the most disturbing clinical symptoms of renal osteodystrophy are muscle weakness and bone pain. The muscle weakness is a clinical manifestation of uremic myopathy which is probably due to vitamin D deficiency. The exact cause of bone pain is not known but may be related to the presence of osteomalacia, osteitis fibrosa, or both. These disturbances may interfere seriously with the daily activity of the patients and may even render them totally disabled. Improvement in these symptoms appears rapidly after initiation of therapy with $1,25(OH)_2D_3$. The improvement in muscle strength may become noticeable within two to five weeks of treatment. A significant amelioration or complete disappearance of bone pain may also occur in some patients within 1 to 3 weeks of treatment, while in others it may take 6 to 28 weeks before a decrease in bone pain becomes evident. This clinical improvement produces a remarkable change in the physical disability of the patients; many of them become symptom free and are able to perform their daily activity without limitation (Fig. 1). Similar observations have been made in children. For example, three children who had ceased to walk for several months prior to therapy began walking within one month and were running after four months of treatment. Treatment of uremic children with $1,25(OH)_2D_3$ may also increase growth velocity; this effect is extremely important, since retarded growth in uremic children is a very common and serious problem.

Therapy with $1,25(OH)_2D_3$ for several months can be associated with a decrease in bone resorption, and treatment for two to three years may result in complete healing of bone resorption.

The effect on bone resorption reflects the degree of success in suppressing the activity of the parathyroid glands. Endosteal fibrosis is either markedly reduced or completely reversed after several months of treatment irrespective of whether serum levels of PTH are decreased or not. This observation raises the possibility that endosteal fibrosis is not entirely the result of excess PTH but could also be related to vitamin D deficiency as well. The osteomalacia in patients with mixed bone disease (osteomalacia and osteitis fibrosa) responds well to therapy with $1,25(OH)_2D_3$. Long-term treatment usually results in marked improvement or healing of the osteomalacia. In patients with pure low turnover osteomalacia, the response to $1,25(OH)_2D_3$ is poor; these patients may respond better to long-term therapy (4 to 6 months) with both $1,25(OH)_2D_3$ and $24,25(OH)_2D_3$ (2.5–10 µg per day). The healing of the bone lesions during treatment with $1,25(OH)_2D_3$ may also be evidenced by improvement in the radiographic findings of the skeleton.

Failure of therapy with $1,25(OH)_2D_3$ to improve clinical signs and symptoms has been reported. The treatment-failure group appears to be heterogeneous and does not display a specific biochemical pattern of bone disease. Although such patients had higher serum calcium concentration than those who responded to treatment, the serum levels of PTH were normal, moderately elevated, or very high, and the bone lesions varied from pure osteomalacia in some to marked osteitis fibrosa in others. Further analysis of the data, however, indicates that there are two distinct subgroups among these patients. The first group consists of patients with severe osteitis fibrosa and marked elevation of serum PTH. In the second group, the patients had normal serum levels of PTH and pure osteomalacia without evidence of hyperparathyroid bone disease. Both of these groups rapidly developed hypercalcemia. As this complication requires cessation of treatment, it would preclude long-term therapy and result in failure to improve the clinical and histologic abnormalities of renal osteodystrophy.

Effect on Renal Function. Data on the effect of $1,25(OH)_2D_3$ on the derangements of divalent ion metabolism in patients with moderate renal failure are limited. Treatment of patients with GFR of 32 to 51 ml/min with 0.5 µg per day of $1,25(OH)_2D_3$ for 6 months raised serum calcium levels, reversed the defect in intestinal calcium absorption, normalized the serum levels of PTH, and healed the bone disease. These observations

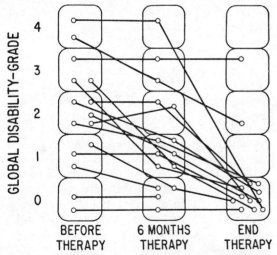

Figure 1 Global disability scoring of the patients before and during therapy with $1,25(OH)_2D_3$. Grade 4, totally disabled, restricted to bed or wheelchair; grade 3, marked disability, pain or weakness restricts activity, walks with aid; grade 2, symptoms reduce activity moderately, walks with aid; grade 1, symptoms only with strenuous activity; grade 0, asymptomatic and no activity restriction. (Reprinted with permission from Goldstein DA, Malluche HH, Massry SG: Management of renal osteodystrophy with $1,25(OH)_2D_3$. Min Elect Metab 2:35, 1979)

suggest that initiation of therapy with $1,25(OH)_2D_3$ early in the course of renal failure could be beneficial for the prevention of the progression of renal osteodystrophy. Such an approach could be justified, however, if treatment with this metabolite has no harmful effect on renal function.

Theoretically, a deleterious effect of $1,25(OH)_2D_3$ on renal function could be caused by action of the metabolite on the structure or function of the kidneys or by other metabolic consequences of the treatment, such as hypercalcemia. It has been claimed that the administration of $1,25(OH)_2D_3$ to patients with moderate renal failure produced a significant reduction in GFR due to direct adverse effect. Analysis of all available and pertinent data does not support the contention that $1,25(OH)_2D_3$ has a direct deleterious effect on renal function. The metabolite could produce a reversible or permanent fall in GFR, however, if sustained hypercalcemia develops during its administration. The use of the proper dosage, the frequent monitoring of serum calcium and creatinine concentrations, and the discontinuation of therapy as hypercalcemia develops are the precautionary measures that should be followed to reduce the likelihood of a harmful effect on renal function.

DIALYSATE AND ITS COMPOSITION

There is evidence for numerous geographic variations in the incidence of skeletal disease in patients undergoing hemodialysis. Various impurities and trace elements, such as fluoride or aluminum, may be responsible for these variations. It is now accepted that water treatment and purification should be employed prior to the preparation of the dialysate.

Variations in the concentration of calcium in dialysate may affect the course of renal osteodystrophy. It should be emphasized that all the calcium present in dialysate is ionized and diffuses freely across the membrane of the dialyzer. This contrasts to calcium in blood; only 60 percent of the total amount is not bound to protein and is able to move across the membrane. Depending upon the gradient, the dialysate calcium level, and the concentration of diffusible calcium in blood, there will be either a loss or a gain of this ion by the patient. The use of dialysate containing 5.0–5.5 mg of calcium/dl is associated with a high incidence of radiographic evidence of bone disease, progressively rising serum levels of alkaline phosphatase, loss of calcium from bones, and persis-

tently elevated serum levels of PTH. For these reasons, dialysate containing such a low concentration of calcium should be abandoned. The use of dialysate containing 8.0 mg of calcium/dl may be hazardous in that it may cause hypercalcemia and enhance soft tissue calcification. Most authorities recommend a calcium concentration of 7.0 mg/dl.

Most centers have used dialysate containing magnesium in a concentration varying between 0.6 and 1.8 mg/dl (0.5–1.5 mEq/l). With the lower dialysate magnesium concentration, predialysis levels of magnesium are usually normal and are slightly below normal immediately after dialysis. Patients treated with dialysate containing the higher concentration of magnesium have moderate hypermagnesemia all the time. There is no evidence that variations in dialysate magnesium concentration *within this range* have an effect on the incidence, course, or severity of skeletal disease, soft tissue calcification, or symptoms related to altered divalent ion metabolism.

PARATHYROIDECTOMY

The various medical therapeutic modalities detailed earlier can result in suppression of the hyperplastic parathyroid glands in uremic patients. However, these measures may not be successful and parathyroidectomy may be the only way to treat the clinical, biochemical, and skeletal manifestations of secondary hyperparathyroidism. Subtotal parathyroidectomy should be considered (1) when persistent hypercalcemia develops; (2) when severe intractable pruritus unresponsive to dialysis is present, especially when the blood levels of PTH are markedly elevated; (3) when marked soft tissue calcification (especially vascular) and radiographic evidence of marked osteitis fibrosa are present, and they cannot be adequately controlled with conservative therapy; and (4) when ischemic lesions of soft tissue with ulcerations and necrosis develop.

The amount of parathyroid tissue to be removed at surgery depends on the size of the parathyroid glands in any particular patient. We recommend that all four glands be first identified; three glands are then removed and weighed. By comparing the size of the fourth gland with those removed, one can roughly estimate the weight of the fourth gland. The surgeon should leave only 150 to 200 mg of this remaining gland. Since the residual parathyroid tissue may undergo further hyperplasia and a second operation may be required, it is recommended that the residual tissue be marked by a metal clip and a long black silk suture. An alterative approach is to remove all four glands and transplant part of a gland in the forearm. If fewer than four glands are identified in the neck, they should all be removed. Rarely, removal of three identified glands will result in a state of permanent hypoparathyroidism. Total parathyroidectomy may be considered in patients who will be maintained with hemodialysis and are not candidates for renal transplantation. The medical and/or surgical treatment of uremic secondary hyperparathyroidism assumes greater significance with the accumulation of evidence indicating that excess PTH in blood may play a major role in uremic toxicity.

The technical problems during the surgical procedure are few. The glands are grossly enlarged and easily identifiable. In the hands of an experienced surgeon the operation is not hazardous, and the patient leaves the hospital within a week. The patients should be treated with dialysis one day prior to surgery.

A major problem during the postoperative period is the control of serum calcium concentration. Its level invariably falls after the removal of three or more parathyroid glands. The magnitude and duration of the hypocalcemia vary from one patient to another. Those with marked periarticular calcification usually maintain the serum levels of calcium between 8.0 and 9.0 mg/dl until the ectopic calcifications disappear. Also, the use of dialysate containing 7.0 mg of calcium/dl causes a rise in serum calcium concentration during dialysis and may alleviate the hypocalcemia during the interdialytic intervals. Profound hypocalcemia may develop in certain patients, especially those with radiographic evidence of bone resorption; treatment of such patients with $1,25(OH)_2D_3$ may reduce the severity of the postoperative hypocalcemia. Tetany may occur in those who develop severe hypocalcemia. When the level of serum calcium falls below 7.5 mg/dl, oral calcium supplementation may prevent a further decrease. The amount of oral calcium needed is usually quite large. The initial treatment should provide at least 2.0 gm of calcium and the dose can be increased at intervals of 3 to 7 days until adequate rise in serum calcium concentration is achieved. If the concentration of serum calcium falls to lower levels and if tetany appears, intravenous calcium should be given in addition to the oral supplements of calcium. In patients with profound and sustained hypocalcemia, $1,25(OH)_2D_3$ may be needed; careful monitoring of serum calcium and phosphorus levels should be undertaken with this therapy. Serum levels of phosphorus almost always fall after parathyroidectomy. Therefore, phosphate binding antacids should be withheld if serum levels of phosphorus decrease to less than 3.0 mg/dl. Also, serum levels of phosphorus should not be allowed to rise above 4.0 mg/dl, because the hyperphosphatemia may aggravate the hypocalcemia in the parathyroidectomized patients.

OTHER THERAPEUTIC MEASURES

The use of beta-adrenergic blocking agents (such as propranolol) may cause a decrease in the serum levels of PTH, but this action is variable and does not completely reverse secondary hyperparathyroidism. Claims that cimetidine may be effective in controlling secondary hyperparathyroidism in uremic patients have not been convincingly substantiated. Occasionally, treatment with diphosphonate (disodium-ethane-1-hydroxy-1, 1-diphosphonate, or DHDP) may cause regression of ectopic calcification resistant to the usual therapy (control of the hyperphosphatemia, suppression of parathyroid gland activity, or parathyroidectomy). Treatment with DHDP by itself may produce osteomalacia.

PARATHYROID CARCINOMA

EUGENE W. FRIEDMAN, M.D.
and ARTHUR E. SCHWARTZ, M.D.

Carcinoma arising in a parathyroid gland is a rare condition. The incidence of primary hyperparathyroidism due to benign adenomas or hyperplasia of the glands is 1 in 1000, which is higher than previously realized; however, no more than 100 primary carcinomas of the parathyroid are recorded, and most reports represent collected series. The incidence is cited as .5 to 4 percent of cases of hyperparathyroidism.

Hyperparathyroidism resulting from benign neoplasms predominantly afflicts females by a factor of 2 or 3 to 1; most reported cases of primary parathyroid carcinoma are evenly distributed between the sexes. We have encountered 7 patients with primary parathyroid carcinoma among 405 patients operated upon for hyperparathyroidism (1.7 percent). Five of these were women.

CLINICAL PRESENTATION

We have treated 7 patients with parathyroid carcinoma. In almost every instance parathyroid carcinoma presented as the metabolic effect of the oversecretion of parathormone. Hypercalcemia is the hallmark of the condition, with bone disease, kidney stones, and parenchymal renal disease occurring in proportion to the severity and length of hyperfunction. Duodenal ulcers, episodes of acute pancreatitis, and mental aberrations were also seen during the course of the disease.

A serum calcium or PTH level higher than those usually seen with adenomas or hyperplasia is usually a feature and may provide a clue that one is not dealing with a benign condition. Parathyroid carcinoma has been associated with serum calcium levels of over 13 mg/dl in most reports. Serum calcium levels in our 6 patients with functioning parathyroid carcinoma ranged from 13 to 20 mg/dl, with an average of 15.2 mg/dl.

A palpable neck mass in the presence of hypercalcemia is often the harbinger of a parathyroid cancer. Whereas it is most unusual to palpate a benign parathyroid adenoma preoperatively (we were able to do so in only 6 percent of our first 112 cases), most observers find a mass in 50 percent of patients with parathyroid carcinomas. The presence of a neck mass was a presenting feature in six of our seven patients, even though two of the tumors were diagnosed as benign adenomas originally and were recognized as malignancies only after they recurred.

FUNCTIONING AND NONFUNCTIONING CARCINOMA

It is extremely difficult to confirm a diagnosis of parathyroid carcinoma without hyperfunction because of the microscopic similarity to tumors of lung, kidney, and thymus. Only a few nonfunctioning parathyroid carcinomas have been reported, but it is reasonable to assume they exist, because other endocrine glands are known to give rise to nonfunctioning tumors. We have one such patient who has never had hypercalcemia or elevated serum PTH levels; however, histologic studies displayed the characteristic clear and oxyphilic cells of parathyroid carcinoma, and metastatic deposits were present in several adjacent lymph nodes.

DIFFERENTIATION OF ADENOMA FROM CARCINOMA

The differentiation of parathyroid adenoma from carcinoma on the basis of microscopic features can be difficult. Abnormal nuclei, cellular atypia, mitoses, and even capsular or blood vessel invasion are not necessarily diagnostic of cancer. As in other endocrine tumors, the criteria for malignancy have been difficult to establish. It is the direct invasion of adjacent structures and metastases to lymph nodes or viscera which confirm the diagnosis.

We are following 3 patients who presented with serum calcium levels of 13.0, 12.5, and 13.1 mg/dl, had parathyroid over 2.5 cm in diameter resected, and in whom specimens showed abnormal features, including bizarre and abnormal nuclear structure with mitoses. These patients remain well and normacalcemic one, four and nine years following surgery, and although the association of large masses and elevated serum calcium levels seemed to indicate malignancy, they are assumed to have had atypical benign adenomas.

The remarkable growth potential of benign parathyroid adenomas and hyperplastic tissue has become apparent in recent years. These tissues, transplanted into the forearm to maintain a normal serum calcium level following total parathyroidectomy, have sometimes shown aggressive local growth and hypercalcemia requiring successive re-excisions; normal parathyroid glands, when transplanted, have not shown this potential. However, there is no convincing evidence that parathyroid carcinomas arise from benign adenomas, or areas of hyperplasia.

FINDINGS AT SURGERY

In almost every case, neck exploration is undertaken with the expectation of finding a benign adenoma or hyperplasia. It is at the operating table that the diagnosis can often be made on the basis of gross findings. In four of our patients, the diagnosis was established at exploration and confirmed by frozen section examination. In another patient the diagnosis was suspected at surgery, and a definitive operative procedure was undertaken even though the frozen section was reported to be "atypical adenoma."

Classically, in parathyroid malignancy, instead of encountering the soft, reddish-brown, smooth-walled mass of a benign adenoma that can easily be dissected free of its adjacent structures, the surgeon is faced with a firm, fibrotic capsule that is adherent to, or invades adjacent structures such as the thyroid lobe, strap muscles, esophagus, carotid vessels or paratracheal tissues and lymph nodes. Less frequently, the diagnosis may not be readily apparent; what appears to be a benign adenoma may be removed, not recognized as a cancer on pathologic examination, only to reveal its true nature later in the form of a recurring mass associated with hypercalcemia. In two of our patients the original parathyroid tumors were reported to be large benign adenomas. These diagnoses were revised to carcinoma eight months and two years later, when recurrent infiltrating masses and hypercalcemia ensued. In retrospect, the large size of the tumors and the marked hypercalcemia were indications of the true nature of the neoplasms. Fortunately, it is often possible to recognize or strongly suspect malignancy at the initial procedure; this offers the surgeon the only real opportunity to resect the lesion completely. There are few, if any, patients who have been cured of recurrent parathyroid cancer. The first exploration offers the surgeon the best chance for a bloc excision, which requires excision of strap muscles if adherent to tumor, resection of the thyroid lobe and isthmus, and clearing of the trachea. Although a 30 percent incidence of neck node metastases is reported, this usually occurs late. Removal of lymph nodes in the tracheoesophageal groove and along the course of the recurrent nerve by an ipsilateral paratracheal dissection as well as resection of the upper mediastinal lymph nodes through the neck incision is advisable at the initial exploration; lateral neck dissection is not usually performed unless metastatic nodes are found.

The statement has been made that all parathyroid carcinomas originate in the lower glands. Although four of our malignancies could be identified as arising in these glands, in three other cases the tumors were either so large or presented in such an indeterminate position that their origin could not be identified. Benign adenomas, in our experience, arise twice as frequently in lower glands as in the upper ones.

COURSE OF DISEASE

Almost all parathyroid carcinomas consist of functioning tissue. The lethal effect of recurrent parathyroid cancer is not due to the invasion of vital structures or to the massive destruction of parenchymal tissues; as in most patients with functioning endocrine tumors, it is the result of uncontrolled hormone overproduction. The cause of death is most often kidney failure from the effects of renal calcinosis. Fatal pancreatitis may also occur. The patient is subjected to the long-term debilitating effect of hypercalcemia on the cardiovascular and musculoskeletal systems. Cardiac arrhythmia is a frequent terminal event. Thus, though cure of the malignancy may not always be possible, the resection of enough functional tumor tissue to reduce the metabolic effects of hyperparathyroidism will help prolong life.

Rates of five-year survival without evidence of disease are reported in the 30 percent range. Although only 8 to 10 percent of patients live beyond 5 years in the presence of recurrent malignancy, and the average length of survival in those who do succumb is only 3 to 4 years, there have been occasional reports of such patients surviving up to 19 years. We have no five-year survivors free of disease, but two of our seven patients remain free of disease two years, three months and three years, eight months after surgery. One patient remains alive with disease nine years after the original surgery.

Local recurrence appears in 30 percent of patients. Metastases to regional lymph nodes or distant organs occur in one-third to one-half of the patients, but the malignancy progresses slowly and metastases appear late in the disease. Widespread systemic involvement is unusual. The lungs, with a 25 percent incidence of involvement, are the most common site of visceral involvement; metastases to neck nodes are ultimately found in 30 percent of patients. Liver and bones are less frequent sites of metastatic dissemination.

MANAGEMENT OF RECURRENT DISEASE

Hypercalcemia associated with elevated serum parathormone levels heralds the recurrence of parathyroid carcinoma. Failure of serum calcium to fall to normal levels postoperatively indicates that tumor has not been completely removed or that metastases are present. Tomograms of the chest and CT scans of the thorax and abdomen may offer some help in localizing the tumor, but without a palpable mass, identification of the site of recurrent disease can be a frustrating problem that may not be readily solved.

Local recurrence of tumor requires re-exploration with an aggressive effort to remove disease widely; if the recurrence is systemic, the decision to resect is more difficult and is best resolved on the basis of whether enough tumor can be safely removed to control hypercalcemia.

The life-threatening aspect of parathyroid carcinoma is usually related to endocrine hyperfunction rather than infiltration from the tumor. It therefore shows good judgment to remove recurrent neoplasm whenever this can be done. There are many reports of successive excisions of recurrent parathyroid carcinoma for control of hypercalcemia which have afforded excellent palliation and extension of life. Resections of localized pulmonary metastases have provided substantial symptomatic relief. The slow growth pattern of parathyroid malignancy facilitates this approach. In one patient, temporary control of hypercalcemia was achieved in spite of the inability to remove recurrent tumor completely. Four successive reoperations have controlled hypercalcemia in another patient, enabling her to remain relatively well with recurrent carcinoma and mild hypercalcemia nine years after the original surgery. The therapeutic value of reoperation for parathyroid cancer can realistically encompass only palliation; permanent cure of recurrent or metastatic parathyroid carcinoma has almost never been achieved. Chemotherapy and radiotherapy have not been found to be effective in controlling parathyroid malignancy.

Since hypercalcemia is mainly responsible for the toxic effect of parathyroid malignancy, agents that lower serum calcium levels can be of great value. Mithramycin, oral phosphates, and thyrocalcitonin are useful on a short-term basis, particularly in preparing a patient for surgery, but none has been helpful in the long-term control of hypercalcemia. As in the case of a functioning adenoma or hyperplasia, only surgical resection of the hyperfunctioning tissue has proved of lasting value in lowering the serum calcium level.

Innovative research is proceeding in the development of parathyroid hormone analogs that would bind to the parathormone receptors but not release cyclic adenosine monophosphate. Such substances would block peripheral parathyroid hormone; they could be of great value in uncontrolled parathyroid carcinoma as well as in the management of the hypercalcemia due to benign neoplasms.

With the advent of routine blood chemistry analyses, the diagnosis of hyperparathyroidism is now usually made by the detection of hypercalcemia in an asymptomatic patient with normal kidney function. Particularly in patients with parathyroid malignancy, in whom serum calcium levels have been higher than in those with benign neoplasms, this offers the hope of earlier diagnosis at a stage when initial bloc resection is easier and can be more effective. As in all cancers, the first chance to cure the disease is the best chance. It is at the first exploration that the surgeon has the best opportunity to remove the tumor completely.

SUMMARY

Diagnostic Features	• Marked hypercalcemia and PTH elevation • Neck mass
Operative Findings	• Large mass (over 2 cm) often, but not always fibrotic and infiltrating adjacent structures
Primary Treatment	• Wide surgical resection: excision of tumor, strap muscles if adherent to tumor, hemithyroidectomy, paratracheal and upper mediastinal node dissection, clearing of trachea. Lateral node dissection is reserved for metastatic disease.
Management of Recurrent Disease	• Aggressive excision of local recurrence • Resection of metastatic disease where possible, to control hypercalcemia • Calcium-lowering agents (mithramycin, saline, oral phosphates, thyrocalcitonin) are of value in preparation for surgery or for palliation, but not in longterm management. • Radiotherapy and chemotherapy are not of proven value.

PAGET'S DISEASE OF BONE

ROBERT E. CANFIELD, M.D.
and ETHEL S. SIRIS, M.D.

Paget's disease of bone is a localized disorder of skeletal remodeling, which appears to be initiated by an increase in osteoclast-mediated bone resorption. It has been reported to occur in up to 3 percent of older individuals in this country. This disease is more common in patients of European ancestry and many investigators have noted a familial association. While the exact etiologic agent is unknown, the primary lesion appears to reside in pagetic osteoclasts that may have been transformed as a consequence of a viral infection earlier in life. This change in osteoclast activity leads to a marked increase in the resorption of bone which is reflected by a rise in total urinary hydroxyproline excretion (UOHP)* as an index of disease activity. There is a compensatory increase in the rate of new bone formation, and this is reflected by a rise in serum alkaline phosphatase (SAP).* The alteration in the skeletal remodeling rate eventually leads to architectural changes characterized by the development of nonlamellar, or "woven," bone that is frequently increased in size, more vascular, and less compact than normal bone.

Skeletal sites commonly affected by Paget's disease include the lumbar and thoracic spine, pelvis, skull, femur and tibia; less commonly the humerus, clavicle, and scapula may also be involved. Frequently, only one or two sites are affected. Thus, depending on the location, extent, and metabolic activity in an individual patient, pagetic involvement of bone may typically cause no symptoms at all or may lead to deformity (for example, skull enlargement or bowing of an extremity), cause a troublesome sensation of heat or frank pain, increase the susceptibility to traumatic or pathologic fracture, produce symptomatic joint dysfunction (especially at the hip or knee), or result in compression or impairment of adjacent neural structures (for example, cranial and spinal nerve or cord compression syndromes). There is a very low incidence (less than 1 percent) of malignant degeneration in pagetic bone with the development of an osteogenic sarcoma.

PURPOSE AND GOALS OF TREATMENT

All of the accepted drug therapies for Paget's disease appear to act by decreasing the bone resorbing activity of pagetic osteoclasts with subsequent restoration of more normal bone histology, and many patients who have specific symptoms resulting from their Paget's disease feel better with treatment. However, given the variability in presentation and symptomatic expression, it is essential that the goals of therapy be individualized for each patient. For example, pharmacologic treatment will not reverse the bowing deformity in a femur or tibia, but there is good evidence that it can prevent the progression and even reverse some

of the neurologic symptoms that occur with spinal cord compression.

In approaching individual patients our goals are to provide relief of current symptoms and to prevent the emergence of new problems or complications. Studies in many centers, including our own, have established that treatment has the potential to relieve certain symptoms, but there are no well-controlled long-term studies to show that therapy will prevent the progression of the disease or the development of new sites of involvement. Therefore, one is left to infer that the evidence for restoration of bone morphology toward normal, the improvement in the biochemical indices of the disease, and specific examples of reversal of neurologic compression syndromes offer promise that treatment for more than immediate symptomatic relief may be worthwhile. Hence, while we incorporate the goal of prevention in our rationale for instituting treatment of patients with Paget's disease, we recognize that there is a paucity of data providing guidelines for this indication.

The studies concerning the efficacy of treatment of Paget's disease of bone which were conducted in a controlled double-blind design not only provided support for symptomatic improvement, they also revealed a high rate of placebo response. In exploring the basis for the subjective benefit in patients taking placebo we gained the impression that individuals with Paget's disease frequently have relatively little comprehension of the nature of their disorder. Thus, when they encounter a treatment program that not only provides a discussion of the character of the desease but also offers a specific treatment, they commonly achieve a marked relief of underlying anxiety that contributes to overall benefit. Therefore patient education and reassurance are important elements of treatment.

INDICATIONS FOR THERAPY

As noted earlier, we believe that the presence of symptoms referable to Paget's disease constitutes the primary indication for therapy. Ours is largely a referral practice made up of symptomatic patients; often in routine practice the disease is discovered incidentally and requires only observation.

In evaluating symptoms it is important to assess the likelihood that reduction in the activity of Paget's disease will provide relief. Bone pain, excessive warmth, arthritic symptoms, and neurologic compression syndromes have all been found

---

*The abbreviation UOHP is used here for urinary hydroxyproline and SAP for serum alkaline phosphatase.

to improve with therapy in many patients. Several studies have documented reduction in cardiac output as a consequence of treatment of Paget's disease, but we only occasionally encounter a circumstance when this makes a difference in the treatment of a patient with congestive heart failure or angina. Hearing loss is a relatively common symptom in patients with skull involvement resulting from eighth nerve compression, otosclerosis, cochlear injury, or any combination of these. Our experience is that this problem is not reversible with treatment; no data are available concerning the effects of therapy on progression. A final point regarding the evaluation of symptoms involves the situation in which new pain develops in a previously quiescent site or there is a recent increase in pain in a symptomatic area. Although this type of complaint most typically reflects changes in underlying pagetic involvement, it must be thoroughly evaluated, as these characteristics may herald an impending fracture or the development of an osteogenic sarcoma.

A second indication for treatment, in our view, is to attempt to slow the pagetic process when it is active in an area of the skeleton where it may progress to produce symptoms in the future. This category includes patients who have involvement of a major weight-bearing bone, such as the femur or tibia, where there is a potential for bowing; those with disease of the vertebral column where there is a risk of spinal nerve or cord compression; those with extensive skull involvement where there is the possibility of basilar invagination; and those with involvement in the immediate vicinity of major joints—especially the hips. In each of these categories we wish to re-emphasize that there are no controlled studies to establish that therapy lessens the likelihood of these potential problems. However, the evidence for reversal of symptoms with treatment, coupled with the improvement that therapy produces in the histologic appearance of lesions as well as the decline of biochemical indices, leads us to counsel treatment for those patients in whom progression could potentially produce troublesome symptoms.

SPECIFIC PHARMACOLOGIC AGENTS AVAILABLE FOR THE TREATMENT OF PAGET'S DISEASE

Three classes of medications that inhibit osteoclast action in Paget's disease are currently in use. Each is capable of producing symptomatic improvement in many patients, and the use of each is associated with decreases in the UOHP and SAP and with restoration toward normal of bone architecture on biopsy specimens. Because of the high rate of bone turnover in this disease, each of these therapies exhibits greater action at the sites of pagetic involvement than on other uninvolved areas of the skeleton.

Calcitonin. Calcitonin is a 32 amino acid polypeptide hormone that is secreted by the parafollicular cells of the thyroid gland in humans and other mammals and by the ultimobranchial body in birds and fish. Its action in decreasing bone resorption is thought to be mediated by recognition at specific receptors that are present in both normal and pagetic osteoclasts.

Early studies of this hormone in therapy for Paget's disease utilized porcine calcitonin, a preparation with a relatively high incidence of the development of neutralizing antibodies. The commercially available calcitonin that has been most widely studied and that is currently used in this country is the synthetic form of the salmon hormone (Calcimar). Administration is usually begun at 100 MRC daily (see below). This preparation is more potent and appears to have a lower incidence of antibody formation in humans. Synthetic human calcitonin may soon be commercially available, and it is of particular value in patients who have developed antibodies to the other forms.

After prolonged periods of treatment with salmon calcitonin the SAP may begin to rise toward pretreatment levels. This may reflect formation of neutralizing antibodies, in which case substitution of the human preparation will restore the effect. However, not all patients who demonstrate this "escape" phenomenon from calcitonin therapy have antibody formation, and it has been postulated that, with prolonged treatment, there is a loss of calcitonin receptors on the target cells and as a result a decrease in responsiveness to this agent.

Salmon calcitonin is expensive because its manufacture requires the synthesis of the entire polypeptide hormone. Side effects, consisting of nausea and occasionally marked cutaneous flushing, may occur in a significant minority of patients following the injection of the medication.

Diphosphonates. The diphosphonates are structural analogues of pyrophosphate. They exhibit a strong affinity for sites of increased bone turnover, a property that has been utilized in bone scanning. When given in larger doses they are bound at areas of high bone turnover, where they are apparently ingested by osteoclasts resorbing bone and then become toxic to these cells. These compounds impair osteoclast action and decrease the excessive rate of bone resorption in pagetic bone, but, to a variable extent, different diphosphonates also interfere with the mineralization of new bone, a fact that limits the dose and the duration of a given course of therapy. They are given orally, but only a small fraction (less than 10 percent) is absorbed from the gastrointestinal tract. Variability in absorption may account for some differences in patient response.

The diphosphonate currently available for the treatment of Paget's disease is the sodium salt of ethane-1-hydroxy-1, 1-diphosphonic acid (commonly referred to as EHDP and sold as Didronel). In a dosage of 5 mg/kg per day (2 tablets totalling 400 mg per day in an average patient) given for a 6-month period, EHDP produces a decrease in both symptoms and biochemical indices and an improvement in bone histology comparable to that seen with calcitonin.

While EHDP has the advantage of oral administration and lower total cost to the patient, it has not been universally accepted as the therapy of choice in all patients with Paget's disease. Early clinical research studies with EHDP employed high dosages (20 mg/kg per day) for long periods of time (6 months or more) and some of the patients reported new pain in pagetic sites. In addition, although a tendency to develop pathologic fractures is part of the natural history of this disease, there appeared to be an increased incidence of this complication in these early studies. We believe that these side effects probably reflected an excessive suppression of bone remodeling that was dose related. As a consequence, we have been careful to limit our routine use of EHDP to low dosages (5 mg/kg per day) and to give the initial course of treatment for no more than 6 months. At these low dosages we have not encountered any serious side effects. It should be noted that higher dosages of EHDP can cause diarrhea, but this is quite unusual at low dosages. EHDP also decreases phosphate excretion in the urine; at low dosages it usually leads to a rise in the serum phosphate of approximately 1 mg/dl. An increase of more than 2 mg/dl may be an indication that the patient is hyperabsorbing the drug from the gastrointestinal tract, and the dosage may have to be reduced.

Mithramycin. Mithramycin is a compound that binds to DNA and inhibits RNA synthesis. Its potent cytotoxic effects on osteoclasts were first appreciated when it was noted that patients receiving this agent as chemotherapy for testicular neoplasms developed hypocalcemia. It is widely used now as an effective treatment for the hypercalcemia associated with a variety of cancers; presumably it inhibits osteoclast-mediated bone destruction.

Mithramycin has significant toxic properties and it must be administered intravenously, preferably over a 4- to 8-hour period. Its use is associated with nausea and transient elevations in the liver enzymes, SGOT, and SGPT in most patients. Less commonly patients develop some degree of reversible nephrotoxicity, and at higher dosages platelet function may be interfered with by this compound.

Despite its side effects, mithramycin is a very useful therapy for Paget's disease in several specific situations, because it is extremely potent and rapidly effective. For example, patients with certain progressive neurologic compression syndromes may experience an improvement in signs and symptoms following mithramycin therapy (see below). It is also sometimes of value in severely affected patients with widespread skeletal disease who are refractory to conventional dosages of EHDP or calcitonin, in which case occasional courses of mithramycin may be given in conjunction with those agents.

APPROACH TO THE INDIVIDUAL PATIENT

Establishment of a Treatment Plan

The initial visit is usually devoted to the history and physical examination and to a careful assessment of the relationship of the patient's symptoms to the location and nature of pagetic lesions. A significant portion of that visit is devoted to assessing the patient's comprehension of the disorder and to explaining the nature of the disease. In this context the patient is introduced to our criteria for recommending therapy, the goals of treatment, and the drugs available.

As part of the initial evaluation we obtain a bone scan to determine the distribution of the disease and radiographs of the affected sites to characterize the lesions, for example, lytic, sclerotic, cortical stress fractures, joint involvement, and so on. A multiphasic screening blood test that includes serum calcium and serum phosphate measurements and indices of renal function is obtained. Duplicate baseline SAP values are determined, and it is important to be certain that the serum was adequately diluted for assay if the reported values are at the upper limits of measurement of the autoanalyzer. Since our practice has a research orientation, we also obtain duplicate UOHP values, because this analysis provides a good reflection of bone resorption. Measurement of UOHP is not necessary in routine practice but, if available, it is recommended.

The second visit is scheduled at a time when all of these data are available, and a decision is made concerning whether or not therapy is to be recommended. At that time the goals of treatment are re-emphasized—especially with regard to the degree of symptomatic improvement that can reasonably be expected. We have already outlined our philosophy about the indications for treatment; one additional point is that we are more inclined to treat a younger individual with relatively minor symptoms that a person in his seventies or eighties. Our rationale is that individuals with Paget's disease have a normal life span and a younger person has a greater potential for progression.

Use of Specific Pharmacologic Agents

Once we have decided to recommend therapy we almost always initiate treatment with EHDP (Didronel) at a dosage of 5 mg/kg per day (2 200-mg tablets per day in the average individual, to be taken on an empty stomach) for a period of 6 months. It is the least expensive therapy and the only one that can be taken orally, so it enjoys the greatest patient acceptance. Ideally, the SAP (and an optional UOHP) is determined at the the end of the six months of medication, and the initial course of treatment is doscontinued at that time. The majority of patients will have had a decline in the biochemical indices (with a reduction by 50 percent of the elevated portion of the SAP and UOHP) and will have experienced some improvement in their potentially reversible symptoms.

While we consider EHDP to be the drug of choice in most situation, there are circumstances in which we prefer to begin treatment with calcitonin (Calcimar). One example involves the patient with a fracture (or radiographic evidence of impending pathologic fracture) through pagetic bone, and another is that of the patient with Paget's disease who is immobolized and develops hypercalcemia, significant hypercalciuria, or both. A third situation is that of the patient with a large lytic lesion or an advancing lytic wedge in a weight-bearing region of the skeleton. Much debate currently exists about the efficacy of EHDP

in the treatment of patients in this last category. Some research groups experience no difficulty, while others find a significant incidence of increased osteolysis and new pain on treatment. Until this issue is resolved by more extensive clinical studies, we believe it is best to utilize therapy with calcitonin for these types of patients. Calcitonin must be injected either subcutaneously or intramuscularly, and we usually begin with a dose of 100 MRC (Medical Research Council) units daily. Some degree of symtomatic and biochemical improvement may be apparent as early as the first few weeks of therapy, if it is to occur, improvement is usually evident after two to three months. As with EHDP, a 50 percent or greater reduction in the elevation of the biochemical values generally results and symptoms are diminished to a variable extent; most of the improvement that is to be gained is achieved by the end of the first six months of treatment. This medication can be continued indefinitely to sustain whatever benefit has been achieved, and usually, following the first three to six months of therapy, the dosage can be lowered without loss of effectiveness to 50–100 MRC units 3 times weekly.

Most patients will therefore be treated with either EHDP or calcitonin as outlined. There are certain situations, however, in which alternative approaches may be necessary. In cases of involvement of the lower thoracic spine which produces progressive neurologic dysfunction due to spinal cord compression, we are inclined to hospitalize the patient and give 25 μg/kg of mithramycin i.v. on alternate days for a minimum of 5 courses. If significant gastrointestinal or other toxicity intervenes, either the dose of mithramycin can be reduced (for example, to 12.5 μg/kg in each infusion) or a longer interval between infusions may be substituted. At the same time that mithramycin therapy is begun we also institute treatment with calcitonin. The goal with mithramycin is to reverse the pagetic process rapidly, and the calcitonin treatment serves to sustain and add to the early benefit achieved with mithramycin. Additionally, since mithramycin tends to lower the serum calcium level, we increase dietary calcium to 1 gm per day and give vitamin D supplements during the course of the mithramycin infusions. Patients with neurologic compression syndromes who are not showing a progressive deficit are in less urgent need of rapid reversal and are treated with either calcitonin or EHDP or both, since there are numerous reports testifying to the efficacy of each of these agents in this situation.

Regardless of the choice of therapy, we believe that after the first six months of treatment it is time to reassess the patient's status. As noted, data regarding objective and subjective benefit are obtained and the laboratory tests are repeated at this time. Except for the need to re-examine lytic disease or fractures, we do not find serial bone scans or radiographs to be of value in determining the benefit of therapy.

Following this evaluation of response to initial treatment, it is important to address the goals of long-term therapy. All of the drugs available only suppress the disease process; they do not cure it. If the first six months of treatment have produced significant relief of symptoms, that outcome testifies to the effectiveness of the treatment program and a commitment to long-term therapy is usually indicated. Many times, however, the physician is left to comtemplate the meaning of a reduction during treatment of the biochemical indices, SAP and UOHP, in a patient with pagetic deformities whose symptomatic expression could not be expected to be reversed. If the abnormal elevation has been reduced by approximately 50 percent, it would indicate that the treatment has slowed the pagetic process significantly. The available data suggest that this correlates with a return of the microscopic elements of bone architecture toward a more normal lemellar pattern. However, we do not believe that a goal of therapy is to reduce the SAP and UOHP to normal values. This is rarely achieved with calcitonin at the usual dosages, and while high dosages of diphosphonates can reduce UOHP to normal levels, it is among this group of patients that we find individuals who exhibit the largest number of disconcerting side effects. Normal bone remodeling requires maintenance of some degree of bone turnover. Thus in Paget's disease we are usually willing to accept a 50 percent reduction in the elevation of the SAP and UOHP as an adequate therapeutic effect.

Unlike calcitonin, which may require continued administration indefinitely at the lowest effective dosage, the essential point of long-term therapy with EHDP is that it must be given in a *cyclic* fashion. If the initial response to this drug was satisfactory we treat with 5 mg/kg per day for 6 months of each year, allowing a 6-month drug-free period to adjust for its effects on normal bone remodeling and on mineralization in the pagetic lesion. The patients are evaluated at six-month intervals and their biochemical indices determined. With this approach SAP may tend to drift back toward the pretreatment value after several years,

probably indicating either insufficient dosage or the emergence of resistance. In some of these individuals we have employed the drug for cycles of 1 month at 20 mg/kg per day followed by a 3-month drug-free interval, the latter to allow for the initiation and completion of one cycle of bone remodeling. While this approach is within the guidelines that have been approved for the use of EHDP, we have had insufficient experience with it to evaluate the long-term effects and the potential for side effects. Patients on the higher dosage of EHDP frequently report that it has a laxative effect and some experience frank diarrhea. When this occurs, we usually discontinue treatment for a few days until symptoms have cleared and then reintroduce the medication for several days at one-half the dose, gradually returning to full dosage.

Some mildly involved patients will have continued relief of symptoms and near normal biochemical indices for a prolonged period after the initial six-month course of low doses of EHDP. Such individuals may be followed at six-month intervals with no further therapy until the SAP again begins to rise or skeletal symptoms recur.

When a patient does not seem to achieve adequate suppression of the disease process with low-dose EHDP therapy, either initially or on a long-term program of cyclic therapy, we recommend that treatment with calcitonin, administered as described earlier, be instituted *in addition* to the EHDP cycles of treatment. Several clinical investigators have reported that, at low doses, these two drugs appear to have an additive effect and our experience is in agreement with this.

Occasionally, a severely affected patient fails to obtain adequate disease suppression even with the combination of EHDP and calcitonin. We have had some success in treating such individuals at approximately yearly intervals with 5 to 7 alternate-day infusions of mithramycin at a dose of 12.5 μg/kg, followed by conventionally administered EHDP or calcitonin or both. The use of the lower dose of mithramycin appears to be efficacious in this setting and leads to far fewer toxic side effects.

Many of our patients ask us whether there is a role for calcium or vitamin D supplements in their treatment. Our position is that normally recommended dietary levels are adequate, taking into account the increased requirement for calcium that has been reported in postmenopausal women at risk for osteoporosis. During lytic phases of Paget's disease patients may have periods of hypercalciuria with an increased propensity toward the development of renal calculi, and we believe that any prolonged use of very high doses of vitamin D might add to the likelihood of that complication.

Although Paget's disease is a localized disorder of the skeleton, the physician should be alert to two potential distrubances in mineral metabolism that may adversely affect the course of the disease. The first is the coincidence of another common problem, namely, a parathyroid adenoma. Hypercalcemia is not a feature of Paget's disease, except in occasional immobilized patients, and its presence should be evaluated because primary hyperparathyroidism can greatly increase the activity of pagetic osteoclasts and the expression of the disease. A second problem that we and several other groups have noted is a tendency for patients with very active Paget's disease to develop secondary hyperparathyroidism, that is, with normal serum calcium values. This presumably arises as a result of prolonged parathyroid stimulation during blastic phases of the disease when there may be a relative calcium deficiency. It is manifested by slight to moderate elevations of serum parathyroid hormone (found in 10 percent of pagetic subjects in one series) and biopsy evidence of a form of hyper-remodeling in uninvolved skeletal sites that is consistent with secondary hyperparathyroidism. The situation in these patients might provide a rationale for supplemental calcium therapy, but we believe this is a subject for extensive clinical investigation before any general recommendations are made.

Other Treatment Modalities

Anti-Inflammatory Agents. Particularly when Paget's disease occurs in the region of large joints, either by directly involving the areas of bone that comprise the joint or by causing a malalignment at the hip or knee (as might occur with bowing of the femur), significant symptomatic arthritis may ensue. The use of specific antipagetic therapy may readily decrease the metabolic indices in such a patient, but mechanical problems, such as bowing or protrusio acetabuli, are often not improved. If supplemental aspirin therapy is insufficient, we have found that considerable symptomatic relief may be afforded by treatment with the nonsteroidal anti-inflammatory agents. For example, naproxen, 250–375 mg twice daily, has been quite helpful in some patients in relieving pain due to mild to moderate hip, knee, or ankle joint dysfunction and variably beneficial for symptoms resulting from spinal stenosis or for low back pain

due to lumbar and sacral involvement by Paget's disease. A trial of these agents is definitely worth undertaking whenever there is a symptomatic arthritic component to Paget's disease, especially if the symptoms are refractory to calcitonin or EHDP therapy. It is also important to note that some patients who fail to respond to one anti-inflammatory drug may do very well with another, so some experimentation among the agents within this class can be tried.

Surgical Intervention. Several of the mechanical complications of Paget's disease can best be approached surgically. Severe joint dysfunction at the hip or the knee may respond only to joint replacement. If performed by orthopedic surgeons with experience in the management of pagetic lesions, these operations can provide relatively good results with respect to pain relief and enhanced mobility. Internal stabilization of a weight-bearing bone that shows signs of an impending fracture is another procedure that is sometimes necessary, particularly when large cortical stress fractures persist or increase over time. Osteotomies of severely bowed limbs may be performed on those patients who have major gait disturbances or have severe pain due to stresses from the malalignment of the bone. This procedure may give symptomatic relief and additionally may lessen arthritis at the joints adjacent to the affected bone or in the opposite leg.

It is important to emphasize that many operations on pagetic bone may be quite difficult because the bone is very soft and vascular, and surgery should be considered only when there is a major mechanical problem causing symptoms that are refractory to medical treatment or that pose a serious risk of future complication, such as fracture. Prior to elective surgery on pagetic bone a course of calcitonin therapy, at a dosage of 100 MRC units daily for up to 3 months preoperatively, may be of value in reducing the increased vascularity around the pagetic tissue, making the surgical procedure somewhat safer with respect to intraoperative blood loss.

Neurosurgical intervention may be required to relieve progressive spinal cord or root compression by pagetic bone if this complication fails to respond to mithramycin, calcitonin, or diphosphonate therapy. Severe basilar invagination occasionally causes obstruction to cerebral spinal fluid flow, producing hydrocephalus and the development of central nervous system symptoms. CT scanning of the skull is an excellent way to evaluate such patients periodically to detect obstructive hydrocephalus. In cases such as these ventricular shunting may be imperative to decrease CSF pressures.

SUMMARY

A great deal of progress has been made in the management of Paget's disease during the past ten years. Many patients with troublesome and painful symptoms can achieve significant relief with the kinds of therapy that have been discussed above. Guidelines for the use of these agents are still evolving, however, and the role of these therapies in the prevention of progression of disease and development of future complications requires better definition. As wider experience is gained in the future many of these questions will be answered.

UROLITHIASIS

CHARLES Y. C. PAK, M.D.

Nephrolithiasis is a common disorder affecting 0.1 to 0.5 percent of the population in the Western world. It may result in considerable morbidity by causing obstruction, hematuria, or infection.

Although the ultimate symptomatic presentation may be the same, it is clear that nephrolithiasis is heterogeneous with respect to composition and etiologic factors. Renal stones typically contain calcium (calcareous calculi); they are less commonly composed of cystine, struvite (magnesium ammonium phosphate), or uric acid (noncalcareous calculi). Many patients with stones have been found to suffer from a variety of physiologic or metabolic disturbances, including hypercalciuria, hyperoxaluria, and hyperuricosuria. Some of these derangements may be endocrinologic in origin, involving altered metabolism of parathyroid hormone and vitamin D.

The above recognition has led to the refined classification and treatment of nephrolithiasis. Thus it has been possible to formulate reliable diagnostic criteria on the basis of underlying metabolic derangements in patients with nephrolithia-

sis. Moreover, treatments could be specifically selected for their ability to "reverse" the particular underlying physiologic disturbances.

This selective approach argues for a thorough diagnostic differentiation of various causes of nephrolithiasis and emphasizes the need for a careful selection of treatment program for each cause of nephrolithiasis. Its feasibility and practicality are considered in detail here.

METABOLIC CLASSIFICATION OF NEPHROLITHIASIS

A simple and logical method of diagnostic differentiation of nephrolithiasis is the categorization on the basis of underlying physiologic abnormalities (Table 1). This classification assumes that these physiologic disturbances are pathogenetically important in stone formation. Although complete validation is lacking, it is generally agreed that excessive renal excretion of calcium, uric acid, oxalate, or cystine may contribute to stone formation by rendering urinary environment supersaturated with respect to stone-forming salts. This classification is based on major or principal physiologic abnormalities. It is recognized that several disturbances may coexist in a given disorder.

THERAPEUTIC CONSIDERATIONS

Improved elucidation of pathophysiology and formulation of diagnostic criteria for different causes of nephrolithiasis have made feasible the adoption of a selective or an optimum treatment program. Such a program should (1) reverse the underlying physiologic derangements, (2) inhibit new stone formation, (3) overcome nonrenal complications of the disease process, and (4) cause no serious side effects.

The rationale for the selection of a certain treatment program according to its ability to reverse physiologic abnormalities as outlined previously is the assumption that the particular physiologic aberrations identified with the given disorder are etiologically important in the formation of renal stones, and that the correction of these disturbances would prevent stone formation. Moreover, it is assumed that such a selective treatment program would be more effective and safe than a "random" treatment. Despite a lack of conclusive experimental verification, these hypotheses appear reasonable and logical.

TABLE 1 Classification of Nephrolithiasis

Calcareous renal calculi	Noncalcareous renal calculi
Hypercalciuria	Uric acid stones
Resorptive	Cystine stones
Absorptive	Cystinuria
Renal	Infection stones
Hyperuricosuria	Infection with urea-splitting
Hyperoxaluria	organisms
Primary	
Secondary	
Inhibitor deficiency	
Renal tubular acidosis	
Other	
No "metabolic" abnormality	

General Treatment Measures

In patients with calcium stones, moderate oxalate restriction should be imposed by discouraging ingestion of dark greens (such as spinach), rhubarb, and chocolate. Ascorbic acid supplementation should be denied because of potential metabolism of vitamin C to oxalate. A high sodium intake should be discouraged; the avoidance of "salty" foods and salt shakers should be advised. All patients with any form of calculi should be encouraged to drink sufficient fluids to achieve a minimum urine output of 2 l/day.

Candidates for Selective Treatments

Specific treatments should be considered for patients with recurrent nephrolithiasis, especially in those with active disease (for example, stone formation or growth within three years of examination).

In patients with a single stone episode, selective treatments should also be considered, if metabolic derangements (such as hypercalciuria) are disclosed and if patients are in the "high-risk" group in which recurrence is likely (that is, young adult white men with a family history of stones).

Selective Treatment Programs

Primary Hyperparathyroidism (Resorptive Hypercalciuria)

Parathyroidectomy is the optimum treatment for nephrolithiasis of primary hyperparathyroidism. Following removal of abnormal parathyroid tissue, urinary calcium is restored to normal, commensurate with a decline in serum concentration of calcium and in intestinal calcium absorption.

Urinary environment becomes less saturated with respect to calcium oxalate and brushite, and its limit of metastability of these calcium salts increases. There is typically a reduced new stone formation rate, unless urinary tract infection is present. Parathyroidectomy is contraindicated in secondary hyperparathyroidism of renal hypercalciuria and in absorptive hypercalciuria.

There is no established medical treatment for the nephrolithiasis of primary hyperparathyroidism. Although orthophosphates have been recommended for disease of mild-to-moderate severity, their safety or efficacy has not yet been proven. They should be used only when parathyroid surgery cannot be undertaken.

Absorptive Hypercalciuria

The presumed principal defect of this condition is the intestinal hyperabsorption of calcium, which accounts for hypercalciuria and calcium nephrolithiasis. This condition may be subdivided into three types. In type I the intestinal absorption and the renal excretion of calcium are increased during a high as well as during a low calcium diet. In type II, normal urinary calcium may be restored by dietary calcium restriction alone, although hypercalciuria is present on a high calcium diet. In type III the principal disturbance is believed to be the renal phosphate "leak," which enhances intestinal calcium absorption from the hypophosphatemia-induced renal synthesis of 1,25-dihydroxyvitamin D.

Absorptive Hypercalciuria Type I. There is currently no treatment program capable of correcting the basic abnormality of absorptive hypercalciuria, although several drugs are available that have been shown to restore normal urinary calcium excretion. *Sodium cellulose phosphate* best meets the criteria for optimum therapy. When given orally, this nonabsorbable ion exchange resin binds calcium and inhibits calcium absorption. However, this inhibition is caused by limiting the amount of intraluminal calcium available for absorption and not by correcting the basic disturbance in calcium transport.

The above mode of action accounts for the two potential complications of sodium cellulose phosphate. First, the treatment may cause magnesium depletion by binding dietary magnesium as well. Second, sodium cellulose phosphate may produce secondary hyperoxaluria by binding divalent cations in the intestinal tract, reducing divalent cation-oxalate complexation, and making more oxalate available for absorption. These complications may be overcome by oral magnesium supplementation (1.0–1.5 g magnesium gluconate twice a day, separately from sodium cellulose phosphate) and moderate dietary restriction of calcium (by avoidance of dairy products) and oxalate. Under such circumstances, sodium cellulose phosphate at a dosage of 10–15 g per day (given with meals) has been shown to lower urinary calcium without significantly altering urinary oxalate or magnesium, to reduce urinary saturation of calcium salts, and to retard new stone formation. This drug therapy is contraindicated in other forms of hypercalciuria because it may further stimulate parathyroid function.

Thiazide exerts the same hypocalciuric action and physicochemical effects in absorptive hypercalciuria as in renal hypercalciuria (see treatment of renal hypercalciuria for action, type, and dosage). Unfortunately, the intestinal hyperabsorption of calcium is not corrected by this treatment in absorptive hypercalciuria, unlike in renal hypercalciuria. The fate of retained calcium, reflected by reduced calcium excretion in the face of high calcium absorption, is not known. Despite this uncertainty, thiazide has been widely used for absorptive hypercalciuria type I, since sodium cellulose phosphate is currently unavailable in the United States.

Absorptive Hypercalciuria Type II. No specific drug treatment may be necessary. Normal urinary calcium may be obtained by a moderate dietary calcium restriction. Because urinary output is often low in this condition, a high fluid intake sufficient to produce urinary volume of at least 2 l per day should be encouraged.

Absorptive Hypercalciuria Type III. Oral administration of *orthophosphate* (neutral or alkaline salt of sodium and/or potassium, 0.5 g phosphorus 3 or 4 times per day) has been shown to lower serum concentration of 1,25-dihydroxyvitamin D. Though not yet proved, this treatment may restore normal calcium absorption in absorptive hypercalciuria type III. The treatment reduces urinary calcium, probably by directly altering renal tubular reabsorption of calcium and by inhibiting calcium absorption. Urinary phosphorus is markedly increased during therapy, a finding reflecting the absorbability of soluble phosphate. Physicochemically, orthophosphate reduces urinary saturation of calcium oxalate but increases that of brushite (calcium phosphate). Moreover, the urinary inhibitor activity is increased, owing probably to the stimulated renal excretion of pyrophosphate, phosphocitrate, and citrate.

Minor gastrointestinal disturbances (including abdominal bloating and diarrhea) may develop during treatment. Though controversial, this treatment program has been reported to cause soft tissue calcification and parathyroid stimulation. In absorptive hypercalciuria type I, orthophosphate does not reduce intestinal calcium absorption, although it lowers urinary calcium.

Renal Hypercalciuria

This condition is characterized by a "primary" impairment in the renal tubular reabsorption of calcium, secondary hyperparathyroidism, and compensatory intestinal hyperabsorption of calcium from the parathyroid hormone-dependent stimulation of 1,25-dihydroxyvitamin D synthesis.

Thiazide is ideally indicated for the treatment of renal hypercalciuria. This form of diuretic has been shown to correct the renal leak of calcium by augmenting calcium reabsorption in the distal tubule, and by causing extracellular volume depletion and stimulating proximal tubular reabsorption of calcium. The ensuing correction of secondary hyperparathyroidism restores normal serum 1,25-dihydroxyvitamin D and intestinal calcium absorption. Physicochemically, urinary environment becomes less saturated with respect to stone-forming salts (calcium oxalate and brushite) during thiazide treatment, largely because of the reduced calcium excretion. Moreover, urinary inhibitor activity is increased by a heretofore undisclosed mechanism.

These effects are shared by hydrochlorothiazide, 50 mg twice a day, chlorthalidone, 50 mg per day, or trichlormethiazide, 4 mg per day. Excessive sodium intake must be avoided because it could attenuate the hypocalciuric action of thiazide.

Concurrent use of triamterene, a potassium-sparing agent, should be undertaken with caution because of recent reports of triamterene stone formation. Amiloride (5–10 mg per day) may be a useful adjunctive agent, since it is potassium sparing and it may augment renal tubular reabsorption of calcium or potentiate the hypocalciuric action of thiazide.

Side effects are mostly due to extracellular volume depletion and hypokalemia. Thiazide treatment should be avoided or stopped in the presence of excessive extrarenal loss of fluids and electrolytes. When hypokalemia is present, it is advisable to provide potassium supplements (40–60 mEq per day) even when patients are asymptomatic. Renal excretion of citrate, an inhibitor of stone formation, may decline when hypokalemia develops. Thiazide is contraindicated in primary hyperparathyroidism because of potential aggravation of hypercalcemia.

Hyperuricosuric Calcium Oxalate Nephrolithiasis

In this condition hyperuricosuria develops, usually from dietary "overindulgence" with purine-rich foods and occasionally from uric acid overproduction. The ensuing hyperuricosuria is believed to cause calcium stone formation from urate-induced calcium oxalate crystallization.

Allopurinol (100 mg 3 times per day) is the physiologically meaningful drug of choice in hyperuricosuric calcium oxalate nephrolithiasis resulting from uric acid overproduction, because of its ability to reduce uric acid synthesis and lower urinary uric acid. Its use in hyperuricosuria associated with dietary purine overindulgence is also reasonable, since dietary purine restriction is impractical. Physicochemical changes ensuing from restoration of normal urinary uric acid include a reduction in urinary saturation of monosodium urate and a commensurate increase in the urinary limit of metastability of calcium oxalate. Thus the spontaneous nucleation of calcium oxalate is retarded by treatment, probably via inhibition of monosodium urate-induced stimulation of calcium oxalate crystallization.

Side effects of allopurinol are uncommon in patients with stones, although hepatotoxicity, bone marrow depression, and rash have been reported. The complication of xanthine stone formation is rare.

In patients with combined disturbances, allopurinol may be given with other agents (for example, allopurinol and thiazide for patients with hyperuricosuria and hypercalciuria).

Hyperoxaluria

Primary Hyperoxaluria. This rare condition is caused by an accelerated oxalate synthesis. Although there is no effective drug for the restoration of normal oxalate synthesis, orthophosphate (0.5 g phosphorus 3 to 4 times per day orally) may be useful in inhibiting stone formation by mechanisms not entirely understood.

Secondary Hyperoxaluria. In ileal disease (surgical resection, intestinal bypass, inflammatory disease), urinary oxalate may be high secondary to intestinal hyperabsorption of oxalate (enteric hyperoxaluria). Other factors that may contribute to stone formation include low urine volume, low urinary acidity (predisposing to uric acid lithiasis), hypocitruria, and hypomagnesiuria. Dietary oxalate restriction should be imposed. A high fluid intake should be encouraged. Oral calcium supplements (250 mg calcium 4 times per day) may

lower urinary oxalate without substantially increasing urinary calcium. Magnesium gluconate (0.5–1.0 g 4 times per day orally) may be tolerated without aggravating diarrhea. Potassium citrate (20–30 mEq 3 to 4 times per day orally) may augment citrate excretion and raise urinary pH. If bone disease is also present, 25-hydroxyvitamin D (50 µg per day) may be given with calcium supplements (250 mg calcium 4 times per day). Should hypercalciuria ensue, thiazide may be added.

Inhibitor Deficiency

Renal Tubular Acidosis. The distal renal tubular acidosis may be associated with nephrocalcinosis and nephrolithiasis. An incomplete renal tubular acidosis may be found in some patients with calcium nephrolithiasis. The exact cause for stone formation in renal tubular acidosis is not known. Acidosis may cause hypercalciuria by impairing renal tubular reabsorption of calcium, at least during the early stages of the disease before a significant renal impairment ensues. Because of high urinary pH, more phosphate is dissociated. Thus urinary environment may become supersaturated with respect to calcium salts, particularly calcium phosphate. There may be a defective renal excretion of citrate and other inhibitors; this defect may therefore facilitate the crystallization process in urine.

Soluble alkali (sodium or potassium bicarbonate or citrate, 20–30 mEq 3 to 4 times per day orally) may correct the acidosis, reduce urinary calcium, and augment urinary citrate. Although the potassium alkali is preferable to the sodium salt, it may cause hyperkalemia if renal impairment is present.

Other. Hypocitruria is present in approximately 50 percent of patients with calcium nephrolithiasis, even in the absence of renal tubular acidosis. The exact cause remains to be elucidated. Oral potassium citrate or bicarbonate (20 mEq 3 to 4 times per day) typically restores normal urinary citrate.

Some patients with calcium nephrolithiasis may have low urinary pyrophosphate. Orthophosphate (0.5 g phosphorus 3 to 4 times per day orally) may increase pyrophosphate excretion. Orthophosphate should not be given to patients with urinary tract infections.

No Metabolic Abnormality

A minority of patients with calcium nephrolithiasis may have none of the disturbances enumerated above. However, many of them have low urine output because of disdain for drinking fluids. A high fluid intake sufficient to produce a volume of at least 2 l per day should be encouraged.

Uric Acid Stones

The critical determinant in the formation of uric acid stones is the passage of unusually acid urine (pH < 5.5) in which uric acid is stable. Uric acid lithiasis is found in gout, secondary causes of purine overproduction (for example, myeloproliferative states and malignancy), and chronic diarrheal syndromes.

The oral administration of soluble alkali may increase urinary pH and create an environment in which uric acid is unstable. While this treatment may inhibit the formation of uric acid stones, it may cause complications by forming calcium stones, especially if alkali is delivered in the sodium form in large amounts. Moderate amounts of alkali (potassium bicarbonate or citrate, 20 mEq 3 to 4 times per day) sufficient to raise urinary pH to a range of 6–6.5 may be helpful in the prevention of uric acid lithiasis, without producing a significant risk of calcium stone formation.

Allopurinol may be used to control hyperuricosuria; a dose of 300 mg per day in 3 divided doses is generally sufficient to restore normal urinary uric acid. Dietary purine restriction is seldom practical. Probenecid is contraindicated because of its uricosuric action.

Cystine Stones

Stone formation is the result of an excessive renal excretion of cystine and the low solubility of this dicarboxylic acid in the normal pH of urine.

The initial treatment program includes a high fluid intake to promote an adequate urine flow (minimum of 2 l per day) and soluble alkali (for example, potassium citrate 20 mEq 4 times per day) to raise urinary pH to approximately 7 in order to lower cystine concentration and raise cystine solubility. If this program is ineffective, d-penicillamine (2 g/day in divided doses) may be used. This treatment reduces cystine excretion by forming a more soluble mixed disulfide with cysteine. Potential side effects include nephrotic syndrome, dermatitis, pancytopenia, and arthralgia. Vitamin B_6 (50 mg per day) should be added to avoid pyridoxine deficiency.

Infection Stones

Urinary tract infection sometimes accompanies nephrolithiasis. When urea-splitting organisms (Proteus, certain species of Staphylococcus, Pseudomonas, Klebsiella) are responsible for infection, stones typically contain struvite (magnesium ammonium phosphate) with varying amounts of apatite.

In some patients, struvite stones may have formed de novo as a consequence solely of infection. In others, specific metabolic disorders associated with the formation of other types of renal stones could be identified; these derangements include hypercalciuria, hyperuricosuria, hyperoxaluria, and cystinuria. Struvite stone formation in the latter instance probably results from metabolic disorder → formation of nonstruvite stone → urinary tract infection with urea-splitting organisms → formation of struvite stone.

The physicochemical basis for struvite lithiasis is probably the same whether such a stone forms primarily or secondarily. The initial event is the formation of ammonia in urine upon enzymatic degradation of urea by bacterial urease. The ammonia undergoes hydrolysis to form ammonium and hydroxyl ions. The resulting alkalinity of urine stimulates the dissociation of phosphate to form more trivalent phosphate ions, and lowers the solubility of struvite. The activity product or the state of saturation of urine with respect to struvite is therefore increased. Stone formation ensues when sufficient oversaturation is reached.

If a longstanding effective control of infection with urea-splitting organisms can be achieved, there is some evidence that new stone formation can be averted or some dissolution of existing stone may occur. Unfortunately, such a control is difficult to obtain with antibiotic therapy. If there is an existing struvite stone, it is difficult to clear the infection completely because the stone often harbors the organisms within its interstices. Even if "sterilization" of urine had been achieved by antibiotic therapy, reinfection could occur by a harbored organism. For these reasons it has been customary to recommend surgical removal of the struvite stones.

In recent clinical trials, acetohydroxamic acid, a urease inhibitor, has been shown to reduce urinary saturation of struvite and to retard stone formation.

PRINCIPLES OF ENDOCRINE THERAPY

PRINCIPLES OF ESTROGEN THERAPY

STANLEY G. KORENMAN, M.D.

CLINICAL INDICATIONS

Estrogens may be employed clinically as replacement for nonexistent ovarian function; to suppress ovarian function; to inhibit implantation of a conceptus; or to inhibit neoplastic growth. Specific indications for estrogen therapy are listed in Table 1. In the estrogen-deficient state the hormone is employed to activate target organs. Since full uterine maturation and regular menstruation in hypogonadal women require progesterone, a progestin is often given to that group. Ovariectomized mature women and postmenopausal women were treated with estrogens alone until recently, but most physicians now prescribe progestins as well.

In contraception and treatment for the polycystic ovarian syndrome the goal is suppression of ovarian function that in one case is normal and in the other is associated with increased estrogen and androgen production and luteal inadequacy. FSH secretion is suppressed early so that the very next follicle fails to mature. At these dosages estrogens

TABLE 1 Indications for Estrogen Therapy

Replacement for absent hormone
  Ovarian agenesis
  Bilateral ovariectomy
  Menopausal state
Suppression of ovarian function
  Contraception
  Polycystic ovarian disease
Postcoital contraception
Reduction of body height
Treatment of cancer
  Breast cancer in late postmenopausal women
  Prostate cancer in men

cause complications based on their effects on peripheral organs, particularly the liver.

For postcoital contraception a high daily dose of an estrogen, such as 5 mg of diethylstilbestrol for 3 to 5 days given within 48 hours of intercourse, will suffice. It is particularly efficacious after a single episode of coitus and is employed all too rarely, because neither the potential patient nor the physician is aware of its usefulness. The estrogens cause intense endometrial proliferation and withdrawal bleeding and thus prevent implantation. Postcoital contraception should be taught in sex education classes. For a more extensive discussion of birth control, see Chapter 85.

Estrogens can be employed to reduce the final height of girls. There are situations in which normal girls have a predicted height in the 95th percentile or greater and the parents are concerned that this will constitute a serious barrier to a satisfactory life adjustment. Fortunately, this attitude has waned. Prior to considering this therapy it is important to determine the lifelong height pattern, whether the adolescent growth spurt has begun, and the degree of sexual maturation of the girl. The therapy is not useful after initiation of the pubertal growth spurt. In that case the parents can be advised that only limited growth remains. Prior to the start of puberty, reductions of 2 to 3 inches in final height may be achieved by continuous estrogen therapy sufficient to initiate sexual maturation. The estrogens accelerate epiphyseal closure, reducing the duration of long bone growth and ultimate height. This is a dubious indication for estrogen therapy.

Estrogens in large doses have been employed in prostate and breast cancer. They produce a "medical orchiectomy" in men refusing castration for metastatic prostate cancer, but they are not useful after failure of orchiectomy. At doses greater than 2.5 mg of diethylstilbestrol, there is evidence for decreased survival rates owing to ischemic cardiovascular disease, making orchiectomy a more desirable therapy. For a more extensive discussion of the hormonal treatment of prostatic cancer, see Chapter 65.

Large doses of estrogens were used for many years as treatment for breast cancer in women more than five years postmenopausal with receptor-positive disease. At the present time the antiestrogen Tamoxifen has replaced estrogens because of its equal effectiveness and its much lower incidence of side effects. For more details on the hormonal treatment of breast cancer, see Chapter 66.

THE CLINICAL BIOLOGY OF ESTROGENS

By now it is widely recognized that all steroid hormones exert their primary actions by binding to a receptor usually located in the cytoplasm of the target cell, and translocation of the hormone-receptor complex to the nucleus where the complex binds to chromatin (the interphase DNA-protein complex). Although the evidence is strong that the hormone-receptor complex initiates transcription (the synthesis of DNA-dependent messenger and ribosomal RNA), the intimate mechanism by which the hormonal signal produces its changes is not known. The products of the new transcripts are responsible for the anatomic and physiologic effects of the hormone in target tissues. Estrogen targets, defined as tissues containing a high concentration of estrogen receptor, include, in addition to the classic reproductive tissues and involved areas of the brain and pituitary, the liver, skin, heart, spinal cord, and gingiva. While the liver might seem to be an unlikely target, in oviparous species it is a major reproductive organ, responding to estrogens by synthesizing the proteins and lipids of egg yolk and of cation transport. Indeed, the hepatic effects of estrogens are responsible for most of the complications of estrogen therapy. Estrogens produce more lithogenic bile by reducing net biliary secretory volume, increasing cholesterol production, and reducing formation of chenodeoxycholic acid. Estrogens increase the production of secreted proteins, including thyroid-, steroid-, and cation-binding proteins, angiotensinogen, and the apoproteins for HDL and VLDL. The increase of angiotensinogen is partially responsible for the increase of aldosterone secretion seen with estrogen therapy. Increase of VLDL apoprotein contributes to the hypertriglyceridemia and increase of HDL apoprotein contributes to the relatively increased HDL cholesterol seen with estrogen therapy. Estrogens stimulate the secretion of clotting factors V, VII, IX, and X, but their principal effect in promoting coagulation is due to the heparin reversible inhibition of the activity of antithrombin III.

Estrogens are known to promote neoplastic transformation in a variety of tissues, including rodent mammary glands. In humans they have been linked to endometrial carcinoma, vaginal adenosis, and hepatic adenomas. A role of estrogens as permissive agents for breast cancer in humans is fairly well established, in that ovariectomy without hormone replacement markedly reduces the incidence of breast cancer, while estrogen therapy returns the incidence to that seen in intact women.

All of the roles of estrogens are influenced by progesterone and by androgens when present in adequate concentration.

CONSEQUENCES OF ESTROGEN THERAPY

The clinical effects of oral contraceptives are considered in Chapter 85.

Clinical consequences of postmenopausal estrogen administration include an increased risk of gallbladder surgery, an increased incidence of endometrial carcinoma, substantial protection against osteoporosis, possible protection against ischemic heart disease, and slightly increased risks of hypertension and of stroke in hypertensives. There appears to be no increased risk of thromboembolism and little evidence of an increased risk of breast cancer, although that important issue is not yet resolved.

ESTROGEN THERAPY IN THE MENOPAUSE

Hormonal intervention should be considered in any woman who has symptoms of hot flashes severe enough to affect her life style; clinical evidence of sex tissue atrophy, including vaginal discomfort and dyspareunia; or who is at high risk for osteoporosis. Postmenopausal osteoporosis is defined for clinical and investigative purposes as demineralization resulting in fractures (usually of the spine, radius, or femur) in older women. Female Caucasians are at great risk for osteoporosis, and other predisposing factors include thinness, cigarette smoking, inactivity, poor calcium and vitamin D intake, and possibly history of ovariectomy. There is no simple laboratory test that predicts the development of fractures, although recent studies have shown very low serum estradiol and testosterone levels in elderly osteoporotic women. Conventional dosages of estrogens have been shown to eliminate menopausal symptoms and to prevent the development of osteoporosis.

Therapy with estrogens or estrogen-containing compounds is absolutely contraindicated in the presence of an estrogen-dependent neoplasm, unexplained vaginal bleeding, current or chronic hepatic impairment, or current or recent vascular thrombosis. It is possible that estrogens have adverse effects in patients with a seizure disorder, hypertension, fibrocystic breast disease, coronary heart disease, familial hyperlipemias, migraine, chronic thrombophlebitis, endometriosis, and gallbladder disease, so the decision to treat should be made with caution in such patients. Since, after the menopause the effect of exogenous estrogen is additive to that of endogenous secretion, evidence of endometrial hyperplasia is a contraindication to therapy. A family history of breast or endometrial carcinoma has also contraindicated menopausal estrogen therapy. The effect of familial association, whether on genetic or environmental grounds, is small in cases of these lesions, which cast doubt on the logic of such arguments, although the patient may wish to exercise caution on this basis.

The dosage and duration of therapy relate to the reason for which it is used. Treatment of hot flashes should be stopped after 18 months or 2 years to determine whether severe symptoms recur. Treatment for sex tissue atrophy and for the prevention of osteoporosis should theoretically be continued for many years.

Available estrogens appear to be equally potent for therapy and also with regard to the development of complications. Since usual dosages appear to inhibit demineralization of bone, the lowest dosage that effectively relieves the clinical symptoms is optimal. Results are inconclusive regarding the putative benefits of interrupted versus continuous therapy. Combination therapy with an estrogen and progestin has been shown to protect against endometrial carcinoma but has the disadvantage of producing vaginal bleeding.

For women with hot flashes, therapy should be initiated with an estrogen dosage adequate to control the symptoms. Thereafter the drug may be given employing the lowest effective oral dose for the first 25 days of each month. In women with a uterus, a progestin in adequate dosage should be added for the last 10 days of the estrogen cycle at least every three months.

Treatment with sequential estrogen plus progestin does not require a preliminary endometrial biopsy, but treatment with estrogen alone does. An aggressive diagnostic approach to vaginal bleeding, whether between treatments or during treatment, is indicated with treatment.

Patients should be followed closely until the therapeutic goal is reached, then at six-month intervals for two years for assessment of blood pressure, serum lipid levels, and evaluation of the clinical state. Thereafter annual follow-up is recommended. In symptomatic women for whom estrogen therapy is contraindicated, the use of oral or depo-progestins alone appears warranted, because control of hot flashes is achieved 70 to 80 percent of the time.

Although oral therapy continues to be the preferred treatment, the clinician should be aware of the development of new agents that may enter the systemic rather than the portal circulation and provide a more balanced effect on the liver and other targets.

Although the use of a progestin is not currently deemed necessary for women lacking a uterus, progestins may reduce the need for estrogens, provide some protection against liver-based complications of treatment, and possibly protect against late breast cancer risk. Therefore, particularly when long-term therapy is contemplated, their use should be strongly considered. Calcium supplements and adequate vitamin D intake or sun exposure should be ensured, and vigorous exercise should be encouraged in all women for the prevention of osteoporosis.

Treatment of clinically apparent osteoporosis was not thought to be successful, but a regimen of estrogens, calcium, and fluoride has recently been reported to increase bone density and reduce the rate of new fractures in such patients. For treatment of osteoporosis also see Chapter 52.

Finally, the choice of long-term therapy of healthy persons which employs drugs carrying a degree of risk should be the result of agreement between physician and patient after both have thoroughly informed themselves as to the risks and benefits. A recent analysis of the costs versus benefits of hormone therapy for menopause found no clearcut advantage with regard to either long-term morbidity or mortality from taking or not taking estrogens. Thus, at present, the decision to undertake hormonal therapy should be made by the informed patient. Each therapeutic initiative should be reassessed regularly in terms of the value of therapy and the appropriateness of the agents, routes, and types of treatment, based on the information in the field and available alternatives.

For additional discussion of estrogen therapy in menopause, see Chapter 86.

PRINCIPLES OF SYSTEMIC CORTICOSTEROID THERAPY IN NONENDOCRINE DISEASE

NICHOLAS P. CHRISTY, M.D.

Over the past thirty years corticosteroids have found a place in the treatment of more kinds of disease than any other class of pharmaceutical agents. The strictly endocrine uses of corticoids in the replacement therapy of adrenocortical insufficiency and suppression of the hypothalamic-pituitary-adrenal (HPA) system in adrenal virilism (see Chapters 27, 31, 32, 33) account for only a small portion of the steroids dispensed annually. Most are given for a broad range of disorders that appear to have no common denominator. The main pathologic disorders ameliorated by these compounds are allergic, inflammatory, and neoplastic diseases in which pharmacologists and cellular biologists now understand, at least superficially, why glucocorticoids are beneficial. But for several other conditions as different as cerebral edema, myxedema coma, and septic shock, the mechanism of therapeutic efficacy remains mysterious.

ACTIONS OF GLUCOCORTICOIDS

The fundamental nature of corticoid action upon virtually all cells seems to provide a basis for explaining the generality of glucocorticoid effects in the organism and for the broad range of pathologic states affected by glucocorticoids. The corticosteroid molecule passes across the cell membrane and binds to a cytoplasmic receptor protein. The steroid-receptor complex enters the nucleus where it stimulates, depresses, or otherwise influences the process of RNA transcription from the DNA template. The rate of synthesis of specific proteins is thus changed; in a sense, the steroid alters the phenotypic expression of genetic information.

This demonstrated sequence of events comes as close as is now possible to a unitary portrayal of the actions of glucocorticoids, but it does not elucidate completely their diverse and divergent effects in different organs and tissues. A corticosteroid effect regarded as primal is inhibition of amino acid incorporation into the protein of peripheral tissues, for example, muscle. Hepatic gluconeogenesis is stimulated, partly by steroid induced increases in the activity and quantity of gluconeogenetic enzymes. Steroids inhibit catecholamine mediated lipogenesis in the fat cells of the extremities, but have the opposite effect on adipose cells of the abdomen and dorsal fat pad. Negative calcium balance is promoted.

Glucocorticoids regulate the circulation through mechanisms not completely understood: There is an inotropic effect on the heart and a series of effects on the microcirculation, all of which may play a part in the protective action of steroids in the shock associated with endotoxin or anaphylaxis. Corticoids suppress every stage of the immune response, cause lysis of lymphocytes and eosinophils, and protect against cellular damage regardless of the noxious stimulus. Capillary leakage is prevented. The hormones stabilize lysosomes, cell membranes, and plasma membranes.

These cellular and tissue reactions to corticosteroids form the basis for the *pathologic* actions of these 11-hydroxy hormones: inhibition of growth, hyperglycemia, hyperinsulinemia and hyperglucagonemia, diabetogenesis, muscle wasting, abnormal fat distribution; and for their *therapeutic* effectiveness in various kinds of circulatory failure, a host of allergic, immunologic, autoimmune and inflammatory disorders, and many neoplastic diseases—particularly those of the lymphatic system or those in which there is an important inflammatory component.

Toxicity of Glucocorticoids

Since glucocorticoids exert a basic action upon cells, that is, they affect an early stage of protein synthesis, it follows that their somatic actions would be many, various, and inseparable from the *toxic* or untoward effects: myopathy, osteoporosis, peptic ulceration, impaired wound healing, hypertension, hypokalemic alkalosis, precipitation of diabetes mellitus, and suppression of the immune response with consequent increase in susceptibility to every kind of infection—viral, bacterial, fungal, and parasitic. Untoward effects not easily predictable from the known actions of glucocorticoids are steroid induced psychosis, pseudotumor cerebri (especially when there is an abrupt change in the dosage or specific type of steroid), glaucoma, and posterior subcapsular cataracts. It is noteworthy that pseudotumor, glaucoma, cataracts, pancreatitis, aseptic necrosis of bone, panniculitis, and vasculitis are almost unique to the iatrogenic form of Cushing's syndrome, a restriction perhaps related to the exclusive use of semisynthetic steroids, not the naturally occurring hormone cortisol, in pharmacotherapeutics.

Actions of Glucocorticoids on the Endocrine System

Glucocorticoids exert a permissive effect on the capacity of catecholamines to stimulate vasoconstriction; this is one mechanism whereby corticoids regulate the circulation and is not a property of mineralocorticoids. The corticoids stimulate hyperinsulinemia, probably secondary to hypergluconeogenesis and hyperglycemia, and hyperglucagonemia, perhaps as a result of the demonstrated hyperaminoacidemia. Because 10 percent of administered C_{21} corticosteroid is metabolized to C_{19} androgens, amenorrhea, hirsutism, and virilism occur in some women receiving corticoids. The C_{19} metabolites are 11-oxygenated (the mammalian organism has no enzyme for removal of $=O$ or $—OH$ from the C-11 position, probably because of steric hindrance); such compounds are weak androgens. Therefore, very large doses of corticoid are required to produce virilism, which appears far less frequently in iatrogenic than in natural Cushing's syndrome, wherein the host's adrenal cortex sometimes secretes large amounts of the more potent 11-deoxy C_{19} androgenic hormones (for example, dehydroepiandrosterone). Administered glucocorticoid inhibits pituitary growth hormone response to insulin hypoglycemia (probably not an important element in steroid induced growth failure) and transiently blunts the adenohypophyseal release of thyrotropin; the consequent "corticogenic hypothyroidism" is chemically demonstrable but not of clinical importance. The steroids promote water diuresis; the mechanisms are not completely understood but may entail both a blunting of neurohypophyseal ADH release and a renal tubular action that is partly dependent upon and partly independent of corticoid-ADH interactions at the level of the renal col-

lecting ducts. Corticoids do not affect aldosterone secretion; the hypokalemic alkalosis induced by glucocorticoids is due to their own intrarenal kaliuric actions and to the potassium loss accompanying the general cellular breakdown associated with the antianabolic property of these agents (K loss is roughly proportional to negative N balance).

Suppression of the Hypothalamic-Pituitary-Adrenal (HPA) System by Glucocorticoids

HPA suppression with adrenocortical failure is the most discussed, most thoroughly studied, and most feared endocrine consequence of long-term corticosteroid administration.* This fear has been much exaggerated in the clinical literature for two reasons. First, three cases were reported in 1952 and 1953 of fatal postoperative shock with apparent addisonian crises and adrenal atrophy following year-long cortisone treatment; these caused great alarm, which still persists. Second, the function of the HPA system can be assessed by fairly simple provocative tests that have been widely used. The voluminous data obtained provide ample biochemical evidence of HPA suppression, but two major uncertainties remain: the relevance of this biochemical lesion to the patient's competence in mounting an appropriate HPA response to a clinical stress, and the length of time clinically important HPA suppression may last after corticosteroids are withdrawn. The available information does not permit definite answers to these two questions, but thirty years' experience validates the following statements.

First, anatomic evidence of a steroid effect upon the adrenal cortex, anterior pituitary, and

---

*It is assumed that the reader is familiar with the negative feedback inhibition exerted by cortisol upon the adenohypophyseal secretion of corticotropin: the higher the plasma level of cortisol, the less ACTH released, and vice versa. Corticoid administration induces adrenal atrophy and failure of adrenocortical response to stress in animals, but it does not prevent the adrenocorticotropic effect of administered ACTH. The cortisol feedback action takes place at two levels: the anterior pituitary corticotroph cells and the CRF (corticotropin releasing factor) secreting neurohumoral cells of the medial basal hypothalamus. In human beings, tests of HPA function usually show blunted responses after long-term administration of natural or semisynthetic corticosteroids; urinary and plasma corticosteroid values tend to be low and rise subnormally during provocative tests with ACTH, metyrapone, insulin hypoglycemia, vasopressin, bacterial pyrogen, and in a very few cases, during the clinical stress of trauma, surgery, or explosive, acute disease.

hypothalamus appears within five days after starting the administration of corticoids. The clinical significance is minor within that short period.

Second, steroids induce a fall in pituitary ACTH release within minutes to hours; this acute decrease is not clinically dangerous.

Third, the "short" synthetic ACTH test with plasma cortisol response provides an adequate assessment of total HPA function; and turns out to yield results that correlate more closely with clinical HPA response to stress than do tests specifically designed to give theoretically more complete information about all the elements of HPA activity. These procedures (metyrapone, insulin hypoglycemia, vasopressin, bacterial pyrogen) are more cumbersome, more time-consuming, and in some instances (the last three) more traumatic. (For details of the ACTH test, see Chapter 64.)

Fourth, careful analysis of such test results has not permitted precise definition of the smallest dosage of steroid or the shortest time of its administration that causes HPA suppression. Nevertheless, the evidence suggests that any patient who has received a glucocorticoid dosage equivalent to 20–30 mg of prednisone/prednisolone daily for 3 to 4 weeks or more should be considered to have *biochemically evident* HPA suppression that may or may not be clinically significant. HPA function remains biochemically intact in patients who have been treated with 4–5 mg of prednisone equivalent daily for 8 years or longer.

Fifth, after prolonged treatment with large doses of glucocorticoid (> 30 mg prednisone equivalent per day), biochemically demonstrable HPA suppression persists for 12 months or more after cessation of steroid therapy. By biochemical criteria, hypothalamic-pituitary recovery occurs first, within 5 to 9 months; adrenocortical response lags, recovering in 9 to 12 months; and the total capacity of the HPA system to react appropriately to clinical stress is not restored until as late as 12 to 16 months following steroid withdrawal.

Sixth, this biochemically detectable HPA suppression can be muted by administering the glucocorticoid as a single daily morning dose; the HPA axis is more susceptible to steroid induced inhibition in the evening. The alternate day schedule of corticoid administration ameliorates or prevents biochemically evident HPA suppression (see below, in the section on Preferred Approach, and Chapter 64).

Seventh, the use of ACTH as a therapeutic agent instead of glucocorticoids is not accompanied by biochemical or clinical evidence of HPA suppression, but ACTH has many disadvantages (see below, in the section on Therapeutic Alternatives, and Chapter 64).

Eighth, it follows from statements four and five above that the high probability of biochemically detectable HPA suppression in patients receiving prolonged, high-dose glucocorticoid therapy compels the use of steroid cover for intercurrent stresses (trauma, surgery, acute illness) to avoid collapse due to acute adrenocortical insufficiency. The physician is theoretically constrained to take this precaution during the treatment period and for a year or more after steroid withdrawal (see the section on Preferred Approach below and Chapter 64).

Ninth, a sufficiently powerful neurogenic stress can break through the negative feedback inhibition imposed by corticosteroids, that is, it can provoke a strong HPA response with a measurable rise of plasma cortisol level in patients whose HPA systems are suppressed by long-term administration of glucocorticoids.

Tenth, *biochemically proven acute adrenocortical failure due to HPA suppression in steroid treated patients has been conclusively demonstrated only a very few times in the entire world literature.* There are several reasons for this. Detailed studies of HPA function are rarely performed during acute medical emergencies. Few investigations have been published relating biochemical behavior of the HPA system to the patient's endocrine response to stress. Such reports as there are indicate that blood pressure and plasma cortisol concentrations show irregular and inconstant correlations: Blood pressure may be low in the face of normal or raised plasma cortisol level, or the converse may be true. Other clinical signs of adrenocortical insufficiency correlate poorly with plasma cortisol values. Finally, the "breakthrough" capacity of the HPA system under stress (see statement nine above) may in many instances preclude adrenocortical failure.

Eleventh, it appears to follow from ten (above) that clinically important HPA failure due to suppression in patients undergoing prolonged high-dose glucocorticoid therapy occurs infrequently, and that plasma cortisol concentration and its response in provocative tests are not the only or necessarily the prime determinants of the patient's overall reaction to clinical stress.

Twelfth, the steroid cover given to such patients for intercurrent clinical crises should therefore be recognized for what it is: a precautionary measure taken in *all* cases to ward off theoretically possible adrenocortical failure with collapse in a *small minority* (see Preferred Approach below).

Finally, flare-ups of the basic disease, corticosteroid dependence (bordering on addiction in some patients), and other manifestations of iatrogenic Cushing's syndrome are more troublesome complications of prolonged steroid therapy than is suppression of the HPA system (see Chapter 64).

PHARMACOLOGIC CONSIDERATIONS

The foregoing review of glucocorticoid action and toxicity applies equally to the naturally occurring hormone cortisol and to its semisynthetic derivatives and congeners. The organic chemists have synthetically introduced many changes into the steroid nucleus and its side chains and have succeeded in producing pharmacologically useful alterations in the ratio of anti-inflammatory (carbohydrate regulating) to sodium retaining effects. Nevertheless, no steroid analogue has been synthesized in which the therapeutically desirable and the seriously toxic effects are divorced. This is perhaps not surprising in view of the basic and therefore general action of glucocorticoids upon early phases of cellular synthesis of protein. Stated briefly, five specific chemical configurations must be present in the steroid molecule for the fullest expression of glucocorticoid and anti-inflammatory action: the 4,5 double bond and the 3-ketone in ring A, the 11β-hydroxyl of ring C, and the 17α-hydroxyl and 21-hydroxyl groups in the 2-carbon side chain at carbon 17 of ring D. Leaving these configurations intact while introducing a double bond at 1,2 of cortisol's ring A (prednisone/prednisolone) augments fourfold the anti-inflammatory potency and reduces by 20 percent the mineralocorticoid activity. 6α-substitution in ring B of prednisolone (methylprednisolone) produces the same two changes, but quantitatively somewhat greater, in the same directions. 9α-fluorination in ring B (9α-fluorocortisol, Florinef) greatly increases all corticosteroid activities, but the enhancement of mineralocorticoid (125-fold) is so much greater than of anti-inflammatory potency (tenfold) that sharp reduction in dosage to fractions of milligrams (0.25–0.5 mg daily or less often) virtually eliminates the latter effect, so that a "pure" salt-active action can be clinically achieved, as in the maintenance therapy of Addison's disease. Even in the presence of the 9α grouping, 16α-hydroxylation (triamcinolone), 16α-methylation (dexamethasone), or 16β-meth-

ylation (betamethasone) in ring D completely does away with the mineralocorticoid effect but only slightly enhances glucocorticoid and anti-inflammatory potency.

The practical result of this chemical manipulation has been the creation of corticosteroid drugs that have diminished salt retaining activity—usually not a life-threatening untoward effect and in any case manageable with modern diuretics—but that also have augmented anti-inflammatory potency along with a roughly proportionate* increase in the characteristic and apparently inseparable capacity of all therapeutically effective glucocorticoids to impair growth and wound healing, promote osteoporosis and diabetes mellitus, and suppress the HPA system. Thus the most troublesome untoward effects of corticosteroid therapy have not been eliminated. To achieve palliation of diseases ranging from acute lymphocytic leukemia to chronic bronchial asthma, the physician and the patient must still accept the risk of the major complications of steroids conferred by their fundamental actions upon the nuclear synthesis of cellular protein.

The chemical changes introduced into the steroid molecule have also given rise to differences in the transport, plasma and biologic half-life, and metabolism of the synthetic analogues as compared with cortisol. They are all less firmly bound to plasma corticosteroid binding globulin (transcortin), yet all are metabolized less rapidly than is cortisol. The influences of these differences on steroid availability at the cellular level and on duration of action are not in harmony with one another nor with observed biologic effectiveness in the treatment of disease. Different indices of potency are affected differently; for instance, the HPA-suppressive action of a single dose of an analogue

---

*It is important to emphasize the fact that the proportionality is only approximate. In general, structural alterations in the steroid molecule enhance anti-inflammatory activity of glucocorticoids in parallel with their carbohydrate activity and other effects on organic metabolism. In the literature of the past two decades it has been fashionable to convey the impression that the anti-inflammatory and HPA suppressive potencies of a given steroid are equal. This is not true. For example, prednisone/prednisolone has an anti-inflammatory action three to five times that of cortisol; the enhancement of HPA suppressive potency is about seven times that of the parent compound. Sources of error in making such comparisons are several. The dose of steroid is critical. Different results emerge from in vitro versus in vivo bioassays. The time at which the assay end point is determined influences the result, and different reactions reach the point of maximal stimulation at different times after application of the steroid.

lasts several hours longer than does the hyperglycemic effect. Doses of prednisone or dexamethasone too small to inhibit HPA function are sufficiently anti-inflammatory to suppress the clinical manifestations of rheumatoid arthritis. *It appears that the enhanced therapeutic effectiveness of the steroid analogues cannot be satisfactorily explained by differences in their metabolism.* Those differences, as set out above, fail to account for the quantitative advantages one sees in the clinic. The more likely explanation is to be found in the cellular receptor. Only at that level does it seem likely that, for example, the *unique* toxicities of the corticosteroid analogues will be elucidated (see Toxicity of Glucocorticoids above). It is noteworthy that the pharmaceutical manufacturers have abandoned the search for a nontoxic corticosteroid. No novel steroids are being introduced nowadays—they have been replaced by a spate of new nonsteroidal anti-inflammatory and brochodilating agents.

The considerations set forth above will determine the use or avoidance of corticosteroids, the dosage, timing, route of administration, and choice of specific compound. In HPA suppressive therapy of adrenal virilism, the aim is simple: to inhibit pituitary ACTH secretion, which can be achieved with a small dose of glucocorticoid. Replacement therapy for Addison's disease and other forms of adrenocortical insufficiency requires by definition only physiologic doses of steroid, enough to sustain the *permissive* actions of the missing adrenocortical secretion upon the rates of cellular biochemical processes. Successful palliation of inflammatory, immunologic, and neoplastic diseases requires larger doses whose toxicity is inescapable, but the fundamental actions of the corticosteroid are the same whether the dose is physiologic or pharmacologic. In the latter instance, the untoward effects only apear to be qualitatively different; most of them are mere exaggerations deducible from the physiologic effects of these potent hormones.

The therapist now has several methods whereby he or she can mitigate but not prevent the complications of glucocorticoid therapy (see Preferred Approach below).

Interactions of Glucocorticoids with Other Drugs. Drug interactions rarely preclude administration of corticosteroids but may necessitate adjustments in dosage. Patients receiving corticoids along with one or more other drugs simultaneously or in close time sequence usually react to them simply as if each was being given independently. With other agents, either the corticosteroid or the other drug shows diminished pharmacologic activity; with still others, such activity is enhanced. Unexpected or unintended effects are also possible.

Fifteen to twenty drug interactions have been reported. Some of these are clinically important. *Two kinds of central nervous system-active drugs* reduce the effectiveness of corticoids: barbiturates as a class and diphenylhydantoin. The presumed mechanism is induction by these agents of hepatic microsomal enzymes that inactivate corticoids. Increasing the dose of steroid may be necessary. A number of *hormones and hormonelike substances* affect corticosteroid action. Estrogens and estrogen-containing oral contraceptives are said to enhance the anti-inflammatory and glucogenic actions of glucocorticoids, perhaps by increasing transcortin binding of the latter and thus delaying their inactivation. This is probably a minor clinical effect and not therapeutically useful or harmful; it has no visible bearing on the steroid treatment of the pregnant woman. Ephedrine diminishes dexamethasone activity; the mechanism is not understood. Corticoid interactions with thyroid hormone are discussed below under Pathologic Considerations. *Antidiabetic agents* oppose the glucogenic effect of corticoids; put another way, corticosteroids blunt the hypoglycemic actions of these drugs. This interaction is of clinical importance and necessitates titrations of dosage. Corticosteroids considerably augment the potassium loss promoted by most *diuretics* (except spironolactone and triamterene) through additive kaliuretic actions on the renal tubule. This also is a significant interaction; doses of both drugs must be monitored and potassium supplements added with more than ordinary care. Among the *antibiotics,* amphotericin B and corticoids work additively, presumably on the renal tubule, to provoke a high degree of potassium loss. The precautions necessary with steroid-diuretic combinations apply. Rifampin reduces corticoid efficacy by inducing steroid-inactivating enzymes in hepatic microsomes. Glucocorticoids have been reported to promote the growth of antibiotic resistant strains of bacteria in patients treated with tetracycline. This is almost certainly not an interaction unique to tetracycline. Corticosteroids appear to operate additively, perhaps synergistically, with the *anti-inflammatory agents* indomethacin and aspirin in causing peptic (especially gastric) ulceration. Doses may have to be reduced or one or the other agent discontinued. The important action of corticosteroids in regulating blood levels of salicylate is dealt with in Chapter 64. Glucocorticoids have no significant effect in evoking hypercoagulability of the blood as was formerly thought; to the contrary, when given together with oral *anticoagulants,* corticosteroids may act additively to promote superficial bleeding because of their subcutaneous tissue wasting actions and adverse effects upon the integrity of dermal blood vessels. *Vitamin A* has been reported to inhibit locally the steroid mediated impairment of wound healing; there is no systemic counterpart. Finally, reduction in dose of a simultaneously administered corticoid may permit excessive activity of the *cytotoxic agent* cyclophosphamide. The mechanism is not certain and further observations are needed to determine the generality of this interaction. If the observation is confirmed, one may have to reduce sharply the dose of Cytoxan if the corticoid is reduced or discontinued.

PATHOLOGIC CONSIDERATIONS

Extreme Physiologic States that Modify Corticoid Action. In *childhood,* the metabolism of corticosteroids is not substantially different from that of adult life, but corticoids markedly inhibit linear growth through their antianabolic properties. The alternate day schedule of hormone administration mitigates this effect (see Preferred Approach below). In extreme *old age,* corticoid metabolism is slowed down; smaller than usual doses are probably indicated. *Postmenopausal women* are exceedingly susceptible to the protein wasting actions of administered corticosteroids, probably because the opposing anabolic activity of ovarian estrogen and androgen is lacking. Easy bruising and a worsening of osteopenia are the familiar consequences. Steroid dosage should be moderated or alternative therapies used where possible. The marked hyperestrogenemia of *pregnancy* greatly increases the binding of cortisol to plasma transcortin. Despite the observed enhancing effect of administered estrogen on the glucogenic and anti-inflammatory properties of cortisol, pregnant women evince no tendency to require less corticosteroid to achieve a given clinical effect. Further, large doses of glucocorticoids have not been convincingly shown to harm the fetus.

Pathologic States that Modify Corticoid Action. Diseases of the liver provide the most vivid demonstrations of pathologic states affecting the therapeutic actions of glucocorticoids. The liver is the principal site of corticosteroid metab-

olism; through a series of microsomal enzymatic and other reactions, the liver reduces the steroid nucleus and its side chains and substituent groups and brings about the formation of sulfate and glucuronoside conjugates, polar metabolites readily excreted in the urine. Any hepatic disease, such as the acute or chronic viral hepatitides, alcoholic hepatitis, poisoning with any hepatotoxic agent, hepatic metastases, or the many forms of cirrhosis, impairs the metabolism and slows the rate of disposition of glucocorticoids. The result is that the slow rate of steroid inactivation permits the same clinical effect to be achieved with about half the expected or premorbid dose of hormone. An interesting detail is that prednisolone is probably preferable to prednisone in patients with major hepatic disease; such people show defective reduction of the 11-keto group to a hydroxyl, a step essential to the biologic effectiveness of a glucocorticoid.

Terminally ill patients show a marked slowing in the rate of corticosteroid metabolism; an administered dose remains in the bloodstream for hours. The detailed implications are not clear.

Hypothyroidism also slows the inactivation of administered corticoids. The effect may be exerted through the liver. As in cirrhosis, a half or less of the expected or previously established dose of corticoid may suffice. There are many reports of iatrogenic Cushing's syndrome occurring in people treated with standard or large amounts of steroid hormone in the face of unrecognized myxedema. Restoration of the patient to a euthyroid state is corrective and the signs of hypercortisolism then disappear. Although corticosteroid metabolism is much accelerated in *hyperthyroidism,* no cogent clinical evidence suggests that unusually large dosages of steroid hormone are needed. It should be noted that corticoids transiently suppress pituitary release of thyrotropin, with a consequent lowering of most indices of thyroidal function. This lesion is biochemically detectable but not of much clinical moment.

Pre-Existing Diseases Made Worse by Corticoids. There are many of these, as stated above. Whether an established disease will be a relative or absolute contraindication to corticosteroid therapy or no contraindication at all is determined by how much is at stake, how long steroid treatment will have to be given, what dosage will be required, and the probable effectiveness of the steroid as a therapeutic agent for the specific disease to be treated in the particular patient. Even the pre-existence of the six major hazards associated with glucocorticoid therapy need not preclude the use of corticosteroids. Hypertension is usually not exacerbated in the absence of renal involvement as signaled by proteinuria. If blood pressure rises significantly, one can usually control it by increasing or changing the antihypertensive agents without stopping the steroids. Patients who have congestive heart failure of any cause may be safely treated with corticoids as long as there is concomitant administration of digitalis and diuretics and employment of the 16-substituted steroids, which are virtually without salt retaining effect. Diabetes mellitus may be precipitated or worsened; this is usually controllable with modifications in the insulin and dietary regimen. The urgency of the clinical need for steroid therapy is a determinant. If an existing peptic ulcer cannot be managed effectively with antacids and cimetidine, the steroid dosage may have to be reduced or stopped. Major complications of ulcer, such as bleeding or perforation, usually mandate reduction of steroid dosage for the sake of the ulcer, but in an emergent clinical situation that dosage may have to be greatly increased for the sake of the "whole" patient and his need for greater adrenocortical support during stress and in the face of HPA suppression (see section above on Suppression of the HPA System by Glucocorticoids). Osteoporosis should not preclude careful administration of steroids. The special predilection of the postmenopausal woman has been discussed. Anabolic steroids have not proved useful in combating the corticoid effects on bone; use of a combined calcium, fluoride, and vitamin D regimen for steroid induced osteopenia may be valuable, but supporting data are not yet at hand. As for major psychologic disorders, the available information indicates that the presteroid personality does not provide a basis for predicting the patient's psychic reaction to corticosteroid therapy. It is known that the emotional disturbances of psychotic patients are unaffected by large doses of corticoids. If the clinical indication is strong, the steroid should be given, regardless of the patient's emotional state. The exception is the addicted subject: persons addicted to other drugs tend to become corticosteroid dependent. As for existing infections, corticosteroids may perhaps be life-saving in some, as in Gram negative sepsis. Disseminated tuberculosis is probably not an absolute contraindication; again, if the clinical need for steroid is compelling enough, it may be cautiously given together with appropriate antituberculous chemotherapy. When specific antibiotics for any infection are available, corticoid treatment may be started or continued along with such agents, but only if the indication for steroids is powerful. Intercurrent infections may require adrenocortical support, as is the case with any clinical stress; the rule is to hold corticosteroid doses to the minimum that will protect against adrenal insufficiency or clinical collapse.

Two disorders of the eye deserve mention. Glaucoma is worsened by corticosteroids. If the clinical need for steroids is great, they may be cautiously continued at the minimum possible dose and with frequent measurement of intraocular pressure and appropriate use of miotic agents. Herpes simplex of the cornea constitutes an absolute contraindication to the use of corticoids, which may promote irreversible opacification of the cornea and blindness.

THERAPEUTIC ALTERNATIVES

Alternatives to systemic corticosteroid therapy are the use of ACTH, corticosteroid therapy administered locally or topically, and the employment of other anti-inflammatory, antiallergic, or antineoplastic agents. Modifications of oral or parenteral dosage schedules as alternative methods are discussed below in the section on Preferred Approach.

ACTH therapy is not a satisfactory substitute for glucocorticoid therapy. The arguments are given in detail in Chapter 64.

The complications of systemic glucocorticoid treatment can be attenuated and sometimes avoided entirely by judicious employment of local, topical, and some forms of parenteral routes of steroid administration. Whenever possible, diseases of the anterior segment of the eye, skin disorders, affections of the bronchi and colon, and many musculoskeletal ailments can be treated effectively by direct application of the corticosteroid (for specific and most appropriate steroid preparations, consult textbooks of pharmacology). The therapist can often circumvent major systemic effects of corticosteroids by prescribing steroid-containing ophthalmic solutions for some cases of iritis; corticoid-containing dermal lotions, ointments, and creams for innumerable skin diseases; steroid aerosols, such as beclomethasone dipropionate, for bronchial asthma and some cases of pulmonary emphysema; corticosteroid enemas for exacerbations of chronic, nonspecific ulcerative colitis; and intrasynovial injection of suitable corticosteroid esters in patients having rheumatoid or osteoarthritis with involvement of only one or two joints. Direct injections of steroid into bursae or musculoskeletal lesions are also feasible.

The physician and patient must be prepared to pay some price for these evasive tactics. If dermal ointments are applied under plastic film, absorption will be considerable and systemic effects may follow. Steroid aerosols and steroid enemas are associated with ample absorption, sooner or later, of glucocorticoid, so that the desired avoidance of untoward effects may be thwarted. The tactic in all these instances should be to space the steroid applications as widely as is consistent with controlling the disease to a reasonable degree. In patients with generalized arthritides, intra-articular injection of corticoids indeed obviates systemic therapy and its complications, but its usefulness is limited by the possibility that such intense local treatment may lead to more rapid breakdown of the joint; therefore, applications of this sort are usually not performed at intervals of less than four to six weeks.

Physicians have begun to adopt the use of other agents to replace corticosteroid therapy. The process has to be one of trial and error, starting and stopping, and frequently having to change direction. In some disorders, the decision to abandon steroids and use something else is easy; in others, it is difficult or impossible. Rheumatologists now agree that systemic treatment of rheumatoid arthritis with glucocorticoids in no way alters the natural history of the disease; the number of disabled joints is the same in patients treated or not so treated. Therefore, a decision to carry out therapeutic trials with such "intermediate" anti-inflammatory drugs as indomethacin or Motrin (ibuprofen), is straightforward. In contrast, treatment of Hodgkin's disease or acute lymphocytic leukemia consists of complex regimens that combine cytotoxic agents, vinca alkaloids, immunosuppressive agents, and corticosteroids in elaborate predetermined dosage schedules; these rigid protocols forbid easy cessation of their glucocorticoid moiety. The general approach would be something like this: In disorders that are not life-threatening, for example, chronic bronchial asthma and rheumatoid arthritis, alternative nonsteroidal therapies, such as various bronchodilating inhalants or indomethacin, should be given a thorough trial, either alone or in combination with other agents. For the serious, sometimes catastrophic diseases in which corticosteroids are used, such as disseminated lupus, the combination of steroids with other drugs (for example, immunosuppressants)

may permit use of lower steroid doses. In these situations, nevertheless, steroid toxicity may not loom large as a disadvantage to the patient when compared with the complications of immunosuppressive therapy or with the consequences of the potentially lethal disease under treatment.

PREFERRED APPROACH

The mechanisms of action of corticosteroids, their untoward actions, and the complications of steroid therapy have been amply discussed. It remains to deal with dosage regimens that blunt the severity of those untoward actions, and assessment of therapeutic response.

To dispose of the last point first, a thorough analysis of the methods whereby the physician estimates the quantitative and qualitative aspects of disease response to corticosteroid therapy would entail an encyclopedic exploration of the subject appropriate to a multivolume treatise on medicine The indices of therapeutic response are, Does the patient survive? Do the objective manifestations of his disease remain in abeyance? For the purposes of this chapter, it is enough to say that there are five major categories of disease in which glucocorticoid therapy is useful in those terms: (1) replacement therapy for the various kinds of adrenocortical insufficiency—here physiologic dosages (the equivalent of 20 mg of cortisol daily) are sufficient (see Chapter 27); (2) suppressive therapy to inhibit pituitary ACTH secretion in the various forms of adrenal virilism (0.5–0.75 mg of dexamethasone or betamethasone nightly, because the adenohypophysis is more prone to steroid suppression of ACTH at night) (see Chapters 31, 32, 33); (3) intensive short-term therapy for catastrophic illness; (4) prolonged high-dose therapy to contain a potentially lethal disease; and (5) chronic low-dose palliative therapy. The following paragraphs will deal with items (3) through (5), which are also analyzed in some detail elsewhere (see Chapter 64).

Corticoid treatment of catastrophic illness is usually desperate and for the most part empiric, having no solid basis in pathophysiology. Such illnesses include thyrotoxic crisis ("storm"), acute cerebral edema of any cause, septic shock, and myxedema coma. Disorders for which glucocorticoids ought to be effective in terms of their known mode of action include hypoglycemic coma, water intoxication, acute hypercalcemia due to vitamin D intoxication or androgen therapy for osseous metastases from mammary carcinoma, and allergic emergencies (for example, anaphylaxis due to bee sting or penicillin hypersensitivity). In all these conditions, whether or not the mode of therapeutic action of corticoids is understood, the hormones must be intravenously administered in large doses as fast as possible. A conventional series of doses would be 100–500 mg of cortisol hemisuccinate given as a single bolus, followed by infusion of the steroid ester at a rate of 100–300 mg in 250–1000 ml of dextrose and water or saline every 4 to 6 hours. Still larger doses of steroid, the equivalent of 2–4 gm of prednisone/prednisolone per day, are said to be required to achieve a favorable effect on blood pressure in septic shock. The point remains controversial; there are no special toxicities associated with these huge doses. Dexamethasone phosphate, available in a concentration of 4 mg/ml is equally effective. Equivalent doses are 1/25 those just described for cortisol. The therapist must remember that, where available, the primary therapeutic agent is more important than the corticosteroid as a life-saving measure. The prime example is allergic anaphylaxis; parenteral epinephrine administration is of more immediate value than steroid injection, which should be viewed as supplementary. As discussed in Chapter 64, steroids, no matter how high the daily dose, can be withdrawn with impunity as abruptly as they were started. In such patients, treated for no more than a few days, the only complications are the occurrence of itching at mucocutaneous junctions, punctate ulcerations of the gastric mucosa (rare), or premature ventricular contractions (very rare).

Therapeutic response in patients with serious disease treated with prolonged high-dose steroids (15–120 mg of prednisone per day) is assessed in Chapter 64. The problems are to keep the manifestations of the disease suppressed on one hand, and to minimize the devastating signs of iatrogenic Cushing's syndrome on the other. The best method yet devised for walking this narrow path is the use of the *alternate day schedule of glucocorticoid dosage*. The rationale is twofold: First, it is taken for granted that the disease can be sufficiently suppressed with inconstant, or, waxing and waning, quantities of administered steroid; and second, it is assumed that this intermittency of exposure to supraphysiologic amounts of glucocorticoid spares the patient serious HPA suppression, physical signs of hypercortisolism, osteopenia, diabetes, psychosis, and so on. Whatever the intellectual

merits of the hypothesis, the method is empirically successful. Most diseases—the notable exception being temporal (giant cell) arteritis with the threat of blindness—respond as well to the alternate day treatment schedule as to daily administration of glucocorticoids in divided doses. Further, patients maintained on this schedule for years show fewer signs of Cushing's syndrome than patients who have received daily steroid, and the indices of function of the immune system and of phagocytic capacity are better preserved.* Children managed by the alternate day scheme have much less impairment of growth than do their coevals treated with steroid every day. HPA suppression is absent or less pronounced, and steroid withdrawal is said to be easier. It is important to use a relatively short-acting corticoid in the alternate day schedule, for example, prednisone/prednisolone or methylprednisolone. If the longer-acting compounds (dexamethasone, betamethasone) are given, their biologic half-life is long enough so that intermittency of exposure to glucocorticoid is not achieved and the organism is not, so to speak, put to rest at intervals; biologically, the regimen is not alternate day. For those patients whose basic disease is not adequately controlled by the alternate day administration of corticoid, the therapist may give a single daily dose in the morning. This modified schedule partially spares the HPA system and controls temporal arteritis in most instances, but does not mitigate the outward signs of Cushing's syndrome.

Simply stated, the alternate day schedule entails giving twice the daily amount of steroid in a single matutinal dose every other day; for exam-

---

*With continuous prolonged high-dose glucocorticoid therapy, the therapist must keep in mind the danger that the anti-inflammatory, antipyretic, and generally supportive properties of corticosteroids may mask infection and, because of the inhibitory effect on wound healing, may permit the spread of an infection that would be walled off in a patient not treated with corticoids. I have seen a woman, treated with high-dose prednisone for nephrotic syndrome and ascites due to disseminated lupus, whose hitherto unsuspected peptic ulcer perforated without clinical signs. There was no fever and the white blood cell count was not elevated. Abdominal signs were minimal. An upright abdominal film done for some other reason showed air under the diaphragm. Bacteriologic study of the ascitic fluid showed generalized peritonitis.

This kind of untoward event is less likely to occur in persons treated by the alternate day method, but the possibility is always present. The physician must still be vigilant, particularly with patients known to harbor a chronic infection that might become active, either because of the steroid therapy or for any other reason.

ple, a patient with lupus nephritis who would ordinarily be given 60 mg of prednisone equivalent daily, receives 120 mg every other morning. For patients already on daily divided doses of steroid, conversion to the alternate day dosage may be accomplished by gradually increasing the steroid dose on odd days, and commensurately reducing it on even days, until double the original daily dose is attained on the odd day, zero on the even. This can usually be completed within two weeks; control of manifestations of the basic disease governs the rate of conversion. The role of the alternate day dosage schedule in the process of discontinuing corticoid therapy is dealt with in Chapter 64. Why this technique is efficacious, controlling the disease while causing fewer and less toxic complications of the administered steroids, is a challenging question that has not yet been answered.

Acute intercurrent medical or surgical emergencies, including sudden exacerbations of the basic disease, prompt the use of the so-called steroid cover during and for a short time after the emergency. The strengths and weaknesses of the arguments for and against this procedure are listed above in the section on Suppression of the HPA System by Glucocorticoids. The suggested protocol, which is modified to suit the needs of individual patients, was originally designed for people receiving prolonged high-dose continuous steroid therapy. For the reasons detailed in previous sections, it is difficult to determine which patients receiving the alternate day or any other intermittent dosage schedule have significant HPA suppression and which do not. Therefore, patients being treated with the interrupted steroid courses should also be given steroid cover.

All patients receiving prolonged high-dose therapy for a serious disease should wear an identification bracelet or carry a card describing the steroid treatment and the need for added hormone during stress—acute medical illness, surgery, or trauma. For minor (office) surgical procedures, no extra steroid should be needed. The same is true for illnesses the patient and his family can treat at home, such as viral gastroenteritis, influenzalike respiratory ailments, or bacterial pharyngitis; for these, the patient must be instructed to continue, not stop, his steroid (as a diabetic person takes more, not less, insulin in similar circumstances). Specific antimicrobial treatment is added as necessary. If the patient is vomiting, the physician may have to administer a parenteral, rapidly acting water-soluble steroid preparation, for example,

cortisol hemisuccinate, either intravenously or (since blood pressure will usually be well maintained) intramuscularly. One hundred mg per day for two to three days should suffice, with immediate return to the maintenance dosage for the underlying disorder. For major intercurrent stresses—a threatening flare-up of the disease being treated with steroids, a major surgical procedure, large-scale trauma—the treatment is entirely intravenous with a daily dose of up to 300 mg of cortisol hemisuccinate (or equivalent) given by infusion around the clock. Higher doses of parenteral corticoid may be needed to maintain blood pressure; there is no contraindication to such doses in the range of several hundred milligrams daily. Gradual reduction of the dose in these patients is not necessary, since their maintenance doses are so high. As the emergency subsides, the patient can be switched to an oral dose of his usual steroid analogue in a range of 30–60 mg of prednisone equivalent. This can then be adjusted as the status of the basic disease dictates. Special and attentive care of surgical wounds usually overcomes the steroid induced impairment of wound healing. For acute infections, it is axiomatic that antibiotics are the central therapeutic agents; steroids are merely supportive.

Patients in this group who have been withdrawn from prolonged high-dose glucocorticoid regimens are conventionally assumed to be at risk for a year or so after withdrawal (see above and Chapter 64). During that time, minor illnesses, minor trauma, and office surgical procedures can be treated with oral doses of cortisone or hydrocortisone, 50–100 mg daily in 2 or 3 doses for 1 to 3 days, tapering carefully to zero within 5 to 10 days. The reduction can almost always be done within that time. For major medical emergencies, daily intravenous infusions containing 100–300 mg of a cortisol ester usually are sufficient; the number of days of treatment at that dosage level is governed by the status of the emergent condition. Transient falls in blood pressure can sometimes be corrected by intravenous injection of boluses of cortisol hemisuccinate, 50–100 mg at a time. The steroid dosage must then be reduced gradually when the patient can be switched to oral cortisone or cortisol. Complete withdrawal of the steroid cover can usually be accomplished successfully within two weeks. If the acute intercurrent illness happens during the period of corticosteroid withdrawal, the emergency dosage plan is the same, except that the corticosteroid tapering is cautiously resumed, when the acute event has run its course, at a level 10 to 25 percent above the dose the patient had been taking just before the emergency.

The treatment plans described above are similar to those for acute adrenocortical insufficiency associated with Addison's disease, except that mineralocorticoid is unnecessary. Since the adrenal cortex may be unresponsive, ACTH as a therapy is contraindicated.

The difficulties in managing patients with rheumatoid arthritis, bronchial asthma, and regional enteritis who are treated with long-term (often lifetime) low-dose palliative corticoid are spelled out in Chapter 64. In this category the dosage is generally below 10 mg of prednisone equivalent daily. The alternate day schedule usually does not work; the patients will not tolerate the recurrent symptoms on the day off steroids. These patients require careful titration of the steroid dosage, which should be set at the level of reasonable palliation, not total relief, to avoid the large doses that would evoke the signs of iatrogenic hypercortisolism. In most instances, the patients also need adjunctive therapy: other anti-inflammatory agents, bronchodilators, anticholinergic drugs. Keeping the corticoid dosage as low as possible is overridingly important in these people, who have a curious propensity to develop corticosteroid dependence, which often makes weaning the patient from the hormone impossible.

The elaborate steroid cover described for prolonged high-dose glucocorticoid regimens is usually not required in patients receiving low-dose palliative steroid treatment. Close observation during acute intercurrent illnesses will show whether modified steroid cover is indicated or not.

SUMMARY

Glucocorticoids exert dramatic therapeutic effects in a bewildering array of diseases. The corticoid action most likely to be primal is the effect on RNA transcription. Altered protein synthesis underlies most but not all physiologic and pathologic effects of these hormones. Since their action is so fundamental, the therapeutic and toxic effects are virtually inseparable. Therefore, the physician who wishes to use them therapeutically must employ methods to mitigate their untoward actions. These methods are to use other therapeutic modalities where possible; where not possible, to give corticosteroids in the minimum effective doses for minimum periods of time; to use local, topical or intralesional applications of corticoid to minimize or at least decelerate systemic exposure to the hormone; and to employ intermittent (for example, alternate day) dosage schedules of steroid administration, which empirically spare the patient the worst of the manifestations associated with iatrogenic Cushing's syndrome, a serious disease in itself.

CORTICOSTEROID WITHDRAWAL

NICHOLAS P. CHRISTY, M.D.

Successful withdrawal of a patient from corticosteroid therapy requires the physician to have a firm grasp of essential background information and to formulate clear answers to several questions. First, one must define "successful withdrawal." Second, one must be fully acquainted with the disease the steroids have been used to suppress. Third, one must be certain why corticoids were used in the first place and why they are now being stopped. Fourth, the physician has to know in detail the duration of steroid treatment, the exact dosage schedule, and the pharmacologic characteristics of the specific corticosteroid the patient has been receiving. Fifth, one must be prepared to identify and then deal with any of the various forms of the "corticosteroid withdrawal syndrome." Finally, it need hardly be said that the physician ought to possess intimate knowledge of all pertinent aspects of the patient's personality and the features of the underlying disease which are peculiar to that patient.

PRINCIPLES

Definition of Successful Steroid Withdrawal

An ideal course of steroid withdrawal would be a smooth and rapid transition from the induced state of "tissue" hyperadrenocorticism to total deprivation of exogenous corticosteroid without recrudescence of the basic disorder and without the emergence of either signs and symptoms of adrenocortical insufficiency due to adrenal suppression or of corticosteroid dependence (see below). This untroubled state of affairs can often be achieved. For example, self-limited, short-lived disorders, such as severe penicillin reactions for which steroid treatment is highly effective, do not recur when corticosteroids are withdrawn. Neither adrenal suppression nor steroid dependence is likely to develop in patients given very small doses—the equivalent of prednisone, 5 mg or less per day, even over periods as long as several years, a dosage schedule often used by gynecologists in treating mild forms of adrenal virilism. Nor does clinically significant suppression or dependence occur with large doses—the equivalent of 60 mg or more of prednisone daily—administered over periods as short as 7 to 10 days, a scheme frequently employed in treating, for example, severe, acute *Rhus* dermatitides (poison ivy, poison oak, poison sumac).

These rules are generally applicable, but it must be recognized that, as with other drugs, patients show wide individual variations in their responses to a given quantity of a given corticoid.

When the ideal smooth withdrawal from steroids cannot be achieved—probably a more common clinical situation—successful management is then defined as gradual stepwise reduction of the corticosteroid dosage, with intermittent increases when and if neessary to control flare-ups of the basic disorder or to palliate the symptoms and signs of adrenal insufficiency or corticoid dependence. This kind of interrupted downward titration demands vigilance on the part of the physician; in practical terms, this means frequent follow-up visits by the patient.

The Underlying Disease

As suggested above, some acquaintance with the disease being suppressed or controlled by the corticoids will enable the physician to make reasonable predictions about the likely course of steroid withdrawal and to gauge the probability that specific signs and symptoms of the disorder in question will ensue. Such acquaintance will, in a sense, alert the physician as to how vigilant he or she must be and will provide the basic information necessary to design appropriate history taking, physical examination, and laboratory tests to detect evidence of recrudescence early, before symptomatically unpleasant or clinically threatening events occur or get out of control.

In inflammatory or noninflammatory disorders which are immediately life-threatening, steroid withdrawal and the rate of steroid dosage reduction are dictated to a degree by the subsidence of the clinical condition. These disorders include, among other medical emergencies, acute adrenocortical insufficiency, allergic crises, shock associated with infection, hypoglycemic coma, water intoxication, central hyperthermia, thyroid storm, and myxedema coma. These conditions, with the exception of adrenal insufficiency, for which steroid therapy is crucial, *may* be improved by high-dose, short-term corticoid therapy, but steroids are not the central mode of therapy. One must of course treat the underlying disease with the appropriate primary modalities as well. Steroid withdrawal can usually be abrupt, without tapering, for the presence or absence of pharmacologic hypercortisolism is not the essential determinant of the patient's recovery.

Most of the patients the physician will encounter who present major difficulties in steroid withdrawal suffer from serious hematologic, inflammatory, and immunologic diseases. This is because the diseases themselves are systemic and more or less catastrophic and because large doses of corticosteroids are administered over long periods of time, usually as the principal means of palliating or suppressing the disease. These diseases include acute lymphocytic leukemia, idiopathic thrombocytopenic purpura, and Hodgkin's disease; ulcerative colitis, chronic active and acute alcoholic hepatitis, subacute hepatic necrosis, temporal (giant cell) arteritis, polymyositis, classic dermatomyositis; disseminated lupus erythematosus; autoimmune hemolytic anemia and severe asthma.

A detailed discussion of all the possible signs, symptoms, and abnormalities of laboratory tests which might mark the resurgence of these disorders during corticoid withdrawal would constitute a virtual textbook of internal medicine. The few essential points to be made are these. In many of the conditions listed above, early signs of recurrence may be straightforward, if rather general. Fever, for example, may characterize, and be the first evidence of, flare-up of leukemia, Hodgkin's disease, lupus, ulcerative colitis, the hepatitides, and the mesenchymal disorders. The physician, knowing this, will regulate the rate of steroid withdrawal in part by the presence or absence of fever. Petechiae of skin and mucous membranes and dermal ecchymoses may mark a recurrence of idiopathic purpura; abdominal pain, diarrhea, and blood in the stool herald the return of colitis. Appearance of such signs mandates slowing the rate of steroid withdrawal and, in most instances, a temporary increase in steroid dosage. For other diseases, one resorts to a combination of clinical and laboratory findings. An example is the nephrotic syndrome of lupus. If ascites appears, the clinical need is obvious, but recurrent peripheral edema may be subtle. If it is, one is forced to measure the daily loss of urinary protein, which is probably a more sensitive and earlier marker for escape of the renal lesion from the suppressive effects of the diminishing quantity of circulating corticosteroid. In the hepatitides that can be treated with steroids, the most prudent course is to monitor hepatic function tests frequently. These are more likely to give early warning of recurrence than are clinical signs, such as fever or jaundice. Resorting to such subtleties is clearly not necessary in asthma; the obvious clinical sign, bronchial wheezing, informs patient and doctor that the disorder is no longer controlled, and the steroid dosage is regulated accordingly.

Some patients with rheumatoid arthritis, many with regional enteritis (Crohn's disease), some with asthma, and the subset of people with disseminated lupus who have arthritis as the principal manifestation, comprise another special group of steroid-responsive entities. These are treated with chronic low-dose palliative doses of corticosteroids. They are troublesome to treat during withdrawal of corticoids not becuase of adrenal suppression but because of apparent flare-ups of the disease upon the slightest reduction in dosage. I have had one patient with regional enteritis whose gastrointestinal symptoms were well controlled with a prednisone dose of 7.5 mg daily; reducing the amount to 5 mg was followed by recurrence of bloody diarrhea. Almost all rheumatologists have treated patients with rheumatoid arthritis who are satisfactorily free of articular pain and stiffness on daily prednisone doses as small as 2.0–2.5 mg of prednisone equivalent, but whose arthritic symptoms become insupportable when the dosage of steroid is cut, not necessarily abruptly, to 1.0 mg or to nothing.

Faced with the problem of withdrawing patients with these four conditions from corticosteroids, the physician is well advised to prepare the patient for a long and tedious period, usually measured in terms of many months to a year, during which the dose of corticoid is diminished very slowly and by minuscule degrees. One must also keep in mind the peculiar tendency of some rheumatoid patients to develop a panmesenchymal reaction, the so-called steroid pseudorheumatism, during steroid withdrawal. Such an occurrence may require the reinstitution of corticosteroids at far higher dosages than the palliative levels that had been used to suppress the basic rheumatoid disease.

Another category of patients, those receiving relatively low dose chronic corticoid treatment to suppress the secretion of ACTH by the adenohypophysis, includes persons with idiopathic hirsutism, presumably due to acquired adrenal hyperplasia (or acquired adrenal virilism), and those with the several forms of congenital adrenocortical hyperplasia with virilism. The first type, found in adolescent or adult women, requires only modest dosages of prednisone equivalent, on the order of 7.5 mg per day or less. These women generally need treatment only during reproductive life, except those few who have associated hypertension. Further, the small dosages do not produce untoward effects, and their withdrawal can be accomplished abruptly without eliciting any of the manifestations of corticosteroid withdrawal syndrome, adrenal suppression, or corticoid dependence.

As for congenital adrenal hyperplasia, most patients can be treated with relatively small daily doses, so that difficulties with steroid withdrawal are generally not severe. This statement must be qualified, however: One must know precisely what type of adrenal enzymatic lesion is present. For the majority of subjects, the disorder is 21-hydroxylase deficiency, with "relative," that is, usually incomplete, lack of cortisol biosynthesis and secretion. Once pituitary-adrenal suppressive therapy with corticoids has brought them successfully through the periods of growth, sexual development, and reproductive function, these individuals do not require further corticosteroid treatment into late adult life and old age. Withdrawal can be carried out abruptly and with impunity. One may wish to add extra steroid cover for intercurrent, severe, acute illnesses in patients still on suppressive therapy (see Chapter 63). For the other forms of congenital adrenal hyperplasia, characterized by more nearly complete cortisol deficiency and by blocked aldosterone biosynthesis or hypertension, corticosteroid therapy is both ACTH-suppressive and a form of adrenal steroid replacement. These patients—those with deficits in 3β-hydroxysteroid dehydrogenase, 17α-hydroxylase, 11β-hydroxylase, and 18-hydroxysteroid dehydrogenase—are committed to a lifelong regimen of steroid medication. Like persons with Addison's disease, these people should never be subjected to steroid withdrawal. (For a more detailed discussion of these disorders, see Chapters 31 and 32.)

A word should be said about patients, other than those just discussed, who are receiving lifelong adrenal replacement therapy. These are people with Addison's disease (primary adrenocortical insufficiency), those who have had surgical total bilateral adrenalectomy (as for neoplastic disease), patients with secondary adrenocortical insufficiency due to hypopituitarism, and those few who are permanently adrenal deficient because of hypothalamic-pituitary-adrenocortical (HPA) suppression caused by prolonged, high-dose corticosteroid administration (see below). The main point to be made about these chronically adrenal deficient patients is that the *replacement* doses of steroid, which are small and not associated with untoward effects, should never be withdrawn. The absolute contraindications to *pharmacologic* doses of corticoids—psychosis, herpes simplex, tuberculosis, and other infectious diseases—are not applicable to the small amounts needed for replacement, namely the equivalent of cortisol, 25 mg per day (the normal daily secretion rate of cortisol normally not exceeding 20 mg). On the contrary, it is worth re-emphasizing the need for *larger* doses of steroid during most acute intercurrent infectious illnesses in these patients, not smaller ones (see Chapters 27 and 63). One other point concerning the secondary adrenal insufficiency states should be made: Unlike Addison's disease and the salt-losing forms of congenital adrenal hyperplasia, significant aldosterone deficiency does not occur. Measurements of plasma electrolytes will therefore be normal in acute emergencies, but these findings do not signify that there is no cortisol deficiency.

The Reasons for Starting and Stopping Corticosteroid Therapy

These are plain enough when the managing physician has made all the decisions him or herself, less so when he or she has inherited a patient from another doctor or another locale. It is essential to familiarize oneself thoroughly with the rationale for the patient's receiving corticoids in the first place. We have seen that the basic indications for corticosteroid therapy may be summarized in this way: supportive-"curative," keeping a serious disease at bay, palliative, ACTH-suppressive, and as replacement. The last two categories are dealt with in Chapters 27, 31, and 32. Knowing which of the other three categories a given patient occupies provides clear signals as to what has been expected of the steroid therapeutically, how long it has been given, and what dosage has been used, large or small. This information in turn permits accurate and detailed predictions concerning the likelihood and specific nature of possible recurrences and the probability of HPA suppression. Whether or not corticoid dependence will supervene appears to be an individual and unpredictable matter.

The rationale for withdrawal of pharmacologic—that is, supraphysiologic—dosages of corticosteroids should be clear and definite. If the corticosteroid is no longer deemed to be therapeutically effective, it should be discontinued. In cases of herpes simplex or apparently disseminated tuberculosis, corticosteroids are thought by most endocrinologists to be absolutely contraindicated and should be stopped as rapidly as possible. The appearance of most other viral, bacterial, fungal, protozoan, and metazoan infections during steroid therapy, which increases host susceptibility to all these infectious diseases, is regarded by most authorities as a relative containdication. The procedure is to weigh the seriousness of the disease for which the steroid is being given against the threat posed by the intercurrent infectious insult. One cannot make a general rule.

As for the untoward effects of steroids themselves (iatrogenic Cushing's syndrome, for example), only a few dictate discontinuance of the drugs. The most definite of these is steroid induced psychosis. Less commonly, the induction of uncontrollable diabetes in a genetic diabetic patient will force one to stop corticoid treatment. The same is rarely true of steroid related severe hypertension, which can usually be controlled by antihypertensive agents even if the steroid is continued at an undiminished dosage. Incapacitating osteoporosis with pathologic fractures is an uncommon indication for withdrawing corticoids, as is pseudotumor cerebri (benign intracranial hypertension). Other untoward effects that may indicate withdrawal are peptic ulceration of the stomach, severe inhibition of growth in children, and crippling impairment of wound healing. The decision to withdraw steroids in each instance is again made by balancing the risks of the untoward effect against the benefit with respect to the underlying disease. As before, there is no simple rule applicable to all cases.

Duration of Therapy, Dosage Schedule, Specific Steroid Used

This information places the doctor in the position of being able to assess the likelihood of clinically significant steroid induced HPA suppression with concomitant inability of the patient's HPA system to respond to clinical stress. It should be apparent that the longer the course of steroid therapy and the higher the dosage, the more likely HPA suppression is to occur. The relation between duration of dosage and magnitude of dose is complex and information is incomplete. A few definite statements can be made. Patients' susceptibility to HPA suppression by steroids is extraordinarily variable. Some patients may receive corticoids for years without impairment in their response to provocative tests of HPA function. Others, treated with prednisone, 15 mg daily for a week, show flattening of the adrenocortical response to ACTH. In general, patients treated with chronic low-dose palliation (as for rheumatoid arthritis), that is, with prednisone equivalent of 10 mg daily or less, show little or no impairment of HPA activity. Most patients with serious diseases treated with prolonged high-dose therapy (leukemia, lupus) have biochemical evidence of HPA suppression. Most people undergoing intensive short-term therapy (as for infectious shock) are not suppressed. People treated with large doses over long periods with the alternate day schedule of corticoid administration (see Chapter 63) have relative or partial preservation of HPA function, but given the present state of knowledge, they must still be considered at risk.

In numerical terms, any patient who has received the corticoid equivalent of 20–30 mg prednisone per day for more than 3 to 4 weeks should be suspected of having biochemical (if not clinically significant) HPA suppression. Since there are so few data relating duration and magnitude of corticoid therapy to rate of recovery of a putatively suppressed HPA axis, a suppressed patient should be considered to have possible HPA suppression, at least biochemically, for a year after cessation of the corticoid. This view is probably too conservative from the scientific point of view, but clinically it is prudent and thoroughly safe.

Further numerical data from stress tests (bacterial pyrogen) indicate that patients given 12.5 mg or more of prednisone equivalent daily for 1 month to 8 years uniformly show HPA suppression, while those receiving 4 mg or less for the same period do not. Suppressed patients are still suppressed one month after withdrawal from steroid therapy but have recovered by five months; alternate day treatment does not suppress the HPA axis. It should be noted that the range of dosage between 4 and 12.5 mg of prednisone equivalent constitutes an area of ambiguity. The prudent therapist will probably consider such patients as having received the 12.5 mg or greater dose.

Thus, for practical purposes, detailed knowledge of duration and dosage schedule permits a fairly accurate calculation of probabilities of HPA suppression.

The only point to be made about the specific corticosteroid used relates to the duration of drug action. Cortisone and cortisol, the "native" hormones, rarely used in pharmacotherapy because of their salt-retaining property in susceptible individuals, have short half-lives in plasma. The semisynthetic corticoid analogues are all less firmly bound to specific plasma corticosteroid binding globulin (transcortin) and albumin than is cortisol, but all have longer plasma half-lives than cortisol; in the cases of prednisone, prednisolone and methlyprednisolone, slightly longer; triamcinolone, somewhat longer; dexamethasone and betamethasone, much longer. Although the relationship between duration of action and plasma half-life is irregular, these properties mean in general that the longer lasting steroids tend to induce a more constant state of "tissue" hyperadrenocorticism, a constancy that is conductive to a higher probability of HPA suppression for an equivalent dose.

The Various Forms of Corticosteroid Withdrawal Syndrome

The specific biologic type of steroid withdrawal syndrome determines its management. This section defines the types and sets out the methods for identifying them.

No Withdrawal Syndrome. Many, perhaps most, patients of the millions receiving steroids undergo withdrawal wihout clinical difficulty. An unknown number may have subtle recrudescences of underlying disease or minor degrees of HPA suppression, but these are not clinically visible to patient or physician. No treatment is indicated.

Hypothalamic-Pituitary-Adrenocortical (HPA) Suppression. The incidence and prevalence of true adrenocortical insufficiency due to

HPA suppression are not known, because the symptoms are often vague and difficult to distinguish from those of corticosteroid dependence, because systematic tests of HPA function are not routinely made, and because not enough data are available to allow firm correlation between tests of HPA function and effective response of the HPA system to clinical stress. Normal biochemical behavior in a provocative test of the HPA system does not necessarily mean a normal adrenocortical capacity to withstand an acute episode of illness, and biochemical evidence of HPA suppression does not always predict inability to make an adequate and appropriate hormonal response to acute illness or trauma or surgery. Nevertheless, tests of HPA response are the only objective guides available, so they should be done where possible and the results cautiously interpreted as if they were predictive (see below).

The symptoms and signs of corticoid induced adrenal insufficiency are much like those of Addison's disease. The most common manifestations are weakness, lassitude, easy fatigability, mental depression, hypotension, postural hypotension, and undue prostration in the face of minor illnesses, such as coryza and mild viral gastroenteritis. Addisonian pigmentation is not seen because pituitary ACTH and "MSH" secretion are suppressed, and hyponatremia and hyperkalemia do not occur because corticosteroid suppression of ACTH has no lasting or quantitatively major effect upon aldosterone production. The nonobjective elements of this clinical picture cannot easily be separated from those of psychologic or physiologic dependence on corticosteroids except by provocative tests of HPA function.

The clinician has a choice of many procedures that test the whole HPA system: insulin hypoglycemia, vasopressin, and bacterial pyrogen, for example. These are cumbersome, stressful, and require hospitalization. The adrenocortical response to ACTH is simpler, less traumatic, correlates well with the other tests of HPA function, and correlates best with the response of the adrenal cortex to clinical stress. The preferred method is to withhold the corticosteroid for 12 to 24 hours, determine baseline plasma cortisol level, at 8 A.M. administer 250 μg of synthetic (proportional to amino acids 1–24) ACTH extra- or intramuscularly, and repeat the plasma cortisol measurement 30 to 60 minutes later. This procedure is safe and virtually devoid of side effects; the unexplained hypotension and prostration during administration

of conventional ACTH to some patients with Addison's disease do not occur. Normal baseline values for plasma cortisol are 7–23 μg/dl, poststimulation values are 19–43 μg/dl, and the normal increment is greater than 6 to about 30. A deficient rise in plasma cortisol level after ACTH should be interpreted as evidence of HPA suppression; a subnormal cortisol response renders the exclusive diagnosis of psychologic dependence on corticoids untenable.

Establishing the presence of HPA suppression rests on four elements: a plausible clinical syndrome, absence of recurrent disease whose symptoms mimic those of HPA suppression, rigorous laboratory demonstration of HPA insufficiency, and relief of the clinical syndrome by *replacement* doses of corticoid, not pharmacologic doses.

Psychologic or Physical Dependence upon Corticosteroids. The diagnosis is made by elimination: recrudescent disease is absent and HPA suppression is biochemically excluded. In those circumstances, a patient who cannot tolerate steroid withdrawal or who demands increased doses, and who evinces weakness, lethargy, mood changes, or delirium when the amount of hormone is being reduced can be considered as corticoid dependent, or, in a sense, habituated. In the presence of anorexia, nausea, weight loss, fine desquamation of the skin of the face, hands, and feet, musculoskeletal aches, arthralgia, and fever the clinician can reasonably suspect physical dependence on corticosteroids. The symptoms and signs are alleviated by *pharmacologic*, not by replacement or physiologic doses of steroid.

The psychologic and subjective features of this type of withdrawal syndrome were originally ascribed to underlying and pre-existing (that is, presteroid) psychologic disturbances. Longer experience has shown that the presteroid personality has no detectable bearing on the likelihood of corticoid habituation, with the single exception that persons known to be or to have been addicted to narcotics tend to become dependent upon steroids as well.

Symptomatic Flare-up of the Underlying Disease. Detection of this kind of withdrawal syndrome depends upon the reappearance of the subjective and objective manifestations of the disease being treated with steroids. The principles and methods are outlined above. If HPA function tests are normal, a given clinical picture cannot be attributed to adrenal insufficiency. Corticoid dependence is not always so easy to differentiate. For

324 / Corticosteroid Withdrawal

example, many of the symptoms and signs listed in the section above on corticoid dependence would be indistinguishable from those of a recurrence of rheumatoid arthritis. But the distinction between disease flare-up and steroid dependence is usually clear and straightforward in patients with asthma and the severe illnesses for which long-term high-dose corticoid treatment is given.

Combination. Finally, probably the commonest form of steroid withdrawal syndrome is a combination of the three syndromes just discussed. The best way to deal with this set of problems is to inject as much objectivity as possible into the clinical setting. This is done by routinely performing the simple ACTH-plasma cortisol test of HPA function and by undertaking careful physical and laboratory investigations for objective criteria of recrudescent disease.

Peculiarities of Patient and Disease

For optimal management of the patient undergoing steroid withdrawal, the physician must be aware of relevant aspects of that patient's personality; his or her tolerance for pain and willingness or unwillingness to undergo a long and tedious process of dosage reduction; the interplay of the patient's illness with his or her family, occupation, and social life; and whether or not there is a history of prior addiction to other pharmacologic agents. The physician must know about absolute and relative contraindications, for example, the status of tuberculin reactivity, which should be monitored every six months, and about the details of possible drug interactions between the corticosteroid and other medications the patient is receiving (see Chapter 63). With respect to the disease being treated with steroids, the therapist must know precisely what symptoms and signs predominate in the particular patient and which manifestations tend to appear earliest during recurrences. For most asthmatics, cough, dyspnea or wheezing, or combinations of these are the straightforward harbingers of recurrence. As suggested above, there is more variety in other diseases. One patient with leukemia may evince easy bruising, and another, fever as the first sign that steroid treatment is failing. Some patients with rheumatoid arthritis may complain of myalgias and stiffness during corticoid withdrawal, others of objective arthritis in two or three joints. Knowledge of the natural history of the disease in the specific patient and of his or her specific reactions to treatment is thus essential to permit early detection of the need for slowing the rate of steroid reduction and for temporarily increasing the dosage of corticosteroid.

THERAPEUTIC ALTERNATIVES

These consist of using other nonhormonal drugs in place of corticosteroids, small or homeopathic doses of steroids, the alternate day schedule of glucocorticoid therapy, or ACTH.

In the severe diseases often treated with long-term high-dose steroids, other immunosuppressive agents may enable the physician to avoid corticoids if there is good reason to do so, that is, if absolute or relative contraindications exist. Immunosuppressives may sometimes suffice in lupus, leukemia, and the hepatitides. In asthma, inhaled steroids may induce less HPA suppression than steroids given systemically; other nonsteroidal inhalants, cromolyn, or other bronchodilators, singly or in combination, may palliate the disease without steroids. As for rheumatoid arthritis, corticosteroids are being used less and less, and other anti-inflammatory agents, for example, indomethacin, are given instead.

Very small doses of corticosteroids may control the manifestations of inflammatory and immunologic diseases, but this is usually not possible. The physician may then resort to larger doses but on the alternate day schedule, which is discussed in Chapter 63. It should be noted here that patients may be converted from the daily to the alternate day schedule in mid-course of their treatment or of steroid withdrawal; this change permits HPA recovery to occur but does not accelerate the process.

Corticotropin (ACTH) has been used in intermittent dosage schedules *during steroid therapy* in attempts to prevent adrenocortical insufficiency due to HPA suppression. Although biochemical HPA response to both insulin and ACTH response tests is usually preserved, the subjective and objective signs of steroid withdrawal syndrome are as severe as with steroid therapy alone. The method has no value.

ACTH given *after a course of steroids* accelerates the return of adrenocortical function, but this return is transitory; the poststeroid hyporesponsiveness can be shown again within a week after the ACTH treatment. One would not expect to improve hypothalamic or pituitary function in these circumstances. In fact, ACTH may sometimes exert a negative feedback inhibitory influence upon endogenous ACTH secretion, and anti-

ACTH antibodies against the native hormone may be formed. This method also appears to be without value.

ACTH given *instead of steroids* has a few advantages. Allegedly there are fewer serious undesirable effects. Growth curves in children are more nearly normal. Some clinicians believe it is easier to withdraw patients from ACTH than from steroids. The HPA system is more likely to remain biochemically intact. But these benefits are outweighed by the disadvantages. ACTH has to be given by injection. No disease responds better clinically to ACTH than to steroid therapy. A moderate number of patients have sustained severe hypersensitivity reactions to ACTH and a few have suffered intra-adrenal hemorrhage. Rarely, acute and catastrophic collapse, presumably due to adrenal failure, has occurred after a prolonged course of ACTH therapy. The maximum amount of endogenous cortisol secretion that can be stimulated by exogenous ACTH is not more than 250 mg per day (or the equivalent of 60 mg of prednisone); many diseases (acute leukemia, lupus nephritis) require more than that. Finally, there is some evidence that exogenous ACTH may interfere with biosynthesis and release of pituitary ACTH. These seem sufficient reasons to discard this method.

PREFERRED APPROACH

Textbooks and treatises on therapeutics provide recommendations and recipes for corticosteroid withdrawal as if the only hazard were HPA suppression, but there are others as well (see above). The foregoing analysis indicates that the disease that has been treated, its recurrence or failure to recur, the therapeutic indications for steroid therapy, the details of the corticosteroid regimen and its duration, the exact type of corticosteroid withdrawal syndrome, and the idiosyncrasies of the particular patient and the particular disease all influence the choice of method for withdrawing a patient from corticosteroids. No single, simple approach will do for all.

General Considerations

The category of disease dictates the intensity and duration of steroid treatment, and that regimen indicates in general the method of withdrawal.

For acute, catastrophic conditions (such as septic shock) treated for no more than two to six days with high-dose steroids (hundreds of milli-grams to grams of prednisone equivalent daily), the physician can stop the steroid therapy as abruptly as it was started. The activity of the precipitating condition dictates the need for tapering the steroid dose (rare), not HPA suppression.

For the serious inflammatory, immunologic, and hematologic disorders (such as disseminated lupus) treated with prolonged high-dose steroid therapy (more than 15 mg of prednisone daily), withdrawal must be gradual because of HPA suppression and the danger of recurrent disease. Further, in these patients acute secondary adrenal insufficiency may be precipitated or exacerbated if the disease flares up during steroid withdrawal. If the patient has not been maintained throughout the course of steroid treatment on the alternate day schedule, it is not useful to switch to it as a prelude to steroid withdrawal, since the process of HPA recovery is not accelerated. The integrity of the HPA system is maintained by the alternate day schedule only when it is employed throughout most of the course.

In the inflammatory disorders (such as rheumatoid arthritis) managed with prolonged low-dose palliative steroid therapy (2–10 mg of prednisone per day), corticoid withdrawal must be gradual because of recurrence of the disease and because of corticosteroid dependence. HPA suppression is probably not much of a factor. The doses have to be decreased by very small steps and very slowly, usually with intermittent plateaus or slight increases in dosage. Withdrawal may take a year or more and a small portion of patients will not tolerate the total elimination of steroid therapy.

As suggested above, the small doses used in chronic inhibition of pituitary ACTH secretion (0.75 mg dexamethasone daily as in congenital adrenal hyperplasia) do not seriously impair the cortisol-secreting facet of HPA function. Gradual lowering of steroid doses is therefore not necessary.

Specific Methods of Corticosteroid Withdrawal

For HPA Suppressed Patients. Patients in this category are chiefly those with a serious disease that has been treated with prolonged high-dose daily steroid therapy. A good rule of thumb is that any patient who looks cushingoid probably has significant HPA suppression. The critical dose of corticosteroid above which cushingoid appearance almost univerally occurs is 15 mg of prednisone daily or the equivalent. Since the dosage range for this category of patients is approximately 15–120 mg of prednisone per day and the duration of treatment more than 3 to 4 weeks, one assumes that all patients in this group are biochemically HPA suppressed, whether the clinical degree of HPA suppression (generally undetectable) is significant or not.

A second rule depends on the reasons for stopping steroid treatment. The rate of withdrawal should be as rapid as possible in the face of major untoward effects of steroids or absolute contraindications to them, such as herpes simplex, varicella infections, or psychosis. If the aim of withdrawal is to take advantage of a strong likelihood that the disease is in remission (when, for example, it has been possible to lower the steroid dosage considerably without recurrence), then the rate of dosage reduction should be gradual. This is the procedure in many instances of disseminated lupus, ulcerative colitis, and acute lymphatic leukemia.

A third precept is that the physician should subdue his or her own excessive anxiety about corticoid withdrawal. With minimal vigilance, no patient dies from this process. Adrenal insufficiency is not of sudden onset and HPA suppression as a cause of death has been proved only rarely. Disease recurrences, with the rare exception of such entities as grand mal seizures due to cerebral microvascular disease in lupus, are not fatal. The aim is to spare the patient avoidable sudden, intense flare-ups of disease. Since corticosteroids seldom eradicate the chronic disorders for which they are used, steroid removal merely allows a condition, hitherto apparently held in check, to show itself. During withdrawal, one wishes to blunt these manifestations as much as possible.

The fourth rule concerning this group of patients is that steroid dependence in a few, HPA suppression in very few, and flare-up of disease in most will govern the rate of withdrawal from steroids. This gradual lowering of dosage is directed toward reducing the probability both of clinically significant adrenocortical insufficiency and of recrudescent illness.

In this category of persons given long-term high-dose steroid therapy, the clinical problem is that the disease (to the extent that one can separate disease from host) tolerates steroid withdrawal poorly; the host (with the same reservation) tolerates withdrawal relatively well.

Method. No prescription can be given which will suit all patients and all diseases. What follows is a practical outline that is generally applicable but must be modified to fit individual needs.

For the patients whose steroid therapy is interrupted because of an acute emergency that contraindicates corticoid administration (generalized viral infection, psychotic break), the principle is to cut the dose rapidly to an amount just enough above the physiologic level (prednisone, 5 mg, or cortisone, 20–25 mg) to sustain a presumably HPA suppressed, that is, adrenal deficient, patient through the stress of the intercurrent illness. Specifically, for the infectious complications, one reduces the steroid dosage from the maintenance level of 15–120 mg prednisone to 10–15 mg prednisone within 1 to 2 days, carefully observing vital signs and the activity of the basic disease. Since disseminated herpetic infection, for example, can be immediately fatal, whereas the steroid-treated systemic diseases are not, one errs on the low side of corticoid administration to minimize the immunosuppressive effect, that is, one lowers the dose still further to 5–10 mg of prednisone daily or 5 mg and 10 mg on alternate days, or less if possible. In managing steroid psychosis, the dosage can be at that level or lower—that is, physiologic—depending on the hyperactivity of the disturbed patient. In the event of severe trauma or a surgical emergency, patients receiving high-dose steroid therapy should be treated with larger doses of parenterally administered corticosteroids, as described in Chapter 63.

For the majority of patients in this high-dose category whose steroids are being eliminated in anticipation of a partial or complete remission, withdrawal can usually be accomplished quite smoothly within four weeks. Before starting withdrawal, the physician carefully notes and records all objective physical signs of the basic disease and obtains the essential laboratory data that will be used as indices of its activity. If one is starting from a dosage range of 15–40 mg of prednisone or equivalent daily, one can reduce the amount of steroid by decrements of 2.5–5 mg every second or third day until a physiologic level, 5 mg daily, is reached within 1 to 2 weeks. This can usually be done with impunity. Beginning at the higher dosage ranges, above 40 to 120 mg of prednisone per day, the dosage is lowered by decrements of 2.5–5 mg every 3 to 7 days. The reduction can be continued through minor recurrences of the basic disease, but if the flare-up is serious or more or less incapacitating, the dosage is raised again to an amount just sufficient to suppress the manifestations and a more gradual reduction is attempted.

It may be necessary to add other therapeutic agents, for example, immunosuppressants or cytotoxic drugs, if these are not already being given. Switching the patient to the alternate day steroid schedule is probably not useful and may only interpose another time-consuming step in an already lengthy procedure. By the third to fourth week, after a steady decrement of steroid dosage or after a series of decrements, brief increments, further decrements, and periods of plateau, the amount of steroid ought to have arrived at a physiologic level, 5 mg of prednisone daily or 0.75 mg of dexamethasone. At this point, after the patient has been shown to tolerate this dosage for 3 to 7 days, the steroid is changed to 20–25 mg of hydrocortisone or cortisone, a physiologic dose of the physiologic hormone, the steroid with the shortest biologic action, given as a single morning dose to allow the maximum opportunity for resurgence of the HPA system.

During the fourth week, an 8 A.M. plasma cortisol determination is made and that day's cortisone dose is withheld. Most patients will then have a cortisol level <10 μg/dl, a value likely to persist for 6 to 9 months after the initiation of corticoid withdrawal. At about the fourth to sixth week, the cortisone dosage is again reduced, to 10 mg of cortisone, given as a single morning dose; this is not enough steroid to foster the continuance of iatrogenic Cushing's syndrome nor to suppress the HPA system, but it is sufficient to provide a cushion against adrenocortical insufficiency under basal conditions. In medical emergencies, such as acute infections, trauma, or surgery, and in minor illnesses or small-scale interventive procedures (endoscopy, dental work), steroid cover is necessary (see Chapter 63). By the sixth to ninth month, the 8 A.M. plasma cortisol level, which is measured about every 2 months, should have returned to >10 μg/dl. Then the physician can assume that basal HPA function has recovered and the morning dose of cortisone can be stopped, but steroid cover for emergencies will still be required.

Nine or more months after the start of withdrawal, the integrity of the entire HPA system should have been restored. There is not much point in performing an ACTH stimulation test until this time, because full HPA capacity to respond to provocative tests may take 9 to 12 months or more. During this period, a synthetic ACTH (Synacthen, Cosyntropin) test is done; when the increment of plasma cortisol is in the range of >6–30 μg/dl HPA recovery is judged to be complete, and steroid cover for medical emergencies should theo-

retically not be required. Nevertheless, the correlation between biochemical tests of HPA function and HPA capacity to react to clinical stress is uncertain, so that for the first 12 to 16 months after the beginning of corticoid withdrawal, steroid cover should be instituted for acute stresses or in the event that manifestations of adrenocortical insufficiency appear.

As stated above, ACTH has no place in the treatment of the corticosteroid withdrawal syndrome or in the management of steroid withdrawal. Since the HPA suppressed patient has an inadequate adrenocortical capacity to respond to endogenous or exogenous corticotropin, ACTH administration will not stimulate enough cortisol secretion to protect the patient from adrenal insufficiency during stress.

For Corticosteroid Dependent Patients. This category includes patients with rheumatoid arthritis and some asthmatics maintained on long-term low-dose palliative therapy. Despite the low dosages (<15 mg of prednisone daily), these people are more difficult to withdraw than those on prolonged high-dose corticosteroid regimens. For unknown reasons, this group evinces a greater tendency to become dependent upon corticosteroids. It is not known whether the dependence is psychologic or physiologic or both. The dangers of corticosteroid withdrawal are less than in the high-dose group, but the likelihood of failure to achieve withdrawal is greater. The clinical problem is that the disease tolerates withdrawal relatively well; the host tolerates it poorly or not at all.

For practical purposes, HPA suppression does not present difficulties during withdrawal, except that the cautious physician will provide steroid cover if medical emergencies supervene during the process. Plasma cortisol measurement and ACTH tests are unnecessary. Particularly in rheumatoid arthritis, reduction of the steroid dosage must be regular and deliberate. The physician has to make every effort to enlist the full cooperation and tolerance of the patient. Decrements in dosage should not exceed 1 mg of prednisone equivalent every 1 to 2 months; at that rate withdrawal may require a year or more. The physician should not try to hasten the withdrawal or attempt alternate day schedules; such maneuvers may precipitate "steroid pseudorheumatism"—more likely a manifestation of corticoid withdrawal than of recurrent arthritis—which requires raising the steroid dosage again, sometimes to levels above the dosage from which one started. For mild to moderate exacerbations, increased amounts of salicylate may be given and indomethacin added. The physician must be careful about salicylates; corticosteroids enhance renal clearance of aspirin, and when the steroid dosage is reduced, blood values of salicylate may rise to the toxic range in some patients. Monitoring of plasma salicylate levels permits appropriate titration of aspirin dosage.

Patients with asthma are almost as difficult to withdraw as are those with rheumatoid arthritis. Reduction of the steroid dose must be gradual, but the decrements need not be as exquisitely small as for rheumatoid patients, and the variety of other effective medications, such as, systemic or inhaled bronchodilators, offers a broader choice in mitigating flare-ups during steroid withdrawal. As in the arthritic subjects, these patients must be persuaded to cooperate fully with the withdrawal procedure.

In this category, the physician must be prepared to fail. An unknown proportion of people with these two diseases cannot or will not tolerate life without corticosteroids. In my opinion, this is because of corticosteroid dependence or habituation, not uncontrollable disease, but a clinical impression of steroid dependence does not give the physician license to adopt a high moral tone toward his dependent—some might say "addicted"—patient. The corticosteroid dependency syndrome, comprising objective and subjective signs, might as well be viewed as an organic illness. The only effective treatment is the lowest possible dosage of steroid, as little as 1–2.5 mg of prednisone daily. Why such small amounts, below the physiologic secretion rate of cortisol in equivalence, should effectively relieve symptoms is not known, but since there is no danger of HPA suppression or iatrogenic Cushing's syndrome with these minute doses, one has no good reason to withhold what the patient will demand in any case.

For Flare-ups of the Steroid Treated Disease. Consideration of recurrent disease during steroid withdrawal is necessarily woven into the foregoing discussions concerning HPA suppression and corticoid dependence. This interweaving emphasizes the difficulty in separating, on clinical grounds, the manifestations of the three elements. This is not difficult in flagrant systemic diseases like ulcerative colitis and disseminated lupus or disorders like asthma, which are marked by some clear and unmistakable sign. But in rheumatoid arthritis, for example, a syndrome—occurring during steroid withdrawal—of weakness, lassitude, muscle aches, joint stiffness with only minimal swelling or redness, and low grade fever can reasonably be interpreted as HPA insufficiency, corticoid dependence, or a mild recrudescence of the rheumatoid process. Serologic tests for mesenchymal disease may be somewhat informative but only rarely provide a definite diagnosis of recurrence. Provocative tests of HPA function may show normal or subnormal biochemical response, but the relation between test and clinical adequacy or deficiency of the HPA system is irregular and obscure. The physician must therefore be prepared to deal with some patients in whom the three threads—status of the HPA system, corticoid dependence, mild flare-up of disease—are almost impossible to disentangle. In such people, the clinical syndrome is relieved by administration of low-dose corticosteroids. This is not intellectually rewarding but leads to a satisfactory clinical result.

SUMMARY

On empiric grounds, the physician cannot withdraw corticosteroids abruptly after long-term administration. Most of the emphasis in the literature has been placed upon the dangers of HPA suppression and how to avoid or mitigate it. This emphasis follows from the fact that biochemical tests of HPA function are the least indefinite and most objective indices we have for assessing a prototypical effect of prolonged steroid therapy; corticoids leave clear tracks upon the HPA system. Nevertheless, the successful handling of patients undergoing withdrawal from steroids depends on the understanding that flare-ups of the systemic disease the steroids have been holding in check and dependence of the patient upon corticosteroids have equal or greater importance in accounting for the manifestations of the corticosteroid withdrawal syndromes and for the difficulties in their management.

ENDOCRINE TREATMENT OF MALIGNANCY

CARCINOMA OF THE PROSTATE

DAVID F. PAULSON, M.D.

The treatment of prostatic adenocarcinoma is based upon the extent of disease at the time of the initial diagnosis. Disease confined to the prostate itself is best treated by removal of the gland and its contained malignancies. Disease that has extended locally beyond the anatomic confines of the gland but does not yet involve lymph node or distant bony parenchymal structures seems to be best treated by radiation therapy. There is no consensus on the treatment of prostatic carcinoma that has spread to the regional lymph nodes but does not yet involve distant bony and parenchymal structures. Disease involving distant bony and parenchymal structures which is either symptomatic or in which the rate of progression can be identified is seemingly best treated initially by androgen deprivation. The discussion that follows focuses upon the treatment of prostatic carcinoma according to the anatomic distribution of disease.

EXTENT OF DISEASE

The treatment for prostatic carcinoma is based on the anatomic extent of disease, and therefore it is appropriate to ascertain the extent of disease prior to treatment selection. Multiple staging systems have been proposed (Fig. 1). All of these systems are similar in that they determine the anatomic extent of the malignancy as either being confined to the gland of origin, having local spread, involving either regional or distant lymph nodes, or involving other bone and parenchymal sites. The anatomic extent of the malignancy is determined best by a sequential application of routine chest and pelvic x-rays, radioisotopic bone scan, and staging pelvic lymphadenectomy. The anatomic extent of prostatic carcinoma can be clas-

Anatomic Extent of Disease

Stage	Stage	AJC Classification	Local Lesion	Prostatic Acid Phosphatase	Lymph Node Extension	Bone Metastases By Bone X-ray
A, Focal	IA	$T_0N_xM_o$	Not palpable, focal	Not elevated	No	No
A, Diffuse	IB	$T_oN_xM_o$	Not palpable, diffuse	Not elevated	No	No
B	II	$T_1T_2N_xM_o$	Confined to prostate	Not elevated	No	No
C	III	$T_3N_xM_o$	Local extension	Not elevated	No	No
D	IVA	$T_{any}N_xM_o$	Any	Elevated	No	No
D	IVB	$T_{any}N_{1-4}M_o$	Any	Any	Yes	No
D	IVC	$T_{any}N_{any}M_1$	Any	Any	Yes/No	Yes

Note: Lymph node extension must be confirmed to determine anatomic extent of disease. All staging categories can be assigned with the exception of IVB ($T_{any}N_{1-4}M_o$) without nodal assessment.

Figure 1. The anatomic extent of the classifications here give an indication of the extent of disease as indicated in the four righthand columns. Under the AJC classification, T stands for the amount of local tumor, N stands for lymph nodes, and M stands for metastatic disease. The subscripts: x stands for not assessed, o stands for none, and the numerical subscripts under N and M indicate the extent of nodal disease or metastatic extention.

sified as (1) tumors that are confined within the anatomic limits of the prostate itself, (2) malignancy that has extended beyond the anatomic limits of the prostate but does not yet involve regional or distant anatomic sites, and (3) disease that has spread to metastatic lymph node, parenchymal, or bony sites. Tumors confined to the prostate may be given either the clinical classification of stage A or stage B. Stage A tumors are identified only by the histologic examination of tissue removed at surgery for clinically benign disease or at autopsy. These occult tumors are confined within the prostate and are neither suspected nor detected prior to the surgery for presumed benign disease. Occult carcinoma is found in approximately 10 percent of all prostates removed for benign disease. The occult stage A tumors are further subclassified by histologic criteria into occult-focal (carcinoma involving less than 5 percent of the prostatic specimen) and occult-diffuse (malignancy involving more than 5 percent of the prostatic tissue). There is ample evidence to indicate that stage A focal disease may be managed by enucleation or transurethral resection of the prostate only. This seems reasonable, as any surgical maneuver that removes the malignancy in its entirety from the involved organ would be as clinically beneficial as a more radical operation. The problem in permitting such a minimal operative procedure to be the definitive treatment for presumably focal disease rests in the inability to identify a small substitute locus of prostatic carcinoma without examination of the entire specimen.

Clinical stage B prostatic carcinoma also is disease confined to the prostate; however, this is disease that is palpable on rectal examination and suspected by the examining physician. Stage B tumors have been subdivided into stage B-1, a nodule on the prostate of no more than 1.5 cm in diameter, and stage B-2, a nodule on the prostate which is greater than 1.5 cm in diameter in 1 lobe or a nodule that involves both lobes of the gland.

Stage C lesions are those found to have crossed the anatomic boundaries of the prostate gland either by rectal examination or by pathologic examination of the excised specimen. Stage D lesions involve regional or distant metastatic sites.

The anatomic distribution of prostatic adenocarcinoma is established through a logical, sequential series of diagnostic staging examinations. The initial test, once there is biopsy confirmation of the presence of prostatic carcinoma in the prostate, should be determination of the serum acid phosphatase level. An elevation of the serum acid phosphatase above the normal level should be taken as indication of disease spread beyond the anatomic limits of the prostate itself, even if the disease cannot be identified in distant bony and parenchymal sites by noninvasive staging maneuvers. The appearance of an elevated acid phosphatase level without identifiable bone disease probably represents early but as yet undetected bony metastatic extension. Patients who have an elevated serum acid phosphatase level but in whom bony metastases cannot be identified, either by routine bone x-rays or isotopic bone scanning, develop bony metastases more often than those who have normal serum phosphatase activity at the time of initial examination.

All patients who do not have evidence of blastic bone disease on the chest x-ray or in the standare KUB should have a radioisotopic bone scan to determine whether or not there is metastatic disease involving the axial or appendicular skeleton. If no disease can be identified in any of the bony structures, attention should then be focused on the pelvic lymph nodes. Patients who have no identified bony disease should be examined for the presence of lymph node extension. The lymphatic spread of prostatic carcinoma occurs through the lymphatic vasculature which exits from the posterior aspect of the prostate. The lymph nodes involved are those of the hypogastric, obturator, external iliac, and presacral lymphatics. The presence of lymph node metastases in these sites is best determined, not by lymphangiography or by computerized axial tomography (CT), but by surgical excision of the lymph nodes of the hypogastric and obturator lymphatics and examination of these lymph nodes under the microscope.

TREATMENT

Treatment of Disease Confined to the Prostate

The treatment philosophy that promotes continued use of radical surgery for disease confined within the prostate is based upon the observation that human malignancies confined to a single anatomic site fare better if that site can be excluded from the host at risk. A recent study by the Uro-Oncology Research Group indicated that radical prostatectomy was more effective in preventing the subsequent appearance of distant disease spread than was radiation therapy when the tumor was initially confined to the prostate.

This multi-institutional randomized trial staged patients on the basis of serum acid phosphatase levels, radioisotopic bone scan, and pelvic lymphadenectomy. In patients in whom the disease was confined to the prostate on the basis of rectal examination and in whom no evidence of distant disease spread could be detected by either routine isotopic bone scan, serum acid phosphatase elevation, or pelvic lymphadenectomy were randomly treated with either radical perineal prostatectomy or external beam radiation therapy using 5000 rads to the full pelvis with 2000-rad boost to the prostate. Treatment failure in this study was defined as the first appearance of metastatic disease identified by either the appearance of acid phosphatase elevation on two subsequent occasions, and/or the appearance of bony metastases confirmed by either radioisotopic bone scanning or routine bone x-rays, and/or the appearance of parenchymal or nodal disease confirmed by either physical examination or other electron beam modalities. The failure rate among patients who received external beam radiation for disease that was apparently confined to the prostate was much higher than the failure rate for patients who were subjected to radical prostatectomy. The histologic grade of tumor in these two treatment groups was identical.

No randomized treatment trials had been used to study the impact of interstitial radiotherapy for disease that was felt to be confined to the prostate. However, a careful evaluation of the results of those treatment groups using either interstitial gold seeds or interstitial radioactive iodine seeds would indicate that, although interstitial radiation may alter to some extent the biology of the disease, it does not eradicate the disease with the same certainty as radical surgery.

Treatment of Disease Extended Beyond the Prostate But Not Involving Regional Lymph Nodes or Distant Metastatic Sites

There are at present no hard data indicating any treatment methodology that significantly improves the survival rate of patients with this stage of disease. It is my present bias, however, that external beam radiation therapy is best for disease that extends beyond the anatomic confines of the gland. However, this position is substantiated not by hard facts but by clinical impression.

Treatment of Disease Involving Regional Lymph Nodes But Not Distant Metastatic Sites

An early review of the disease course in a series of patients at Duke Medical Center who underwent radical prostatectomy indicated that the time between initiation of therapy and recognition of its failure for patients who had radical prostatectomy and node positive disease was short; 50 percent of the patients with node positive disease showed evidence of distant disease spread in less than two years. These observations led to the development of an institutional trial in which patients with regional lymph node metastases and negative isotopic bone scan were, after pelvic lymphadetomy, assigned to treatment with either radical prostatectomy, external beam radiation therapy (5000 rads to the full pelvis and periaortic nodes, with a 2000-rad boost to the prostate), or delayed androgen deprivation therapy. In this institutional trial, 11 patients underwent radical perineal prostatectomy, 20 patients received radiation therapy, and 13 patients were assigned to delayed androgen deprivation with treatment being withheld until progression of disease was noted. Again, time-to-failure curves were used to permit the early identification of treatment effect unencumbered by the imposition of a second treatment. The time to first evidence of treatment failure was similar for each of the treatment groups. The median time to first evidence of treatment failure was less than two years for all of the treatment groups. It was then asked whether there was a difference in the time to failure between patients who had only one positive lymph node and patients who had more than one positive lymph node. An eight-month difference in the time to failure could be identified in patients having only one positive lymph node as compared with those having more than one positive lymph node.

This institutional study provided the impetus to examine this problem in a large multi-institutional randomized trial. In this trial, patients who had no evidence of bone disease on isotopic scanning and no evidence of parenchymal disease involving either the lung or liver, but who had node positive disease on the basis of pelvic lymphadenectomy, were subjected to either external beam radiation therapy, 5000 rads to the full pelvis and periaortic lymph nodes to the level of L-1, with a 2000-rad boost to the prostate; or to delayed androgen deprivation. Again, time to first evidence of treatment failure was used as the end point of this study. This trial indicated that some marginal benefit was achieved with external beam radiation therapy over delayed androgen deprivation.

Treatment of Disease At Distant Metastatic Sites (Androgen Deprivation)

The management of prostatic carcinoma that is anatomically distributed at sites distant from the prostate is very controversial. The observation that adult prostatic epithelium atrophies when the sustaining physiologic effect of the androgenic hormones is removed has led to the therapeutic application of androgen deprivation or suppression in the management of metastatic prostatic adenocarcinoma. Androgen deprivation, which should be promoted as the treatment of choice in metastatic prostatic adenocarcinoma, is based on the assumption that malignant prostatic epithelium is androgen dependent, as is nonmalignant prostatic tissue. A reduction in the androgenic support of prostatic epithelium can be accomplished therapeutically by (1) removal of the primary source of circulating androgens, (2) removal or suppression of hypothalamic luteinizing hormone with a reduction of testicular testosterone production, (3) direct inhibition of androgen synthesis on the cellular level, (4) a blocking of androgens or their effect at the cellular level.

Removal of the Primary Androgen Source. The serum testosterone levels in the normal male range between 400 and 1000 ng percent. Bilateral orchiectomy will reduce plasma testosterone levels by approximately 90 percent. In the adult male there is no detectable increase in plasma testosterone levels from the subsequent activation of secondary androgen sources following removal of the testicle. The subsequent appearance of endocrine-unresponsive symptomatic disease after bilateral orchiectomy is not associated with any demonstrable elevation in circulating plasma, androstenedione, dehydroepiandrosterone, or testosterone levels, indicating that the symptomatic recurrence is not associated with an increase in circulating androgens or their metabolic end product. These studies would lead one to believe that the application of a secondary treatment designed also to reduce androgen levels will not save patients whose disease progresses after orchiectomy. The published experience of high-dose estrogen trials supports this hypothesis.

Hypothalamic Suppression. Estrogens establish androgen deprivation at a hypothalmic level

by occupying the hypothalamic binding site of testosterone and thus inhibiting the release of luteinizing hormone-releasing factor, with subsequent suppression of the luteinizing hormone release by the pituitary and a reduction in testosterone production by the testicle. Plasma testosterone levels in males treated with 1 mg of diethylstilbestrol or its equivalent may vary not only among subjects, but also with respect to serial values obtained during longitudinal observations on a single subject. In these patients serum testosterone levels may not reach the anorchid levels that can be achieved by bilateral orchiectomy. However, 3 mg per day of diethylstilbestrol will suppress testosterone levels into the castrate range. Doses exceeding 3 mg per day will not suppress serum testosterone farther.

Inhibitors of Androgen Synthesis. Certain selective inhibitors of androgen synthesis will produce a pharmaceutical orchiectomy. Some of these agents are available for clinical trial but none has been released with this specific indication. The most familiar drug is aminoglutethimide. This agent will block side-chain cleavage of cholesterol and its subsequent hydroxylation, thus inhibiting the production of both testosterone and aldosterone. Cyproterone acetate blocks 17, 20-desmolase and thus interferes with androgen synthesis. Spironolactone will suppress plasma testosterone levels by 90 percent and plasma androstenedione and dehydroepiandrosterone levels by 40 to 60 percent. Aminoglutethimide, Cyproterone acetate, and spironolactone have all undergone evaluation with regard to the treatment of prostatic carcinoma that has progressed after initial androgen deprivation. None of these agents has been found effective in reversing the clinical course in this patient population.

Antiandrogens. Antiandrogens block the effectiveness of the androgenic substance at the target level by interfering with the intracellular events that mediate androgenic action. The antiandrogens can inhibit both endogenously secreted and exogenously administered androgenic hormones. All effective compounds tested to date act through a common mechanism by inhibiting the formation of the receptor-dihydrotestosterone complex. Cyproterone acetate is the most potent of the steroidal antiandrogens. It is well absorbed locally, and it not only produces target organ inhibition, but also interferes with gonadotropin release and presumably inhibits steroidogenesis.

Controversies in Androgen Deprivation Therapy. There is much controversy regarding the best mechanisms for androgen deprivation in prostatic carcinoma. This controversy has been engendered by the clinical observation that androgen deprivation will provide dramatic symptomatic relief with possible disease progression and the statistical observation that survival of the prostatic cancer patient is probably not enhanced by androgen deprivation. The uncertainty results from several factors, including the form of androgen deprivation selected, the dose level of exogenous estrogens that may be administered to interfere with hypothalamic stimulation of testosterone production, and the timing of therapeutic intervention in the course of disease. The accepted clinical assumption is that survival must necessarily be prolonged as a consequence of any treatment that appears so effective in reducing the debilitating symptoms of disease progression.

The wide variation in estrogen dosages and in disease staging in the majority of publications to date prevents rational assessment of the relative benefits and hazards of estrogen control. The Veterans Administration Cooperative Urologic Research Group (VACURG) was established specifically to examine questions raised in many previous publications. This Group produced a landmark study in which four treatments were examined in a randomized trial. Placebo; placebo plus orchiectomy; diethylstilbestrol, 5 mg daily; and orchiectomy plus diethylstilbestrol, 5 mg daily were evaluated in 1093 stage C and stage D prostatic cancer patients. In stage C prostatic disease, treatment with placebo and orchiectomy plus placebo was demonstrated to be significantly better than orchiectomy plus estrogen with respect to overall survival. However, less than a 10 percent difference between the worst and the best treatment groups could be detected nine years after initiation of the trial. In stage D disease, in which the risk of death from cancer was significant, no difference in overall survival rates among any of the four treatment groups could be detected. When stage C and stage D disease were combined and survival curves established, dependent upon death from prostatic cancer alone, diethylstilbestrol, 5 mg daily, and orchiectomy plus estrogens were both more effective than orchiectomy plus placebo or placebo alone. Subsequent studies by this same group indicated that 1 mg of diethylstilbestrol daily was as effective of 5 mg daily in controlling cancer deaths in either stage C or stage D disease, but that in stage C disease, in which there was less competing risk of death from malignancy, there were fewer cardiovascular deaths on the 1 mg dosage than on the 5 mg dosage. These higher dosages

were both superior to placebo or 0.2 mg of diethylstilbestrol daily in controlling death from malignant disease. Thus it would appear that there is a dose-dependent association between the negative effects of diethylstilbestrol on the cardiovascular system and the therapeutic effect of controlling malignancy. The minimal difference in these trials between placebo and the use of estrogens was initially felt to demonstrate that androgen deprivation using diethystilbestrol had minimal impact on the course of disease. However, within the VACURG studies, patients treated with placebo actually were placed on estrogens when disease progression was identified. Thus the placebo treated groups were, in truth, not placebo treated groups but were treated with delayed androgen deprivation. Thus this study would indicate that delaying androgen deprivation until such time as progression of the disease within the specific host can be identified does not adversely affect survival. The minimal impact on overall survival produced by the various endocrine treatments would therefore indicate that the predictors determining the relative cardiovascular and cancer risks within a specific patient have not yet been established. Thus there seems to be little advantage in initiating androgen deprivation prior to the onset of symptoms of bone pain or evidence of active progression, such as weakness, anemia, or progressive outflow of ureteral obstruction. Considerable controversy exists as to the form that androgen deprivation should take. It seems ideal to select a level of androgen deprivation that (1) incurs least risk of disease, and (2) establishes adequate disease control. Orchiectomy would seem to ensure removal of the source of persistent androgen production and would obviate the need for faithful exogenous estrogen consumption—and thus eliminate the associated cardiovascular risks accompanying exogenous androgens. Diethylstilbestrol, 1 mg daily, does not produce uniformly anorchid levels of serum testosterone but has demonstrated fewer cardiovascular hazards than administration of 5 mg daily. Diethylstilbestrol, 3 mg daily, does produce anorchid levels of serum testosterone; however, the relative cardiovascular hazard of this dosage level has not been established in randomized trials. Diethylstilbestrol, 5 mg daily, also produces anorchid levels of serum testosterone, but it is associated with a cardiovascular hazard greater than that with the 1 mg dose. Orchiectomy seems the surest way to reduce serum testosterone while providing the least cardiovascular hazard. Simultaneous administration of diethylstilbestrol, 1 mg daily, or its equivalent is postulated to provide additional control at the cellular level, but this has not been proved. When estrogen therapy with or without orchiectomy is administered, certain biologic effects can be anticipated. Gynecomastia always occurs, and this may be both physiologically and psychologically painful. Radiation of the breast (900–1200 rads) in a single or divided dose prior to the initiation of exogenous estrogens will prevent this problem and should be considered in each male patient before initiation of androgen deprivation therapy using exogenous estrogens. Dependent edema can be managed with diuretics. The use of Coumadin or aspirin to reduce thromboembolic hazards of Estradiol is an attractive treatment adjunct, but its efficacy is as yet unproven.

ENDOCRINE THERAPY OF METASTATIC BREAST CANCER

C. KENT OSBORNE, M.D.
and WILLIAM L. McGUIRE, M.D.

Breast cancer is the leading cause of cancer deaths in women in this country. More than 100,000 cases are diagnosed each year and about a third of those women die annually from this disease. Although new treatment strategies have had only a minimal impact to date on survival of this disease, over the past decade several advances have dramatically changed and improved the management of these patients. Many of these advances have been derived from basic laboratory research into the factors controlling breast cancer cell growth.

This is especially true in the area of hormone-dependent breast cancer. It has been known for nearly one hundred years that alteration of the hormonal milieu in certain women with metastatic breast cancer causes tumor regression. Since the normal mammary gland is influenced by a variety of hormones, it is not surprising that certain cancers derived from this gland might also retain this "hormone dependence." However, only about one-third of women with breast cancer have hormone-dependent tumors and respond to hormonal manipulation. Furthermore, until recently the basic mechanisms involved in endocrine-induced tumor regression have been poorly understood.

Prior to 1970, before the development and widespread use of effective cytotoxic chemotherapy, endocrine therapy was the primary mode of treatment for most women with advanced breast cancer. Because of the relatively low response rates to endocrine therapy, cytotoxic chemotherapy has become increasingly popular as a primary treatment for patients with this disease. With modern chemotherapy, 60 to 70 percent of patients now have an objective response, with median durations of remission approaching one year. Yet such therapy is not without significant morbidity. Furthermore, those patients who might have had a durable remission with a simpler, less toxic endocrine therapy are lost by the routine use of primary chemotherapy. In the last several years, the pendulum has begun to swing in the opposite direction and there has been renewed interest in endocrine therapy. This is due to at least two developments. First, the development of the estrogen and progesterone receptor assays now allows physicians to select accurately those patients most likely to respond to endocrine therapy. Second, the development of new forms of endocrine therapy, such as the antiestrogens and medical adrenalectomy, have further reduced the hazards associated with endocrine therapy and have reduced the need for such high-risk ablative procedures as hypophysectomy and surgical adrenalectomy.

In this chapter we briefly review the current status of the use of steroid hormone receptor assays in selecting appropriate patients for endocrine therapy. In addition, we review the many therapeutic alternatives in the hormonal management of breast cancer and outline our preferred method of management.

SELECTING THE APPROPRIATE PATIENT

In the past, clinical criteria, such as menopausal status, age, sites of tumor involvement, and disease-free interval after primary surgery, were used to select patients for endocrine therapy. These criteria have proven inaccurate, as only 30 to 40 percent of patients selected respond to initial endocrine management. Recently, the biochemical mechanisms involved in estrogen stimulation of the breast have been more precisely defined.

Estrogen enters the cytoplasm of the cell and binds to its specific receptor molecule. This complex then translocates to the nucleus, stimulates transcription of messenger RNA, which translates for the synthesis of new proteins. These new proteins are then responsible for the estrogenic effects on the cell, such as enhanced growth or alteration of other metabolic pathways. One important protein that is under estrogen control is the progesterone receptor.

When these mechanisms became apparent, it was first hypothesized that quantification of the initial step in the pathway, estrogen receptor (ER), might indicate that a tumor cell had the machinery for "endocrine dependence" and would respond to endocrine therapy. Later it was suggested that measurement of progesterone receptor (PgR), an end product of estrogen action, might be an even better marker for hormone dependence. Both hypotheses have proven correct (see below) and have given the clinician a tool for more accurate selection of patients for endocrine therapy.

Understanding these pathways is of more than academic interest. Standard assays measure the presence of receptor in tumor cytosol. Thus in patients undergoing tumor biopsy for receptor who have recently been treated with estrogens or antiestrogens, ER will be in the nucleus, resulting in a false negative assay. Because of a prolonged half-life, these drugs may have to be discontinued for several weeks before ER can be accurately determined. In premenopausal women, PgR may similarly be difficult to detect during the luteal phase of the menstrual cycle when endogenous serum progesterone is high. Finally, postmenopausal women may have a false negative PgR because of insufficient estrogen to stimulate PgR synthesis. These factors need to be considered when interpreting assay results.

When the assays are performed and interpreted correctly, they are useful in predicting the endocrine responsiveness of an individual patient's breast cancer. No matter which endocrine therapy is used, 50 to 60 percent of patients with ER + tumors will respond, whereas less than 10 percent of those with ER − tumors respond. Although this assay is not perfect, it is a significant improvement compared with the old clinical criteria for selecting patients for endocrine therapy. Furthermore, quantifying ER, rather than simply designating a tumor positive or negative, offers even better discrimination. Tumors with a high ER concentration

(greater than 100 fmol/mg protein in our laboratory) respond more frequently than do tumors with an intermediate ER value. Retrospective data suggest that PgR is a better marker for endocrine responsiveness than ER (Table 1). In fact, those tumors containing both receptors have a very high response rate to endocrine therapy.

It should be emphasized that receptor status is useful only in predicting response to endocrine therapy and not in deciding which endocrine therapy to use. *All* endocrine therapies (either additive or ablative) are more likely to cause tumor regression in ER + patients. Since the mechanisms by which certain endocrine therapies induce tumor regression are not clear, and since they may or may not involve the estrogen-response pathway, ER and PgR may simply be serving as markers of tumor differentiation. Perhaps more differentiated tumors retain the ability to respond to a variety of changes in the hormonal milieu. Histologic correlations, in fact, demonstrate that ER is more likely to be present in tumors with morphologic evidence of tumor differentiation. The relationship between ER and tumor differentiation may also partially explain why patients with ER + tumors have a better prognosis for prolonged survival than those with ER − tumors. In any event, the ER and PgR assays now permit physicians to individualize therapy with considerably more confidence than in the past.

THERAPEUTIC ALTERNATIVES

Endocrine therapies have been used most extensively for the palliation of women with advanced metastatic breast cancer. Current clinical trials have also been designed to evaluate the use of endocrine treatment as an adjunct to surgery in patients with primary breast cancer. These studies, however, must mature for several more years be-

TABLE 1 PgR Status and Response to Endocrine Treatment*

Receptors	Response Rate (%)
ER −, PgR −	10/102 (10%)
ER −, PgR +	6/13 (46%)
ER +, PgR −	26/92 (28%)
ER +, PgR +	83/109 (76%)

*Pooled data from nine institutions

Note: ER = estrogen receptor, PgR = progesterone receptor

fore firm conclusions can be drawn and recommendations made. Thus this review focuses on the hormonal management of advanced disease. For discussion purposes the many therapeutic alternatives are divided into ablative and additive therapies.

Ablative Therapies

Ablative treatments involve the destruction or surgical removal of endocrine organs, such as the ovaries, adrenals, and pituitary gland. These glands presumably secrete hormones that directly or indirectly stimulate growth of endocrine-dependent breast cancers. Adrenalectomy and hypophysectomy, although effective therapies, are being performed less often today because of their immediate and long-term morbidities; the development of the ER assay and the rejection of ER− patients for consideration for major endocrine surgery; and the development of other effective treatments, such as antiestrogens and medical adrenalectomy.

Ovarian Ablation

Ovarian ablation is the conventional first-line therapy for premenopausal women and women less than one year postmenopause (last menstrual period). Ablation can be accomplished by surgical ovariectomy or by ovarian irradiation. Results are equivalent, but the former method is preferred by most oncologists because the endocrine effects are immediate and the operation is safe. Tumor response is delayed by several weeks to months with radiation castration, which limits its usefulness in patients in whom a rapid antitumor effect is desirable. Radiation castration may be used in those patients who are not surgical candidates for reasons unrelated to their breast cancer.

Tumor regression with castration occurs in about 20 to 40 percent of patients not selected by ER or PgR status. Very young women and those in the perimenopausal period may respond less frequently than the average premenopausal woman. Castration is of no value in the truly postmenopausal patient.

Complete tumor regression (disappearance of all clinically evident disease) is uncommon with castration, as it is with all endocrine therapies. Those patients achieving partial regression, which typically lasts for about 12 months (longer in certain patients), have a significant improvement in survival rates compared with nonresponding patients.

The complications of ovarian ablation are few and are primarily related to the risks of surgery, as well as the induction of menopausal symptoms. The latter should not be treated with replacement estrogens becausse of the potential for stimulating tumor growth.

Surgical Adrenalectomy

Surgical adrenalectomy and hypophysectomy are sometimes referred to as "major" ablative endocrine therapies because of the greater potential for treatment-related mortality and long-term morbidity. These treatments may induce the longest remissions of metastatic breast cancer, but comparable results can probably be obtained by the proper sequence of other, less toxic hormonal manipulations. Unfortunately, there are few studies that adequately examine the proper sequence of ablative and additive treatments in selected patients with receptor-positive tumors. Response durations in patients treated with major endocrine ablation average 12 to 24 months, with some patients benefiting for several years.

Adrenalectomy traditionally has been used in premenopausal women who have been previously ovariectomized, and in postmenopausal women. The adrenal secretes estrogen "precursors," such as androstenedione, which may rise after menopause. These precursors are converted to estrogen in peripheral tissues, such as fat, resulting in a blood estrogen level that presumably is sufficient to stimulate certain breast cancers. Adrenalectomy removes the source of the estrogen precursors, with a further reduction in circulating estrogen. Interestingly, estrogen can still be detected in women subjected to castration and major ablative surgery.

The response rate to adrenalectomy is similar to that observed with castration. The best responses are seen in patients who have previously responded to castration and in patients more than five years postmenopause. Curiously, an occasional response to adrenalectomy is observed in patients failing castration. We do not recommend major ablation in such patients, because the potential risks outweigh the potential benefits in this setting. Although combining ovariectomy and adrenalectomy in premenopausal patients may increase the initial response rate, there is no evidence for prolonged survival rates compared to those achieved with their sequential use, and the combined approach is not recommended.

The complications of surgical adrenalectomy relate to the morbidity and occasional death associated with a major surgical procedure. Furthermore, patients and physicians must deal with the permanent threat of adrenal insufficiency and crisis. Patients must be maintained on daily steroid replacement, usually 37.5 to 50 mg of cortisone acetate daily. Mineralocorticoid (9a-fluorohydrocortisone) is also frequently required to prevent hypoaldosteronism. Obviously, adrenalectomy should not be considered in noncompliant patients. Major ablative surgery will probably become a very uncommon procedure owing to the recent development of medical adrenalectomy (see below).

Pituitary Ablation

The other form of major ablative endocrine therapy is pituitary ablation. This may be accomplished by surgical techniques (usually transsphenoidal hypophysectomy) or by implantation of radioactive rods or pellets (usually yttrium). The expertise required for either technique has limited the use of this form of endocrine therapy to major centers.

The mechanism of tumor regression seen with hypophysectomy is not totally clear. Traditional thinking suggests that the mechanism is similar to that described for adrenalectomy: reduction in serum estrogen level. There is no good correlation between tumor response and levels of pituitary hormones. Changes in serum prolactin are not likely to be related to tumor regression, since patients having incomplete hypophysectomy or stalk section, with elevated prolactin levels, are just as likely to benefit as those with complete ablation. The observation that certain patients may respond to hypophysectomy after adrenalectomy, and vice versa, suggests that alternative mechanisms may also be involved.

Hypophysectomy is generally considered in the same groups of patients as described for adrenalectomy. It has been used in premenopausal patients who have previously responded to castration, and in postmenopausal patients as first-line therapy or second-line therapy after treatment with estrogens or antiestrogens. Studies comparing adrenalectomy with hypophysectomy tend to show a slight edge for the latter in terms of response rate and duration of response. However, this difference is of little, if any, clinical significance. The decision as to which therapy to choose is based primarily on the surgical expertise available in a given institution.

The complications of hypophysectomy are numerous and include diabetes insipidus, meningitis, rhinorrhea, hemorrhage, loss of vision, impairment of taste, pituitary insufficiency, and death. Fortunately, these complications are uncommon when the procedure is performed by an expert surgeon, and the mortality rate is less than 5 percent in most studies. After hypophysectomy most patients require cortisone, thyroid, and vasopressin replacement therapy.

Additive Therapies

The pharmacologic administration of hormones has been used to treat patients with breast cancer for more than 30 years. The mechanisms by which most of these hormones induce tumor regression are not well defined. Additive therapy remains popular because of its high therapeutic index.

Estrogens

Pharmacologic estrogen therapy has been the mainstay of treatment for postmenopausal women with breast cancer. Its mechanism of action is not known. It is puzzling that both reduction of estrogen by ablative therapy and the administration of high doses of estrogen can cause tumor regression. Objective responses to estrogens have been reported in premenopausal women, but these are uncommon and this therapy is usually reserved for the postmenopausal patient.

The response rate to estrogen therapy is similar to that described for the ablative therapies (Table 2). About one-third of all patients will benefit with an average duration of 12 to 18 months. An occasional patient will respond for as long as five years or more. The best responses are seen in women more than five years postmenopause. The response rate may vary depending on the site of tumor involvement. Soft tissue disease (breast, skin, lymph nodes) responds best, whereas visceral disease responds poorly. Patients with massive liver involvement or brain metastasis rarely benefit from estrogens or any other endocrine ther-

TABLE 2 Response to Estrogen and Androgen Therapy According to Site of Involvement

Site	% Response	
	Estrogen	Androgen
Soft tissue	40	22
Bone	25	20
Visceral	20	18

apy. Although subtle differences in response rate according to site of disease exist among the various hormonal therapies, the most important factor in predicting response is the tumor receptor status.

Diethylstilbestrol, 15 mg per day, or ethinyl estradiol, 3 mg per day, are the most commonly used estrogenic preparations. With nearly all endocrine therapies, but particularly with estrogens, there may be transient stimulation of tumor growth, sometimes with hypercalcemia, immediately after initiating treatment. This "tumor flare" is not an indication to discontinue treatment, since it is usually transient, and many patients will subsequently enjoy tumor regression. With additive therapy, tumor regression may not be evident for several weeks, and the maximal effect may take several months. In patients whose tumors are progressing on estrogen therapy after a period of improvement, a second response may be obtained (20 percent) by simply stopping the hormone. Patients without life-threatening or rapidly progressing disease should be evaluated for this estrogen withdrawal response prior to initiating a new treatment.

Although the tumor response to estrogen therapy can be gratifying, these drugs are not without complications. About 10 percent of patients require discontinuation of the drug because of untoward effects, usually anorexia, nausea and vomiting. Estrogens may be difficult to administer and may be contraindicated in some patients with severe underlying cardiovascular disease in whom fluid retention, congestive failure, or thromboembolism may occur. Other side effects include skin pigmentation, breast engorgement, and vaginal discharge or bleeding.

Androgens

Androgens are conventionally used as second- or third-line therapy in postmenopausal women with advanced breast cancer. They are occasionally used in premenopausal women, but responses are less frequent than with ovariectomy. The mechanism of androgen-induced regression of breast cancer is not clear. Androgens in high concentrations can bind to estrogen receptor, fueling speculation that they might interfere with estrogenic stimulation of the cell.

Many androgen preparations have been studied, but the most frequently used are fluoxymesterone, 10 mg orally twice a day, and testosterone propionate, 100 mg intramuscularly 3 times per week. Tumor flare and withdrawal responses are observed less frequently with androgens than with estrogens.

About 20 percent of unselected patients respond to androgen therapy (Table 2). This figure is higher if treatment is confined to patients who have responded to a previous endocrine therapy. Occasionally patients who have failed with a previous endocrine therapy will have tumor regression from androgens.

In addition to objective tumor regression, androgens exhibit an important palliative effect through their anabolic activity. Symptomatic improvement of pain, increase in appetite and weight, and improved sense of well-being occur frequently, even in the absence of objective tumor regression.

Androgens also have several annoying side effects. The most distressing to the patient are related to virilization (hirsutism, temporal hair loss, acne). Fluid retention and cardiovascular toxicity are less severe than with estrogens. Cholestatic jaundice and increased libido may also be noted.

Progestins

This form of additive hormonal therapy does not have the popularity of estrogens or androgens despite the fact that progestins have significant activity in breast cancer. Response rates may not be as high as with some of the other first-line regimens, but beneficial effects are common in patients who have previously responded to one or more ablative or additive endocrine therapies. Thus progestins are excellent second- or third-line agents in the management of breast cancer. A recent surge in the popularity of progestins may be due to the preliminary observation that extremely high-dose therapy may be as effective as some of the conventional first-line endocrine therapies.

With conventional-dose progestational therapy, objective tumor regressions are observed in about 20 percent of patients, similar to the activity of androgens. The average response duration is about nine months. Responses are more frequent in patients previously responding to an endocrine therapy and in patients with ER+ tumors. Older postmenopausal women have the highest response rate, although responses are also observed in premenopausal patients who have had ablative therapy.

The most commonly used agents for progestational therapy are megestrol acetate, 40 mg orally 4 times a day, and medroxyprogesterone acetate 100–400 mg per day. Side effects are uncommon with these regimens. Some patients have mild fluid retention, increased appetite, and weight gain.

The use of high-dose parenteral medroxyprogesterone acetate has become increasingly popular in Europe. Response rates appear to be higher than with conventional-dose therapy, and randomized studies suggest that results are equivalent to the best first-line therapies. Further study is required to assess accurately the role of high-dose therapy in the management of breast cancer. These preparations are not yet available in this country.

Corticosteroids

Adrenal steroids administered in pharmacologic doses are widely used in the treatment of breast cancer, although usually in combination with cytotoxic chemotherapy. They have also been used as a third- or fourth-line additive endocrine therapy, with objective responses occurring in about 5 to 10 percent of patients. The mechanism of tumor inhibition is unclear, but it may be mediated by a direct toxic effect on the cell, or by inhibition of adrenal steroid hormone synthesis. Their usefulness is limited by the unacceptable toxicity associated with chronic administration. Short-term corticosteroid therapy is useful in the management of cerebral edema associated with brain metastasis, in the management of hypercalcemia, and in the management of the end-stage patient for its general stimulatory effect.

New Endocrine Therapies

In the past decade, two new endocrine therapies, the antiestrogens and "medical" adrenalectomy, have been developed. These therapies have already had a major impact in the endocrine therapy of breast cancer, and they are almost certain to have an even greater impact in the near future.

Antiestrogens

Antiestrogens, initially developed as antifertility drugs, were later found to have significant activity in human breast cancer. These drugs, like estrogens, can bind to estrogen receptor and translocate to the nucleus. Although the nuclear events involved with estrogen stimulation and antiestrogen inhibition are poorly understood, the ultimate effect of the antiestrogen in hormone-dependent tumors is inhibition of growth.

Several antiestrogens have been developed, but only one, tamoxifen, is available in this country. The optimal dose of tamoxifen has not been

accurately determined, but 10 mg orally twice a day is the most frequent schedule employed. The half-life of tamoxifen and of its biologically active metabolites is more than several days, suggesting that a single daily dose should suffice. The prolonged half-life also presents a common clinical problem. Since tamoxifen binds ER and translocates receptor to the nucleus, receptors will be unavailable for assay by standard techniques. Patients undergoing repeat tumor biopsy for ER within two months of stopping the drug are likely to have a false negative ER assay.

The objective response rate to tamoxifen in advanced breast cancer is reported to be 40 to 50 percent. This is somewhat higher than that reported for other endocrine therapies, but it is important to point out that tamoxifen has been studied in an era when ER assays were available to select appropriate patients. Nevertheless, tamoxifen is among the most active of endocrine treatments. Randomized studies demonstrate that tamoxifen treatment is equivalent to the ablative and first-line additive hormone therapies in terms of response rate and response duration (12 to 18 months).

Tamoxifen has been best studied in postmenopausal patients. Response rates are reported to be higher in older postmenopausal patients, although this is probably a function of an increased percentage of ER+ tumors in elderly patients. Antiestrogen therapy is effective in previously untreated postmenopausal patients. Interestingly, tamoxifen is also active as a second-line therapy in patients previously treated with pharmacologic estrogens or pituitary ablation. This suggests that these therapies inhibit tumor growth by totally different mechanisms. Tamoxifen may not be effective in patients previously treated by medical adrenalectomy (see below).

Antiestrogen therapy is also effective in premenopausal women both before and after castration. In patients with intact ovaries, the serum estrogen level gradually rises with tamoxifen therapy and may reach concentrations sufficient to reverse the inhibitory effect. Such patients may then benefit from bilateral ovariectomy. A trial of tamoxifen has even been touted as a clinical test to select appropriate patients for castration. Antiestrogens are also effective in premenopausal women who have previously responded to castration, presumably by blocking the effects of the residual estrogens of adrenal origin.

Perhaps the most important aspect of tamoxifen therapy is the remarkable absence of side effects. The drug is rarely discontinued because of intolerance. An occasional patient has nausea or vomiting, atrophic vaginitis, uterine bleeding, or menopausal symptoms. Transient thrombocytopenia has been reported. Tumor flare, hypercalcemia, and even withdrawal responses occur rarely. The high level of antitumor activity coupled with the low level of toxicity has made tamoxifen therapy the first-line treatment of choice in most postmenopausal patients.

Medical Adrenalectomy

As described earlier, major ablative endocrine therapy is very effective in patients with endocrine-dependent breast cancer. Because of the potential for morbidity and mortality, however, its use has been limited to selected patients.

Aminoglutethimide, originally promoted as an anticonvulsive agent, was found to be a potent inhibitor of adrenal steroid hormone biosynthesis. Subsequently, the drug has also been found to be a potent inhibitor of the aromatase reaction necessary for the peripheral conversion of adrenal androgens to estrogen. After administration of the drug to postmenopausal women, or to premenopausal women after castration, there is a prompt fall in serum estrogens as well as other adrenal steroids. The fall in glucocorticoids necessitates the use of hydrocortisone replacement therapy, which also prevents the compensatory rise in ACTH that might otherwise be sufficient to overcome the block in steroidogenesis. This medical adrenalectomy regimen of aminoglutethimide, 1000 mg daily, plus hydrocortisone, 40–60 mg daily (or dexamethasone 2–3 mg daily), has now been studied in several institutions in patients with advanced breast cancer.

Thirty to 40 percent of unselected patients respond to medical adrenalectomy. Median response duration is from 12 to 18 months. Similar to other endocrine therapies, the response rate is higher in patients with ER + tumors. This regimen has now been compared with both major ablative procedures (surgical adrenalectomy and hypophysectomy) as well as additive therapy with tamoxifen. Objective response rates and response durations are equivalent in all studies. For unclear reasons, aminoglutethimide produces responses twice as frequently as tamoxifen in patients with predominant bone metastases. Furthermore, patients frequently respond to medical adrenalectomy after an initial response to tamoxifen, whereas the converse is uncommon. This suggests that the proper sequence of hormonal therapy in postmenopausal women should be tamoxifen followed by medical adrenalectomy.

TABLE 3 Side Effects of Aminoglutethimide When Used for Medical Adrenalectomy

	Percentage of Patients
Lethargy	43
Skin rash	30
Postural dizziness	16
Drug fever	2
Ataxia	11
Nystagmus	6

This sequence is also supported by toxicity information. Aminoglutethimide is considerably more toxic than tamoxifen, although many of the side effects occur acutely and are rapidly reversible with chronic administration (Table 3). In the majority of patients, these side effects abate within one to six weeks of therapy. Discontinuation of therapy is required in only 5 percent of patients. Importantly, adrenal suppression induced by aminoglutethimide is rapidly reversible after discontinuing the drug.

Thus, aminoglutethimide plus hydrocortisone, although more toxic than tamoxifen, is a tolerable regimen with considerable activity in human breast cancer. The drug is not yet commercially available in this country for use in breast cancer, and its exact role in the sequential management of endocrine-responsive breast cancer is not totally defined. However, in the near future, medical adrenalectomy should make the need for major ablative surgery rare.

PREFERRED APPROACH

With a large variety of equally effective endocrine therapies available, it is difficult to recommend a standard or preferred approach. The decision of which endocrine therapy to choose in a given situation depends upon several factors, including patient age and menopausal status, the overall medical condition of the patient, and physician preference or expertise.

Before discussing specific recommendations, several general concepts need emphasis. First, endocrine therapy generally should not be considered in ER − patients because of the small chance of benefit. Chemotherapy is usually recommended as initial therapy in these patients. Second, endocrine therapy should be considered for initial therapy in most ER + or ER unknown patients, especially if PgR is known to be positive. An exception might be the patient with advanced life-threatening pul-

TABLE 4 Sequential Therapy for Premenopausal Women

First line:	Bilateral ovariectomy or tamoxifen
Second line:	Tamoxifen or bilateral ovariectomy
Third line:	Medical adrenalectomy* or major surgical ablation
Fourth line:	Androgens, progestins
Fifth line:	Glucocorticoids

*Treatment of choice when approved by Food and Drug Administration

TABLE 5 Sequential Therapy for Postmenopausal Women

First line:	Tamoxifen
Second line:	Estrogens
	Medical adrenalectomy* or major ablative surgery
	High-dose medroxyprogesterone acetate*
Third line:	Androgens
	Low-dose progestins
Fourth line:	Glucocorticoids

*When approved by Food and Drug Administration

monary or liver disease in whom a rapid tumor response is required. These patients should receive chemotherapy, although some physicians might empirically combine chemotherapy with endocrine therapy. However, the combined approach has not yet been proved superior to the sequential use of these modalities. Third, after initiating an endocrine therapy, the patient should be observed for 6 to 12 weeks, in the absence of frank progression, before deciding on alternative therapy. Tumor regression may be quite delayed in certain patients. Fourth, patients failing an initial endocrine therapy should usually be considered to have endocrine unresponsive tumors that require chemotherapy. Only a few of these patients will respond to a second endocrine therapy. Perhaps an exception might be the patient with very indolent disease in whom time lost from a fruitless second endocrine therapy would be unimportant. In contrast, patients responding to an initial hormone therapy should be carefully considered for sequential second- or third-line therapies, especially if a repeat tumor biopsy is ER+. Such patients have an excellent chance of additional remissions, although the remission durations tend to become shorter with each treatment. Nevertheless, certain patients can be controlled for many years with this approach. Finally, therapy should not be stopped because of "tumor flare" (unless it is life-threatening). Many patients will eventually have tumor regression with continued therapy.

With these principles in mind, a general schema for the sequential use of endocrine therapy for premenopausal and postmenopausal patients is shown in Tables 4 and 5, respectively. The specific choice within a given strata depends upon the factors discussed above. Major surgical ablation should become nearly obsolete when medical adrenalectomy with aminoglutethimide and hydrocortisone becomes widely available. Glucocorticoids alone are rarely used except for palliation of the preterminal patient. Additional well-designed studies will be required before more definite statements can be made regarding the appropriate sequential or combined use of the many modalities of therapy available for patients with advanced breast cancer.

ENDOCRINE TREATMENT OF ENDOMETRIAL MALIGNANCY

RODRIGUE MORTEL, M.D.
and WILLIAM A. NAHHAS, M.D.

Endometrial carcinoma is now the most common invasive malignancy of the female genital tract. The majority of patients with this disease have tumors confined to the uterus (FIGO stages I and II) and are amenable to standard therapy utilizing surgery, irradiation, or more commonly, a combination of both. However, a significant number of patients develop recurrent or metastatic disease and require systemic therapy. Such therapy usually consists of progestational agents, cytotoxic drugs, or both.

That endometrial carcinoma is a hormonally dependent tumor is evidenced by its well-known association with unopposed estrogen stimulation. In fact, the administration of large doses of estrogenic hormones to rabbits has induced endometrial hyperplasia and carcinoma. Hyperplasia has also been produced in organ culture when explants of normal endometrium were incubated with estrogenic compounds. In humans, endometrial carcinoma has occured in association with various endocrinologic disorders, many of which are related to continuous prolonged unopposed estrogenic stimulation. Ovarian abnormalities associated with increased estrogen production often coexist with endometrial carcinoma. In addition, an increased risk of endometrial carcinoma has been noted in women suffering from anovulation, obesity, and diabetes, as well as in those receiving unopposed exogenous estrogen medication.

The antiestrogenic properties of progestational agents constitute the basis for their use in endometrial carcinoma. However, not all patients respond to these agents, and, based on clinical criteria alone, selection of patients who will benefit from progestational therapy has not been possible.

Target tissues contain specific intracellular receptors for steroid hormones, and receptor concentration in tumors has been suggested as a possible indicator of hormone responsiveness. Based on this concept, the determination of hormone receptor concentration has been of clinical value in the management of patients with carcinoma of the breast. Patients whose breast tumors contain a high concentration of estrogen and progesterone receptors are more likely to respond to hormonal manipulation.

Since the uterus is a sex-steroid-responsive target organ, many investigators have explored the usefulness of measuring sex steroid receptor concentration in endometrial cancers as a means of predicting hormone responsiveness. It was postulated that patients whose endometrial tumors contain a high progesterone receptor concentration would be more likely to respond to progestational agents. Antiestrogenic substances such as Tamoxifen are also being investigated as therapeutic agents because of their binding affinity to estrogen receptors.

THERAPEUTIC ALTERNATIVES

Local Recurrences

Radiation therapy has been utilized in the treatment of pelvic recurrences following surgery for endometrial carcinoma. Pelvic exenteration has occasionally been resorted to in patients previously treated by radiation therapy. However, the natural history of this disease is such that very few patients are candidates for ultraradical pelvic surgery. The results of pelvic exenteration in endometrial carcinoma have been poor.

Metastastic Disease

Radiation therapy has been of limited value in the treatment of metastatic endometrial carcinoma. Symptomatic relief from painful bony lesions occasionally, can be achieved by localized radiation therapy. Cytotoxic agents have been utilized following failed progestational therapy. More recently adriamycin and cis-platinum have been used as primary therapy for metastatic disease. The response rates have been similar to those obtained with progestational agents.

PREFERRED APPROACH

Progestational Agents

Although cytotoxic chemotherapy achieves response rates similar to those obtained with progestational agents, the use of progestins has been the preferred approach because of the relative absence of side effects and the ease of administration. Various preparations, such as medroxyprogesterone acetate (Depo Provera) and hydroxyprogesterone caproate (Delalutin) have been used. More recently, oral progestational agents have been investigated. These include megestrol acetate (Megace) and medroxyprogesterone acetate (CT Provera). The response to these various medications has been similar.

Mechanism of Action. The mechanism by which progestational agents affect endometrial carcinoma is not completely understood. Although mediation via the pituitary gland has been suggested, there is still no experimental evidence of such an effect. Direct effect on endometrial tissue, however, is likely, since these agents—administered systemically or locally—have been shown to produce cellular changes in the form of maturation, glandular regression, and stromal decidual reaction. These cellular changes occur in endometrial carcinomas that are responsive to progestational therapy, but they are not observed in nonresponsive lesions.

Tissue culture studies provide further support for a local endometrial effect. In fact, endometrial cancers incubated with progestational agents show necrosis of cells compared with control cultures. Moreover, recent studies on the relationship of progesterone receptor content and the response of endometrial carcinoma to progestational therapy provide further evidence that the action of progestational agents is mediated via the intracellular progesterone receptor.

Dosage and Route of Administration. Most authors agree that "large" doses of progestins have to be used and that the dosage that produces an objective response should be maintained indefinitely. Although there is no experimental evidence to support the concept of a loading dose when using progestational agents our regimen consists of the administration of medroxyprogesterone acetate, 1000 mg i.m. every week for 4 weeks, followed by 400 mg i.m. every week for the next 8 weeks. At the end of 12 weeks of treatment, therapy is continued utilizing megestrol acetate, 80 mg daily. If the tumor remains stable or shows evidence of regression, this medication is continued indefinitely. However, therapy is discontinued if there is evidence of progressive disease. Patients in whom weekly intramuscular injections are undesirable, are treated with megestrol acetate, 80 to 160 mg per day, or by oral medroxyprogesterone acetate, 50 mg 3 times a day. All agents are used for a minimum of 12 weeks before a decision is made regarding response. Oral medications should be avoided in patients with intestinal obstruction, and proper care must be exercised in the administration of intramuscular injections to prevent local abscess formation.

Assessment of Response. In patients with measurable disease, lesion size should be assessed in the largest diameter and its perpendicular. Changes in these diameters or in pleural and ascitic fluids are utilized as parameters of response. In patients with no measurable disease, response is determined by the progression-free interval.

Objective response to therapy with progestational agents can be characterized as follows:

Complete response means disappearance of all disease for at least one month.

Partial response means 50 percent or greater reduction in the product of perpendicular diameters for each lesion, 50 percent regression of ascites or pleural effusion for at least one month or both.

Progressive disease is evidenced by a 50 percent or greater increase in the product of perpendicular diameters of any lesion documented on two separate examinations at least two weeks apart, the appearance of any new lesions, or a 50 percent or greater increase of an effusion.

Stable disease is disease not meeting any of the above criteria.

Subjective response is assessed by observations relating to the patient's performance status and regression of symptoms of disease. A general feeling of well-being in the absence of objective tumor regression is also considered a subjective response.

Response Rate. A 30 percent to 35 percent response rate to progestational therapy has been noted, especially in older patients with well-differentiated tumors that recurred long after initial treatment of their cancer.

Side Effects. Even though the lack of side effects has been considered one of the most attractive aspects of the use of progestational agents in endometrial carcinoma, patients receiving these drugs occasionally experience adverse reactions.

Local Reactions. Such reactions include discomfort at the injection site, local dermal reaction, inflammation, and abscess formation.

Systemic Reactions. Systemic side effects include allergic reactions, fluid retention, chills, gastrointestinal complaints, and transient episodes of chest symptoms immediately following injection. The chest manifestations are thought to be due to inadvertent intravenous injection of the oily solution. Other complications include nausea, vomiting, and insomnia. Embolic phenomenon have rarely, been observed.

Tamoxifen

Tamoxifen is a compound that has shown antiestrogenic activity in the chick oviduct and other experimental models as well as in humans. It has also shown estrogenic properties by increasing the progesterone receptor concentration when added to breast cancer cells in culture. Moreover, in patients with endometrial carcinoma, increase in progesterone receptor concentration has been noted following short-term administration of tamoxifen. This compound also induces steroid binding globulins.

Mechanism of Action. The role that estrogens may play in the origin of endometrial cancer has led to the experimental use of the antiestrogenic effects of tamoxifen in the treatment of patients with this disease. Tamoxifen is thought to manifest its antiestrogenic properties in the following manner. It binds with high affinity to the cytoplasmic estrogen receptor. The tamoxifen-estrogen receptor complex is then translocated into the nucleus, leading to new protein synthesis. One protein that is not synthesized is the estrogen receptor itself. Since the cytoplasmic estrogen receptor is not replenished, estrogen can no longer bind to its own receptor.

Dosage and Route of Administration. Tamoxifen is administered orally in a continuous daily dose of 20 to 40 mg.

Response Rate. Tamoxifen has not been used as primary therapy for metastatic endometrial carcinoma. A few investigators have attempted its use following failure of progestational agents. Response rates of 30 to 50 percent have been noted, with duration of remission shorter than that obtained with progestins.

Side Effects. Tamoxifen is usually well tolerated. The most common side effects are related to the antiestrogenic properties of the drug and include hot flashes and vaginal discharge. Nausea and vomiting have been reported in approximately 10 percent of patients. These side effects are rarely severe and usually do not require discontinuation of treatment. Less frequently reported adverse reactions include vaginal bleeding, menstrual irregularities, and skin rash. Pumonary emboli have been noted in a few cases during tamoxifen administration, but a causal relationship with drug treatment has not been clearly established. Other infrequent adverse reactions are hypercalcemia, peripheral edema, distaste for food, pruritus vulvae, depression, dizziness, lightheadedness, and headache. Leukopenia and throbocytopenia have occasionally been observed, but it is uncertain if these effects are really due to Tamoxifen therapy. No hemorrhagic tendency has been recorded.

Combination Chemotherapy

Progestational agents have definite value in the treatment of patients with advanced or metastatic endometrial carcinoma. However, one drawback of pregesterone therapy is the decrease of progesterone receptor concentration in the tumor. This may explain the relatively short duration of remission following initial response to progestins. Any substance that can rescue the progesterone receptor can theoretically increase the magnitude or duration of response, or both.

It is well documented that estrogen induces progesterone receptor synthesis in endometrial tissue. Consequently, some investigators utilized the combination of estrogen and progesterone in the treatment of patients with endometrial carcinoma in the hope of priming the tumor with estrogen and improving its response to progestational agents. However, because estrogen has mitotic action on the endometrium and because of its implication in the origin of endometrial hyperplasia and adenocarcinoma, the reluctance of most clinicians to use this combination may be warranted.

Tamoxifen, on the other hand, increases progesterone receptor concentration in endometrial cancer but does not appear to enhance endometrial cell division. It is therefore plausible that the sequential or combined use of progestational agents and tamoxifen may be beneficial in increasing the magnitude or duration of response, or both, in patients with metastatic disease.

Adjuvant Therapy

The response rate achieved by progestational agents in metastatic or recurrent endometrial tumors has caused investigators to consider their use as adjuvants to either surgery or radiation therapy in the management of patients with early disease. Large sloughing tumors were found to shrink and become less vascular after the administration of progestational agents. Likewise, small lesions were reported to disappear after treatment with progestins either systemically or by injection into the uterine cavity. In addition, destruction of tumor was enhanced by the administration of progestational agents preceding intracavitary radium application. In spite of these local effects of progestins on endometrial tumors, most clinical studies performed in the United States failed to confirm improved survival rates with the use of adjuvant progestational therapy.

Primary Therapy

Progestational therapy has occasionally been used as primary treatment in patients with early endometrial cancer. Most of these patients have either been very young or had other medical conditions that precluded the use of more conventional therapy, such as irradiation and surgery. Such patients should be carefully followed with regular endometrial sampling every three months, and conservative therapy should be abandoned in the face of nonresponsiveness or persistent disease.

TESTICULAR DISORDERS

HYPOGONADISM: ANDROGEN THERAPY

REBECCA Z. SOKOL, M.D.
and RONALD S. SWERDLOFF, M.D.

The goal of androgen replacement therapy is to simulate the physiologic actions of endogenous testosterone in the male. Testosterone exerts its actions on a number of androgen sensitive tissues. Essentially, androgens stimulate the development of male secondary sexual characteristics; maintain normal male libido and sexual potency; stimulate a pubertal growth spurt, which directly or indirectly results in fusion of long bone epiphyses; and exert a protein anabolic action that results in an increase in protein synthesis by the muscle cells. Androgen therapy cannot correct ambiguous genitalia that occurred as a result of abnormal early fetal development, and it has never been given in sufficiently high doses to maintain spermatogenesis in man. In fact, through its inhibitory effects on the hypothalamic-pituitary axis, androgen therapy suppresses spermatogenesis. While androgens may be given for their anabolic and erythropoietic effects, the most common clinical indication for androgen treatment of men is androgen deficiency (hypogonadism).

BIOCHEMISTRY

Testosterone, a 17β-hydroxylated C19 steroid, is the principal androgen produced by the Leydig cells of the testes. Testosterone exerts its action on its target tissues either by a direct effect or after intracellular conversion by 5α-reductase to dihydrotestosterone (DHT). Both testosterone and dihydrotestosterone act directly on skeletal muscle kidney and the seminiferous tubules. DHT is responsible for the androgenic actions on the reproductive organs, and skin.

An important consideration in androgen pharmacology is the availability of non-5α-reduced androgens, such as testosterone, as substrate for aromatization to estrogens. Thus testosterone can be aromatized to estradiol, whereas DHT and fluoxymesterone cannot. Endogenous testosterone circulates largely bound to a carrier protein, sex-hormone-binding globulin, which serves to prolong its half-life. The unbound component of testosterone is biologically available but is rapidly degraded by the liver, and its metabolites are predominantly excreted in the urine.

PREPARATIONS

Androgen replacement preparations are theoretically available in three forms (Fig. 1): (1) crystalline unmodified testosterone, (2) the 17-alkylated testosterones, and (3) the esterified testos-

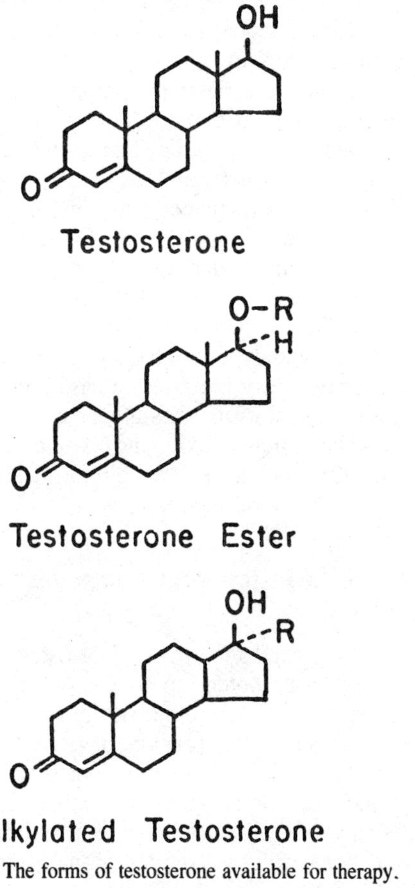

Figure 1 The forms of testosterone available for therapy.

terones. Only the latter two forms are approved by the FDA for use in the United States. There are three routes of administration: oral, subcutaneous pellet implantations, and intramuscular injections.

Crystalline Testosterone

In the United States, crystalline T is available only in aqueous suspension for intramuscular injection (50 mg every 3 weeks) or as subcutaneous pellets (300 mg every 4 to 6 months). In general, unmodified testosterone is rapidly metabolized and its androgen effects are minimal. Recent data from Johnsen's laboratories in Denmark have indicated that oral free testosterone given in daily doses of 400 mg (200 mg b.i.d.) produced eugonadal serum T levels in all hypogonadal subjects studied, and normalized sexual function in the majority of subjects. Even though some subjects were treated for up to seven years, no side effects were noted.

Alkylated Testosterone Preparations (Table 1)

The alkylated testosterones are available for administration by all three routes. These compounds are less polar than crystalline T and are therefore absorbed more slowly. Initially it was believed that alkylated androgens had minimal androgenizing effects, and they were prescribed primarily for their anabolic actions. This postulate was based on animal studies. Observations in humans have indicated that their androgenicity in man is greater than that observed in animals. Two compounds, methyltestosterone and fluoxymesterone, are widely promoted as androgenic agents. Their popularity is primarily based on their availability in oral form. The alkylated compounds are potentially hepatotoxic and should not be prescribed except in unusual circumstances (see the section on side effects).

Esterified Testosterone Compounds (Table 2)

In general the esters of testosterone are considered to be potent androgens that do not result in hepatotoxicity or other severe side effects. The two longer acting preparations, testosterone enanthate and testosterone cypionate, are the compounds of choice for hypogonadal replacement therapy. They are available only as intramuscular injections. Another shorter acting ester of testosterone, testosterone propionate, is available in both an injectable and a buccal form. The testosterone esters are more lipophilic and are therefore absorbed much more slowly than crystalline testosterone when injected in oil. After these conjugates are de-esterified, the product is metabolized identically to endogenous testosterone. Because of the similarity in structure, it is postulated that the kinetics of all the enanthate and cypionate compounds are similar. Studies to assess the pharmacokinetics of testosterone enanthate have been conducted in our laboratories, and our results indicate that after intravenous injection of TE or T, these compounds disappear from the blood in an almost identical pattern. The plasma clearance rate for testosterone is 0.8 1/min and for testosterone enanthate is 1.0 1/min. After an intramuscular injection of TE, the compound is metabolized both at the injection site and after its absorption into the blood. Testosterone enanthate and testosterone circulate in the blood at relatively high levels for up to 120 hours. Both compounds then gradually disappear from the plasma over the next 21 days. Schulte-Beerbühl and associates compared the kinetics of testosterone enanthate and testosterone cypionate when these compounds were injected in equivalent doses. These injections yielded identical serum testosterone concentrations and suppressed LH and FSH levels similarly.

Testosterone undecanoate (organon) is another oral androgen preparation being investigated in Europe. This compound is lipid soluble and is absorbed into the intestinal lymphatics. It allegedly does not result in hepatotoxicity and has been used in the treatment of hypogonadal men. Preliminary data indicate that testosterone levels after a single oral dose of testosterone undecanoate peak between 2 and 4 hours and return to baseline by 24 hours. Chronic therapy with testosterone undecanoate (dosages ranging from 90–240 mg in 3 divided doses per day) will result in testosterone levels in hypogonadal men which fall in the low eugonadal range. The drug may be impractical in that relatively high doses are required three times a day.

DOSAGE

Adult Replacement Therapy

The theoretic goal of androgen therapy in the treatment of hypogonadism in the adult male is to maintain testosterone at physiologic levels. Unfortunately, the preparations available today usually do not meet this goal in that most preparations and regimens produce unsteady circulating hormone levels. Studies performed in our laboratories on

TABLE 1   The Alkylated Testosterone Compounds*

Alkylated Testosterones

Generic Name	Popular Trade Names	Original Classification	Chemical Structure
Methyltestosterone	Many	Androgenic	(structure)
Fluoxymesterone	Halotestin	Androgenic	(structure)
Mesterolone	Androviron Proviron	Androgenic	(structure)
Methandriol	Stenediol	Anabolic	(structure)
Methandrostenolone (Methandienone)	Dianabol	Anabolic	(structure)

Alkylated Testosterones

Generic Name	Popular Trade Names	Original Classification	Chemical Structure
Norethandrolone	Nilevar	Anabolic	(structure)
Oxandrolone	Anavar	Anabolic	(structure)
Oxymetholone	Anadrol	Anabolic	(structure)
Stanolone	Androlone	Anabolic	(structure)
Stanozolol	Winstrol	Anabolic	(structure)

*Adapted from Goodman, L. S. and Gilman, A. (eds), The Pharmacological Basis of Therapeutics, MacMillan Publishing Co., Inc., New York, 1975.

TABLE 2   The Esterified Testosterone Compound*

Esterified Testosterones

Generic Name	Popular Trade Names	Original Classification	Chemical Structure
Testosterone Propionate	Oreton Propionate	Androgenic	
Testosterone Enanthate	Delatestryl	Androgenic	
Testosterone Cypionate	Depo-testosterone	Androgenic	
Dromostanolone Propionate	Drolban	Anabolic	
Nandrolone Decanoate	Deca-durabolin	Anabolic	

*Adapted from Goodman, L. S. and Gilman, A (eds), The Pharmacological Basis of Therapeutics, MacMillan Publishing Co., Inc., New York, 1975.

eugonadal and hypogonadal men who received a 200-mg intramuscular injection of testosterone enanthate showed that in the eugonadal subjects, serum testosterone peaked at supraphysiologic levels at 6 hours and returned to baseline by day 9. In the hypogonadal subjects studied, peak supraphysiologic levels were reached at 24 hours and fell below eugonadal levels by day 9. LH and FSH levels returned to baseline by day 14 in both groups. When a 100-mg dosage of testosterone enanthate was administered to eugonadal subjects peak levels were also reached in 24 hours, but the values were not as high as those after the 200-mg injection. In this case testosterone levels returned to baseline by day 7, two days earlier than with the 200-mg dose. Serum LH and FSH returned to baseline by day 11.

Other data in the literature concur with these observations. In a study designed to evaluate the effects of androgen on sexual behavior in hypogonadal men, Davidson and colleagues administered either 100 mg or 400 mg of testosterone enanthate or a placebo to hypogonadal men once a month for approximately 5 months. Although they did not have data on serum hormone levels immediately after injection, they did note that the levels had returned to the hypogonadal range by 2 weeks after the 100-mg dose and by 4 weeks after the 400-mg dose. They also reported that sexual activity manifested a dose-response relationship in all subjects. More erections were observed in the period after the high dose treatment than after the low dose, and more occurred after the 100-mg treatment than after the placebo. They concluded, based on the serum hormone levels and sexual activity responses, that even high doses of testosterone enanthate should be given no less frequently than once every three weeks. Snyder and Lawrence published a study that evaluated the treatment of hypogonadal men with testosterone enanthate in dosages of 100 mg per week, 200 mg every 2 weeks, 300 mg every 3 weeks, and 400 mg every 4 weeks. The treatment period ranged from 12 to 16 weeks. Based on their data, they concluded that 200 mg every 2 weeks or 300 mg every 3 weeks appeared to be the most effective regimens in terms of the suppression of serum LH concentrations to normal and the frequency of administration. Taking into consideration the limitations of the compounds currently available, we conclude that replacement therapy for hypogonadal men should be 150–200 mg of testosterone enanthate every 10 to 14 days.

Although similar detailed studies have not been published on the pharmacokinetics of testosterone cypionate, its chemical structure is very similar to that of testosterone enanthate and the dosage regimen for this preparation would therefore also be 150–200 mg every 2 weeks. Testosterone propionate is a shorter acting testosterone ester and must be given in a dosage of 50 mg 3 times weekly. This makes it a less desirable choice for androgen replacement therapy.

Pubertal (Adolescent) Replacement Therapy

Replacement therapy for the teenage boy is somewhat complicated by the concurrent therapeutic goal of avoiding early epiphyseal closure that would result in short stature. The traditional approach has therefore, been one of low-dose therapy of 100 mg every month for the first year of treatment, with an increase to 200 mg every month during the second year of treatment. Based on our data on the kinetics of testosterone enanthate, a more physiologic regimen would be 50–100 mg every 2 weeks for the first 2 years.

Micropenis Therapy

Two approaches to testosterone therapy for the treatment of micropenis have been described. Smith and others advocate a dosage of 25 mg of intramuscular depot testosterone every 3 weeks for 3 months (4 doses) as the regimen for an infant, and 25 mg every 3 weeks for 3 months for the prepubertal child. Others have advocated the topical application of testosterone cream. We treated a 12-month-old child with micropenis with 5 percent testosterone cream applied to the phallus b.i.d. After one month of treatment, the baby developed some pubic hair with increased wrinkling and pigmentation of the scrotum. Stretched penile length had increased from 2.4 cm to greater than 3.5 cm. There was no acceleration in bone age. Prior to treatment, the serum testosterone level was 58 ng/dl. Four and 16 hours after the last application of testosterone cream, the testosterone levels were 600 ng% and less than 10 ng%, respectively. Thus the effect of this cream is most likely via systemic absorption of testosterone. We know of no systematic data on different concentrations of topical testosterone administration. In more recent trials of children with micropenis, we have used lower concentrations (2.5 percent and 1.25 percent), which have less tendency to accelerate pubic hair development. Although topical absorption may be more variable than absorption following an intramuscular injection, ease of administration of topical compounds is a significant advantage. This approach is limited owing to the nonavailability of testosterone creams to the practicing physician.

SIDE EFFECTS

Hepatotoxicity (Table 3)

A number of hepatotoxic effects have been reported with the use of the 17-alkylated testosterone compounds, but not with the use of testosterone esters. These include changes in hepatic enzymes, abnormal BSP retention, and cholestatic alterations. Hepatomas and peliosis hepatis have also been implicated. It is important to note that the vast majority of the patients reported with the latter two complications had pre-existing serious medical illnesses that may have predisposed them to these tumors.

Alterations in Erythropoiesis

When administered in large doses (that is, 1 gm/week), androgens stimulate erythropoiesis. They have also been noted to increase leukocyte and platelet counts. In a study conducted in our laboratories, men received weekly or bimonthly injections of 200 mg of testosterone enanthate for up to 10 months. Mild but significant increases in WBC, RBC, hematocrit, and hemoglobin concentrations were noted. These effects correlated with dose-frequency schedules. Negligible changes in MCV, MCH, and MCHC were observed. Despite the significant increases in blood parameters, all values remained within the normal population range and no clinical manifestations were observed.

TABLE 3 Summary of Studies Evaluating the Possible Hepatotoxicity of Androgenic and Anabolic Compounds

Author	# of Subjects	Drug Given	Dosage mg/day	Duration of Therapy	Abnormalities Noted			
					BSP Retention	Total Bilirubin	SGOT	Alkaline Phosphatase
Wynn, et al.	19	Methandienone	10-100	<70 days	12	0	4	0
	14	Methandienone	10-100	>70 days	11	0	6	1
Kory	47	Norethandrolone	25 or 50 mg	6 months	35	2	0	2
Werner	6	Methyltestosterone	60 mg	8 days to 4½ months	Not tested	6	Not Reported	6
Schaffner	27	Norethandrolone	60 mg	3-5 weeks	17	9	6	0
Marquarat	8	Norethandrolone	30 mg	5 weeks	8	0	Not Reported	8
	6	Methyltestosterone	30 mg	5 weeks	6	0	"	
	7	Methandrostenolone	15 mg	5 weeks	7	0	"	
	7	Fluoxymesterone	15 mg	5 weeks	7	0	"	
	5	SC-7294	200 ng/wk	5 weeks	5	0	"	5
	5	SC-6507	30 mg	5 weeks	5	0	"	
	8	Norethandrolone IM	30 ng	2 weeks	8	0	"	
	8	Norethandrolone Oral	30 ng	2 weeks	8	0	"	
Westaby	60	42 - Methyltestosterone	150 mg	2 weeks to	Not Reported	1	20*	1
		18 - Methyl T + TE	150 mg (750 mg/study)	5 years				

*Serum appartate amino transferase

350

Effects on Testis Size

Based on data collected from normal volunteers, we have noted that chronic testosterone enanthate treatment results in a significant decrease in testicular volume which is directly related to the decrease in sperm count. Testicular volumes return to normal after treatment is discontinued. These results agree with those published by a number of other groups who administered either TE or testosterone propionate to normal volunteers.

Gynecomastia

Because testosterone is aromatized to estradiol, patients who are treated with exogenous androgens have increased circulating levels of estradiol as well as testosterone. Fortunately, the blood testosterone:estradiol ratio remains above normal, perhaps explaining the relatively unusual incidence of gynecomastia and/or breast tenderness despite supraphysiologic estradiol levels during the first few days after each testosterone ester injection.

Spermatogenesis

As stated, exogenous testosterone suppresses spermatogenesis. It is important to note that chronic testosterone therapy in patients with hypogonadotropic hypogonadism will not adversely alter the subsequent responsiveness of these tests to gonadotropin or GnRH therapy.

Effects on Prostate

Prostatic growth is primarily androgen dependent. Therefore testosterone replacement therapy is contraindicated in patients with prostatic carcinoma. Those patients with a diagnosis of benign prostatic hypertrophy should be monitored with frequent rectal examinations.

Miscellaneous

Weight gain secondary to sodium retention and protein anabolism, oily skin, and mild acne have also been reported. In one of our studies, 25 of 39 volunteers complained of these skin changes, while 11 subjects noted a weight gain.

While improvement in libido is expected in the majority of hypogonadal men, there are no data to suggest that greater than normal sexual drive or performance is attained with supraphysiologic levels.

Glucose, Cholesterol, and Lipid Metabolism

Although it has been suggested that testosterone therapy alters glucose, lipid, and cholesterol metabolism, detailed clinical studies of these possible side effects are not available. Animal studies have produced conflicting results.

In our study using TE as a contraceptive agent, we found no significant abnormalities in serum cholesterol or triglyceride concentrations, nor in GTT or insulin levels. Data collected by other groups corroborate this finding.

DELAYED PUBERTY IN THE MALE

HOWARD E. KULIN, M.D.

Delayed puberty is a common problem confronting the general practitioner, pediatrician, or internist. The condition is probably as common in both sexes, but more boys are referred to physicians for advice and possible treatment. The concern is primarily psychologic, since the great majority of patients are, in fact, perfectly normal and will eventually reach full adult stature and sexual development. Unfortunately there is no good diagnostic test to separate these normal individuals with physiologic or constitutional delay in adolescence from some patients with specific deficiency disorders of the hypothalamic-pituitary-gonadal axis. Because of this diagnostic dilemma, short-term trial therapy with replacement androgens may be used to help identify those patients with bona fide endocrine disease. This type of therapy is quite different from the administration of replacement androgens to a boy of pubertal age who is known to be deficient in ndogenous testosterone production.

The specific disorders associated with delayed puberty are convenient to consider on the basis of luteinizing hormone (LH) or follicle stimulating hormone (FSH) levels, that is hyper- or hypogonadotropic hypogonadism. Delayed puberty due to primary gonadal disease is relatively unusual in the male and most commonly is due to anorchia or other congenital variations of diminished testicular reserve. In contrast, the bulk of patients are hypogonadotropic and most of these boys, as already stated, will have constitutional delay in puberty. It is the diagnosis of patients with true pituitary hormone loss—either isolated hypogonadotropism or multiple tropic hormone deficiency—that may be difficult in the boy of adolescent age. A reasonable amount of procrastination may be judicious, but by the time a boy has reached the age of 14 with little significant change in secondary sex characteristics, physician referral is required. Some patients will respond positively to reassurance but many will need treatment, either for just a short period or, pending diagnosis, to replace deficient hormone production.

THERAPEUTIC ALTERNATIVES

In the absence of functioning Leydig cells, replacement androgen must be provided. In the absence of endogenous gonadotropins or hypothalamic releasing factors, however, substances that stimulate the gonad provide alternative therapeutic modalities. While luteinizing hormone releasing factor (LRF) has been given on a long-term basis and can induce adult male levels of testosterone, this form of treatment is neither practical nor widely available. The short half-life of LRF makes a daily or multiple daily administration schedule necessary if the drug is used.

Human chorionic gonadotropin (hCG) has long been available as a means of stimulating endogenous androgens in the male. Multiple weekly injections have usually been employed, but recent investigations suggest that a weekly injection of hCG (approximately 1500 IU) may be an adequate growth promoting regimen. While it makes good physiologic sense to stimulate endogenous testosterone, if possible, there is no clear advantage to initiating puberty by these means. The relatively frequent injections are a disadvantage, and hCG has become very expensive. In addition, patients with hypogonadotropic eunuchoidism associated with bilateral cryptorchidism may have a testicular defect that limits the levels of testosterone which can be stimulated by hCG.

Exogenous androgens are the mainstay in treating the adolescent boy who needs virilizing substances. A safe and fully effective orally active drug is not available in the United States. Prompt degradation by the liver necessitates a modification of the testosterone molecule, most commonly

methyl or ethyl substitutions in the 17α position. Such changes may make oral therapy practical, but liver abnormalities appear in a small but significant number of patients so treated. Routine testosterone assays cannot be used to monitor levels of such substances.

Another means of prolonging the duration of action of the testosterone molecule is esterification of the 17β-hydroxl group of the steroid. One such drug—testosterone undecanoate—is orally active and currently undergoing clinical trial. Most esters have to be injected, however, and the long-acting cypionate or enanthate as usually administered at intervals of two to four weeks. These latter substances are the drugs of choice for the replacement of androgens in a child of pubertal age.

PREFERRED APPROACH

The aim of androgen therapy for the boy of pubertal age is to promote secondary sex characteristics and normal linear growth. An additional objective in the patient with constitutional delay in adolescence is to speed the pace of hypothalamic maturation. There is no question that this latter effect will occur with any of the sex steroids, and even the weekly estrogenic antiestrogen, clomiphene citrate.

The pubertal growth spurt is a relatively late manifestation of normal male puberty, usually occurring between ages 12 and 15. Endogenous testosterone levels range between 50 and 170 ng/dl at the time of the most rapid gain in height during puberty. The growth spurt is the result of the synergistic effects of increasing androgen levels working in the presence of growth hormone.

The secondary sex characteristics of importance in the initiation of puberty are penile size and pubic hair. Treatment with exogenous androgens will also cause an increase in scrotal rugations and pigmentation, but the size of the testes will usually remain unchanged. Enlargement of the testis during testosterone administration connotes the advance of normal pubertal processes. Pubic hair may also appear relatively late in male puberty. The appearance of axillary and facial hair and voice change are most variable and of little clinical use in following the onset of puberty. Facial hair, in particular, requires high-dose parenteral therapy, is very variable, and is a decidedly late development in the pubertal process. Excluded from this discussion is the onset of sperm-producing capabilities.

The primary side effect to be avoided in the

initiation of puberty with sex steroids is acceleration of bone maturation in excess of chronologic gain. The epiphyses are very sensitive to androgens, but the usual means of assessing such changes are relatively insensitive ones. That is, the proper interpretation of bone age is dependent on the skill of the individual reading the appropriate x-rays, an awareness of the age-related standard deviations of such a measurement, and the fact that it usually takes months to ascertain changes. The underlying dictum of treatment is to use as little replacement hormone as possible and to realize that remarkably little androgen is needed to promote growth and the onset of secondary sex characteristics.

Short-term Trial Therapy

Fifty to 100 mg of testosterone enanthate or cypionate administered intramuscularly every 3 to 4 weeks is an appropriate drug dosage for this regimen. Depending on patient preference and availability of instruction, the injections may be given either by physician or parent. Therapy is administered for three to four months and then stopped for a similar time period. During the latter interval the boy is to be observed for further changes of puberty and for spontaneous increments in gonadotropin and serum testosterone levels. The accurate assessment of testicular size is the most important parameter to follow. If no significant progression is noted, an additional course of injections should be instituted.

Though changes in the first months may be small, many patients find these advances reassuring enough to let some time pass without additional treatment. The needs of the adolescent under such circumstances must be appreciated. Several intermittent courses of low-dose testosterone can be administered until either spontaneous puberty is well along or the need for long-term exogenous therapy is confirmed. In rare cases normal puberty may be delayed until the late teenage years, and such a lag time in drug intervention is unwarranted. This regimen has no harmful effect on either the potential for full somatic growth or subsequent testicular function.

Long-term Replacement Hormone Therapy

A somewhat different approach is taken for patients in whom the diagnosis of permanent hy-

pogonadism has been made. Such individuals will need long-term treatment, and all attempts to duplicate the events of spontaneous puberty should be made. In this regard careful attention must be paid to somatic growth and corresponding gains in bone maturation.

Direct administration of long-acting androgen preparations in the form of testosterone enanthate or testosterone cypionate, 50–100 mg i.m. every 3 to 4 weeks, is the preferred mode of therapy. This regimen is convenient, relatively inexpensive, and hormone levels can be easily monitored. Gonadal enlargement is usually not seen in those patients with scrotal testes. The lower dose regimen should be chosen to preserve maximum growth potential; again, remarkably little testosterone is needed to induce considerable change in phallic size, scrotal maturation, and pubic hair.

By the second or third year of treatment an intramuscular dose of testosterone, 100 mg very 3 to 4 weeks, is appropriate. Over four to five years the amount of long-acting testosterone is gradually increased to adult male maintenance levels of 200 mg i.m. every 2 to 3 weeks. Bone age monitoring throughout this period is imperative with a view to ensuring that skeletal age does not exceed chronologic age. The amount of testosterone needed to produce facial hair growth varies greatly from individual to individual. Despite the natural desire of the adolescent boy to achieve this end, the pubertal process must not be speeded up at the risk of excessively fast bone maturation.

Side effects of long-term treatment are directly related to dosage and duration of therapy. For the adolescent boy the most troublesome side effect of drug administration is gynecomastia. This effect is a result of the fact that testosterone analogues, as well as testosterone itself, can be aromatized in peripheral tissue to estradiol. Significant sodium retention is not a problem.

It is important to bear in mind the differences between initiating puberty in the male and achieving full adult virilization. Libido, like facial hair, is very variable in its relation to a given testosterone level. A heightened feeling of well-being, reported by some adult men who have had their testosterone levels increased from low-normal levels, is not a prominent objective in treating the adolescent boy.

Testicular prostheses should be implanted in the agonadal patient diagnosed in the peripubertal period. Most urologists feel that surgery is easier after some scrotal stimulation by testosterone. For psychologic reasons this aspect of puberty in the male should also not be unduly delayed.

PROS AND CONS OF TREATMENT

There is little argument about the need to treat the boy who does not have the potential for endogenous testosterone production. Any controversy exists only with respect to the timing and pace of the induced process. I feel it is important to reproduce the timing of normal puberty as closely as possible and still not compromise eventual adult stature. Long-acting parenteral testosterone is, by far, the drug most pediatric endocrinologists choose.

The administration of any drug to someone who may not need it is a larger bone of contention with regard to short-term trial therapy. Because this regimen is safe if appropriately monitored, the psychologic gains stand out. The continuing diagnostic dilemma posed by the significant number of boys who have delayed puberty makes this approach a valid one.

HYPOGONADOTROPIC HYPOGONADISM IN MEN

RICHARD J. SHERINS, M.D.

Although gonadotropin deficiency is relatively uncommon, it is an important diagnostic entity, because therapy is now available to restore fertility. Choice of treatment depends upon many factors, including the patient's goal. For some individuals only full virilization is requested, while for others restoration of spermatogenesis is also desired. One choice of therapy depends not only on the degree of gonadotropin deficiency, but also upon the age of the patient.

Hypogonadotropic hypogonadism can occur either as a selective deficiency of FSH and LH secretion or as a component of panhypopituitarism in which one or more of the other pituitary tropic hormones is absent. Selective deficiency of FSH and LH secretion is most commonly due to the absence of hypothalamic gonadotropin releasing hormone (GNRH), a syndrome in which there is no pituitary destruction.

DIAGNOSIS AND PATIENT SELECTION

Since disorders of the hypothalamic-pituitary gonadal axis can arise before puberty, during puberty, and in sexually mature adults, the approach to the patient depends on when the problem occurs. Gonadotropin deficiency frequently presents as delayed puberty. In the presence of panhypopituitarism, or when a pituitary tumor produces signs and symptoms of growth, thyroid or adrenal deficiency, or visual disturbances and sella abnormalities, a diagnosis of hypogonadotropic hypogonadism is easily established. However, in the absence of other hormonal deficiencies, the diagnosis of hypogonadotropism in a young patient presents a diagnostic dilemma, because it is very difficult to distinguish between boys with constitutionally delayed puberty and those with true hypogonadotropic hypogonadism. This distinction is critical, since proper therapeutic intervention requires a correct diagnosis.

While the norms for the major pubertal milestones have been well established, these serve only as rough guides in determining whether puberty in a teenage boy is significantly delayed. Of all the physical signs of sexual maturation, increase in testicular size (greater than 3.0×2.0 cm, 6 ml) is the earliest, occurring on the average at 11 (9–13) years of age. A Prader orchidometer is a useful tool for measuring testicular volume to determine whether there is progressive increase in testicular size over a 6 to 12 month period. Growth of the testes normally precedes the appearance of pubic hair by approximately two years, and thus it is an early, sensitive index of the onset of puberty. By contrast, rapid growth in height normally does not occur until approximately age 14 in most boys, and height gives no indication of the gonadal status.

Growth of testes is the most reliable index of pubertal progression, since the laboratory tests currently available are far too insensitive to show early pubertal changes. Serum LH, FSH, and testosterone levels in young hypogonadotropic boys are indistinguishable from levels in normal prepubertal males of comparable age and degree of sexual maturation. Similarly, the LH and FSH response to GNRH administration is low in both groups, and LH and FSH concentrations do not increase following clomiphene administration, since a positive response to clomiphene does not occur until midpuberty. By contrast, in being able to demonstrate testicular growth over 6 to 12 months one can reassure the patient that he has entered puberty and can predict the onset of his virilization.

Since most teenagers (and their parents) are very concerned about a delay in sexual maturation, it is often desirable to hospitalize a boy with suspected hypogonadism for several days to carry out special tests, rather than waiting to assess testicular growth. By drawing multiple blood samples every half hour throughout the night, one can determine whether there is nocturnal release of LH, an event that normally takes place in early puberty. In addition, the prolactin response to chlorpromazine administration (1 mg/3 kg body weight i.m.) can be measured, since recent studies show that the prolactin concentration in truly hypogonadotropic subjects does not increase, while in normal pubertal subjects with a comparable degree of sexual maturation prolactin levels rise more than 15 ng/ml.

In an occasional patient with gonadotropin deficiency, the testes are larger than 6 ml, virilization is moderately advanced, nocturnal release of LH is present, and prolactin release can be stimulated, but the individual fails to complete his sexual maturation or to show further progressive testicular growth. This entity has been called the "fertile eunuch syndrome" because germ cells are present on testicular biopsy, and rarely sperm are present in a scant ejaculate. This variant occurs because there is enough testosterone produced within the testes to initiate spermatogenesis, but secretion of the androgen into the peripheral circulation is inadequate to stimulate full virilization or appropriate early closure of the epiphyses and thus eunuchoid proportions develop. Such individuals actually have partial gonadotropin deficiency; hypogonadotropic hypogonadism is really a spectrum of disorders ranging from complete to partial insufficiency.

Approximately half of the patients with selective gonadotropin deficiency have an inherited disorder with associated "midline defects," such as anosmia, harelip, cleft palate, cryptorchidism, microphalus, seizures, or cerebellar ataxia. While the presence of one of these signs or a positive family history may suggest the diagnosis of Kallmann's syndrome, the occurrence of such a somatic abnormality in a young subject does not always confirm the diagnosis of hypogonadotropic hypogonadism, because the midline defects and the hypogonadotropism are inherited independently.

Teenage boys with isolated growth hormone deficiency are in an unusual situation with regard to confirming a diagnosis of hypogonadotropic hypogonadism. In the untreated state, individuals with isolated growth hormone deficiency do not mature sexually until considerably later in life, often mid- to late twenties; but once completed, sexual maturation is normal and patients are fertile. Similarly, we have noted that such subjects enter puberty spontaneously soon after growth hormone replacement is instituted. Therefore, one should not conclude that there is associated hypogonadotropism in short, sexually immature boys with growth hormone deficiency, unless thyroid and/or adrenal insufficiency are also present. This distinction has important therapeutic implications. For the very young patient, growth hormone administration is begun well before sexual maturation is of concern and signs of puberty can be observed prospectively; however, for the individual who is not brought for medical care until his teens, it is not always clear whether to institute androgen replacement. In general, in boys with isolated growth hormone deficiency it is wise to wait 6 to 12 months to determine if there is any spontaneous gonadal enlargement after beginning growth hormone administration, and then to proceed with androgen replacement if necessary. It is not desirable to withhold androgens if puberty does not begin spontaneously, since recent evidence in the teenager shows that the rate of growth and the ultimate height achieved are enhanced when both hormones are given together.

Gonadotropin deficiency can also occur in sexually mature men. This is usually the result of the presence of a pituitary tumor or one of the rare causes of pituitary destruction such as sarcoidosis, infection, amyloidosis, hemochromatosis, or interruption of the vascular supply following head trauma. Since loss of gonadotropin secretion is one of the earliest manifestations of pituitary destruction, impotence and loss of libido may occur prior to the onset of visual field impairment or other signs of adrenal or thyroid insufficiency. There is usually a reduced plasma testosterone level in the face of normal or low serum LH and FSH levels. It is important to distinguish an adult male patient with hypogonadotropic hypogonadism from the occasional patient complaining of impotence and/or infertility who also manifests a low testosterone level secondary to a congenitally low concentration of testosterone binding globulin.

INDICATIONS FOR TESTICULAR BIOPSY

Testicular biopsy can be helpful in confirming a diagnosis of hypogonadotropic hypogonadism, because the testes of patients with *complete* absence of LH and FSH release have seminiferous tubules of less than 25 μ in diameter and devoid of any germ cells, similar to testes of a 7-month fetus. By comparison, the testes of males with *partial* gonadotropin deficiency have larger seminiferous tubules which contain germinal elements in proportion to the degree of gonadotropin insufficiency. However, the testicular biopsy is usually reserved for special cases, such as when it is unclear whether a palpable scrotal mass is a testis, when there is cryptorchidism, or in cases with unusual phenotypic features. One reason for this caution is the fear that, with small testes, the epididymis might be incised accidentally, leading to epididymal obstruction. In addition, testicular biopsy often removes too much tissue, leaving signigicantly fewer tubules for maximum testicular growth following gonadotropin replacement. Most importantly, however, biopsy is not required to make the diagnosis or to judge progress of treatment. This is not to say that the testicular biopsy may not be helpful in the rare patient who has been treated with gonadotropin but who fails to produce sperm in the ejaculate. Here the testicular biopsy is requested as an adjunctive procedure to scrotal exploration because the prime purpose of the surgery is to exclude epididymal obstruction coexisting with the hypogonadotropism.

TREATMENT WITH ANDROGEN

As mentioned previously the choice of treatment depends on a number of factors, including the age of the patient and the degree of gonadotropin deficiency. In the case of an adolescent it is most practical to give testosterone first to stimulate virilization and to switch to gonadotropin replacement later when fertility is desired. When a boy suspected of having gonadotropin deficiency is less than 14 years of age, it may be particularly difficult to be confident of the diagnosis (as described above), and repeated physical examinations are necessary to determine whether there is progressive sexual maturation. Between the ages of 14 and 15 the patient—and his family—may be quite anxious regarding any apparent delay of puberty, and it is often necessary to institute androgen replacement to avoid serious psychosocial problems. Since there is now abundant evidence that androgen replacement does not preclude a proper testicular response to gonadotropin later, even after 10 to 12 years of treatment, one should not hesitate to begin androgen therapy. Certainly after the age of 15 all boys should be treated with androgen so that their social, emotional, and sexual adjustment can occur at the appropriate chronologic age.

Testosterone enanthate and testosterone cypionate are the most effective preparations available to initiate sexual maturation. Both are long-acting testosterone esters suspended in oil to retard absorption. Intramuscular injection provides a peak level 48 to 72 hours after administration, which then slowly declines for the next 3 to 6 weeks. While the rate of decline is highly variable, 200 mg every 2 weeks is optimal for most boys. Certainly testosterone administered every fourth week is inadequate to stimulate full virilization. I feel that it is not so much the dose but rather the frequency of administration which is most important in providing sustained adequate androgen levels.

Patients should be taught to administer their own medication to reduce the number of office visits required for their care. For the "needle-shy" individual (less than 1 in 100 patients in my experience), injections may be given by a nurse or by family members. Only on rare occasions is it necessary to use oral androgens because the patient refused parenteral treatment. The primary disadvantage of oral androgens (fluoxymesterone, methyltestosterone) is that their absorption is variable and low. At best, oral androgens provide minimal virilization compared with the results of repository testosterone administration. In addition, oral androgens result in a low but significant incidence of cholestatic hepatitis, probably because of their modified chemical structure and the fact that they transit through the liver prior to their distribution in the systemic circulation. Such side effects have not been reported with the use of intramuscular testosterone.

Full virilization requires four to five years of testosterone replacement, a time interval similar to that of normal pubertal progression. It is surprising how many patients and physicians expect the rate of progress to be faster. Many frustrations and anxieties can be avoided by seeing the patient every four to six months to review progress. Reasonably frequent follow-up also provides an opportunity to review compliance, to detect problems in sexual adjustment, and to advise counseling when necessary. In general, the majority of patients take their medication correctly, very likely because of the gratification they obtain watching their body develop and enjoying normal libido and potency.

TREATMENT WITH GONADOTROPINS

Because maximum stimulation of spermatogenesis requires three to four years of gonadotropin replacement, this aspect of treatment begins when a patient reaches his early twenties. In the patients who have already been treated with androgen to stimulate virilization, treatment is discontinued for 8 to 12 weeks to reassess testicular function and to determine if the patient can initiate any spontaneous gonadotropin release. A very rare individual enters puberty spontaneously after the age of 20. While androgen replacement might be expected to suppress gonadal development, in actuality, testosterone injections every two weeks do not completely block gonadotropin release or growth of the testes in normal boys.

Initiation of spermatogenesis requires LH to stimulate the Leydig cells to secrete testosterone in high concentrations within the testes. FSH administered alone or in combination with exogenous androgen does not initiate spermatogenesis in hypogonadotropic men. Therefore, human chorionic gonadotropin is administered as 2000 IU i.m. 3 times a week when this phase of treatment is begun. This dose of hCG will fully virilize a hypogonadotropic male who has never been treated with androgen, and the rate and extent of virilization will be indistinguishable from those achieved with testosterone injections.

In patients with complete hypogonadotropic hypogonadism, hCG will increase testicular size to approximately 8 ml but will not advance it further despite completion of virilization. Growth of the testes is due to an increase of early germinal elements within the seminiferous tubules, but they do not advance beyond the spermatid stage without supplemental FSH. By contrast, patients with partial gonadotropin deficiency usually achieve full spermatogenesis and adequate sperm output when hCG is administered alone. In the latter subjects completion of spermatogenesis most likely occurs with hCG alone because there is adequate endogenous production of FSH. However, we have found that it may take 12 to 18 months of continuous hCG administration before sperm appear in the ejaculate.

Patients should be examined every fourth month to assess testicular growth and plasma testosterone levels. Ejaculates should be evaluated every month to determine when sperm first appear in the ejaculate. After 18 to 24 months of hCG administration, if there is no further testicular growth and the patient remains azoospermic, FSH (human menopausal gonadotropin) is added to the regimen. Both medications can be mixed in the same syringe. From our studies we know that virtually all patients will complete spermatogenesis when given 75 IU FSH (1 vial) 3 times a week; however, half of them do so using only 25 IU, and almost all of the remainder require only 38 IU 3 times a week once the testes have been primed with hCG. The cost effectiveness of using lower dosages of FSH is obvious. The lower dosage is continued for at least six to nine months before increasing the dosage, since it takes at least three to six months to determine confidently if there is any growth of the testes or appearance of sperm in the ejaculate.

After treatment most patients with complete hypogonadotropic hypogonadism achieve a testicular size of 12–15 ml and sperm output between 2 and 5 million per ejaculate. This low level of sperm production is adequate to impregnate an otherwise normal healthy ovulating spouse. By contrast, patients with partial gonadotropin insufficiency achieve higher levels of sperm output. In fact, a normal ejaculate can be produced with hCG alone in many such patients. The more limited testicular growth and sperm output achieved in men with complete hypogonadotropism suggest that growth factors other than gonadotropin may be missing. The ability of men to impregnate their spouses with only 2 to 5 million sperm per ejaculate indicates that our concept of the minimally adequate number of sperm required for impregnation should be revised; sperm number and sperm function are not equivalent.

In patients receiving both hCG and FSH, once maximum stimulation of the germinal tissue and sperm output has been achieved, the FSH can be stopped and sperm production will continue in the majority of patients as long as the hCG is continued at the same dosage of 2000 IU 3 times a week. However, continued sperm production requires excellent patient compliance because irregularity in hCG administration leads to a prompt decline in sperm output. In such cases FSH can be readministered to restore the subject's full spermatogenic potential.

Use of human chlorionic gonadotropin and human menopausal gonadotropin in stimulating spermatogenesis has not been associated with any side effects, and the same drugs, used in thousands of women for ovulation induction, likewise have not been associated with any allergic reactions. The medications appear to be quite safe. Patient discomfort from the parenteral injection is minimal, patient compliance is usually excellent, and teaching the patient to self-administer the medication measurably increases the cost effectiveness of the therapy.

In the future, treatment of hypogonadotropic men may also include the use of GNRH, since the pituitary of the patients with selective hypogonadotropic hypogonadism is normal and longitudinal administration of the releasing factor leads to normal secretion of LH and FSH. However, optimum administration of GNRH requires that it be given approximately every 2 hours subcutaneously or intravenously, which is, at the moment, impractical. In the near future, however, automated hormone delivery systems will probably be available which will make this feasible.

TREATMENT WITH BROMOCRIPTINE

Treatment of men with hypogonadotropic hypogonadism in association with prolactin producing hypothalamic or pituitary tumors requires special consideration. While gonadotropin replacement (usually hCG alone) will restore Leydig cell function and spermatogenesis despite high prolactin levels, bromocriptine offers an effective alternative in many instances. This drug is a dopamine agonist that lowers the prolactin concentration. It has worked very effectively in women with amenorrhea and galactorrhea associated with prolactin-producing adenomas by reducing the prolactin concentration and stimulating return of normal cyclic menses. Similarly, bromocriptine can restore gonadotropin secretion and normal gonadal function in men with prolactin-producing tumors. Bromocriptine is usually well tolerated when taken with meals at dosages below 7.5 mg per day; however, it can cause dizziness, fainting, hypotension, headache, nausea, and vomiting. Recent studies indicate that this agent may also be cytotoxic to prolactin-producing tumors, which results in a decrease in tumor size. Treatment must be individualized, since the tumors themselves, or the surgical ablative procedure used to remove the bulk of the tumor, may leave insufficient normal pituitary tissue to provide adequate gonadotropin re-

lease after administering the drug. Therefore, bromocryiptine is the drug of choice for the primary problem; gonadotropins or androgens are utilized if necessary.

INFECTIONS OF THE MALE REPRODUCTIVE TRACT
RICHARD E. BERGER, M.D.

GONOCOCCAL URETHRITIS

Gonococcal disease has continued to defy most existing control measures, and continues to increase in both developed and undeveloped countries. Trends in sexual behavior, population mobility, and the development of β-lactamase producing *Neisseria gonorrhoeae* have all been factors in the spread of gonococcal disease. Forty to 90 percent of men will contract gonorrhea from a single exposure.

More than half of the men who carry *N. gonorrhoeae* in the urethra are asymptomatic. They may therefore be a large reservoir for the transmission of gonorrhea, which may go undetected or be detected only after complications, such as epididymitis, develop. Pharyngeal or rectal infection is also common in men who practice oral or anal intercourse. These sites, as well as the urethra, should be cultured in appropriate patients.

The diagnosis of gonococcal urethritis is easily made by Gram stain of the urethral smear. In men with typical Gram negative intracellular diplococci, the diagnosis of gonococcal urethritis can be confirmed by culture in almost 100 percent of cases. In cases with atypical smears or negative smears, cultures are required to rule out gonococcal disease. Gram stain has no place in the diagnosis of pharyngeal or rectal infections, in which cultures are required. Cultures are also required on follow-up examinations to rule out recurrence.

After the diagnosis of gonococcal urethritis

has been made, the patient should be treated with appropriate antibiotic therapy. This treatment usually consists of 1 gm of probenecid orally followed in 1/2 hour by 3.5 gm of ampicillin orally or 3 gm of amoxicillin orally, or 4.8×10^6 units of aqueous procaine penicillin i.m., or cephoxatin, 2 mg i.m. Patients treated with procaine penicillin should be observed for a procaine reaction for about 30 minutes. All patients treated with a large single dose of a penicillin derivative should also be observed for anaphylaxis for at least 30 minutes. One-dose therapy with any of these regimens has the advantage of requiring no long-term compliance by the patient. Therapy may also be given with tetracycline, 500 mg orally 4 times per day for 5 to 7 days, either at one or following single dose therapy. A loading dose of tetracycline is not required. This regimen offers the advantage of effectiveness against incubating *Chlamydia trachomatis,* which will cause postgonococcal urethritis. *C. trachomatis* is present in approximately 40 percent of men with gonococcal urethritis. All of these regimens offer better than a 90 percent cure rate for simple gonococcal urethritis. Trimethoprim-sulfamethoxazole, nine tablets daily for five days, is an alternative treatment. Neither the ampicillin, amoxicillin, spectinomycin, nor trimethoprim-sulfa-methoxazole regimens is effective for pharyngeal gonococcal infection. Patients should be recultured approximately five days after treatment to ensure cure. Treatment failure may be due to reinfection, noncompliance with the regimen, or the presence of penicillinase-resistant strains. All nonresponsive patients should be tested for penicillinase resistance, and if it is found, treated with spectinomycin, 2 gm i.m.

The sexual partner of the man with gonococcal urethritis should always be treated concurrently. Many women with gonococcal infection are asymptomatic; however, infection may lead to serious sequelae, such as salpingitis. Treatment is the same as for the patient.

NONGONOCOCCAL URETHRITIS

Nongonococcal urethritis (NGU) is the most common genitourinary tract infection in men. Because of difficulties in diagnosis, lack of recognition of this syndrome as a sexually transmitted disease, and changes in social mores, NGU has increased faster than any other sexually transmitted disease. The most common etiologic agent in nongonococcal urethritis is *Chlamydia trachomatis.*

NGU may be the least serious of all diseases caused by *C. trachomatis.* However, improper treatment of NGU may lead to serious complications in men and in their sexual partners, such as epididymitis, Reiter's syndrome, and salpingitis. Proper treatment of NGU caused by *C. trachomatis* is therefore essential.

The diagnosis of nongonococcal urethritis requires both the diagnosis of urethritis and the exclusion of gonococcal disease. The patient should be examined 4 hours after last voiding. An endourethral swab is placed approximately 2 cm into the urethra and a smear taken for Gram stain and, if possible, culture for *C. trachomatis.* The appearance of greater than 4 WBCs on oil immersion high-powered field ($\times 1000$) is evidence of urethritis. Gonococci are not seen, but cultures should be obtained to rule out gonococcal disease. If the criteria for urethritis are not met and suspicion is still high because of typical symptoms, the patient should be examined in the early morning prior to urination. Many more cases of NGU may be diagnosed on such examination.

Once the diagnosis of NGU has been made, treatment should be instituted. Treatment usually consists of tetracycline, 500 mg orally 4 times per day for 7 days, or doxycycline, 500 mg orally 2 times per day for 7 days. Erythromycin, 500 mg orally 4 times per day for 7 days, is also effective. The sexual partner should be treated with the same regimen. All types of NGU initially respond to tetracycline. *C. trachomatis* is uniformly sensitive to tetracycline. Most strains of *Ureaplasma urealyticum,* another probable cause of urethritis, are also sensitive to tetracycline. For recurrent urethritis, erythromycin, 500 mg 4 times per day for 3 weeks, is recommended. Nonchlamydial, nonureaplasma urethritis, which is of unknown origin, is the most resistant to therapy. In the case of recurrence, reinfection should be ruled out. Patients should also have another urethral smear to ensure that inflammation is truly present. After a second recurrence, cyctoscopic and/or radiographic evaluation of the patient's urethra for structural abnormalities is indicated.

PROSTATITIS

Prostatitis is an abused diagnosis often given to several clinical syndromes, and it has little meaning in terms of selection of therapy. For proper therapy to be selected, patients must be subclassified into the syndromes of acute bacterial prostatitis, chronic bacterial prostatitis, idiopathic prostatitis, and prostatodynia.

Men with *acute bacterial prostatitis* often present with high fever, difficulty voiding, and burning upon urination. They may appear acutely ill. Rectal examination reveals a very tender, tense prostate. Massage of the prostate should not be performed for fear of precipitating sepsis. The etiologic agent responsible for the prostatitis can almost always be isolated from midstream urine culture. Initial therapy should consist of hospitalization and administration of broad-spectrum antimicrobials. Ampicillin, 1 gm every 4 hours, and tobramycin, 80 mg i.v. every 8 hours, are good initial choices. Cephalosporin or amikacin may also be used. When the culture and sensitivity results have returned, therapy with a specific agent should be instituted. The patient can be placed on oral antibiotics after he has been afebrile for 48 hours. When infection is improperly treated, or when treatment is delayed, abscess formation in the prostate and/or epididymitis may occur. If abscess formation occurs in the prostate, the preferred treatment is transurethral drainage. Appropriate antibiotic therapy for acute bacterial prostatitis should be continued for six weeks. Most of these men can be cured by appropriate antibiotic therapy and seldom develop a chronic condition.

Chronic bacterial prostatitis is probably the most common cause of recurrent bacteriuria in adult men. Men with this syndrome often present with recurrent bouts of cystitis or bacteriuria with a common urinary pathogen because of failure to eradicate the etiologic organisms form a prostatic focus. They seldom complain of perineal, testicular, or suprapubic pain, although these symptoms may be present. Examination of the prostate usually yields results within normal limits, although in some patients prostatic stones may be felt.

The diagnosis and therefore the proper treatment of chronic bacterial prostatitis requires that the pathogenic organisms be localized to the prostate. Localization is performed when the patient is free of bacteriuria and off antimicrobials. The patient cleanses his glans penis with soap and rinses it off with water. He then voids the first 10 cc of urine into a sterile container. A midstream urine specimen is then obtained in a second container and the patient told to hold the rest of his urine in his bladder. The physician then performs a rectal examination and prostatic massage. The expressed prostatic secretions are collected in a third sterile container. The patient is then asked to void the first 10 cc of postmassage urine into a fourth container. Quantitative cultures and sensitivity tests

are then performed on all specimens. The patient must have at least a tenfold increase of bacteria in his expressed prostatic secretions and/or post massage urine over his first-void urine in order to justify the diagnosis of chronic bacterial prostatitis.

Therapy for chronic bacterial prostatitis should, if possible, be based on culture and sensitivity results obtained from prostatic localization. Carbenicillin is currently the only drug approved by the FDA for use in chronic bacterial prostatitis. It is given in dosages of 2 tablets orally 4 times per day for 30 days. Oral trimethoprim-sulfamethoxazole is also commonly recommended because of its ability to penetrate into prostatic fluid. Treatment should be with 2 tablets twice daily for 12 weeks. Prolonged therapy (6 to 12 weeks) has a better cure rate than short-course (10 to 14 days) therapy. If resistant organisms are present, a course of aminoglycoside may be warranted. Infection may recur months after therapy has been discontinued. In cases in which the bacteriuria cannot be cleared, even with an adequate course of antimicrobials, the patient should be placed on chronic antibacterial prophylaxis. Prophylaxis usually consists of trimethoprim-sulfamethoxazole, one tablet orally once per day. This will usually prevent bacteriuria and symptoms.

If the patient has many prostatic stones, removal by transurethral prostatectomy may cure the infection. Since the outer prostate is the most likely portion of the prostate to be infected, this procedure cannot be expected to improve the majority of patients.

Men with *chronic "idiopathic" prostatitis* present with perineal, inguinal, suprapubic pain sometimes associated with urinary difficulties of slow stream and hesitancy. The etiologic agent in this syndrome is unknown. Cystitis is not present. Localization cultures as for bacterial prostatitis reveal that no pathogenic organisms can be localized to the prostate. Examination of the expressed prostatic secretions, however, reveals abundant white blood cells. Urethritis must be excluded by urethral smear and culture for *N. gonorrhoeae*. If urethritis is found, these patients should be treated for urethritis and not receive the diagnosis of prostatitis. Although some men with idiopathic prostatitis seem to respond to antibiotic therapy, periodic recurrence of symptoms is the norm rather than the exception. Initial therapy should be with tetracycline, 500 mg orally 4 times per day for 2 weeks, or doxycycline, 100 mg orally 2 times per day for 2 weeks. Some men show improvement on this regimen even though no infection can be demonstrated. The physician should inform the patient that he has a benign condition that will not lead to any serious sequelae. The patients should not be told they have a "chronic" infection. Some of these men have underlying neuroses and may develop an obsession with what they consider to be a serious transmissible infection. Some may benefit from psychiatric counseling.

The syndrome of *prostatodynia* presents in the same fashion as chronic idiopathic prostatitis. However, no purulence can be noted in prostatic secretions. Prostatic localization cultures are negative. These patients should also be reassured about the lack of serious consequences of their condition. In patients with a slow urinary stream and hesitancy, phenoxybenzamine, 10 mg orally daily, to relax the bladder neck and sphincter can sometimes be of benefit. Certain patients may also benefit from a course of a prostaglandin inhibitor, such as aspirin, 2 tablets orally every 4 hours. The benign nature of this condition argues against instituting any therapy with potential long-term side effects. Patients may also benefit from psychologic counseling or biofeedback techniques.

ACUTE EPIDIDYMO-ORCHITIS

Acute epididymitis is an acute infection of the epididymis that often involves the testicle. Proper therapy depends upon the etiologic agent.

In men under age 35, the sexually transmitted organisms that cause urethritis, *N. gonorrhoeae* and *C. trachomatis,* are the most common causes of acute epididymitis. These men present with relatively acute onset of scrotal pain. They do not usually complain of symptoms of urethritis; however, a urethral discharge can often be demonstrated. In infection with *N. gonorrhoeae*, typical Gram negative diplococci are seen on Gram stain on the urethral smear. In infection with *Chlamydia trachomatis,* Gram stain of urethral smear may show more than 4 polymorphonuclear leukocytes per high-powered oil immersion field, or first-void (first 10 cc) urine may show pyuria. Men with gonococcal epididymitis should start receiving 1 g of probenecid orally followed by 4.8×10^6 units of aqueous penicillin i.m., or 3.5 g of ampicillin, or 3.0 g of amoxicillin orally. Therapy should then be continued with either tetracycline, 500 mg orally 4 times per day, or doxycycline, 100 mg orally twice per day for 10 days. The patient's sexual partner should also be treated.

Therapy for nongonococcal epididymitis associated with NGU presumably caused by *C. trachomatis* should be with tetracycline, 500 mg or-

ally 4 times per day for 10 days, and with oral doxycycline, 100 mg orally 2 times per day for 10 days. Erythromycin, 500 mg 4 times a day for 10 days, may also be effective. The patient's sexual partner should also be treated.

In men over the age of 35, the most common causes of epididymitis are the usual urinary pathogens (for example, *E. coli*). In this age group the incidence of sexually transmitted disease is decreasing and the incidence of acquired urinary abnormalities predisposing to urinary tract infections is increasing. Therapy can be rationally based on the culture of the patient's midstream urine. In the absence of infected urine, or in men with polymicrobial bladder infection and urethral catheters, aspiration cultures of the epididymis may be of benefit to obtain culture and sensitivity results. Pending sensitivity results, the patient should be started on broad-spectrum parenteral antibiotics. Ampicillin, 1 gm every 4 hours, and tobramycin, 80 mg every 8 hours, are good choices. Trimethoprim-sulfamethoxazol is a good choice for outpatients. Therapy may be prolonged.

All patients with epididymitis should be placed on bed rest. The lymphatics of the infected epididymis drain poorly when the patient is in the upright position. Ambulation may therefore lead to increased swelling and decreased clearance of the toxic products of local infection. Bed rest should be maintained until the patient is free of pain and tenderness. Gradual ambulation may then be begun. Patients can usually be expected to improve after 48 to 72 hours. Acute relief of pain is easily obtained by infiltrating the spermatic cord at the external ring with 5 cc of 0.25 percent marcaine.

Delay in treatment or inappropriate therapy may result in abscess formation, testicular infarction from inflammatory thrombosis of the testicular artery, or both. If the patient fails to improve with appropriate therapy, these complications should be considered. Radionuclide testicular scan, ultrasound, or both will confirm the diagnosis. Scrotal exploration must be undertaken in these cases. Orchiectomy is almost always necessary to drain an abscess adequately.

PRIMARY SYPHILIS

Primary syphilis often presents as a painless rubbery ulcer in the genital region. Diagnosis is confirmed by dark field examination of scrapings of the base of the ulcer, rapid plasma reagent test (RPR), or the VDRL test (Venereal Disease Research Laboratory). Treatment consists of benzathine penicillin, 2.4 million units i.m. in a single visit. Penicillin-allergic patients may also be treated with tetracycline, 500 mg 4 times a day for 15 days. Of course, sexual contacts should also be treated in a similar fashion. About half of the patients treated with penicillin will experience a Jarisch-Herxheimer reaction. It usually can be managed with aspirin.

CHANCROID

Chancroid is a disease caused by *Haemophilus ducreyi*. Ulcers caused by these organisms usually occur around the coronal sulcus. They usually heal in two to three weeks. Treatment is with erythromycin 500 mg orally four times per day, or trimethoprim-sulfamethoxazol 60/800 mg orally two times per day for at least ten days. Fluctuant material should be aspirated from lymph nodes as needed. Sexual partners must also be treated.

LYMPHOGRANULOMA VENEREUM

Lymphogranuloma venereum is caused by *C. trachomatis* immunotypes L-1 to L-3. Diagnosis is suspected on finding a lesion on the penis and inguinal adenopathy. Diagnosis is made on finding microimmunofluorescent antibody to specific LGV types of *C. trachomatis* in the serum. Treatment is with sulfamethoxazol 800 mg orally two times per day, or with tetracycline, 500 mg orally 4 times per day for at least two weeks. Treatment of sexual partners is also required.

HERPES SIMPLEX, TYPE II

Herpes simplex is an acute, self-limited, pustular eruption often found on the penis. It frequently causes recurrent attacks. Transmission of this disease usually occurs in periods of active pustule and ulcer formation. Currently there is no available treatment to cure herpes simplex infection. Dyes plus light, ether, and topical antivirals have not been helpful. Acyclovir ointment, 5%, may decrease the duration of pain and viral shedding in primary infection but will not decrease recurrences. Therapy should be aimed at patient comfort and education about the disease and its spread. Patients should be informed that they should not have intercourse during periods of at-

tacks. The best therapy involves keeping the lesions clean and dry. The use of jellies may contribute to the local spread of organism.

MUMPS ORCHITIS

Mumps orchitis may appear in adult males five to ten days after the appearance of parotiditis. It is usually unilateral but may be bilateral. Testicular atrophy occurs in approximately 50 percent of the cases. Sterility may occur as a consequence. Treatment of mumps orchitis is symptomatic; bed rest, scrotal support, and pain medications are advised. Gamma globulin, diethylstilbestrol, and steroids have been advocated; however, their efficacy is unproved.

Surgical treatment by incising the tunica albuginea of the testicle in order to relieve pressure has also been advocated, but this therapy is probably never indicated.

NONSPECIFIC INFECTIONS AND MALE INFERTILITY

E. coli and other common urinary pathogens that may cause bacterial prostatitis and cystitis may decrease sperm function and motility. If they are cultured from the semen or urine, antibiotic treatment is determined by culture and sensitivity testing. Prolonged therapy may be necessary for chronic bacterial prostatitis.

Both gonococcal and nongonococcal urethritis in the male may be related to infertility. Both of these infections may lead to epididymitis and to vasal or epididymal occlusion and/or testicular atrophy. Furthermore, both *C. trachomatis* and *N. gonorrhoeae* have been shown to produce salpingitis and tubal occlusion in the female. These infections should therefore be treated to prevent possible infertility.

Therapy for epididymitis should be instituted early and patients kept on bed rest in an effort to reduce the inflammation and subsequent testicular atrophy and infertility.

Idiopathic prostatitis has often been implicated as the etiologic agent in infertility in males who have no other obvious cause. White blood cells may be seen in the semen or in expressed prostatic secretions. However, no pathogens can be recovered. The relationship of this syndrome to infertility is obscure. However, select patients may benefit from empiric doxycycline therapy, 100 mg orally 2 times per day for 3 to 6 weeks. These men may have a decrease in pyospermia with treatment even if no pathogens can be isolated from the semen. However, proof that this therapy affects fertility is lacking.

VARICOCELE

HARRIS M. NAGLER, M.D.
and LARRY I. LIPSHULTZ, M.D.

The clinical significance of the scrotal varicocele remains a topic of confusion and controversy. All physicians accept the fact that a patient with a varicocele may be normally fertile; however, there seems little doubt that varicoceles are frequently associated with impaired testicular function. Eight to 22 percent of normal males are reported to have varicoceles, whereas 21 to 39 percent of men undergoing evaluation for infertility will demonstrate this same vascular abnormality. The variability of the gonadotoxic effect of the varicocele, as well as the unpredictable improvement of semen quality and subsequent fertility after varicocelectomy, make the relationship between the varicocele and infertility a complicated issue. Before this relationship can be better defined it is necessary to gain a clearer understanding of both the etiology and the pathophysiology of the varicocele. The primary purpose of this chapter, however, is not to explore the currently proposed mechanisms by which the varicocele exerts its deleterious effects on spermatogenesis, but rather to outline a rational approach to the infertile male with a scrotal varix.

ANATOMY

Several anatomic considerations should be reviewed when discussing varicoceles. The testicle has three venous drainage routes: (1) The left internal spermatic vein (gonadal vein), the major drainage of the left testis, enters the left renal vein; the right internal spermatic vein drains directly into the vena cava; (2) the deferential vein which follows the course of the vas deferens enters the superior vesical vein and subsequently the hypogas-

tric vein; and (3) the cremasteric (external spermatic) vein separates from the cord structures at the level of the external ring and drains via the pudendal vein. These alternative pathways allow for adequate drainage and testicular preservation after interruption of the internal spermatic vein during varicocelectomy. However, aberrant flow in these normal structures, as well as the presence of various anomalous venous pathways, may be the cause of a "recurrent" varicocele after a seemingly complete ligation of the internal system alone.

Three major types of varicoceles have recently been differentiated on the basis of venographic studies. In the first group, abnormalities *within* the internal spermatic system give rise to the varicocele. Generally it is thought that either congenital absence or incompetence of the valvular mechanism in the proximal portion of the left internal spermatic vein may lead to a varicocele. There are several explanations for the origin of this valvular inadequacy. These are (1) congenital absence of the valves in the internal spermatic vein, (2) increased hydrostatic pressure from the long vertical course of the left internal spermatic vein, (3) a "nutcracker phenomenon" created by the superior mesenteric artery partially occluding the left renal drainage and leading to increased pressure within the spermatic vein, and (4) intrinsic ectasia of the pampiniform plexus promoting venous stasis with dilatation and subsequent valvular incompetence. Moreover, it has been recently demonstrated that the proximal part of the internal spermatic vein may remain competent in a patient with a varicocele. In these cases, the varicocele occurs secondary to a *renal-spermatic vein communicating shunt,* allowing reflux into the distal dilated portion of the internal spermatic vein.

In a second group of patients with varicoceles the etiologic abnormality appears to be a *distal* "nutcracker" phenomenon. This involves obstruction of the left common iliac vein owing to compression by the common iliac artery and results in dilatation of the *external spermatic* venous drainage. In this setting pelvic varicosities may develop and produce concurrent right scrotal varices. The third group of patients with scrotal varicoceles seems to have both internal and external spermatic vein abnormalities. These observations individually or in concert may explain the observed predominance of the left-sided lesions. They also offer a potential mechanism of failure after what appears to be an adequate and complete internal spermatic vein ligation, especially if a high retroperitoneal approach has been used.

DIAGNOSIS

It is important to realize that the size of the varicocele does not appear to correlate with its gonadotoxic effect. A corollary of this is that "subclinical" varicoceles that is, systems with retrograde flow but lacking *palpable* evidence of vascular ectasia or dilatation, either right, left, or bilateral may have the same detrimental effect on fertility. The impact of the subclinical varicocele, which is reported to occur in 45 to 75 percent of infertile men, has not been adequately studied. Recent venography studies have noted right-sided "subclinical" varicoceles in 70 percent of men with clinical left-sided varicoceles.

If indeed a small varicocele has the same clinical implication as a large varicocele, then the pursuit of even a small lesion must be rigorous. In light of these considerations it is clear that to outline a therapeutic approach to the varicocele, one must include a diagnostic approach as well. There are several maneuvers that should be employed during the physical examination to assure an accurate and complete diagnosis.

The patient should first be examined in the erect position. Bilateral cord structures are palpated and compared. A Valsalva maneuver is carried out while the examiner palpates both right and left cord structures concurrently. Asymmetry both prior to and after a Valsalva maneuver should lead one to suspect the presence of a varicocele. A discrete pulse wave appreciated with a Valsalva maneuver indicates a varicocele. Cremasteric muscle contraction at the time of the Valsalva maneuver, which results in shortening and thickening of the cord, may mimic venous engorgement; consequently, an attempt to differentiate this artifact should be made. Stabilizing the testicle with some traction applied to the cord structures will minimize the confusion caused by cremasteric musculature contraction. The patient is then moved to a supine position; a diminution of cord "thickness" may indicate the presence of a varicocele rather than a cord lipoma. If after these manuevers there is still uncertainty, a helpful technique is to control the cord structures between the thumb and forefinger with the patient in the supine position. The patient is directed to stand up, and compression is then removed while palpating the cord structures distally. Retrograde filling can at times be appreciated by this manuever.

The fact that lesions may indeed be bilateral at times makes reliance solely on cord asymmetry an unreliable diagnostic criterion. The measurement of testicular dimensions is worthwhile in evaluation of infertility; asymmetry may be a clue to an underlying scrotal varix. The Doppler pencil probe stethoscope may be utilized to assess retrograde blood flow in those patients whose physical examination is equivocal even after the above maneuvers. However, the diagnosis of a varicocele should not be based solely on Doppler examination. The doppler is used to *confirm* one's diagnostic impression.

The routine use of venography in diagnosis of subclinical varicoceles is at best premature. The significance of the subclinical varicocele identified in this manner is as yet undefined and the procedure is not without risk. In the patient with "recurrent" varicocele, it is useful to perform venography to determine if the recurrence is due to anomalous vasculature or to a technical surgical failure.

THERAPEUTIC APPROACH

Assessment of Sperm Function

The anatomic identification of the varicocele, though at times difficult, is only the beginning of a clinical approach to its identification. The physiologic significance of the identified anatomic abnormality must be determined. Unfortunately, the pathophysiology of altered spermatogenesis that occurs in the presence of varicoceles has not been delineated; therefore, no pathognomonic "markers" exist which may be quantitated to identify the "significant" varicocele. The semen analysis itself is the test that most often draws attention to the presence or absence of the varicocele. In the presence of "normal" semen parameters the varicocele is often ignored. However, when abnormalities in spermatogenesis are noted (density, morphology, or motility) the coexisting varicocele is generally implicated as a significant etiologic factor. Two difficult questions then arise: (1) Is the varicocele causing the semen abnormalities, and (2) more importantly, does the couple's infertility result from the semen abnormalities? The functional significance of the observed semen abnormalities can and must be carefully assessed to avoid unnecessary as well as unsuccessful surgery. The mere presence of a varicocele in the male partner of an infertile couple is not an indication for varicocelectomy. Furthermore, andrologic evaluation is incomplete without including an evaluation of the female.

Briefly, the ovulatory status of the woman

must be established. This can often be determined by basal body tempature (BBT) monitoring with or without hormonal confirmation. The adequacy of the luteal phase may be determined by BBT in conjunction with an endometrial biopsy or appropriately timed serum progesterone determinations. These latter two studies assess the *ovulatory* effectiveness. The *cervical factor* must also be assessed. There must be sufficient normal mucus at the time of ovulation to be conducive to sperm penetration and survival.

The well-timed periovulatory postcoital test allows one to assess the quality of the cervical mucus, as well as the functional quality of the sperm. The postcoital test provides in vivo testing of sperm function. An abnormal postcoital test in the presence of normal cervical mucus will reinforce the functional significance of abnormalities identified by semen analysis. A satisfactory postcoital test, however, may direct one to the further study of possibly abnormal *pelvic factors,* such as inflammatory tubular disease, endometriosis, uterine abnormalities, and so on. The bovine mucus penetration test is being investigated as a potentially more objective and reproducible method of assessing sperm function. This method would be advantageous because it could be performed and quantitated without the constraints of the ovulatory cycle. As yet, this newly popularized assessment of sperm function, the cross-species sperm penetration test (SPA), is not widely available and remains somewhat investigational.

The above studies help to define the functional significance of abnormalities in the semen analysis. If sperm are demonstrated to be functionally abnormal and a varicocele is present, it is generally recommended that the varicocele be surgically repaired. Sixty to 80 percent of patients who undergo correction of a varicocele will have improved semen characteristics; 35 to 55 percent of these patients will initiate a pregnancy. These statistics are better than the statistics reported for any medical regimen. Therefore, when a varicocele is identified in the above setting, varicocele repair is recommended.

SURGICAL APPROACH

There are three approaches to the correction of a varicocele. The scrotal approach is mentioned only for the sake of condemnation. It is a more difficult procedure and is more likely to be followed by complications. It should be avoided.

The inguinal, or Ivanissevitch, approach has undergone several modifications; however, in all such modifications the internal spermatic veins are ligated within the course of the inguinal canal. Most often general or regional anesthesia is employed. Recent reports of varicocelectomy under local anesthesia have also been published. The inguinal canal is approached in the standard fashion using a hernia incision or modification thereof. The external oblique aponeurosis is opened and the cord is mobilized. A Penrose drain is placed beneath the cord structures and clamped to the drapes at either end. This elevates the cord into the wound. The inguinal nerve is isolated from the cord structures and a mosquito clamp is utilized to exclude it from the area of dissection. With the spermatic fascia incised, the dilated veins are individually dissected, clamped, and ligated using silk sutures. This approach also affords access to the external spermatic (cremasteric) vein. It leaves the cord at the level of the external ring to join the pudendal and ultimately the saphenous vein. The external vein should also be ligated if it is enlarged and incompetent. Its abnormal flow may contribute to the failure of a varicocele repair when only the external spermatic vein is removed. Though it is not mandatory, a portion of the venous segment is often submitted for pathologic confirmation. When identifying the internal spermatic vein, one should attempt to progress perpendicularly across the cord in one plane to prevent multiple ligations of a single vessel. The Penrose drain beneath the cord structures aids in this process. Care is taken to identify and spare the vas deferens. The vas should not be skeletonized, as this may injure the accompanying artery, removing collateral blood supply to the testicle. This is of paramount importance if the testicular artery itself becomes injured during the procedure. Care is taken to divide venous structures without incorporating the surrounding cremasteric fibers to minimize the potential of testicular damage. The cord is then repositioned within the canal and the external oblique aponeurosis is closed with chromic catgut. Scarpa's fascia is reapproximated with plain catgut sutures, and the skin is closed with a subcuticular closure. Collodion is applied to the wound and the patient is generally discharged on the same evening or the day after surgery. Antibiotics are not employed. Local anesthesia and well-equipped outpatient surgery units are becoming increasingly popular, making overnight hospitalization less common.

The inguinal approach to the correction of

varicocele is rarely associated with complications. The most common, though still infrequent, complication is the formation of a hydrocele. This is rarely of clinical significance. The most devastating complication is damage to the vas or testicular artery. The latter may result in testicular atrophy. Both of these complications are most distressing for a patient in whom an operation was performed to improve fertility. Careful identification of cord structures should prevent both of these complications.

The Poloma retroperitoneal approach divides the internal spermatic vein as it passes through the internal spermatic ring into the retroperitoneal space. The incision for this approach is made at the level of the umbilicus. The retroperitoneal space is entered and the peritoneal envelope is retracted medially. The internal spermatic vein is readily identified on the posterior aspect of the peritoneal reflection. It is then dissected free and ligated as previously described. Although this procedure is quite simple, the potential for postoperative complications is greater and the advantage is insignificant when compared with the inguinal approach. However, the retroperitoneal approach is useful in patients who have had prior inguinal surgery, for hernia repair, previous varicocele surgery, and so on. If preoperative venography reveals reflux via the internal spermatic vein, this approach may be used to avoid the violated inguinal canal and thus decrease the potential for testicular atrophy or vasal disruption. Except for these well-defined circumstances, we prefer to use the inguinal approach for primary varicocelectomy.

Recently there has been much discussion about percutaneous venographic techniques for varicocele correction. The rate of morbidity associated with venography has been reported to be anywhere from 0.5 to 9 percent. The reported morbidity rate from varicocelectomies has been reported to vary from 1 to 3 percent; none of the complications is considered major. There have been more procedures and more extensive follow-up for surgical correction of varicocele than for transvenous occlusion; any comparison between the two techniques would therefore be invalid at this point. It is clear, however, that the morbidity rate after the surgical approach is minimal and the complications minor. Certainly the complications that could arise after transvenous occlusion of the spermatic vein are potentially serious. Peripheral migrations of balloons, coils, and so on have been reported with other applications of transvenous or transarterial occlusion techniques. There is no reason to expect that this cannot occur with transvenous varicocelectomy. Indeed, in a preliminary series of 50 patients there was one balloon migration to the lungs. Though this did not appear to have any clinical significance, the potential for serious morbidity remains. The safety and validity of this procedure must be confirmed through further studies before universal application and the abandonment of the time-tested surgical varicocelectomy can even be considered. As local anesthesia is being utilized more frequently, the safety of outpatient varicocelectomy becomes even more difficult to impugn.

Until such time as the pathophysiology of the varicocele is more clearly defined, it is unlikely that we will be better able to assess the prospective contribution of the varicocele to any given patient's decreased fertility. It is imperative that a thorough evaluation of both partners, individually as well as together, be carried out prior to committing a patient to a surgical procedure. If however, sperm function, is judged abnormal as outlined above in the presence of a varicocele, a surgical varicocelectomy will afford the best opportunity for a pregnancy. Correction of a scrotal varicocele remains the most reproducible and effective method of treating the thoroughly evaluated male with infertility.

MALE INFERTILITY OF UNDETERMINED ETIOLOGY

H. W. G. BAKER, M.D., Ph.D.

DIAGNOSTIC CONSIDERATIONS

Initial assessment of the male partner of an infertile union is directed at separating the small number of men who can be treated successfully and the larger number who are irreversibly sterile, from the bulk who are subfertile and have conditions for which there are currently no clearly defined effective treatments.

Treatable Conditions

Gonadotropin deficiency (Chapter 70) and coital disorders (impotence, Chapter 76; retrograde ejaculation; Chapter 40) are covered in other chapters. Obstruction of the ejaculatory ducts by cysts or inflammatory scarring is rare but can be corrected by surgery. Suggestive findings are normal testicular size, palpable vasa, normal serum follicle stimulating hormone (FSH), and azoospermia with low semen volume and fructose concentration. Epididymal disorders causing obstructive azoospermia or partial obstruction with oligospermia are also potentially treatable by bypass surgery. Patients with epididymal obstructions have normal testicular size and serum FSH levels and they may have slightly enlarged and tender epididymal heads and histories of epididymitis, scrotal surgery, or bronchiectasis.

Irreversible Sterility

Untreatable conditions causing sterility are azoospermia due to primary seminiferous tubular failure, vasal agenesis, zero sperm motility, and total teratospermia. Primary tubular failure is suggested by reduced testicular size and elevated serum FSH levels. Agenesis of the vasa deferentia should be discovered during examination of the scrotum. Zero sperm motility often results from structural defects in the sperm tails, such as absent dynein arms, and this may be associated with other evidence of the immotile cilia syndrome, such as bronchiectasis. Total teratospermia, in which all sperm show the same abnormality, such as pinheads or absent acrosomes, is rare but must be recognized to avoid fruitless attempts at treatment.

Oligospermia and Asthenospermia

Many infertile men have none of the above disorders. They have abnormalities in their semen—oligospermia (mean sperm concentration less than 20 million/ml, usually with poor sperm motility and increased abnormal morphology of mixed type), or asthenospermia (mean sperm concentration above 20 million/ml but motility less than 60 percent with poor forward progression). Results of semen analyses in these men are often highly variable, and at least three tests should be performed over a six- to eight-week period. Causes for the poor semen quality, such as mumps orchitis or undescended testes, are found in some patients, but these conditions do not have any specific prognostic significance. Prognosis depends more on average sperm concentration. Associated disorders, such as varicoceles, genital tract infections, sperm autoimmunity, and chronic ill health, may be relevant in some patients. Treatments for varicocele and genital tract infections are discussed in Chapters 71 and 72. Sperm antibodies causing agglutination and immobilization of sperm are found in the sera of many men who have undergone vasectomy reversal, in some following orchitis or trauma to the scrotal contents, and in a few for unknown reasons. These antibodies may contribute to the infertility of patients with oligospermia. But with normal sperm output, additional evidence of the presence of antibodies in semen is required; in particular, lack of sperm penetration of normal midcycle cervical mucus. Sperm agglutination and low motility with very poor progression and shaking may be noted in the semen analysis. Chronic illnesses or their treatments, for example, hepatic cirrhosis, renal failure and cytotoxic therapy for malignancies, are well known to impair testicular function. Provided the illness is controlled, the infertility can be dealt with in the same way as for other patients.

About three-quarters of men seen for infertility fall into this group. We will review various treatments used in the past and outline our current approach to management of men with poor semen quality.

THERAPEUTIC ALTERNATIVES

Many treatments have been recommended for oligospermia and asthenospermia on the basis of anecdotal experience or uncontrolled trials in which improvement in semen quality or pregnancies occurred. The natural variability of semen analysis results has been neglected, as has the fact that men with such disorders are subfertile rather than sterile and have some chance of producing a pregnancy without treatment. Furthermore, there is usually no sound basis for the treatments. Some of these treatments were used in Melbourne, and results are summarized in Table 1. Pregnancy rates were calculated by life table analysis, which takes into account the time factor—when the pregnancies occurred and the duration of follow-up of unsuccessful couples.

TABLE 1   Treatments of Uncertain Value for Oligospermia and Asthenospermia

Treatment	Melbourne Experience (Logrank Test)			
	Number of Courses	Number of Pregnancies	Expected Pregnancies	Relative Pregnancy Rate
Testosterone "rebound"	33	6	7.92	0.76
Mesterolone	49	7	12.93	0.54
hCG	10	2	2.15	0.93
Clomiphene	50	5	10.66	0.47
Antibacterial agents	95	25	18.83	1.33
Bromocriptine	13	3	3.15	0.95
Varicocelectomy	201	70	57.37	1.22
AIH	61	10	11.76	0.85
None	583	102	105.22	0.97

Note: Logrank χ^2 = 11.37 p NS. Side effects or complications of the treatments were uncommon, although there were some instances of acne with testosterone rebound; dyspepsia, diarrhea, or rashes with antibacterial agents; nausea with bromocriptine, hydroceles following varicocelectomy; and anxiety and inability to produce semen during AIH (artificial insemination with husband's semen).

Drug Treatments

Androgens and Human Chorionic Gonadotropin (hCG).   Androgens in low dose (methyltestosterone, 10–50 mg per day; mesterolone, 50–75 mg per day; fluoxymesterone, 5–20 mg per day) or hCG (1500–3000 IU twice or thrice weekly) have been given for 3 or more months in the hope that spermatogenesis might be stimulated or sperm maturation and motility improved by direct actions of androgens on the germinal epithelium and epididymis. Androgens are also used in high doses (testosterone enanthate, 250 mg every 2 weeks for 3 months) to suppress gonadotropin secretion and spermatogenesis temporarily. Following treatment, a rebound rise in sperm output above pretreatment values is supposed to occur. In Melbourne, 92 courses of androgen or hCG therapy produced pregnancy rates no greater than those achieved by untreated men with similar degrees of subfertility. Sperm concentrations were significantly suppressed during treatment with high-dose testosterone and hCG, but there was no significant "rebound" and sperm motility was unchanged.

Gonadotropins and Antiestrogens.   Extracts of human urinary or pituitary gonadotropins containing FSH and variable amounts of luteinizing hormone (LH) or pregnant mare serum gonadotropin have been injected alone (FSH 75–600 IU) or with hCG twice or thrice weekly for several months in attempts to stimulate the seminiferous epithelium of men with idiopathic oligospermia. Gonadotropin releasing hormone has also been used in small uncontrolled trials. In our opinion the results were unremarkable, and such expensive treatments should be reserved for patients with gonadotropin deficiency.

The antiestrogens, clomiphene citrate (25–50 mg per day) and tamoxifen (20 mg per day) also increase circulating levels of FSH and LH. Treatment for three to six months is claimed to increase sperm output in men with idiopathic oligospermia and normal pretreatment serum gonadotropin levels. However, the trials were inadequately controlled. Fifty patients treated with clomiphene in Melbourne showed no significant change in semen quality, and the pregnancy rate was not significantly different from that for untreated infertile men.

Antibacterial Agents.   Erythromycin (0.75–1.5 g per day), doxycycline (100 mg per day), trimethoprim with sulfamethoxazole (160 mg and 800 mg per day) or other antibacterial agents that enter prostatic fluid are often prescribed in prolonged courses (28 days or more) for infertile men with asthenospermia, leukocytes in the semen, or symptoms of inflammation of the prostate or genital tract (see Chapter 71). Courses of therapy with these agents in 95 patients, most of whom had asthenospermia, produced a slightly but not significantly better pregnancy rate than that for untreated patients.

Glucocorticoids.   Men with sperm antibodies have been treated with immunosuppressive doses of glucocorticoids, for example, prednisolone, 0.75 mg/kg per day for 4 months, or methylprednisolone, 96 mg per day for 5 days repeated at 2- to 3-month intervals. Antibody titers were often reduced, sperm motility and penetration of cervical mucus improved, and some pregnancies occurred. Marked improvement in sperm output has been noted in rare patients with severe oligospermia and sperm antibodies. However, no controlled trials have been reported. Also, such treatment has unpleasant and potentially serious side effects.

Other Drugs. Thyroxine, glucocorticoids in low doses, vitamins, minerals, and amino acids have been recommended for men with oligospermia or asthenospermia, but there is no reason to believe they might help in the absence of a specific deficiency state. Bromocriptine has not proved useful for infertile men with normal or slightly elevated prolactin levels. Pathologic hyperprolactinemia appears to be uncommon in men with oligospermia or asthenospermia.

Surgical Treatments

Varicocelectomy. Spermatic vein ligation is commonly advised for infertile men with varicoceles of various size (see Chapter 72). However, it is not certain that this procedure improves semen quality and fertility. From a follow-up of subfertile couples in Melbourne, it would appear that the presence of a varicocele is associated with a better chance of fertility whether or not it is surgically corrected.

Vasoepididymostomy. Because results of conventional vasoepididymostomy are so poor, the possibility that oligospermia might be due to partial epididymal obstruction is usually not investigated. However, new microsurgical procedures in which the epididymal tubule is anastomosed end to end to the vas appear to have much higher success rates. Thus the detection of men with partial obstructions may become more important in the future (see Chapter 77).

Other Methods

Coital Techniques. Some infertile couples are told to abstain from intercourse until the midcycle period of the wife's menstrual cycle because sperm concentrations usually rise with abstinence and fall with frequent ejaculation. However, the influence of ejaculatory frequency on sperm concentration is much less in oligospermic than in normospermic men, and many couples attempting this technique miss midcycle. Another method is the split ejaculate withdrawal procedure whereby only the first part of the ejaculate is deposited in the vagina. While the first part of the ejaculate often contains a higher concentration of sperm and has better morphology and motility than later parts, this is not invariably so and should be checked by a split ejaculate semen analysis. Although they have not been studied adequately, we believe these coital techniques are unlikely to improve fertility. In addition, they often distress the couple.

Artificial Insemination with Husband's Semen (AIH). Pregnancies may occur following AIH with oligospermic or asthenospermic semen, but it is not clear that AIH provides a better pregnancy rate than natural insemination. Until AIH can be shown to be beneficial in controlled trials, it should be reserved for situations in which natural insemination is impossible, for instance, in cases of impotence or anejaculation and when the husband's semen was collected and stored before vasectomy or other treatment causing sterility.

In Vitro Fertilization. As human ova can be fertilized in the laboratory with as few as 100,000 sperm, in vitro fertilization and embryo transfer may become a method of treatment for oligospermia in the future, provided the rate of implantation, currently about 10 percent can be improved.

General Advice

Many infertile men are told to avoid smoking, alcohol and unnecessary drugs, sauna and spa baths, stress at work, and unbalanced diets. While such exhortations are reasonable for general health purposes, compliance is not reliably associated with improved semen quality and fertility.

PREFERRED APPROACH

Our present strategy for managing subfertile men with oligospermia and asthenospermia has developed through disillusionment with empiric therapies, and is mainly advisory. The lack of proof that such treatments improve fertility is explained to the couple. Their chances of achieving a pregnancy are estimated and alternative methods for starting a family are discussed. We restrict drug treatments, varicocelectomy, and AIH to patients who volunteer to be included in controlled trials.

Prognosis for Fertility

A method for estimating the chances of conception occurring in a given time has been developed from a life table analysis of 250 pregnancies in 788 subfertile couples followed in Melbourne over the last 10 years. Overall, 25 percent achieved a pregnancy within one year and 30 percent within two years, but certain factors were associated with higher or lower pregnancy rates. The major prognostic factors were mean sperm concentration, duration of infertility, and age of wife. The lower the sperm concentration, the longer the duration of infertility, and the older the wife the worse the outlook. Also, the presence of a varicocele and previous pregnancies in the union were associated with better chances. We use these factors to predict the likelihood of a pregnancy occurring with each couple, and we emphasize the lack of treatments proven to increase pregnancy rates.

Alternatives and Planning

Following discussion of prognosis, the alternatives of adoption, artificial insemination with donor semen (AID), or childlessness are mentioned. In Melbourne there are few children for adoption, waiting lists are long, and guidelines for acceptance of adopting parents stringent. Thus couples are advised to consider entering a waiting list early unless they are sure they would never want to adopt. At present, AID has an overall success rate of 70 percent in one year, which is clearly superior to the chances with the average subfertile men (25 percent in one year). For many couples the major decision is whether or not to have AID, and when. They must balance the desire to have their own children against the uncertainty of success, while bearing in mind the declining chance with time. We suggest that plans for the future be made at an early stage. For example, the average couple with three years primary infertility, a healthy wife aged 30, and a husband with mild oligospermia have a 25 percent chance of pregnancy in one year and 30 per cent in two years. A reasonable plan is for them to continue trying for one or two years, during which time the husband might enter a therapeutic trial, and if no pregnancy occurs the wife will have AID. Similar couples might decide this chance of success is too low and use AID sooner. Others are not interested in AID; they may wish to continue trying for a much longer period and are prepared to accept childlessness.

Female Factors

Unless the couple do not wish to pursue treatment, investigations of the wife are reviewed and further consultations with gynecologists expert in the management of infertility are arranged as necessary. In Melbourne, between 10 and 20 percent of wives of subfertile men have tubal or ovulatory disorders. Because pregnancy may occur with poor semen quality, easily correctable problems in the wife, such as anovulation, should be treated vigorously.

Timing of Intercourse

We believe it to be important that the couple have some understanding of the physiology of fertilization, particularly indications of ovulation and the requirement that coitus occur near the time of ovulation. We suggest they have intercourse at least every 48 hours over 8 to 10 days spanning ovulation. This should ensure the presence of the maximum possible number of sperm in the cervical mucus and female genital tract at the time of ovulation. Intercourse need not be restricted to this time, however, and may occur more frequently during midcycle and at other times as desired.

Reduction of Anxiety and Acceptance of Infertility

Infertility presents a severe psychologic trauma to most couples. Denial, grief, and hostility reactions are common and many patients take months or years before they come to terms with their infertility. The fact that no clear explanation of the cause and no effective treatment can be offered to the majority of infertile men causes further frustration. Stress and anxiety increase with each unsuccessful treatment. Furthermore, a significant proportion of couples end up with no children despite trying everything, including AID. We try to be frank yet empathetic when dealing with these difficult aspects of infertility. We request that both partners be present when results of investigations, prognosis, and alternatives such as AID are discussed, and we also mention the possibility of their seeking another opinion about their case and the availability of self-help groups for infertile couples.

PROS AND CONS OF TREATMENT

The aim of treatment of subfertile men is to improve fertility. The Melbourne results suggest methods commonly used in men with poor semen quality—drugs, varicocele operations, and AIH—do not produce higher pregnancy rates than occur with no treatment. However, retrospective analysis may be subject to serious bias. Therefore adequately controlled prospective trials are required. Multicenter trials of spermatic vein ligation for varicoceles, AIH for oligospermia and asthenospermia, and prednisolone for sperm autoimmunity have been initiated, and a trial of erythromycin for asthenospermia is nearing completion in Melbourne.

In the future, clinical research may indicate that certain treatments do improve fertility. Alternatively, logical approaches to therapy may arise from basic research on the pathophysiology of disorders of spermatogenesis or sperm maturation. In the meantime, we believe drug and surgical treatments should not be used indiscriminately in men with oligospermia and asthenospermia.

CRYPTORCHIDISM

JULIAN FRICK, M.D.

The term cryptorchidism should be used to describe only the abdominal variety of this anomaly, but it is often used when referring to all varieties of imperfectly descended testes. The testes fail to reach their normal destination in the base of the scrotum at birth in 1 to 3 percent of all males, and of these cases about 10 percent are bilateral. Right- and left-sided involvement are about equal. In one-third of premature newborn males the testes are not descended; by the end of one year only 1 percent remain in the abdomen and half of these will descend at puberty if given the time. If this does not occur the likelihood of subsequent descent is slim, and there is a danger that the normal function of the tubular compartment will be permanently impaired.

It is generally recognized that in cases of maldescent of testis the incidence of traumatic lesions, testicular torsion, and malignant tumors is greater as compared with cases of scrotal testis. Malignancy developing in undescended testes after orchidopexy has been observed. Since orchidopexy does not protect against subsequent malignancy, and since the gonads become irreversibly infertile when the operation is performed after puberty, the argument in favor of prolonged observation cannot

be sustained. In addition, many physicians believe scrotal testes contribute to the appearance of the external genitalia, which is important for normal sexual behavior.

CONSIDERATIONS REGARDING THE BASIS FOR TREATMENT

Cryptorchidism may be caused by one of several mechanisms, including (1) delayed onset of androgen secretion by the testis, (2) inadequate production of androgen by the testis, and (3) target organ insensitivity to the action of androgen. These etiologic factors have been identified in a few well-documented genetic disorders. These include hypogonadotropic hypogonadism or Kallman's syndrome, which results from deficient gonadotropin production due to the lack of luteinizing hormone releasing hormone; inadequate production of androgen due to a defect in any one of five enzymes required for the conversion of cholesterol to testosterone; and androgen insensitivity (testicular feminization, Reifenstein's syndrome), which is secondary to an androgen receptor defect.

It is recognized that, in addition to endocrine factors, the following anatomic factors, either singly or in combination, may predispose to cryptorchidism: (1) an unusually long mesorchium; (2) mesorchioperitoneal adhesions preventing testis descent; (3) an abnormal persistence of the plica vascularis, which may anchor the testis too high; (4) short spermatic vessels or vas deferens; (5) a small inguinal canal; (6) testicular fusion; (7) an absent, unusually long, or inactive gubernaculum; (8) cremasteric hyperactivity interfering with descent; (9) maldevelopment of the inguinal canal with relative or absolute atresia; or (10) scrotal maldevelopment with absence of a testicular cavity.

There is considerable doubt about the effect of maldescent on the testis. There is no conclusive information as to whether the morphologic changes that are observed in the undescended testis are due to cryptorchidism per se or to the same factors that led to maldescent. This matter is of great importance, because the interpretation of the available evidence will guide the clinician in the choice and timing of treatment.

It is evident from several studies that the number of germ cells and the fertility potential of a testis are reduced if it remains in an undescended position after the age of 2 years; however, it must be emphasized that the etiologic factor in the cellular degeneration is not clear. It is possible that the factors that led to these changes may be primary and therefore the cause of the nondescent, or it may be that both are due to some other deficiency. It is known that even before the age of 2 the number of germ cells in the undescended testis is reduced. In unilateral cryptorchidism there is also reduction in germinal elements in the contralateral fully descended testis. In addition, there is no evidence that orchidopexy prevents germ cell deterioration even if performed at the age of 2.

One factor that has probably confused the complex problem of undescended testis is the possibility that there might be a difference in pathology between an upper scrotal retention and the truly cryptorchid testis (Fig. 1). In almost 80 percent of testes retained in the upper scrotal region unassociated with a hernia, the macroscopic appearance suggests that it is a healthier organ than the inguinal or abdominal testis. Also, a testis that is diverted from its course during normal descent should be intrinsically normal, whereas the truly cryptorchid testis might show some evidence of a developmental failure.

GUIDELINES FOR TREATMENT

It is commonly agreed that early treatment should be undertaken, but the question is still open as to when and what treatment should be performed. The choice of therapy often depends upon a physician's background: Pediatricians prefer an endocrine approach, while urologists and pediatric surgeons prefer orchidopexy. In our department the therapeutic objectives are: (1) to encourage maximum fertility, (2) to prevent damage to the organ from trauma caused by its abnormal position, (3) to achieve a satisfactory cosmetic result (which in itself will contribute greatly to the psychologic outlook), and (4) to forestall malignant changes. Unless early hormonal and surgical therapy succeeds in bringing the testicle permanently into its normal scrotal position, aspermatogenesis becomes a virtual certainty.

We emphasize early treatment; this advice is based on an extensive histologic study of cryptorchid testes. We strongly advocate treatment within the first two years, especially in bilateral cryptorchidism. If this is not possible, therapy should be undertaken by the fourth or fifth year to obtain maximum benefits. When there is a demonstrable hernia, the condition is considered surgical from the outset. When no demonstrable hernia is present a trial of hormonal therapy should be undertaken;

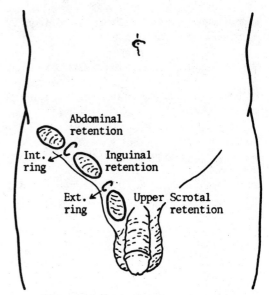

Figure 1 Sites of congenital ectopic testes.

in our experience this will promote normal, permanent descent in about 30 to 40 percent of the cases.

When treatment is delayed until puberty, as is still advocated by some physicians, there is an increased risk of one or a combination of the following: (1) torsion of the spermatic cord, (2) trauma to testis in the inguinal canal, (3) strangulation of an associated hernia, (4) infertility, and (5) neoplastic transformation. In the rare cases of spontaneous testicular descent following puberty, the organ will appear immature or congenitally defective and in all likelihood will be sterile. Almost 90 percent of men with bilateral cryptorchidism after puberty are infertile. The ability to use endocrine therapy (gonadotropins, LHRH or its analogues) makes it possible to determine prior to puberty if the testicle will descend spontaneously.

Conservative, or Nonsurgical, Treatment

Ever since it was discovered that the descent of the testis in the preadolescent monkey could be induced prematurely by injecting gonadotropic hormones, attempts have been made to treat humans using this approach. When hernia is absent and the testicle, or both testes, is imperfectly descended or migratory, the patient may be given a trial of hormonal therapy as (1) definitive treatment, (2) a diagnostic test, or (3) a preparatory step for surgery. It is fairly clear that neither the real cryptorchid testis nor the testis associated with a hernia is likely to be influenced by hormonal therapy. Following treatment with hCG or LHRH or one of its agonists, the interstitial compartment of the testis is stimulated and testosterone secretion increases. Excessive or prolonged treatment may produce pubertas praecox and may stimulate closure of epiphyseal centers, resulting in short stature in adult life. Our conservative therapeutic approach is designed to avoid these side effects, and it includes three possibilities: gonadotropin preparations, native LHRH, and synthetic analogues of LHRH. Our experience with these compounds is summarized below.

hCG treatment. Our treatment schedule with hCG is 1500 units twice a week for 6 weeks. We are successful in inducing descent of testes in about 40 percent of boys treated. In almost all the treated cases there is an increase in penis size and, in about 40 percent there is an increased frequency of erection during the treatment period. These signs disappear, when the treatment is stopped.

Plasma testosterone measurements reveal that in most of the cases HCG administration produces a marked elevation of serum testosterone. Androgen levels after HCG administration may be slightly lower in the bilateral group. At present there is no way to determine whether the lower response in boys with bilateral cryptorchidism is responsible for the failure of descent or is the result of the ectopic location of the testicles.

LHRH Treatment. LHRH controls the release of LH and SH and can be used for conservative treatment of cryptorchidism. A daily dose between 20 μg and 40 μg intramuscularly should be sufficient; larger daily amounts may lead to a down regulation of LH, as demonstrated in some studies. One of the disadvantages of this treatment might be the necessity for the daily intramuscular administration. (It should be noted that LHRH must be used under an IND in the United States.)

LHRH Analogues. We have used the synthetic peptide [D-leu 6, des-gly-10 ethylamide] LHRH dissolved in an aqueous solution (25 μg in 0.2 ml) delivered through the nasal route in 18 boys, age 3 to 12. The boys were divided into two groups, and the results are summarized in Table 1. The boys in group I received 50 μg of the analogue every 48 hours; the dosage used in patients in group II was 50 μg every 24 hours. In the group of 8 patients treated nasally with 50 μg every 48 hours for 36 days, testes descended in 3 cases. When treatment was effective in boys with bilateral cryptorchidism both testes descended. In the second group (50 μg administered every 24 hours) the therapy was successful in 2 of the 5 boys with unilateral, and in 2 of the 5 boys with bilateral cryptorchidism (Table 1).

TABLE 1   Testicular Descent after Therapy with Synthetic LHRH Analogue

| Groups* | No. of subjects | Age in years | Undescended testes | | |
| | | | Unilateral | | |
			Right	Left	Bilateral
I	8	3–11	1	1	6 (3)†
II	10	3–12	3 (1)†	2 (1)†	5 (2)†

*Group I: 50 μg every 48 hours; group II: 50 μg every 24 hours

†In parenthesis is the number of descents after therapy with synthetic LHRH analogue.

In 44 percent of the boys unilateral or bilateral descent was obtained immediately after the end of therapy. We have seen no correlation between plasma hormone levels of the patients who had a descent and those who did not respond to therapy. No undesirable clinical side effects were seen following intranasal administration of synthetic LHRH analogue for 36 days. The treated boys did not mention any effects that could be related to the hormone application. The testicle, examined very carefully throughout the observation period, did not change in size or consistency.

Based on our experiences with different potent LHRH analogues, we recommend the following therapeutic regimen for the treatment of cryptorchidism in those patients who may respond to this type of therapy: 50 μg of a synthetic hormone administered either as nasal drops or spray, 3 times per week for 4 to 6 weeks to induce testis descent. (It should be noted that LHRH agonists must be used under an IND in the United States.)

Surgical Therapy

Operative intervention is a necessity in cases complicated by hernia or when endocrine therapy fails to achieve the desired result. The mainstay of treatment for the imperfectly descended testis is an operation designed to remove the structures preventing descent and to place the testis securely in the scrotum to preserve the integrity of the vas deferens and the testicular blood supply. It should be emphasized that even a skilled and experienced surgeon faces a greater risk of operative damage to the structures in the spermatic cord and vas deferens in a child below the age of 2 years. It is probable that more testes are lost through clumsy surgery than by delaying the operation. Furthermore, the evidence that fertility is improved by surgery in early childhood is by no means conclusive, and those who elect to operate on boys under the age of 2 must carry the extra burden of responsibility of preserving the delicate structures they encounter.

Although there are a number of operative methods we prefer the following, which we have used in more than 90 percent of our cases: An inguinal incision is made through the membranous layer of the superficial fascia. The external oblique aponeurosis is incised parallel to its fibers through the external inguinal ring so as to open the inguinal canal. The testis and spermatic cord are mobilized and lifted out of the inguinal canal by dividing the cremasteric muscle fibers and fascia and the cremasteric vein. The hernia sac, if one is present, is then divided, excised, and closed after it is carefully separated from the vas deferens and testicular vessels. This will lengthen the cord, but additional length must be obtained by dividing the fibers that run into the base of the cord from the retroperitoneal tissue. After this extensive mobilization, the testis, including the cord, is brought down to the lowest part of the scrotum after a scrotal tunnel is formed using the index or little finger (depending on the age of the child), and fixed for five days on the inner side of the thigh with a pull-out suture through the scrotal skin. The inguinal incision is then closed in layers. Postoperative complications, seen in about 10 percent of the boys, include temporary swelling of the scrotum, hematoma formation, and wound infection. The operative results are good in 85 percent of our cases; in the remaining cases we encounter either a recurrence or a less than ideal displacement of the testis into the scrotum.

When a testis is congenitally atrophic or malformed, it should be removed. Orchiectomy is preferable to leaving the testis in the groin or abdomen. An additional compelling reason for removal is the danger of neoplastic change. Some patients in whom orchiectomy has been performed may have psychogenic problems. The cosmetic appearance of the scrotum may then be improved with Silastic prostheses.

Treatment of abnormally mobile testicles consists of a simple scrotal orchiopexy, which securely anchors the gland to the lowest part of the scrotum. This alone will prevent torsion of the spermatic cord.

In some rare cases with intra-abdominal testes it may be necessary to transplant the testicle to the scrotum using microvascular techniques. The use of the operating microscope has made possible the anastomosis of blood vessels as small as $\frac{1}{3}$ mm in diameter. Between 1 and 5 percent of cryptorchid testes are intra-abdominal and cannot be properly brought down into the scrotum by conventional methods because of the risk of testicular ischemia. A small percentage of these may be suitable for a microanastomosis of the spermatic vessels to the inferior epigastric vessels in the groin.

TESTICULAR TUMORS

ROBERT B. GOLBEY, M.D.

Germ cell tumors of the testes constitute only a small fraction of the malignant tumors in males, but the importance of effective treatment is magnified by the fact that most of the patients are young men with a potentially long and productive survival if cured.

The optimal management of patients with testicular germ cell tumors is truly multi-modal. Regardless of the stage of the disease at presentation, the goal of initial treatment is cure. Vital decisions must be made early, involving surgery, pathology, diagnostic radiology, radiation therapy, and chemotherapy. Reliable biochemical laboratory data, particularly relating to the serum tumor markers, are essential to the decision-making process. Because of the relative rarity of the disease and because of the rapid evolution of new and better techniques, adequate experience and skill in dealing with this complex problem may not be available in every community. If this is the case, consideration should be given to the early referral of the patient to a cancer treatment center for consultation and/or continued care.

In the past decade the cure rate in patients with advanced testicular germ cell tumors (TGCT) treated with steadily improving chemotherapeutic regimens has risen from 10 percent to more than 60 percent. When surgery is used in selected high-risk situations, as an adjuvant to the drug treatment, cure rates in excess of 80 percent can be achieved in patients with advanced disease. These results in stage III patients are leading to significant changes in the accepted management of stage I and II disease.

STAGING

The normal lymphatic drainage of the testicle is directly to the para-aortic nodes in the retroperitoneal space. It then proceeds upward to the thoracic duct, which may drain into a Virchow node in the neck before entering the systemic circulation. Drainage through the mediastinal nodes does occur, but is less common.

This pathway of lymphatic dissemination is the accepted basis for the staging of the disease. In the past a simple staging system sufficed:

Stage I: Disease confined to the testicle
Stage II: Disease in the retroperitoneal nodes
Stage III: Disease beyond the retroperitoneal nodes

About one-third of the patients will be in each of these stages when first seen. Stage I is potentially curable by orchiectomy alone; however, only pathologic examination can identify the micrometastases that are sometimes present in the regional nodes. For this reason, clinical stage I patients have been routinely treated identically with stage II patients with a radical retroperitoneal lymph node dissection or radiation therapy to this area, depending on the histology of the tumor. About 85 percent of the stage I patients and approximately 50 percent of the stage II patients are in fact cured by these "local" measures. The failures are usually because of unrecognized hematogenously disseminated systemic metastases, and like the recognized stage III disease, can only be treated effectively with systemic chemotherapy.

Occasionally an elevated serum tumor marker remains elevated after the removal of all recognized disease. This is an indication for an intensified search for the unrecognized foci of tumor or for treatment at stage III with chemotherapy.

In recent years, the TNM staging system has provided a notational system allowing a more meaningful grouping within the same three basic stages. The most important change is in the following characterization of the retroperitoneal nodes:

N_0—Nodes not involved.
N_1—Micrometastases present.
N_2—Gross nodal involvement of less than 5 nodes. No nodes larger than 2 cm.
N_3—More than 5 nodes. Largest is more than 2 cm.
N_4—Extranodal extension.

N_0 is necessary for stage I. N_1 and N_2 are "good-risk" stage II patients, and N_3 is "poor-risk" stage II, whereas N_4 should be considered Stage III and treated as such.

The problem of staging is further complicated by the fact that one must deal at various times with clinical staging, surgical staging, and pathologic staging with their varying degrees of validity. The evidence provided by serum tumor markers must be superimposed upon the anatomic stage.

HISTOLOGY

In addition to differences in staging, patients with testicular germ cell tumors also present with a variety of cell types in their tumors, which have a definite influence on prognosis and on the treatment plan.

Depending on the state of differentiation of the multi-potential germ cell at the time it becomes neoplastic, a variety of histologic types of tumor can result, and since differentiation can continue even after the cell becomes neoplastic, variations in cell type can be seen during the course of the illness. The possible cell types are: seminoma, embryonal carcinoma, yolk sac tumor, choriocarcinoma, and teratoma. A given tumor may be pure or it can contain a mixture of any or all of the aforementioned elements. The development of effective broad-spectrum chemotherapy has enabled us to use similar treatments for several of the types. Therefore, in this paper we will discuss the management of (1) pure seminoma, and (2) nonseminomatous germ cell tumor (NSGCT). Pure choriocarcinoma and adult teratoma will be mentioned as separate problems. Group 2 (NSGCT) encompasses embryonal carcinoma, yolk sac tumor, and all mixed tumors, including the one frequently referred to as teratocarcinoma.

MARKERS

A third important factor in the management of these patients is the status of the serum tumor markers. The presence and the level of elevation of the β subunit of chorionic gonadotrophin (hCGβ) and of alpha feto protein (AFP) has diagnostic, prognostic, and therapeutic implications. These proteins are produced by, and are specific for, certain cell types, and their serial measurement can be a useful indicator of the efficacy of treatment or, in the follow-up period, of the regrowth of disease. If both are present, they do not invariably move in parallel, since some treatments can eliminate one cell type while another cell type continues to grow.

Lactic dehydrogenase (LDH) is a third useful marker. It is not specific for tumor and consequently has no diagnostic value, but in this young and usually healthy population of patients, in whom other causes of LDH elevation are uncommon, it is a useful and reliable indicator of tumor bulk and of progression or regression. In pure seminoma, where hCGβ elevations are rare and AFP elevations are not seen, serial determinations of LDH can be particularly helpful. In patients who have been rendered free of evidence of disease, including the return of all tumor markers to normal, the serial determinations of tumor markers during the follow-up period is mandatory. A rising LDH titer can precede the clinical detection of recurrent disease by several months, and the level is a rough indicator of the tumor burden regardless of cell type. Rising hCGβ and/or AFP titers have the same significance and also give an indication of the cell type that is regrowing.

MANAGEMENT

The traditional management of TGCT up to the early 1970s was capable of curing about 50 per cent of the patients of all stages. Orchiectomy plus retroperitoneal lymph node dissection, or plus radiation therapy to the primary lymphatic drainage area, cured 85 per cent of stage I and 50 per cent of stage II cases. Chemotherapy was used in patients who could not be cured by local measures (stage III) or who were not cured (stage I and stage II failures). Of this 50 per cent with advanced disease, about 10 per cent were cured with the relatively simple chemotherapy of the era.

Since the early 1970s chemotherapy for this disease has improved markedly and rapidly. A number of different chemotherapeutic regimens have been developed and advocated. The best of them are now capable of producing almost exactly comparable therapeutic results. There are differences in morbidity, in dosage schedules, and in number of drugs used, but the similarities are more conspicuous and more important. The most effective programs use diamminedichloro cis-platinum in high dosage, vincaleukoblastine, and bleomycin with or without other drugs.

The availablity of these highly active drug regimens for advanced disease and the salvage they afford most, if not all, patients who suffer recurrence after local therapy have encouraged a search for the minimal therapy, with minimal morbidity and risk of mortality, necessary for cure.

The usual presentation of these tumors is pain and/or swelling of one testicle in a young adult. Frequently an initial diagnosis of epididymitis is made and antibiotic therapy begun. If the response is not prompt and complete, urologic consultation should be obtained. The diagnosis is established and the initial therapeutic step completed by orchiectomy. The orchiectomy should be radical and should include an inguinal incision, with high ligation of the cord. When tumor is suspected, or its presence is merely possible, a scrotal incision is absolutely contraindicated as is a transscrotal needle biopsy. These procedures should not be performed because of the danger of seeding the wound, and also because any involvement of the scrotum opens another lymphatic pathway for the spread of tumor to the groin and inguinal nodes, and requires a more extended surgical procedure. Serum tumor markers should be drawn promptly, even if a trial of antibiotic therapy is to be undertaken. If the specific markers (AFP, hCGβ) are positive, a diagnosis has been made. However, if they are negative, the diagnosis has not been ruled out. Certainly at some point before the orchiectomy all three markers should be obtained. Occasionally a patient, with or without a testicular complaint, complains of painful breasts and/or gynecomastia. This too requires that serum markers be drawn, and the testes be carefully evaluated. (Usually the hCGβ is elevated and the tumor contains major components of choriocarcinoma.) If the physical examination does not reveal a testicular tumor, sonography of the testes is sometimes helpful in localizing the primary tumor.

After the tumor has been removed by radical orchiectomy, pathologic examination of multiple representative sections is necessary to identify all the cell types present. The serum tumor markers should be repeated, and the results, if positive, should be correlated with the known histology of the tumor and with the other staging procedures being done at the same time. A high titer of hCGβ suggests that choriocarcinoma is present. If the titer is low, chorio elements may not be microscopically detectable in seminoma or embryonal carcinoma, although they usually can be identified if appropriate immunoperoxidase staining techniques are used.

Alpha feto protein is produced by the cells of the yolk sac tumor, but since this tumor is sometimes difficult to differentiate from embryonal carcinoma it may be present when only embryonal carcinoma is identified under the microscope.

The biologic half-life of hCGβ is one hour. The half-life of AFP is about 2 weeks. These differences must be considered when one interprets the significance of any post-therapy decline in the measured titer. If, after orchiectomy, the work-up for metastatic disease is negative and the marker titer falls along the normal curve, it suggests, but does not prove, that all disease has been removed. If, however, the fall in titer lags behind the normal decay curve, one can be sure that all disease was not removed or destroyed. While the markers are being evaluated, a staging work-up should also be done. This should include PA and lateral chest roentgenograms, retroperitoneal lymphangiogram (LAG), abdominal computerized transaxial tomography (CAT), blood count, and a routine chemical screening profile to evaluate liver and renal function.

The status of the lungs is crucial for the detection of hemotogenous metastases. Involvement of the brain and liver is not seen, unless there has been prior or concurrent involvement of the lungs. Therefore, if the routine roentgenograms are negative, one should obtain a chest CAT scan or lung tomograms. If any of the chest examinations are positive, brain, liver, and bone scans are necessary. If distant metastases are not found, the status of the retroperitoneal nodes becomes the determining factor for choice of therapy. Lymphangiogram is the single most useful test. It can detect enlarged nodes, but can also show structural alteration in normal-size nodes. The CAT scan supplements this by detecting enlarged nodes, but also by revealing extranodal masses, hepatic involvement, hydronephrosis, and other anatomic details. These examinations provide vastly more accurate clinical staging than was possible when only the IVP was available. With the information these tests provide, clinical staging is possible, and the treatment plan should be defined even though it may have to be refined as more precise pathologic staging becomes possible.

Stage III

Stage III includes all patients in whom disease was detected beyond the resectable retroperitoneal nodes. It also includes all patients with pure choriocarcinoma regardless of the extent of the disease and those with N_4 nodal involvement as defined earlier.

Pure choriocarcinomas are included in this group because they usually have hematogenous metastases, even before nodal involvement is apparent, and sometimes even before the primary tumor in the testicle is detectable. N_4 nodes, by definition, are not curable surgically, and the record of radiation therapy is not good in the treatment of these bulky tumors. They are usually teratocarcinoma (embryonal carcinoma and teratoma). This group of patients has the worst prognosis of all identifiable subgroups with germ cell tumors. Their best hope is to shrink the tumor with intensive chemotherapy and to then resect the remaining tumor.

The initial treatment of stage III patients is with chemotherapy. If brain metastases are present, they should be treated adjuvantly with surgery if they are solitary and accessible (usually embryonal carcinoma) or with radiation therapy if they are multiple (usually choriocarcinoma) or inaccessible for surgery. As with the N_4 group, all sites of bulky metastases (mass greater than 10 cm in diameter) should be explored after three or more courses of chemotherapy and any residual disease resected, whether or not there was an apparent complete response to chemotherapy.

Stage II

Stage II includes all patients with disease detected only in the retroperitoneal nodes, which are potentially resectable. They are divided into good-risk and poor-risk groups, depending on the size and number of involved nodes, as defined earlier.

The patient with a poor-risk stage II pure seminoma should be treated with the same chemotherapy as is recommended for stage III patients. Subsequent adjuvant radiation therapy may or may not be indicated. This is still a moot point and is under investigation. Current information should be sought when the problem arises.

Stage III "good-risk" patients should be treated with radiation therapy delivered to an "inverted Y" port including the iliac and para-aortic nodes. A dose of approximately 3,000 rads should be adequate. For all patients with seminoma, LDH titer should be followed serially. If it does not return to normal and remain normal after the completion of treatment, more study is required.

Stage II "poor-risk" nonseminomatous germ cell tumor patients should have a radical retroperitoneal lymph node dissection. If the resection is complete and the markers return to normal, the patient should have a course of adjuvant chemotherapy. If the resection is not complete, or if any of the markers remain abnormal, they should be treated with a full course of chemotherapy as recommended for stage III.

Stage III "good-risk" NSGCT patients should be treated in the same way as the "bad-risk" patients, except that if the resection is complete and the markers normalize, the adjuvant chemotherapy should be omitted. Careful follow-up is all that is indicated. A small percentage of these patients subsequently manifest hematogenous metastases and require stage III type chemotherapy. If detected early by a rising marker titer or minimal pulmonary metastases, the vast majority can be cured. Adjuvant chemotherapy in all cases could probably prevent these recurrences, but it seems preferable, at present, to intensively treat those few people who demonstrate the need for it than to less intensively treat a lot of people, most of whom do not need it.

Stage I

Stage I patients are those who have no evidence of tumor after orchiectomy, including normal serum tumor markers. In the past, and currently, the conventional management of these patients is identical with that of the "good-risk" stage II patients, in both the seminoma and nonseminoma groups. For the seminoma patients, there is little incentive to change this procedure, since the morbidity of the administered radiation is minimal. In the nonseminoma group, however, the functional sterility that is a usual result of radical retroperitoneal lymph node dissection makes it desirable to avoid this surgical procedure if the patient's ultimate change of survival is not compromised.

Randomized studies looking at retroperitoneal lymph node dissection (RPLND) versus close observation are under way, but they may never be satisfactorily completed because of an understandable reluctance of patients to participate. On the basis of past experience and the scanty available data, it is known that even after a satisfactory RPLND, 15 percent of the patients have hematogenous metastases requiring chemotherapy. If no RPLND is done, a few more patients who were understaged by clinical methods develop nodal metastases, which also requires chemotherapy and possibly a node dissection. If the staging was extremely carefully and thoroughly done and was

unequivocally negative, the risks of not doing the node dissection seem justified if the patient can be relied on to be conscientiously followed up with x-ray studies, markers, and physical examination for at least 3 years (year 1, monthly; year 2, every other month; year 3, every third month). The prompt initiation of chemotherapy should be effective in most cases of recurrence.

This stage I area requires more information. Before deciding on a course of action, pros and cons must be carefully discussed with the patient. It is his decision to make as to which risks and which morbidity he finds more acceptable. There is no present role for adjuvant chemotherapy in stage I disease.

Chemotherapy

Chemotherapy has been referred to nonspecifically throughout this chapter. This is because at present several different drug programs exist that can produce similar results and because tomorrow there may well be a better modification available.

Currently our preferred drug treatment is code named VAB-6:

VAB-6

Day 1	Cyclophosphamide	600 mg/m² IV
	Vinblastine	4 mg/M² IV
	Actinomycin D	1 mg/M² IV
	Bleomycin	30 mg/M² IV
Day 1–3	Bleomycin	20 mg/M²/day × 3 days by 24-hr infusion
Day 4	Cis-Platinum	120 mg/M² IV c̄ hydration and mannitol diuresis

Days 1–4 repeated q 3–4 weeks × 3.
Bleomycin is omitted for the third course.

Originally this protocol included a maintenance phase that continued for one year. This has been eliminated without detriment. For adjuvant therapy, only the first two cycles are employed. For stage III therapy, there are three cycles, followed, if necessary, by adjuvant surgery, to remove any known residual disease or to resect the site of originally bulky disease (N_4). When there is remaining tissue resected at surgery, one-third of the cases show necrotic tissue only, one-third of the cases show that the malignant tumor has been converted into an adult teratoma, and the final one-third show residual viable malignant tumor. If all residual tumor is removed, the treatment is concluded for the first two groups. The third group receives two more courses of VAB-6, one with and one without bleomycin. If the tumor was not completely resected, the treatment is a failure and experimental secondary therapy is begun.

A sometimes difficult exception to this generalization arises when the remaining nonresectable tissue is adult (histologically benign) teratoma, and the tumor markers are all normal. The transition from malignant germ cell tumor to adult teratoma occurs rarely as a spontaneous event, but is now seen frequently in the wake of aggressive chemotherapy. The resulting tumor is not sensitive to radiation or to presently known drug combinations. The only effective treatment is surgical removal; however, if the surgical risks of resection are great, and the histology is well established, it may be preferable to leave the disease in place. Although the slowly growing tumor may produce morbidity (depending on its location), long-term survival is possible with nothing more than observation and symptomatic support. The decision to resect or not to resect requires the judgment of a highly experienced surgeon.

The chemotherapy just described is relatively safe, but does have the potential for significant morbidity. It should be given only by someone thoroughly familiar with the administration and potential toxicity of the individual drugs employed.

IMPOTENCE

MARC GOLDSTEIN, M.D.
and C. WAYNE BARDIN, M.D.

Impotence is a disorder that involves men primarily in the third to ninth decades of life. The etiologic factors are hormonal, vascular, pharmacologic, and psychiatric (Table 1). A careful search must be made to uncover the origin of this complaint so that proper therapy can be instituted. Impotence affects many men at some time in their lives. In many instances it is short-lived and clears spontaneously with improved health or sense of well-being.

TABLE 1 Causes of Impotence

Endocrine	*Vascular*
Pituitary disease (tumors, etc.)	Diabetes mellitus
	Arteriosclerosis
Hyper- and hypoadrenocorticism	Pelvic irradiation
	Ruptured pelvis
Hyper- and hypothyroidism	Peyronie's disease
Diabetes mellitus	
Renal failure	*Drugs*
Hepatic failure	Estrogen
Primary testicular (Klinefelter's, mumps orchitis, etc.)	Antiandrogens
	Narcotics
	Sympathetic inhibitors
	Antihistamines
Neurologic	Antihypertensives
Diabetes mellitus	Dilantin
Demyelinating diseases	Phenothiazines
Trauma to, or congenital anomalies of, the cord and spine	Amphetamines
	Tricyclic antidepressants
Pernicious anemia	*Inflammatory*
Tabes dorsalis	Prostatitis
Temporal lobe epilepsy	Urethritis, cystitis
Post-surgical (radical prostatectomy, cystectomy, abdominal-perineal resection, aortic aneurysmectomy, sphincterotomy, ruptured urethra, ruptured pelvis)	Seminal vesiculitis, orchitis
	Epididymitis
	Psychogenic
	Depression
	Extreme stress

ANDROGEN DEFICIENCY

When androgen deficiency occurs in the adult, it is usually a result of testicular failure. In contrast to ovarian function, spermatogenesis and testosterone production do not suddenly decline at a certain time of life unless some pathologic process intervenes. In contrast to spermatogenesis, there are relatively few diseases that selectively decrease testosterone production. When Leydig cell function is impaired and total serum testosterone levels decline, symptoms similar to those occurring in postmenopausal women appear which are related to androgen withdrawal. In addition to having hot flashes along with decreased libido and sexual potential, approximately one-half of these men experience increased irritability, inability to concentrate, and episodes of depression. The entity has been designated by some authors as the male climacteric. This condition is often associated with testicular or pituitary pathologic factors that have been present for some years. Leydig cell function may have been declining over a period of time and has finally become symptomatic. The conditions associated with the male climacteric include Klinefelter's syndrome, pituitary tumors, idiopathic Leydig cell failure, mumps orchitis, and testicular atrophy secondary to reduced blood flow.

The age of onset is variable and depends upon pathogenesis. In patients with Klinefelter's syndrome who had relatively good Leydig cell function early in life, androgen production may decline sometime after age 40. In patients with mumps orchitis, the signs of androgen deficiency may not occur until the seventh or eighth decade. Although testicular blood supply can be interrupted at any time following surgery in the inguinal canal, older men appear to be more vulnerable to this complication.

Establishing the correct diagnosis is less of a problem when the aforementioned pathologic processes are present and the clinician is alerted to the possibility of androgen failure by the presence of small atrophic testes. Ideally, the diagnosis is established by determining plasma testosterone concentrations. The presence of a value less than 100–150 ng/dl is usually diagnostic. However, it should be noted that the plasma testosterone concentrations at which symptoms will appear is highly variable from patient to patient. In some men the signs of androgen deficiency will develop with a testosterone concentration of 200 ng/dl, whereas in others, apparently normal sexual function is possible with 100 ng/dl.

Treatment of Patients with Androgens

The principles of androgen therapy have been outlined in Chapter 68. If patients have no evidence of prostatic hypertrophy and are under 60 years of age, testosterone enanthate or cyclopentyl propionate, 200 mg i.m. every 2 to 3 weeks, can be administered for maintenance. If there is evidence of prostatic disease, a more rapidly acting testosterone preparation is recommended. This will permit rapid withdrawal should difficulty with urination develop. In this regard, testosterone propionate 50 mg i.m. 3 times a week, may be satisfactory, or fluoxymesterone, 5 mg orally daily, may be recommended.

HYPERPROLACTINEMIA

Men with pituitary tumors secreting prolactin may present the physician with symptoms of visual impairment, headaches, or other complaints associated with an intracranial mass. A number of these individuals, however, present because of loss of libido and potentia. In the past, these symptoms were attributed to compression atrophy of normal pituitary with attendant hypogonadotropism. More recently, it was realized that many of these men do not respond to androgen replacement as might be expected in a patient with typical androgen deficiency. These observations, coupled with studies in animals, have suggested that prolactin may have a direct behavioral effect on the brain. In addition, increased prolactin may decrease LHRH secretion, which in turn may result in hypogonadotropism. As a consequence, therapy must be directed at lowering serum prolactin levels either by surgery or by use of bromocriptine (see Chapters 9 and 10 for details). Once serum prolactin levels have been brought into the normal range, the addition of androgen replacement therapy may be warranted if serum testosterone levels are not above 250 ng/dl. Hyperprolactinemia is often found in impotent men on chronic dialysis. Treatment with bromocriptine has restored potency in approximately 50 percent of these individuals.

PSYCHOGENIC IMPOTENCE

Exclusion of organic causes of impotence should precede exploration of psychogenic origins. Just a few years ago it was commonly stated that 90 to 95 percent of impotence is psychogenic in origin. Improved methods of diagnosis currently result in the finding of organic etiologic agents in at least 50 percent of impotent men. Use of nocturnal penile tumescence monitoring, penile Doppler flowmetry, and careful neurologic and psychiatric evaluation help distinguish between organic and psychogenic causes of impotence. Functional and organic etiologic factors are frequently present in the same patient. Close collaboration between the urologist and psychiatrist is necessary to manage such patients successfully.

Difficulty may arise in attempting to differentiate patients with pathologic Leydig cell failure from patients with psychogenic impotence such as can occur in depression. In major depressive disorders, patients have a dysphoric mode or loss of interest and one or several of the following: anorexia, sleep disturbance, loss of energy, loss of libido, guilt, psychomotor agitation and suicidal ideation. A variety of data suggest that major depressive disorders represent a disturbance that in some way is related to a deficiency of brain neuroadrenergic or serotoninergic activity. This suggestion is supported by the contention that these patients often respond rapidly to antidepressant medication or electroshock therapy and not to conventional psychotherapy. Situational depression, even though it is felt to have a different origin, nonetheless has many of the same symptoms, including impotence. The endocrinologist should be alert to the individual who presents with this symptom as the first manifestation of depression arising out of a threatening situation, such as a myocardial infarction, coronary bypass surgery, or loss of a job. Potency usually improves following treatment with antidepressants or psychotherapy.

When psychogenic impotence is of short duration (less than three months), a high spontaneous cure rate can be expected. Reassurance, marital counseling, or both is often all that is needed. In impotence of short or intermediate duration (less than one year), intensive sex behavior therapy results in 75 to 80 percent success rates. Impotence of long duration in men over the age of 50 results in a poor cure rate with sex therapy, and these patients may be candidates for a penile prosthesis.

DRUGS

A wide variety of drugs have been implicated as a cause of impotence. The most commonly prescribed offenders are antihypertensives (especially sympathetic inhibitors), tricyclic antidepressants, major and minor tranquilizers, narcotics, and estrogens. If medication induced impotence is suspected, withdrawal of the drug for at least one month constitutes an adequate test. Substitution of other drugs with a different mechanism of action frequently results in return of potency. When drugs cannot be withdrawn or substituted and psychogenic factors have been excluded, implantation of a penile prosthesis may be considered.

Drug abuse is a very common cause of impotence among young men. Heavy use of alcohol or marijuana derivatives inhibits cerebral function and, secondarily, sexual performance. Chronic alcoholism can lead to impotence secondary either to peripheral neuropathy or to elevated blood estrogen levels secondary to hepatic decomposition. The fact that heavy marijuana use is associated with gynecomastia and infertility suggests that this agent also alters endocrine function.

NEUROGENIC IMPOTENCE

When correctable endocrine and metabolic conditions have been excluded as a cause of impotence, a careful search must be made for other etiologic factors. A neurologic examination, including bulbocavernus reflex, cremaster reflex, tactile perineal sensation, cystometry, and electromyography, will often suggest a correct diagnosis. If the neurologic deficit results from a medical condition, such as pernicious anemia or tabes dorsalis, appropriate therapy may restore potency. The vast majority of patients with impotence secondary to neurologic deficits, however, have irreversible lesions resulting from disease or trauma to the spinal cord, peripheral neuropathy (seen most frequently in diabetics), or previous pelvic surgery. In these cases, implantation of a prosthetic device is the most appropriate solution.

IMPOTENCE OF VASCULAR ORIGIN

Impotence due to vascular insufficiency may be suspected on the basis of history and physical examination. Work-up would include careful palpation of peripheral pulses, Doppler recording of penile pulses, and simultaneous recording of penile and brachial artery pressures. Other diagnostic modalities may be employed, including penile thermography and arteriography with selective injection of the internal pudendal arteries. Specific vascular lesions, such as those seen with Leriche's syndrome, are often surgically correctable. Impotence resulting from diffuse small vessel disease (frequently seen in diabetics) is best managed with a prosthetic device. Fibrosis of the tunica albuginea due to Peyronie's disease or penile trauma often results in severe penile curvatures precluding vaginal penetration. These curves are successfully corrected by a plastic operation on the corpora. When impotence results from fibrosis of the cavernous bodies, such as occurs with advanced Peyronie's disease, recurrent priapism, or cavernositis, a prosthetic implant is the only solution.

INFLAMMATORY CAUSES OF IMPOTENCE

Inflammatory processes involving the primary or secondary sex organs often cause temporary impotence. This usually presents as pain in the affected organ during intercourse or ejaculation. Appropriate antibiotic therapy, as discussed in Chapter 71, usually results in complete resolution and return of potency. Severe bilateral orchitis may result in androgen deficiency, in which case androgen replacement therapy, as described previously, is indicated. Severe cavernositis can result in fibrosis of the corporal bodies. In these cases a prosthetic device must be implanted.

SURGICAL THERAPY OF IMPOTENCE

The Chinese implanted pieces of ivory into the penis over 3000 years ago to treat impotence. More recently, a variety of prosthetic devices have been successfully implanted in thousands of impotent men. When treatable medical causes of impotence have been excluded or when the impotence is psychogenic but refractory to long-term sex behavior therapy, implantation of a prosthetic device is indicated. Surgical treatment of impotence is contraindicated in patients with poor libido, emotional instability, poor general health (such as severe angina, uncontrolled diabetes), or in immunosuppressed patients at high risk for infection. In patients with combined causes of impotence, maximal medical or sex therapy or both should be tried before resorting to a prosthesis.

Rigid or Semi-rigid Devices

Silicone prostheses are implanted in the corpora cavernosa and result in a permanent erection. New devices of this type are either hinged or malleable and permit easier concealment. The advantages of this prosthesis include low cost, relative ease of implantation, and the "always ready" feature. Disadvantages include difficulty in concealment, possibility of erosion through the penis, and ability of the partner to detect the presence of a prosthesis.

Inflatable Prosthesis

This type of device consists of two hollow silicone tubes connected to a fluid reservoir and an inflate-deflate pump. A silicone tube is placed in each corpora, the reservoir is placed behind the rectus muscles, and the pump is placed in the scrotum where it is activated and deactivated by the patient. The advantages of the inflatable prosthesis include simulation of natural erections and flaccidity, easy concealment, and the fact that the partner cannot detect the prosthesis, and erosion is uncommon. Disadvantages of this prosthesis are high cost, increased likelihood of mechanical failures, and greater difficulty and length of the surgical procedure.

Among the complications possible with both implants are infection (requiring removal of the prosthesis), erosion (also requiring removal), hemorrhage (unlikely), and gangrene of the penis (rare). Both types of prosthesis have proved to be highly satisfactory in managing impotence. Patient-partner acceptance of a prosthesis has been excellent in properly selected surgical candidates. Satisfaction rates between 80 and 95 percent are regularly reported. Mechanical failure necessitating reoperation occurs about 30 percent of the time with inflatable devices. Continuing improvements in design and techniques of implantation are resulting in a steady decline in the incidence of mechanical failures. To date, prosthetic penile implants provide a highly acceptable and effective method of treating organic impotence.

Vascular Surgery

In the past ten years attempts have been made to correct penile vascular insufficiency by surgical revascularization. Early approaches involved anastomosis of an inferior epigastric artery directly to the corpora cavernosa. Although initial success was reported, unphysiologic hemodynamics led to thrombosis of this anastomosis in almost all cases. Other patients developed priapism, necessitating ligation of the inferior epigastric artery. A more physiologic, but difficult, approach involving microsurgical anastomosis of an inferior epigastric artery to a superficial or deep penile artery looks promising and is currently being evaluated in the United States and Europe. In patients with a specific vascular lesion demonstrable by arteriography, such as transection of a pudendal artery after pelvic fracture or Leriche's syndrome, vascular surgery bypassing the occluded vessels has frequently been successful.

VASECTOMY AND VASECTOMY REVERSAL

MARC GOLDSTEIN, M.D.

Vasectomy was advocated and used in the late nineteenth and early twentieth centuries as a treatment for benign prostatic hyperplasia, rejuvenation, and eugenic sterilization. These uses have long since been discredited. In the preantibiotic era, however, vasectomy was legitimately performed prior to invasive urologic procedures to reduce the likelihood of postoperative epididymitis and orchitis. The now routine use of perioperative antimicrobial therapy effectively prevents these complications and has resulted in the virtual abandonment of therapeutic vasectomy.

Interest in vasectomy is now largely confined to its use for permanent contraception. Each year approximately half a million American men undergo vasectomy as their form of birth control, and at least 12 million have already made that choice. The surgical occlusion of the excurrent ducts of an organ with important exocrine and endocrine functions, on such a vast scale, has naturally stimulated intense interest in its consequences. Although a significant body of evidence has accumulated regarding the long-term effects of vasectomy in animals, marked species differences make much of this evidence difficult to interpret. In addition, there are few case-controlled studies in man, and truly long-term studies (over ten years) are still in progress.

MEDICAL INDICATIONS FOR VASECTOMY

Legitimate therapeutic uses of vasectomy have been confined to surgical interruption of the ascending pathways of infection which, in the preantibiotic era, frequently caused epididymitis and orchitis following prostatectomy and urethral instrumentation. The use of perioperative antimicrobials has reduced the incidence of epididymitis following prostatectomy without prophylactic vasectomy to 1–3 per 500 cases. This approximates the incidence of epididymitis following vasectomy performed for sterilization. Thus there is little reason for its continued use in conjunction with invasive urologic procedures.

Vasectomy is, however, indicated in men with recurrent epididymitis or epididymo-orchitis who fail to respond to appropriate long-term antibiotics. Since most of these men have sterile urine and epididymal aspirates, it has been suggested that reflux of urine via the ejaculatory ducts incites a chemical epididymitis. The efficacy of vasectomy in preventing recurrence indirectly supports this notion. Diagnostic epididymal aspiration, incidentally, can cause sperm granuloma and obstruction even when done with a thin needle, and therefore it should never be performed on potential fathers.

VASECTOMY FOR PERMANENT CONTRACEPTION

Surgical Techniques

Vasectomy can be safely performed as an outpatient procedure and with minimal discomfort using local anesthetics. Exposure of the vas deferens high in the scrotum avoids inadvertent epididymal damage. Bilateral incisions of 0.5–1.0 cm or a single incision high on the median raphe provide equally good exposure. Once the vas has been identified and stabilized, infiltration of local anesthetic into and around the cephalad side of the perivasal sheath prevents the dull ache and nausea that frequently occur when the vas is placed under tension. Blind infiltration of cord structures prior to visualization of the vas is to be avoided because of the danger of damage to the $\frac{1}{3}$ mm testicular artery. The deferential artery and vein, with accompanying nerves, can usually be dissected free of the vas and spared. Preservation of these structures minimizes bleeding complications and may enhance the success of subsequent reversal attempts by preserving the innervation and blood supply necessary for normal vas function.

Once the vas has been identified, a 1 cm segment is removed for pathologic identification and the lumina of both ends are occluded. Simple suture ligature occasionally results in necrosis and sloughing of the ends if placed too tightly. The recanalization rate using this technique averages about 1 percent. I have used this method for over 300 vasectomies with a single failure. Two large series of over 1000 vasectomies each have now been reported without any failures. In one of these series the vasa were doubly occluded with metal clips and one end sealed in its sheath. In the other method, described by Schmidt and which I now use, the vasal lumina were occluded internally with an electrocautery needle and the testicular end was sealed in its sheath. Although failure rates with these methods are probably less than 0.25 percent, vasectomy should never be considered 100 percent foolproof.

Since vasectomy failure can be effectively prevented without removal of long segments of vas, excision of more than 1 cm for the pathologist's examination is unnecessary and could complicate a subsequent reversal attempt.

Once the ends of the vasa have been secured and bleeders ligated or coagulated, suture closure of the scrotal wounds is optional. The author prefers to leave the 0.5 cm incisions open. This helps prevent hematoma formation. The wound seals itself in 24 hours and is virtually invisible in a week. Plain gauze dressings are held in place by a snug fitting athletic supporter, which is worn for a week. An evening in bed and two days around the house precede a return to light work on the third postoperative day. Heavy lfting, sports, and sex can be resumed in a week.

Short-term Complications

Hematoma is the most common early complication of vasectomy. It occurs in approximately 1 percent of the cases and even less frequently in more experienced hands. Hematomas can grow to frightening size, sometimes requiring surgical evacuation and an extended hospital stay.

Infection is rare after vasectomy performed under sterile conditions. Prophylactic antibiotics are unnecessay. I performed 150 vasectomies with tetracycline prophylaxis and 237 without and have seen no hematomas or infections in either group.

Epididymitis is a rare complication of vasectomy, occurring in 1–3 of every 500 cases. Whether this is a true infection, or a congestive epididymitis resulting from the acute increase in intraepididymal pressures after vasectomy, is best determined by an empiric trial of tetracycline, 500 mg 4 times a day for 3 weeks, and thrice daily sitz baths. If this treatment fails, a trial of metronidazole is indicated in light of recent reports that trichomonads are often found in the epididymal fluid of patients at the time of vasectomy reversal. If these drug treatments fail, one is dealing with a congestive epididymitis that usually resolves in 6 to 12 weeks with no treatment. In perhaps 1 out of every 100,000 vasectomies chronic orchialgia occurs, probably as a result of unvented high intraepididymal pressures. Occasionally vasectomy reversal, or perhaps purposeful creation of a sperm granuloma on the testicular side of the vas, is necessary to relieve the pain.

Time to Achieve Azoospermia

The disappearance rate of sperm from the ejaculate correlates better with the number of ejaculates than with the time interval after vasectomy. Eighty to 90 percent of men will be azoospermic after 12 to 15 ejaculations. Eighty percent will be azoospermic six weeks after vasectomy regardless of ejaculatory frequency. Since sperm stored in the abdominal side of the vas and ejaculatory ducts lose their motility three weeks after a vasectomy, the appearance of motile sperm after this interval indicates recanalization.

Vasectomy Failure

As noted above, vasectomies fail about 1 percent of the time when ligatures are used to occlude the vas, and less than .25 percent of the time when multiple clip or fulguration techniques are used. The vast majority of failures result from recanalization. This is usually associated with sperm granuloma formation at the site of a leak of sperm from the testicular side of the vas. One of the multiple interconnecting epithelialized channels within the granuloma penetrates to the abdominal side of the vas, re-establishing patency. Usually sperm counts are low after a recanalization and azoospermia ultimately ensues.

If this fails to occur within three months of the vasectomy, the procedure must be repeated. Although recanalizations have been reported up to 17 months after vasectomy, the vast majority occur within 6 weeks. Recanalization is also very rare after azoospermia has been achieved.

Surgical error resulting in division or ligation of a structure other than the vas deferens occurs less than once in a thousand vasectomies. Supernumerary vasa are even rarer.

LOCAL EFFECTS OF VASECTOMY ON THE MALE REPRODUCTIVE TRACT

Sperm Granuloma

I discuss this first because its presence or absence seems to be of critical importance in modulating the local effects of chronic obstruction on the male reproductive tract. The sperm granuloma's complex network of epithelialized channels provides additional absorptive surface that helps vent the high intraluminal pressures in the obstructed excurrent ducts. Numerous animal studies have correlated the presence or absence of sperm granuloma at the vasectomy site with degree of epididymal and testicular damage. Species that always develop granulomas after vasectomy have minimal damage to the seminiferous tubules. Silber's studies of men undergoing vasectomy reversal have revealed a similar correlation between degree of vasal dilation and epididymal damage, and the presence or absence of a sperm granuloma.

Sperm granuloma, however, is a double-edged sword. Its presence increases the likelihood of recanalization and vasectomy failure. In fact, attempts were made to develop a more reversible vasectomy procedure by leaving the testicular end of the vas open, thus assuring the formation of a sperm granuloma at the vasectomy site. This technique had to be abandoned because of unacceptably high failure rates. Occasionally sperm granulomas are painful and must be surgically removed. Furthermore, a sperm granuloma represents a violation of the blood-testis barrier and may therefore contribute to the stimulation of antisperm antibody formation after vasectomy.

Although sperm granulomas are palpable in only about 6 percent of men after vasectomy, they are present microscopically in at least 30 percent of men undergoing reversal. It is likely that, given enough time, virtually all men will develop sperm granulomas either at the vasectomy site, epididymis, or rete testis.

Testis

In some animals spermatogenesis is reduced after vasectomy, but this effect varies considerably from species to species. Seminiferous tubular damage is directly related to the ability of the epididymis and remaining vas to distend and resorb testicular fluid and sperm. These adaptations protect the testes of rats, rabbits, and monkeys for at least 18 months. The unavoidable sperm granulomas that form at the vasectomy site in these species provide further testicular protection against pressure-induced damage. Dogs, which have limited distensibility of the vas deferens and epididymis and do not form granulomas, develop marked seminiferous tubular damage after vasectomy.

In humans, micropuncture studies have revealed that the markedly increased pressures that occur on the testicular side of the vas and epididymis after vasectomy are not transmitted to the seminiferous tubules. Therefore, little disruption of spermatogenesis occurs in humans. Biopsies up to 15 years after vasectomy show the testes to be normal by light microscopy. Electron microscopic studies have revealed some thickening of the basal lamina and scattered areas of disrupted spermatogenesis in portions of the biopsy specimens, but the majority of sections examined in monkeys and men are normal.

In all species studied, Leydig cell structure and function are unaltered by vasectomy, and circulating levels of gonadotropic and steroid hormones show no significant changes.

Rete Testis and Epididymis

The brunt of pressure-induced damage after vasectomy falls upon the rete testis and epididymis. These delicate tubules become markedly distended and adapt to reabsorb large volumes of testicular fluid and sperm products. It is likely that, given enough time, all vasectomized men will develop blowouts in either the epididymis or rete testes. Sperm granulomas will then form at the site of rupture and usually lead to secondary epididymal or rete testis obstruction. For this reason reversal surgery is less successful as the time interval from the original vasectomy increases. As noted previously, the presence of a sperm granuloma at the *vasectomy site* vents some of the high pressure ordinarily transmitted to the epididymis and rete, and therefore confers some protection against damage to these structures.

Vas Deferens

In animals and humans alike, vasectomy causes significant dilation of the vasal lumina on the testicular side. The external diamater of the vas is unchanged, however, indicating loss of vasal musculature with time. As with other pressure-induced phenomena, there is significantly less luminal dilation when a sperm granuloma forms at the vasectomy site. In crudely performed vasectomies, damage to the deferential vessels and nerve supply may further compromise vasal function. These changes are of consequence only if reversal is sought.

The abdominal side of the vas deferens remains unchanged after vasectomy. There is no evidence of atrophy or epithelial changes in the defunctionalized segment.

Seminal Vesicles and Prostate

These accessory sex organs provide 90 to 95 percent of the volume of seminal fluid discharged during ejaculation, and this function continues unchanged after vasectomy. Therefore, the taste, quantity, and appearance of the ejaculate is virtually the same after vasectomy.

LONG-TERM SYSTEMIC CONSEQUENCES OF VASECTOMY

The long-term local effects of vasectomy on the male reproductive tract have been clearly described in many species, including man, and most of the evidence is in agreement. The potential systemic effects of vasectomy, thought to be antibody mediated, are poorly understood. There are few good long-term studies in either animals or man, and much of the evidence presented below is highly controversial.

The unique surface characteristics of sperm, as well as the delay in their appearance until puberty, make them potential targets for recognition as foreign by the immune system. The presence of a blood-testis barrier, maintained by the Sertoli cell tight junctions of the seminiferous tubules, normally prevents the exposure of sperm antigens to the systemic circulation. The integrity of this barrier is maintained from the rete testis to the urethra by an unbroken epithelial lining. If this barrier is violated by surgery, such as vasectomy, or any operation or injury that allows sperm leakage outside the barrier, antibodies to sperm antigens can form in the blood. Most human studies indicate that a majority of men will have detectable antisperm antibodies in the blood after vasectomy. Although some of these studies indicate that antibody titers diminish two or more years after vasectomy, others suggest that they persist. Although sperm granulomas are thought to be associated with higher titers of antisperm antibodies after vasectomy, firm evidence of this is lacking.

In several animal species experimental immune orchitis has been induced using adjuvant-bound heterologous sperm antigens. However, definitive evidence for vasectomy induced deposition of immune complexes exists in only two species. In the rabbit, sperm antigen associated immune complex deposits have been found in the testes of 50 percent of vasectomized animals, and in the kidneys of 8 percent. In monkeys, such deposits are found in less than 5 percent of vasectomized animals. Neither circulating immune complexes nor deposits are increased after vasectomy in man. Furthermore, studies in animals and man have failed to find any association between antisperm antibodies and immune complex mediated diseases, such as lupus erythematosus, scleroderma, rheumatoid arthritis, or glomerulonephritis.

The most provocative studies implicating sperm-antibody mediated immune complex damage after vasectomy concern the association between atherosclerosis and vasectomy in cynomolgus monkeys. Nancy Alexander and colleagues at the Oregon Regional Primate Research Center have reported significantly more frequent and extensive atherosclerosis of the major vessels of previously vasectomized monkeys fed a high cholesterol diet. A smaller but still significant increase was found in vasectomized monkeys fed a normal diet. Although immunoglobulin and complement were demonstrated in plaques from some of the vasectomized animals, the antigens and antibodies involved have not yet been positively identified. These small but controlled studies have stimulated an intensive search for possible cardiovascular effects of vasectomy in men.

Over a dozen recent reports have failed to find any evidence of excess cardiovascular disease, hospitalization, illness, or biochemical alteration in vasectomized men. Six of these studies employed matched controls. The largest examined over 6000 men who had undergone vasectomy 3 to 10 years previously. A more recent but as yet unpublished study specifically looked for circulating immune complexes in the blood and arteriolosclerotic retinopathy in men five years after vasectomy. No differences were found between the vasectomized men and strictly age-matched controls.

These early reports indicate that the risk of any serious systemic aftereffects of vasectomy is not large. Detection of small risks, however, will require studies of larger populations over longer periods of time.

VASECTOMY REVERSAL

Although the number of American men who undergo vasectomy has stabilized at about one-half million annually, the number requesting surgical reversal has grown dramatically. Recent estimates indicate that 2 to 6 percent of vasectomized men will ultimately seek reversal. In this country divorce with subsequent remarriage is by far the most common reason given for requesting reversal. In undeveloped countries the death of a child is the most common reason. In Bangladesh, for example, 5 percent of all couples who choose sterilization experience the death of a child within one year after the operation.

Prior to the refinement of microsurgical techniques, results of vasectomy reversal were relatively poor, with pregnancy rates varying from 5 to 50 percent. The technical problems inherent in creating an accurate leakproof anastomosis of structures with a luminal diameter of only 1/3 mm are formidable. Employment of internal splints frequently resulted in granuloma formation at the site of splint removal and obstruction.

In 1968, Fernandes, Shah, and Draper reported a 95 percent success rate in reversing vasectomy in dogs using × 25–40 magnification and fine suture materials. In 1977, Sherman Silber, using microsurgical techniques, reported a 71 percent pregnancy rate in humans. Shortly thereafter Earl Owen, an Australian microsurgeon, reported similar results. Silber's current claim of 82 percent pregnancy rates in couples followed for at least five years is truly remarkable. His experience with over 1500 reversals is the largest by far. Table 1 shows the clear superiority of microsurgical techniques for vasectomy reversal.

Surgical Technique

Microsurgical vasectomy reversal is an extremely difficult operation, requiring general or spinal anesthetic and taking anywhere from 2 to 6 hours to perform. Once the scarred ends of the vasa are identified through scrotal incisions, the patency of the abdominal side is ascertained by passage of a monofilament nylon thread or injection of saline. If large segments of vas have been removed or damaged, the incision may have to be extended into the groin or pelvis to obtain adequate vasal length for a tension-free anastomosis. After patency of the cephalad side of the vas has been ascertained, the testicular side is serially transected until free flow of fluid from its lumen is detected under × 10–25 magnification. This fluid is examined for the presence of sperm. If morphologically normal sperm are present in this fluid, a vasovasotomy is performed under × 25–40 magnification. The inner mucosal layer is approximated using 4 to 6 interrupted sutures of 22 μ diameter monofilament nylon swaged to a 100 μ diameter needle. The placement of eight to ten sutures of the same material in the outer muscular layer completes the anastomosis. The identical procedure is repeated on the opposite side.

In 30 to 50 percent of reversals, rupture of the epididymis and sperm granuloma formation have produced secondary obstruction. Under these circumstances the epididymis is serially transected at higher levels until free flow of fluid and normal sperm are found. A vasoepididymostomy is then performed in a fashion similar to that described above. Vasoepididymostomy is considerably more difficult than vasovasotomy. It requires identification, under high power magnification, of the single epididymal tubule among the many transected that maintains continuity with the proximal excurrent ducts. In addition, the epididymal tubule is considerably smaller and more delicate than the vas deferens. Nevertheless, in the hands of a skilled microsurgeon, the results of a specific vasoepididymal anatomosis can be very good.

Drains are left in the scrotum for a day or two and the patient can usually be discharged on the second or third postoperative day. Normal activities, including intercourse, may be resumed in two weeks.

FACTORS THAT INFLUENCE THE SUCCESS OF REVERSAL SURGERY

Time Interval since Vasectomy

Generally, the longer the interval between vasectomy and reversal, the greater the chances of epididymal or rete testis blowout and secondary

TABLE 1   Pregnancy Rates After Vasectomy Reversal

	Conventional Techniques			Microsurgical Techniques	
1931	Hasner	40%	1977	Silber	71%
1948	O'Connor	25%	1977	Owen	62%
1967	Phadke et al.	55%	1978	Fitzpatrick	64%
1977	Urquart-Hay	45%	1980	Lee and McLoughlin	54%
1978	Lee	25%	1981	Shessel and Politano	70%
1978	Fallon et al.	40%	1982	Soonewalla	62%
1978	Middleton et al.	39%	1982	Silber*	82%
1978	Soonewalla	43%			
1980	Lee and McLoughlin	46%			

*Unpublished personal communication

obstruction. If epididymal obstruction is found, the more difficult vasoepididymostomy must be performed. Under these circumstances pregnancy rates will be 10 to 15 percent lower. Furthermore, intervals of over ten years since the original vasectomy are frequently associated with epididymal obstruction at the level of the caput. If an anastomosis must be performed high in the caput epididymis, poor or absent motility usually results in spite of adequate sperm counts. At least 1 cm of functional epididymis is necessary for adequate sperm maturation. If the rete testes is obstructed bilaterally, the situation is hopeless.

Sperm Granuloma

As noted previously, the presence of a sperm granuloma at the vasectomy site confers protection against pressure-induced damage to the epididymis and is associated with significantly higher success rates for reversal surgery. Sperm granulomas at the level of the epididymis or rete testis, on the other hand, produce secondary obstruction and indicate a poorer outcome.

Antisperm Antibodies

There is little convincing evidence that the results of reversal surgery correlate with the presence or absence of antisperm antibodies in the blood. Even when antibody titers to sperm antigens in the blood are high, such antibodies are rarely found in the semen.

Quality of the Vas Fluid

When fluid samples from the testicular side of the vas contain normal sperm or clear fluid, the prognosis is good. If no sperm or only sperm parts or thick cloudy fluid is found, the vas must be transected higher up or the epididymis explored.

Microsurgical Technique

This is probably the single most important factor in determining the success of reversal surgery. Hundreds of hours of laboratory practice are necessary to acquire the requisite skills. The unpredictable necessity for a vasoepididymostomy places an even greater premium on technical expertise.

RECOVERY OF FERTILITY

Although some pregnancies occur in the first three to six months after reversal, typically they occur between six months and a year. It must be emphasized, however, that many pregnancies have been recorded two to five years after reversal. Furthermore, second or third attempts at reversal, often requiring vasoepididymostomy, are frequently successful.

Finally, although a longer time interval since vasectomy means a lower overall success rate, there is no way of accurately predicting the outcome until the actual time of surgical exploration. Vasography does not reliably demonstrate the epididymal lesions that most frequently compromise success.

GYNECOMASTIA

STEVEN A. BRODY, M.D.
D. LYNN LORIAUX, M.D., Ph.D.

Breast enlargement in the male, gynecomastia, is a common clinical finding. It occurs normally in 70 percent of pubertal boys and can be found in as many as 80 percent of healthy men, depending on their age. Gynecomastia may also be the initial manifestation of serious illness (Table 1). Thus the appropriate treatment of gynecomastia depends upon an accurate diagnosis of the underlying disorder. The discussion that follows considers the treatment of gynecomastia in the context of the more common disorders with which it is associated.

GENERAL CONSIDERATIONS

The diagnosis of gynecomastia is made on the basis of palpable glandular tissue in the breast. This may be in the form of a subareolar "button" or a soft tissue mass with a more diffuse contour. Breast enlargement is unilateral in 40 percent of cases. Glandular breast tissue can usually be distinguished from simple adipose tissue by palpa-

TABLE 1   Classification of Gynecomastia

Physiologic Gynecomastia
  Neonatal
  Pubertal gynecomastia
  Senescent gynecomastia
Drugs—see Table 2
Hypogonadism
  Primary (hypergonadotropic) hypogonadism
    Vanishing testis syndrome
    Klinefelter's syndrome
    Testicular damage or atrophy (mumps orchitis, leprosy,
      trauma, irradiation, chemotherapy, castration)
  Secondary (hypogonadotropic) hypogonadism
    Kallmann's syndrome (uncommon prior to treatment)
    Fertile eunuch variant
    Hypothalamic-pituitary (uncommon prior to treatment)
Feminizing Neoplasms
  Testis
    Leydig cell tumor
    Germinal cell tumors
  Adrenal
    Feminizing adrenocortical adenoma or carcinoma
  hCG-producing nontesticular tumors
    Hepatoblastoma
    Pinealoma
    Bronchogenic carcinoma
Metabolic and Chronic Diseases
  Hyperthyroidism
  Cirrhosis
  Refeeding gynecomastia
    Hemodialysis
    Neoplasms in remission
    Successfully treated heart failure
Idiopathic
  Persistent pubertal Macromastia

---

tion, comparing the texture of the breast mass with adjacent areas of subcutaneous fat. Breast tisssue usually has a finely nodular texture not characteristic of subcutaneous fat. Neurofibromas, lipomas, hemangiomas, and breast carcinoma can all cause breast enlargement, but they do not have this characteristic texture. The findings of expressible serosanguineous fluid, axillary adenopathy, or fixation of the skin to underlying structures suggest malignancy and are indications for biopsy.

The Tanner criteria for staging breast development in girls are useful in classifying and following patients with gynecomastia. Tanner staging also has prognostic importance in that breast enlargement to a Tanner stage III or greater rarely regresses completely.*

The pathogenetic factor in gynecomastia,

---

*Tanner stage III is a conical breast comprised of glandular, fat, and fibrous tissue. The areola is enlarged beyond the breast bud stage.

---

when it is understood, appears to be an alteration in the circulating levels or biologic effectiveness of sex steroids, favoring estrogenic over androgenic effects.

PHYSIOLOGIC GYNECOMASTIA

Neonatal gynecomastia is a transient phenomenon that occurs in most male neonates and appears to be a consequence of the estrogens of pregnancy. It usually disappears within a few weeks of birth. *Pubertal gynecomastia* occurs in about 70 percent of adolescent boys. Serum levels of sex steroid hormones and the development of secondary sex characteristics are normal. Pubertal gynecomastia should be considered a normal feature of puberty. The gynecomastia disappears in two to three years in the majority of boys. The condition requires no therapy. *Pubertal macromastia* is a term used to describe the situation in which pubertal breast changes reach a Tanner stage III or greater and fail to regress completely. Cosmetic surgery will generally be required for this group of patients. *Senescent gynecomastia* is often found in men in the seventh and eighth decades of life. Histologic examination of the breast reveals ductular proliferation in as many as 80 percent of men in this age group. The cause appears to be a combination of decreased testosterone production in conjunction with an increase in peripheral aromatization of testosterone to estradiol. No specific treatment is indicated.

DRUG-RELATED GYNECOMASTIA

Several drugs cause gynecomastia and constitute a common cause of symptomatic gynecomastia in adults. In addition to steroid hormones, spironolactone, cimetidine, digitoxin, and op'DDD have been closely linked with gynecomastia (Table 2). Digitoxin is a weak estrogen agonist; digoxin has not been shown to have this effect. Spironolactone and cimetidine are antiandrogens and probably cause gynecomastia via this mechanism. Withdrawal of the offending drug will stop the progression of breast enlargement and may lead to regression if the process has not advanced too far.

Most men receiving estrogen therapy for prostatic carcinoma develop symptomatic gynecomastia. Pretreatment orthovoltage irradiation of the breasts, 900–1500 rads over 3 days, will prevent gynecomastia in 90 percent of these men.

TABLE 2 Drugs Associated with Gynecomastia

Clear association
  spironolactone
  cimetidine
  digitoxin
  op'DDD
  cyproterone acetate
  human chorionic gonadotopin
  birth control pills
  testosterone

Anecdotal association
  digoxin
  methyldopa
  reserpine
  isoniazid
  ethionamide
  tricyclic antidepressants
  phenothiazines
  diazepam
  hydroxyzine
  heroin
  marijuana

HYPOGONADAL STATES

Both primary and secondary hypogonadism can be associated with gynecomastia. Klinefelter's syndrome, with an incidence of about 1 in 200 live births, is the most common cause of gynecomastia in this group. The incidence of gynecomastia in patients with Klinefelter's syndrome is about 40 percent. Although adequate sexual maturation can be achieved with exogenous testosterone administration, this usually fails to improve the gynecomastia. Cosmetic surgery is the treatment of choice.

FEMINIZING NEOPLASMS

Feminizing tumors of the adrenal gland and Leydig cell tumors of the testes, both of which are rare, cause gynecomastia by direct secretion of estradiol or its precursors. hCG secreting neoplasms can also cause gynecomastia. Examples of hCG secreting tumors include hepatoblastomas, choriocarcinomas, hypothalamic dysgerminomas, and other extragonadal tumors, such as oat cell carcinomas of the lung. hCG secreting tumors appear to cause gynecomastia by enhancing testicular aromatase activity which results in increased testicular secretion of estradiol.

The appropriate therapy for these patients is surgical or chemotherapeutic ablation of the neoplasm. If the underlying lesion proves refractory to treatment and the breast swelling and tenderness are disabling, the estrogen antagonist Tamoxifen may be beneficial. Doses of 10 mg twice daily can reduce pain and swelling in as little as 2 weeks. Side effects include nausea, vomiting, peripheral edema, and transient thrombocytopenia.

METABOLIC AND CHRONIC DISEASE

Hyperthyroidism is associated with clinically apparent gynecomastia in about 40 percent of cases. The breast enlargement, if not greater than Tanner stage II, responds to treatment of the underlying disorder.

Cirrhotic liver disease can be associated with several signs of hyperestrogenism, including gynecomastia. Improvement of liver function is the goal of therapy. Refeeding gynecomastia occurs in debilitated patients recovering from serious systemic disease such as uremia or heart failure. Like pubertal gynecomastia, it usually abates spontaneously within a year to two and no specific treatment is indicated.

GYNECOMASTIA IN PREPUBERTAL BOYS

The most common cause of gynecomastia in prepubertal boys is exposure to estrogen containing medication such as birth control pills or vaginal creams. Meat from DES treated animals can also be a source of estrogens. Feminizing adrenal cancer is the only other condition that causes gynecomastia in boys without concomitant pubertal changes such as pubic and axillary hair.

hCG secreting tumors and Leydig cell tumors can cause gynecomastia in boys in this age group, but these tumors are always associated with other pubertal changes such as pubic hair and phallic enlargement. The treatment of gynecomastia in these conditions is directed at the underlying abnormality.

Male pseudohermaphroditism can be associated with gynecomastia. The causes include androgen resistance (Reifenstein's syndrome), androgen biosynthetic defects (17-hydroxylase, 17-20 desmolase, and 17-ketosteroid reductase deficiency), and mixed gonadal dysgenesis. True hermaphroditism is also a cause of gynecomastia associated with ambiguous genitalia. The gynecomastia found with these conditions usually requires surgical reduction.

SURGICAL TREATMENT

Breast development of Tanner stage III or greater, like the female postmenopausal breast, will not significantly regress when the hormonal stimulus is removed. Reduction mammoplasty is the only effective treatment for these patients. Surgical correction is particularly important to counter the self-consciousness and embarrassment that invariably accompany this disorder in adolescents.

The important variables affecting the ultimate cosmetic result of the surgical procedure are the Tanner stage of the breast and the amount of redundant skin that must be removed. Whenever possible, incisions should be confined to the border of the areola without displacement of the nipple. When the areola must be reduced in size or transplanted, or redundant skin must be removed by incisions extending away from the areola, the results will rarely be satisfactory.

The use of the periareolar incision presents a greater technical challenge for the surgeon but yields the best cosmetic result. In the hands of a skilled plastic surgeon, the procedure can at times be performed on an outpatient basis.

ANDROGEN RESISTANCE SYNDROMES

JAMES E. GRIFFIN, M.D.,
MARK LESHIN, M.D.
and JEAN D. WILSON, M.D.

Male pseudohermaphroditism is characterized by incomplete virilization in 46,XY chromosomal males with bilateral testes. Although a defect in testosterone formation may be the cause of the defective virilization, the majority of individuals with male pseudohermaphroditism have normal testosterone synthesis and a presumed defect in androgen action at the target cell level. Two types of hereditary resistance to the action of androgen can be separated on genetic, phenotypic, and endocrinologic grounds. One is an autosomal recessive disorder in which there is either deficient activity or a qualitative abnormality in the 5α-reductase enzyme that converts testosterone to dihydrotestosterone. Patients with this form of male pseudohermaphroditism have male internal urogenital tracts, predominantly female external genitalia, and normal male levels of plasma testosterone, estradiol, and luteinizing hormone. The second form of androgen resistance is composed of a group of X-linked disorders that can be divided on genetic grounds into at least four distinct subtypes: (1) normal-appearing women (complete testicular feminization); (2) phenotypic women with some virilization (incomplete testicular feminization); (3) phenotypic men with incomplete virilization of the external and internal genitalia (Reifenstein's syndrome); and (4) infertile but otherwise phenotypically normal men (the infertile male syndrome). The defect in most of these patients appears to affect either the amount or the function of the cytoplasmic receptor that binds testosterone and dihydrotestosterone, but in some cases a postreceptor abnormality may be operative. Affected individuals characteristically have normal to elevated levels of plasma testosterone, luteinizing hormone, and estradiol.

Since no specific therapy is available to circumvent or reverse the abnormal development that takes place during embryogenesis, management involves appropriate gender assignment in the newborn and the prevention or treatment of adverse secondary effects of the mutations (Table 1).

GENDER ASSIGNMENT IN THE NEWBORN

The majority of newborns with problems of gender assignment have congenital adrenal hyperplasia, mixed gonadal dysgenesis, or dysgenetic testes. Occasional patients with androgen resistance present as problems of gender assignment. Neonates with either complete testicular feminization or the infertile male syndrome have unambiguously normal female or male external genitalia respectively, and therefore do not constitute problems of gender assignment. In contrast, patients with 5α-reductase deficiency, incomplete testicular feminization, or Reifenstein's syndrome may be brought for treatment during the newborn period because of ambiguous genitalia. Attempts to make a precise diagnosis of the cause of the male pseudohermaphroditism (distinguishing between one of the androgen resistance syndromes and de-

TABLE 1   The Androgen Resistance Syndromes and Their Therapy

Syndrome	Usual Predominant Phenotype	Problem in Gender Assignment	Need for Castration	Mastectomy for Gynecomastia	Hormonal Therapy
5α-Reductase deficiency	Female	Unusual	Prepubertal if female	Gynecomastia not present	Estrogens at puberty if female
Complete testicular feminization	Female	No	Postpubertal	Not appropriate	Estrogens after castration
Incomplete testicular feminization	Female	Rare	Prepubertal	Not appropriate	Estrogens at puberty
Reifenstein's syndrome	Male	Unusual	None	Usually	Androgens not helpful
Infertile male syndrome	Male	No	None	Occasionally	Androgens not helpful

fects in testosterone formation) and to localize the site of impairment in androgen action should be made early in life. In some instances it may be useful to know the response to chorionic gonadotropin stimulation to help predict response to androgen therapy (for example, those with deficient increase in plasma testosterone are generally androgen deficient and respond well to androgen therapy). In most instances a decision regarding sex of rearing can be made before the infant leaves the hospital.

In those patients with milder defects in virilization a male gender assignment can be made, thus permitting phenotypic sex to correspond to chromosomal and gonadal sex. This is unfortunately not practical in patients with severe defects in virilization. In patients with androgen resistance, infertility is probably inevitable and thus does not enter into the decision of appropriate gender of rearing. The central problem is thus the question of whether there will be adequate growth of the phallus to allow normal male sexual function after the time of expected puberty. The major predictor of adequate virilization at puberty, and consequently the major determining factor in assigning gender in patients with androgen resistance, is the degree of masculinization of the external genitalia that occurs in utero. If the phallus is of sufficient size at birth that the child has the potential of adequate male sexual function as an adult, the individual should be raised as male. If the phallus is inadequately developed the child should be reared as a female, regardless of the etiologic factors. In many patients the phallus is bound by a chordee, which makes interpretation of phallus length difficult. Perhaps more important than length of the newborn phallus is the diameter. We generally consider a phallus less than 0.5 cm in diameter just proximal to the glans as being inadequate in size. The feasibility of repair of coexistent hypospadias also must be estimated in conjunction with a pediatric urologist before making final gender assignment.

Once gender assignment is made the indicated surgery should be performed. For patients raised as males this may involve orchiopexy and staged hypospadias repair, depending on the specific phenotype. These procedures are usually begun when the child is 1 to 2 years of age or older and the genitalia have increased somewhat in size. Patients who are to be raised as females usually require a clitoral resection and castration. Castration is usually performed at the time of clitoral resection and should always be performed prior to the time of expected puberty to prevent any further virilization. Surgical reduction in phallus size in a child reared as female can usually be accomplished in the first few months of life.

SURGICAL MANAGEMENT OF THE OLDER CHILD OR ADOLESCENT

In contrast to the newborn with ambiguous genitalia in whom a decision can be made about gender assignment, it is inadvisable in children beyond the newborn period to attempt alteration of the assigned sex of rearing, regardless of the anatomy of the external genitalia. Even if the child is too young to appreciate the change, adverse psychologic effects on parents and other relatives are usually conveyed to the subject. A possible exception to this dictum is the fraction of patients with 5α-reductase deficiency who are identified in adolescence after some virilization has occurred and who appear to be experiencing a change in gender role from female to male, a phenomenon that has been described in this syndrome in the untreated state. Following appropriate psychiatric evaluation in such patients it might be more appropriate to allow virilization to proceed and support the patient emotionally through such a change.

Females

Most patients with androgen resistance who are raised as females require two procedures in addition to those related to the size of the phallus as discussed above: removal of the testes and construction of a vagina. The most serious complication of intra-abdominal testes due to all causes, including complete testicular feminization, is the development of tumors. The frequency of tumor development is about four times greater in abdominal than in inguinal testes, but only about one in 64 undescended testes becomes malignant. Although the natural history of testicular tumors in subjects with testicular feminization is not entirely clear, some behave as true malignancies. Therefore it is generally accepted that testes in women with complete testicular feminization should be removed. Since these patients undergo a normal pubertal growth spurt and feminize successfully at the time of expected puberty, and since tumors rarely develop in cryptorchid testes until after this time, it is customary to delay castration until after secondary sexual maturation is completed. If, however, hernia repair is indicated in the prepubertal years or if the testes are in the inguinal region or the labia majora and cause discomfort, some physicians prefer to remove the testes at the time of herniorrhaphy. Women with incomplete testicular feminization and 5α-reductase deficiency most likely have an incidence of tumor development similar to that seen in women with complete testicular feminization. Furthermore, subjects with incomplete testicular feminization and those with 5α-reductase deficiency who are raised as females undergo orchiectomy shortly after coming to medical attention to remove the risk of tumor development and also to prevent further virilization.

The need for and the method chosen for construction of a vagina in women with androgen resistance depends on the phenotype of the external genitalia, that is, whether a pseudovagina is already present. If this is the case, a nonoperative technique to increase vaginal depth is often sufficient to result in a vagina adequate for intercourse. The Frank procedure involves application of pressure with a test tube-shaped dilator (or series of dilators of increasing size) to the pseudovagina for a brief period daily to increase vaginal depth gradually. If the Frank technique is not successful it may be necessary to utilize an operative procedure (vaginoplasty) in which an artificial vagina is created by placing a skin graft over a preformed mold into a space created in the proper location. Either method can result in the formation of a functioning vagina and the development of a vaginal endothelium that shows cornification similar to normal vaginal epithelium in response to estrogens. Construction of a vagina can usually be delayed until the time of sexual maturity, since maintenance of adequate vaginal depth and patency requires continued use of a dilator and mold, respectively, or regular sexual intercourse.

Males

The management of patients with androgen resistance who are raised as males involves repair of defects of the external genitalia, treatment of gynecomastia, and correction of cryptorchidism. Surgical procedures that may be necessary to repair developmental defects of the external genitalia include relief of chordee and correction of hypospadias. Because of the difficulty involved in staged repair of hypospadias it may not be possible in every instance to bring the opening of the urethra to the end of the glans. Since these patients are almost always infertile on the basis of their primary androgen resistance, and since normal sexual function is not dependent on a complete repair of the hypospadias, the decision regarding repair of the hypospadias must be made on an individual basis after consideration of the specific defect and the likely difficulty of its correction.

Gynecomastia in patients with androgen resistance is indistinguishable histologically from other forms of estrogen-induced gynecomastia. In men with Reifenstein's syndrome and in occasional infertile men, gynecomastia develops as the result of both increased estrogen production and the androgen resistance. Since most Reifenstein subjects have male gender assignment and male gender identity, the gynecomastia may be disfiguring as well as psychologically disturbing. The only form of therapy available is surgical removal. Carcinoma of the breast has not been described in men with androgen resistance.

Cryptorchidism is frequent in the Reifenstein syndrome and should be corrected surgically. As in other forms of cryptorchidism there is less likelihood of damage to the testes if the orchiopexy is performed prior to sexual maturation. We generally recommend such a correction before the age of 6 years. There is an increased risk of malignancy in all cryptorchid testes, but the frequency is sufficiently low that removal of a testis that can be relocated into the scrotum is not indicated.

HORMONAL THERAPY

Estrogen treatment is indicated in all phenotypic women following removal of the testes. If the testes are removed prepubertally, estrogen therapy is begun sufficiently early (11 to 13 years) to ensure normal linear growth and breast development. Patients in whom castration is performed after pubescence may develop vasomotor menopausal symptoms as well as other consequences of estrogen withdrawal, such as premature osteoporosis. These problems are prevented by estrogen replacement in the form of ethinyl estradiol (20–50 μg daily) or conjugated estrogens (0.625–1.25 mg daily). Lower estrogen doses are adequate for induction of initial sexual maturation. Since an endometrium is not present, progestin therapy is not required.

Supplemental androgen therapy is without benefit in promoting virilization in men with Reifenstein's syndrome and is not ordinarily needed in subjects with 5α-reductase deficiency who are raised as men. Whether dihydrotestosterone treatment of men with 5σ-reductase deficiency would promote more complete development of secondary sex characteristics is not known.

PSYCHOLOGIC PROBLEMS

It is unwise to inform patients at any age in life that their chromosomal sex and phenotypic sex are discordant. When castration is indicated, the patient and her parents should be told that as a result of a hereditary defect the gonads are abnormal, that the resulting infertility is not treatable, and that because of the potential for tumor development the gonads should be removed at a suitable time. With appropriate counseling and reassurance, most persons with androgen resistance whom we have managed have made an adequate psychologic adjustment. Women with testicular feminization usually have a completely feminine outlook and make successful adoptive mothers. Men with Reifenstein's syndrome usually have an unequivocally male psychosexual orientation and function well as adoptive fathers. The adult men with Reifenstein's syndrome have some emotional problems related to inadequate ejaculate volume. The one group of patients with androgen resistance in whom psychologic problems are most likely to occur are those patients with 5α-reductase deficiency who are not identified until the time of sexual maturation when virilization has proceeded in a child raised as female and some change in their gender role may have taken place. Decisions regarding castration and clitoral resection in such patients should be made only after careful psychologic evaluation. Patients who undergo such shifts from female to male gender role—and their families—require a great deal of emotional support.

OVARIAN DISORDERS

DELAYED PUBERTY IN GIRLS

MICHAEL B. FOSTER, M.D.
and FRANK S. FRENCH, M.D.

Boys with delayed puberty seldom have a significant physiologic derangement at the root of their problem, whereas similarly affected girls very often do. Underlying this maxim is the relative infrequency of pubertal delay in girls as compared with boys. Suspicion should therefore be aroused whenever a girl reaches the age of 13 years without displaying the development of breast buds. Conditions that result in delayed onset of puberty may be divided into four general categories: (1) gonadal dysgenesis, (2) conditions associated with an altered balance between caloric intake and energy expenditure, (3) hypopituitarism, and (4) constitutional delay of adolescence.

Gonadal dysgenesis may occur either with a normal complement of sex chromosomes or with an abnormality of the sex chromosomes. Girls with Turner's syndrome (45,XO) or one of its variants are almost always short and generally have complete lack of pubertal development. However, girls with sex chromosome mosaicism may be taller than the mean for girls with classic Turner's syndrome, and those with XO,XX mosaicism may occasionally undergo spontaneous pubertal development, rarely including spontaneous menarche. The term pure gonadal dysgenesis is applied in the case of phenotypic females who have dysgenetic gonads with either a 46,XX or 46,XY karyotype. These girls generally have normal stature but fail to show a pubertal growth spurt, development of secondary sex characteristics, or menarche. Although stimulation of pubertal development is the major therapeutic consideration in all types of gonadal dysgenesis, management of growth failure is a significant additional problem in girls with Turner's syndrome.

Girls who experience pubertal delay as the apparent result of an imbalance between caloric intake and energy expenditure comprise an increasingly large fraction of girls presenting with this complaint. Whether girls with anorexia nervosa can be properly included in this category is open to question. The remaining patients in this group experience a problem that is in large part volitional and derives from their serious commitment to physical fitness and vigorous training for athletic endeavors, such as gymnastics, track, competitive swimming, and ballet dancing. Whether the clinical presentation takes the form of amenorrhea or pubertal delay depends largely on the age at which the training is begun. Susceptibility to derangements of this nature is not uniform among female athletes, and the appropriate therapeutic approach is educational rather than pharmacologic. Once the source of the problem has been identified, a decision must be made as to whether training at the present level is necessary for the desired level of performance, and if so, whether the patient desires athletic excellence more strongly than physiologic normalcy.

Female patients with growth hormone deficiency frequently experience delay in the onset of puberty even when the GH deficiency is thought to be isolated rather than part of the syndrome of panhypopituitarism. Although a delay in the skeletal maturation associated with puberty has the advantage of allowing a longer period of effective therapy with human GH, the psychologic impact of sexual infantilism in this group is similar to that in patients with gonadal dysgenesis. Consequently, induction of puberty generally becomes a therapeutic goal sometime during the teenage years. The salient difference between girls with hypopituitarism and those with Turner's syndrome is that human growth hormone is a currently available and effective treatment for short stature in the hypopituitary patient. Treatment for pubertal delay in hypopituitarism must be carried out in such a way as to avoid compromising the final adult height. A discussion of the treatment of hypopituitarism is included elsewhere in this volume (See Chapter 5).

Occasionally girls are encountered who display short stature, delayed puberty, and a retarded bone age but who are otherwise healthy, have a normal karyotype, and have normal prepubertal gonadotropin levels indicating normal ovarian function. Such girls have been classified as having constitutional delay of adolescence. These girls have predicted adult heights in the normal range and can anticipate normal reproductive function. Although some investigators have suggested that treatment with human growth hormone, possible combined with low dose estrogen therapy, might provide a means of easing the psychologic burden imposed by short stature and the delayed sexual development, this therapy has not yet been thoroughly evaluated in clinical trials. Intervention is usually limited to counseling and periodic evaluations at intervals of six months to one year to assure that growth and development are progressing normally.

TREATMENT OF GONADAL DYSGENESIS

An appropriate strategy for treatment of girls with gonadal dysgenesis should encompass four goals: (1) successfully establishing a female gender role; (2) augmentation of the growth rate; (3) development of female secondary sex characteristics; (4) and, establishment of regular menstrual cycles. This list presents the approximate temporal sequence in which the goals are approached, although there is a need for considerable flexibility in order to accommodate those patients who develop a psychological need for secondary sexual development. Further, it must be kept in mind that the principles of treatment for gonadal dysgenesis cannot be applied to the other three diagnostic categories mentioned above.

Establishing a Female Gender

The ultimate goal of the hormonal treatment of gonadal dysgenesis is to provide for normal psychosocial development. Adequate hormonal therapy is only a first step toward achieving this goal. We have found a vital role for a team of health professionals in performing psychologic and developmental evaluations and in recommending specific measures that assist the patient in progressing toward the establishment of a secure self-image as a female. One of the problems that has arisen in our patients is parental concern over tomboyish behavior, particularly in partially masculinized patients. Examination of the child's relationship to her parents and other members of the family has often proved helpful in pointing out ways of allaying the parents' worries and of establishing more effective role modeling for feminine development. Another problem is the feeling of inadequacy resulting from the lack of reproductive capability. The option of adopting children and the potential, although remote, for in vitro fertilization of donor-supplied ova and subsequent implantation in uteri of agonadal patients may serve to alleviate these feelings. Lastly, many patients with gonadal dysgenesis encounter scholastic difficulties in dealing with abstract concepts, the classic example being the introduction to algebra in junior high school. Collaborating with school guidance personnel and taking advantage of flexibility in the curriculum as well as the availability of alternative teaching techniques have proved helpful in most cases. Realistic educational goals must be set if the patient's self esteem is to be preserved.

Augmentation of Growth

Short stature is a common finding in gonadal dysgenesis associated with abnormalities of the sex chromosome, but it is generally absent in pure gonadal dysgenesis. Unless there is a prohibitive need for rapid feminization, the initial therapy in girls with Turner's syndrome and its variants is directed toward acceleration of the growth rate. Long-term, large-scale trials of human GH in high doses have not been carried out in these patients. Current therapy is thus limited to the use of anabolic steroids. The only anabolic agent in use in our clinic is oxandrolone, although others are available. Treatment is begun between 10 and 12 years of age, with a goal of approximately 2 years of treatment before estrogen is added. The dose of oxandrolone is 2.5 mg per day, which is usually sufficient to increase the height velocity without inducing unacceptable virilization. However, mild acne and slight stimulation of the clitoris may occur. Clitoral size should be carefully measured and recorded before starting treatment in order to document that enlargement did not precede treatment. Care must be taken to avoid excessive androgen stimulation, since virilization in a girl whose feminine image is not well established could be psychologically damaging. Whether oxandrolone increases ultimate stature or merely accelerates the height velocity without altering the final height is unresolved. Regardless of which is true, substantial psychologic benefit is to be gained during adolescence by stimulating an obvious physical change toward normalcy. Oxandrolone therapy is monitored by serial bone age determinations at twelve-month intervals.

Sexual Development

In general, the patient's concern regarding the development of an adequate feminine phenotype centers on the breast. The hormonal control of breast development is a complex and poorly understood process. Prolactin, estrogen, progesterone, growth hormone, insulin, cortisol, and thyroid hormone have all been ascribed roles in the normal process of breast development. However, an oversimplifed scheme is that prolactin is necessary for estrogen and progesterone to exert their effects. In the presence of prolactin, estrogen acts to stimulate ductal development and progesterone acts synergistically with prolactin to induce lobuloalveolar development in the estrogen stimulated breast. Growth hormone appears to act similarly to prolactin, and insulin, cortisol, and thyroxine seem to have mainly permissive roles. Replacement therapy is based on the presumption of adequate levels of the other hormones and therefore includes only the administration of estrogen and progesterone.

Estrogen replacement therapy is usually begun between 12 and 13 years of age unless delay is desired to allow a more prolonged period of prepubertal growth. Initially a low dose of conjugated estrogens (0.3 mg per day Premarin) or crystalline micromized estradiol-17β (0.25 mg Estrace) is given continually in a single daily dose. If signs of breast development are not apparent in three to six months the dose is doubled. A slight acceleration in growth rate may occur during this phase of treatment. Estrogen alone is continued for 6 to 12 months or until breakthrough vaginal bleeding occurs, at which time a progestin is added and a cyclic schedule begun. Estrogen is taken for the first 21 days of the monthly cycle, and from day 7 to 21 a progestin, such as medroxyprogesterone acetate, 5–10 mg daily, or norethindrone acetate, 2.5 mg daily, is taken together with estrogen. Both hormones are discontinued from day 22 to the end of the month, during which time menstrual bleeding should occur. There is evidence now that the use of progestin replacement in adequate doses for 14 days during the cycle improves the completeness of endometrial sloughing, diminishes the complication of endometrial hyperplasia, and reduces the long-term risk of endometrial cancer. The therapeutic goal should be to achieve adequate breast development and maintain normal menstrual cycles with the smallest possible dose of estrogen. After 1 to 2 years on the lower dose feminine development can be completed by raising the cyclic dose of estrogen to conjugated estrogens, 1.25 mg daily, or crystalline estradiol 17β, 1.0 mg daily. If additional estrogen is required for full development it can be added to the cyclic regimen noted above as an estrogen-progestogen combination pill containing 30–50 mg of ethinyl estradiol with norethindrone acetate, 1.5–2.5 mg, given from day 7 to 21 of the cycle. Alternatively, large doses of estrogen (conjugated estrogens, 2.5 mg, or crystalline estradiol 17β, 2.0 mg) can be given from days 1 to 21 of the cycle with a progestogen from days 7 to 21. Caution should be observed in continuing large doses of estrogen for more than several months. Adequate estrogen replacement should be judged not only by breast enlargement but also by estrinization of the vaginal mucosa, abundance of vaginal secretions, and enlargement of the uterus as determined by pelvic or rectal examination.

Surgical Treatment

Surgical exploration is not indicated in girls with gonadal dysgenesis, with one exception. Girls with gonadal dysgenesis who have a Y chromosome bearing cell line should have gonadal tissue or fibrous streak gonads removed because of the increased risk of developing gonadoblastoma in the dysgenetic tissue. Although timing of the surgery is not critical, an argument can be made for performing the gonadectomy prior to the usual age of onset of adolescence. With dysgenetic gonads in place, clitoral enlargement, which is often present at the time of diagnosis, will become more pronounced or the gonadotropin and testosterone levels rise further. In addition, gonadoblastoma may develop before puberty and the risk of tumor development increases with advancing age.

HYPOGONADOTROPISM

CHARLES M. MARCH, M.D.

Treatment plans for ovarian deficiency secondary to hypogonadotropism may be readily designed after answering four questions: (1) Has the diagnosis been established with certainty? (2) Is the etiologic agent a serious or life-threatening condition that requires specific therapy and/or contraindicates other treatment modalities? (3) Are other factors present which prevent the use of a particular treatment regimen? (4) What are the patient's desires?

The overall prevalence of amenorrhea among women in the reproductive years is 1 percent (if amenorrhea is defined as 12 months without menses) or 2 percent (for 6 months). About two-thirds of these women will have gonadotropin and estrogen levels within the normal range for the follicular phase of the menstrual cycle. Approximately half of the remaining one-third of amenorrheic women will have estrogen deficiency secondary to hypogonadotropism. The lack of ovarian follicular function in the amenorrheic woman may be presumed on the basis of any symptom or sign of estrogen deficiency. However, the most specific proofs are a serum estradiol concentration below 40 pg/ml (usually the value is much lower) and the lack of withdrawal bleeding following the intramuscular injection of progesterone in oil or the oral administration of a progestin. The latter sign is of course possible only in the woman with a uterus and in whom the diagnoses of cervical stenosis and intrauterine adhesions have been ruled out. The other half of estrogen deficient women have ovarian failure, and therefore the second requirement for the diagnosis of hypogonadotropism is a serum FSH concentration that is low or within the normal range. Random serum FSH and LH levels may be within the normal range and the patient will still have hypogonadotropism because the episodic pulsatile discharge of FSII and LII is absent. Therefore the total production rate of these hormones is reduced. Those with elevated FSH levels have ovarian failure and hypergonadotropism.

Other testing is necessary in this group of patients to rule out the presence of hypothalmic and/or pituitary neoplasms that might demand surgical intervention or radiation therapy, disorders such as estrogen dependent neoplasms that would contraindicate a specific treatment regimen, associated conditions that would dictate that one specific modality be utilized, and any coexisting illnesses that would preclude or contraindicate pregnancy.

Finally, the patient's wishes—maintenance of "well-being," relief of estrogen deficiency symptoms, or pregnancy—will dictate which treatment modality to select.

ESTROGEN REPLACEMENT THERAPY

Treatment regimens can be set up according to the patient's wishes, provided there are no contraindications to one or another treatment method or to pregnancy. The sole exception to this principle is the patient whose hypogonadotropic hypogonadism is secondary to hyperprolactinemia.

The general management of these patients is covered in Chapters 9 and 10. However, approximately two-thirds of amenorrheic women who have hyperprolactinemia will also be found to have estrogen deficiency. These women are at high risk for the development of osteoporosis. Although the regimen of calcium supplementation, sodium fluoride ingestion (if preliminary studies are confirmed), and exercise outlined below should be used in these women, the addition of estrogen may be dangerous. Whether or not a prolactin-secreting pituitary tumor has been demonstrated, these women do have pituitary lactotroph hyperfunction that may be potentiated by estrogen treatment. Therefore treatment with bromocryptine is appropriate. The duration of treatment is uncertain but may have to be lifelong. For those who do not wish to conceive, a barrier method of contraception should be prescribed.

Treatment for those without hyperprolactinemia who do not wish to conceive is geared toward prevention of osteoporosis and relief of estrogen deficiency symptoms. Maintenance of total calcium ingestion of 1.5 to 2.0 g per day and a vigorous exercise program will prevent or minimize the extent of bone loss. Preliminary studies have indicated that the addition of fluoride at a dosage of 40–60 mg per day has a further beneficial effect. The high rate of side effects with fluoride treatment prevents its widespread use until alterations in treatment schedules reduce their frequency and severity. This approach is probably satisfactory for patients who are obese and for those who are black. However, estrogen replacement is an important adjunct for other women. Among those who have serum estradiol (E_2) levels of 25–40 pg/ml and thus are not severely estrogen deficient, the use of estrogen supplementation is not as urgent as it is for women with E_2 levels below 10–15 pg/ml. Many amenorrheic women, especially those whose amenorrhea is related to weight loss, exercise, stress, or combinations thereof, prefer not to ingest any medications, especially "hormones." Thus it may be prudent to limit strong encouragement to the most severely estrogen deficient women.

Most symptoms of estrogen deficiency can be relieved only by estrogen replacement. One exception to this is hot flashes. A common misconception is that signs of vasomotor instability are limited to those with ovarian failure. The frequency and severity of hot flashes are less among hypogonadotropic women but they do occur. These symptoms can be controlled by medroxyprogesterone acetate, 20–30 mg per day in divided doses. This regimen is useful for women in whom estrogen replacement is contraindicated. However, two possible side effects of progestin therapy are depression and aggravation of the estrogen deficiency signs (decreased breast size, further genital atrophy with increasing dyspareunia).

Other estrogen deficiency symptoms require estrogen therapy. The intramuscular administration of estrogen results in widely fluctuating serum estrogen levels, is frequently associated with abnormal bleeding, and achieves pharmacologic rather than physiologic estrogen levels. This method has no role in the therapy of the hypogonadotropic woman. Although not widely used in the United States today, estrogen replacement by subcutaneous implantation of one 25-mg estradiol pellet does have significant advantages over other treatment modalities. Serum E_2 levels are maintained between 50 and 100 pg/ml for 5 to 9 months with little fluctuation; the normal premenopausal estradiol to estrone ratio of greater than 1 is maintained; and hepatic protein and lipid levels are not altered. A drawback of this therapy is that it may be difficult to remove the pellet should complications mandate removal; there is also the theoretic problem of spontaneous resolution of the hypogonadotropism occurring together with an unexpected pregnancy. The theoretic objection of unopposed estrogen stimulation of the endometrium can easily be prevented by the use of medroxyprogesterone acetate, 5 mg per day for the first 10 calendar days of each month.

The prime method of estrogen replacement consists of oral estrogens. Conjugated estrogens, 0.625 mg per day, are prescribed on days 1 through 25 of each month. On days 16 through 25, medroxyprogesterone acetate, 5 mg per day, is added. Although as little as 2.5 mg per day has been shown to turn off endometrial estradiol receptors, histologic patterns are more normal when the higher dose is used. Progestational therapy should continue for at least ten days. Five or seven days of treatment are insufficient to prevent the development of endometrial hyperplasia and to prevent abnormal bleeding. Withdrawal bleeding often occurs in both these women and in those treated by pellet implantation. Although spontaneous recovery with ovulation and pregnancy occurs infrequently in these cases, it must always be considered if withdrawal bleeding does not occur. Contraception should therefore be prescribed for these women. Although both contraception and estrogen replacement may be accomplished by oral

contraceptive use, this is not advised. The estrogen dose is much higher than needed, and further hypothalamic-pituitary suppression serves no purpose and may delay partial or complete recovery. Diethylstilbestrol, micronized estradiol, estrone sulfate, ethinyl estradiol, and other oral estrogens offer no advantages over conjugated estrogens and may have pharmacologic effects upon hepatic proteins. The intravaginal application of estrogens may also be used. Absorption via the vaginal epithelium is excellent and both local and systemic benefits will occur. Therefore, progestins should also be used for those receiving topical therapy.

INDUCTION OF OVULATION

The use of ovulation inducing drugs should be limited to women who wish to conceive. Brief trials with these drugs for "testing" purposes have no prognostic value and may lead to complications or an unwanted pregnancy. The mechanism of action of clomiphene citrate requires the displacement of estradiol from its hypothalamic receptor sites by clomiphene. Hypogonadotropic amenorrheic women are estrogen deficient, and therefore this mechanism cannot operate. Nevertheless, occasional ovulations occur, and thus a brief trial with clomiphene is indicated. Treatment is begun with a daily clomiphene dose of 250 mg, which is continued for 5 days. A simulated LH surge is afforded by giving 10,000 I.U. hCG i.m. 5 to 8 days after stopping clomiphene administration. The exact day of hCG administration is selected by determining the cervical score. As estrogen production by the developing follicle(s) increases, its effect upon the cervix causes an increase in the amount of cervical mucus, an increase in its ferning capacity, an increased spinnbarkeit, and an increase in the size and vascularity of the external cervical os (Table 1). Each of these 4 parameters is graded from 0 to 3. When the cervical score reaches or exceeds 8, hCG is given. If ovulation occurs this regimen is continued. If the patient does not ovulate (as determined by a flat basal body temperature curve), treatment with human menopausal gonadotropins (HMG) is initiated.

Because treatment with gonadotropins is expensive and complicated, an extensive investigation should be performed prior to beginning therapy. A semen analysis should reveal a volume in excess of 2 ml; a sperm density of greater than 20 million per ml; at least 60 percent active, directionally motile sperm 2 hours after collection; and

TABLE 1   Modified Cervical Score

	Score			
	0	*1*	*2*	*3*
Cervical Mucus				
Amount	None	Minimal	Moderate	Profuse
Spinnbarkeit	None	3 cm	6 cm	8–10 cm
Ferning	None	Minimal	Partial	Complete
Cervical Os	Closed	Minimally Open	Partially Open	Gaping

greater than 60 percent with normal morphology and no extraneous material or other cells. If these criteria are not met, the semen analysis should be repeated. If the second analysis is not normal, the husband should be referred to a urologist who has special interest in reproductive disorders.

A hysterosalpingogram is also necessary. A water-soluble iodine medium (such as Sinografin) should be instilled slowly under fluoroscopy with image intensification. Good views of the uterine cavity and both fallopian tubes should be obtained. If an endometrial cavity defect is discovered or if the patient has an iodine allergy, hysteroscopy is necessary.

The final pretreatment study is laparoscopy under general anesthesia using a double puncture technique and with chromopertubation using a dilute solution of indigo carmine. If a pelvic pathologic disorder is found it should be corrected before beginning gonadotropin therapy. Some investigators recommend other studies prior to beginning HMG administration, including immunologic studies and the zona-free hamster egg sperm penetration assay. These have some value, but the low frequency of positive findings does not warrant their routine use.

If any abnormalities are found which cannot be corrected completely, the likelihood of pregnancy is reduced and treatment may be undertaken with that understanding.

Extensive counseling of the couple prior to therapy is mandatory. They should have a stable relationship. Therapy with HMG is inconvenient and stressful for both partners, so each one must provide support for the other. They should be advised that the chance of conceiving in any one course of therapy is approximately 25 percent, a rate similar to the conception rate in spontaneous ovulatory cycles. Of all patients who conceive during therapy, the average number of treatment courses needed to achieve a pregnancy is three. Sixty percent of all patients treated with HMG will

conceive. These data, together with a thorough explanation of the risks and sequelae of multiple gestations and hyperstimulation, will ensure that the couple is well informed prior to therapy.

Treatment with HMG involves the attempt to mimic as closely as possible the follicular development that occurs in a spontaneous cycle. An index of this development is provided by the rising level of estradiol. Therefore, treatment should be undertaken only in centers where estrogen levels in serum or in urine may be obtained rapidly on a daily basis. Individuality of response is the hallmark of gonadotropin therapy. The amount of medication required to induce adequate follicular development, as well as the duration of therapy, varies greatly not only from one patient to another, but also from one course of treatment to another in the same patient. However, as a general rule, "progesterone-negative" amenorrheic patients require significantly more medication than do those who are "progesterone-positive" (have withdrawal bleeding after progesterone treatment). For this reason, treatment must be tailored individually to each patient. Three different treatment regimens are used for the administration of HMG: HMG only, sequential clomiphene-HMG, and sequential estrogen-HMG.

Patients who have oligomenorrhea and those who have amenorrhea and withdrawal uterine bleeding following adminstration of progesterone in oil should receive pretreatment with clomiphene citrate, 200 mg per day for 5 days. On day six of this regimen, HMG is administered. In this group of patients clomiphene will induce partial follicular maturation, and the duration of treatment and the dose of HMG required will be reduced by one-half compared to treatment with HMG only.

However, the hypogonadotropic estrogen deficient amenorrheic woman will not benefit from clomiphene pretreatment. She should be treated with estrogen before HMG therapy is begun. Conjugated estrogens, 1.25 mg per day, are given for

25 consecutive days, and medroxyprogesterone acetate, 5 mg per day, is given on days 21 through 25 of estrogen treatment. This regimen is continued for two months. Following the second withdrawal menses, HMG is begun. The purpose of this therapy is to prime the endometrium and endocervix so that both may respond normally to the estradiol and progesterone stimulation that will follow the gonadotropin stimulation. The value of stimulating the endocervix to produce mucus prior to beginning HMG therapy is clear. Despite high serum E_2 levels, cervical mucus production is often poor among these chronically estrogen deficient women. The pregnancy rate during HMG induced ovulations is significantly higher during cycles in which estrogen therapy preceded gonadotropins, compared to that achieved by therapy with gonadotropin only (Table 2).

During each patient's first course of therapy, treatment is begun with a daily dose of 2 ampules HMG (150 IU FSH and 150 IU LH) given intramuscularly. On the first day of treatment a serum estradiol (E_2) level is obtained and a pelvic examination is performed to assess the quality and quantity of cervical mucus and to verify that there is no ovarian enlargement or tenderness. The semiquantitative cervical score is determined, then a pelvic ultrasound is performed using a real time sector scanner (for example, ADR Model 2140) with attention directed toward the ovaries, specifically toward the number and size of ovarian follicles. These estrogen deficient women usually have quiescent ovaries, and little or no follicle development can be seen on the first treatment day. The same dose of HMG is continued daily. The ultrasound and serum E_2 level test are repeated in three or four days. If the E_2 concentration remains unchanged, the dose of HMG is increased by a factor of 0.5 and continued at this new level for another 3 or 4 days. The stepwise increase every 3 or 4 days by a factor of 0.5 is continued until the dose that will initiate a rise in serum E_2 levels is found. At this point, this "ideal dose" is maintained. When an ovarian follicle reaches 14 mm in 1 diameter, estrogen measurements may be discontinued and scans are performed daily. Treatment is continued until the dominant follicle reaches or exceeds 18 mm. This correlates with an E_2 level of 700–1000 pg/ml among estrogen deficient patients and 1000–1500 pg/ml among normoestrogenic patients. The latter have higher E_2 levels because multiple follicles usually develop during treatment.

As an adequate degree of follicular develop-

TABLE 2   Effect of Pretreatment on Gonadotropin Pregnancies

With Estrogen	13/30 (43.3%)
Without Estrogen	4/60 (6.7%)*

*$p < 0.01$

ment is achieved, the rapidly rising estrogen levels will stimulate cervical mucus production. When there is an increase in the amount of cervical mucus, as well as an increase in spinnbarkeit and ferning, a fractional postcoital test is performed. In this way, the adequacy of the sperm transport is verified. If the sperm transport is abnormal, a cervical cup insemination utilizing the husband's semen is performed 24 to 36 hours after the injection of hCG. When optimal levels of estrogen are reached, and provided the ovaries are not tender or enlarged, 10,000 IU of hCG are given 24 to 36 hours after the last injection of HMG. The couple is instructed to have intercourse at least every other day, including the last day of HMG therapy, as well as 24 to 36 hours after the hCG injection. Four days and 8 days following the first injection of hCG, 3000 IU of hCG are given to maintain the corpus luteum. The supplemental hCG is withheld if the ovaries are enlarged or tender. Eight days after the first detection of hCG, a serum sample is obtained for measurement of the progesterone concentration. After an estrogen deficient patient has been treated for one cycle, her clinical response (cervical mucus production, ferning, and spinnbarkeit, as well as changes in the configuration of the cervix) is correlated with her daily estrogen levels. If the clinical changes were able to predict the rising estrogen levels, the frequency of serum samples may be markedly reduced during subsequent courses of treatment.

By utilizing this protocol, we have been able to achieve ovulation in 99 percent of our courses of therapy. This high rate surpasses that in other published reports and reflects careful patient selection as well as strict adherence to the protocol. Only 6 percent of our pregnancies have been multiple gestations and none has been of a number greater than triplets. Minimal ovarian enlargement (5–10 cm), which resolved spontaneously, occurred in 7 percent of our treatment cycles. This same regimen should be used in hypogonadotropic women who have hyperprolactinemia and who do not respond to bromocryptine.

To summarize, treatment with HMG is complex. In the absence of a carefully planned protocol and strict adherence to it, and in the absence of careful monitoring techniques, treatment with human menopausal gonadotropins may lead to complications. However, with appropriate protocol and monitoring techniques, almost all patients treated may expect to ovulate safely. Pregnancy rates of approximately 60 percent, with a very low rate of multiple gestations and other complications, may be expected. Although the rate of spontaneous abortion is increased somewhat, no increase in the incidence of congenital anomalies has been reported.

Future therapy for patients with hypogonadotropism who wish to conceive may involve gonadotropin releasing hormone (GnRH, LRF, LHRH). Except for those patients who have Sheehan's syndrome or who have undergone hypophysectomy, GnRH should induce ovulation. The most efficient method of treatment may be with a cigarette package-size pump that injects a small amount of GnRH intravenously at 90-minute intervals. This method has resulted in a few pregnancies in preliminary trials and has the theoretic advantage of a lower rate of multiple gestations because the pituitary-ovarian system of interaction is kept intact. If future studies are confirmatory, GnRH will become a valued addition to our therapeutic armamentarium.

The management of the hypogonadotropic patient should be individualized according to the guidelines outlined. These protocols result in a satisfactory outcome for almost all women.

DYSMENORRHEA

DAVID R. HALBERT, M.D.

Therapy for primary dysmenorrhea has changed considerably over the last ten years. With the recognition that abnormalities in prostaglandin production seemed to play an etiologic role in the eventual production of pain, usage of antiprostaglandin agents was a logical extension of pioneering work by Pickles and others.

Significant dysmenorrhea affects as many as 40 percent of all women at least sometime in their menstrual lives. Various estimates of time lost from school and work leave little doubt that this common discomfort has considerable social and monetary impact. The degree of discomfort suffered at least one or two days each month varies, but certainly significant numbers of menstruating women experience total disability when the pain is at its worst. The role of psychosomatic factors, once overemphasized in older texts, is almost passé and a more sympathetic physician approach has developed, encouraged by the discovery that organic factors cause dysmenorrhea in most women. Factors of individual reactivity to pain must still be considered in treating patients.

PATHOPHYSIOLOGY

The pathophysiology of abnormalities in prostaglandin production by the endometrium seems to point to the involvement of the prostaglandin $F_2\alpha$, and possibly other precursors or metabolites which are produced in excess or retained in the endometrial cavity when menses begin. The accumulation of arachidonic acid, as well as the prostaglandin synthetase system for the conversion of arachidonic acid to prostaglandins in endometrial cells, increases dramatically after ovulation as menses near. Endometrial cellular necrosis occurring about 12 hours before visible bleeding seems to be the triggering event for lysosomal breakdown and the rapid conversion of arachidonic acid to active prostaglandins. The release of prostaglandin $F_2\alpha$ and perhaps other prostaglandins leads to their local action on myometrium with intense smooth muscle contractions.

Whether the final pathway of pain production involves simply intense muscle contraction or muscle ischemia perhaps similar to anginal pain, or whether it involves a prostaglandin effect on uterine nerve endings also is unclear. Various techniques of intrauterine pressure monitoring have demonstrated increased frequency and intensity of uterine contractions occurring concomitantly with pain, and also that antiprostaglandin agents gradually slow and stop both contractions and pain.

Studies of endometrial prostaglandin production using techniques of menstrual dressing extraction, endometrial jet wash, tissue assays, and cervical caps all show significantly elevated levels of prostaglandin $F_2\alpha$ in dysmenorrheic women compared with pain-free controls. There are, however, some women who do not show these elevations of prostaglandin with painful menses, and clinically only 70 to 85 percent of women respond well to antiprostaglandin therapy. There are obviously other factors, as yet undefined, that cause menstrual pain for some women.

Several mechanisms of prostaglandin excess may be operative. Overproduction is probably responsible for some dysmenorrhea, but prolonged uterine retention of necrotic debris and menstrual effluvia containing high levels of prostaglandins may be responsible for myometrial stimulation. It is also probable that myometrial vascular absorption of prostaglandins results in some of the distant systemic effects of smooth muscle contraction now recognized as part of the primary dysmenorrhea syndrome. These effects are bowel hypermotility manifested by nausea, vomiting, and stool frequency, as well as vasoactive phenomena like fainting, flushing, paleness, dizziness, and headache. Dilation of the stenotic cervix, most often during childbirth but occasionally with therapeutic dilation of the cervix, seems to be very effective in providing pain relief for some, presumably because of freer egress of prostaglandin-containing menstrual products.

DIAGNOSTIC CONSIDERATIONS

Therapy for primary dysmenorrhea depends in part on recognition of this entity as having different organic pathologic factors from those responsible for secondary dysmenorrhea. There is significant overlap of symptoms between primary and secondary dysmenorrhea. Fortunately, the advent of laparoscopy has allowed a much freer identification of endometriosis and the residual of pelvic infection. There are probably also many women experiencing pain from both primary and secondary dysmenorrhea. A woman's partial response to antiprostaglandin drugs may in fact represent total relief of her primary dysmenorrhea and little if any relief of secondary dysmenorrhea.

The syndrome of primary dysmenorrhea involves crampy pain a few hours prior to the onset of flow or with flow; the pain generally lasts a few hours, perhaps as long as 48 hours. Some pain is relieved with the onset of flow. Nausea occurs in 50 percent, vomiting in 25 percent, and stool frequency or diarrhea in 35 percent of dysmenorrheic women. Other vasoactive phenomena, including paleness, dizziness, fainting, and headache, are less frequent, but when they occur compound the misery. Antiprostaglandin therapy seems particularly effective in blocking the intestinal hypermotility, especially if the patient is pretreated with antiprostaglandin agents a day or more prior to expected menses.

Secondary dysmenorrhea is more likely to produce continuous rather than crampy pain, to last longer through the menstrual period, and to be associated with pre- or postmenstrual soreness or with pain at other times of the cycle. There may be a history of pelvic infection. Acquired dysmenorrhea occurring from a woman's late twenties onward may suggest adenomyosis or endometriosis. Dyspareunia as well as painful bowel or bladder function, especially with menses, is suggestive of endometriosis. Pain with body movements suggests an organic cause. Failure of usually successful antiprostaglandin agents, including oral contraceptives, is suggestive of secondary dysmenorrhea and should encourage an aggressive laparoscopic approach. Identification of endometriosis or pelvic infection usually leads to quite different therapy to relieve the pain. When appropriate, sometimes only hysterectomy and pathologic examination of the uterus will finally reveal adenomyosis.

It is presumed that almost all secondary dysmenorrhea will not respond to antiprostaglandin agents. That presumption may or may not be correct; clinicians believe, at least theoretically, endometriosis occasionally may respond to antiprostaglandin agents. As expected, elevated prostaglandin levels have been found in peritoneal fluid of patients with endometriosis.

TREATMENT OF PRIMARY DYSMENORRHEA

Probably all of the antiprostaglandin drugs currently available will help at least some patients with dysmenorrhea. Aspirin has the advantage of not sedating or interfering with critical functioning in daily situations, such as work, school, or driving. Agents blocking the prostaglandin synthetase system are most effective when started one to three days prior to the onset of flow. Indomethacin, 25 mg t.i.d. 1 to 3 days prior to menses, was tried; about 70 percent of patients obtained relief, but an unacceptably high frequency of central nervous system side effects, such as headaches and peculiar psychic effects, has limited its applicability.

Ibuprofen, 400 mg t.i.d., and naproxen sodium 275 mg with 2 tablets to start and 1 q.i.d. or t.i.d., have been advocated both for use with the onset of menses and for pretreatment before a period. Most patients will find their own best timing of doses with a little experimentation.

Pretreatment schedules are difficult in patients with irregular periods. The idea of an "impact" dose followed by a maintenance dose if pain persists has been found effective with both naproxen sodium and mefenamic acid. At the present time, we advise the administration of mefenamic acid (2 250-mg capsules) at the onset of pain or period, followed every 6 hours by 250 mg. This approach seems attended by few side effects.

Side effects of newer antiprostaglandin agents are minimal. Gastrointestinal irritation seems to be the most frequent, particularly if patients take double doses of a drug or take it more frequently than recommended when pain relief is not as complete as desired. Fortunately the duration of therapy is short, tending to minimize side effects, even if the patient does take more than recommended doses. Other modalities for pain relief should be used in patients with asthma and prior ulcer disease.

The majority of patients using oral contraceptives have long been known to obtain relief from dysmenorrhea. Combination oral contraceptives work better than sequentials. A decrease in prostaglandin production in patients on pills has been shown, both by a direct effect in the endometrium as well as by a reduction in the mass of the endometrium to be expelled at menses. Recently, decreased myometrial reactivity in patients on oral contraceptives has been demonstrated when prostaglandin $F_2 \alpha$ was given intravenously or instilled directly into the endometrial cavity. This effect was seen at all phases of the cycle. Other mechanisms explaining the success of the pill in treating dysmenorrhea may be possible and should be explored.

If the patient with dysmenorrhea needs contraception, a strong case for considering the pill can be made. A recent study has shown that dysmenorrhea and its potential relief were factors in choosing to use a pill among 20 percent of young women requesting contraception. As a result of public concern for possible pill side effects engendered by frequent articles in lay literature, there is sometimes resistance to trying the pill. It is reasonable to consider the pill as a therapeutic drug to control dysmenorrhea even if contraception is not a consideration. Young patients and their parents accept this if other antiprostaglandin drugs have been tried and proved ineffective. This is particularly true if patients are significantly incapacitated. In so doing, the risks and potential side effects are balanced against pain relief and the ability to function. No studies exist comparing antiprostaglandin agents and the pill in relief of dysmenorrhea in the same individual. If relief is incomplete both may be used. The ability to live, work, and study through menses without the soporific effect of analgesic drugs should be emphasized in proper perspective.

With new therapeutic approaches to dysmenorrhea much unnecessary discomfort can be prevented. Even now many patients are unaware of how much of their dysmenorrhea could be alleviated. Equally important, the existence of a group of patients failing to respond at all to medical management eventually becomes apparent. No studies indicate what percentage of these patients have endometriosis or other causes of secondary dysmenorrhea. It is likely to be well above the average incidence in normal patients or in all patients initially presenting with dysmenorrhea. With the ability to coagulate endometriosis through the laparoscope or to treat it medically with Danacrine or surgery, there is a real need to be aggressive with laparoscopy for those facing many years of discomfort or incapacitation.

POLYCYSTIC AND SCLEROCYSTIC OVARIES

MARVIN A. KIRSCHNER, M.D.

The polycystic, sclerocystic, or androgenizing ovary syndrome represents a spectrum of abnormalities ranging from idiopathic hirsutism to polycystic ovaries to hyperthecosis. Although the pathogenesis of these abnormalities is not entirely clear at this time, it appears that chronic hypersecretion of LH and suppressed FSH is associated with overgrowth of stromal or lutein cells, excess androgen production, and blighted ovarian follicles. The spectrum of histologic changes ranges from no or minimal abnormalities, to severe sclerotic changes and stromal cell overgrowth associated with major excesses of androgen production.

Women with polycystic ovaries (PCO) generally seek medical advice for the following reasons: (1) menstrual abnormalities (oligo- or amenorrhea); (2) infertility; (3) control of hirsutism; (4) obesity. Of these problems, menstrual disturbances are most easily treated. Infertility problems generally have a favorable prognosis. Hirsutism and obesity are the more difficult of these problems to control adequately.

TREATMENT OF MENSTRUAL DISTURBANCES

In a small percentage of women with polycystic ovary syndrome, oligo- or amenorrhea may be the only symptomatic abnormality; however, in the majority of cases hirsutism is present along with the menstrual disturbances. For those women with PCO who are fortunate enough to have only menstrual abnormalities, reassurance as to the benign pathophysiology of the disorder and favorable outlook for future pregnancy will generally suffice. Such women can be counseled that their reproduction system is "intact" and that when fertility is desired, the outlook is favorable, although pharmacologic measures may be required.

Women with PCO should be cautioned that oligo- or amenorrhea *does not* necessarily mean they cannot ovulate at any given time. Such women cannot safely use rhythm methods for contraceptive purposes, since ovulatory timing may be quite erratic. Should pregnancy not be desired, usual contraceptive measures may be used.

PCO patients with menstrual abnormalities who desire monthly menstrual periods can be offered oral contraceptives. Combination contraceptives containing minimal estrogens and adequate progestins taken for 21 days will produce withdrawal bleeding, as in normal women. Such drugs will, of course, cause anovulation and can serve as contraceptives as well. Further, oral contraceptives represent reasonably effective therapy for control of hirsutism.

Oral contraceptives should not be given to women with previous history of breast nodules, endometrial carcinoma, or jaundice of pregnancy, nor should they be used in women beyond the age of 40. Periodic follow-up office visits are useful to be certain that oral contraceptive usage is not associated with development of hypertension, diabetes, or thromboembolic phenomena.

TREATMENT OF INFERTILITY

Patients with anovulation due to PCO who have been unsuccessful in becoming pregnant after six months can be considered as candidates for pharmacologic therapy. Generally such patients respond favorably to ovulation-inducing drugs such as clomiphene or human menopausal gonadotropin (HMG) in combination with human chorionic gonadotropin (hCG). Despite the "relative ease" of inducing ovulation in such women by means of pharmacologic agents, the author strongly urges gynecologists and endocrinologists *not* to treat an anecdotal case, but rather to refer such patients to a center with day-to-day experience and a complete laboratory set-up to provide proper assessment of hormonal parameters during the treatment regimen.

In patients with milder forms of PCO or idiopathic hirsutism who have oligomenorrhea, treatment with glucocorticoids can be associated with normalization of their ovulatory pattern and normal menses. Such treatment with low-dose glucocorticoids can result in normal conception and a subsequent normal pregnancy.

In the majority of PCO patients with anovulation not corrected by glucocorticoids, induction of ovulation can be achieved with a 70 percent success rate by use of clomiphene citrate given for a five-day period on days five through nine following onset of menstrual flow. In women who are amenorrheic, an endometrial slough can be brought about with medroxyprogesterone acetate, 10 mg o.d. for 5 days. Five days after the onset of menses, the course of clomiphene can be started. Clomiphene should be used in the lowest possible dose required to achieve ovulation so as to prevent superovulation that would result in multiple pregnancies. Clomiphene is started at a dose of 50 mg daily for 5 days. Careful assessment of serum estrogens in response to the clomiphene guides the dosage schedule. Other clinical parameters of hormonal response, such as vaginal cytology, cervical mucus changes, or both, are not sufficiently sensitive indicators of estrogen effect to monitor the course of drug therapy. If serum estrogens do not show a significant rise over the ten days following the administration of clomiphene, then ovulation is unlikely at this dosage, and the next course of therapy should be increased to 100 mg o.d. for 5 days, 150, and as high as 200 mg o.d. given in 5-day courses. If serum estrogens show modest responses to the clomiphene dosage (elevations of 500–1000 pg/ml), sexual exposure should be advised q.o.d. from days 7 through 15 following the onset of clomiphene therapy. Ovulation will occur approximately ten to fifteen days after the onset of clomiphene therapy, and a pregnancy rate of approximately 30 percent may be anticipated. If pregnancy does not occur despite an adequate estrogen response and subsequent progesterone elevation (indicating ovulation had occurred), the same dosage should be recommended for the next one to two months in the hope of achieving fertilization. If serum estrogens show an unexpectedly great increase in response to the clomiphene dosage, superovulation is a distinct possibility and the couple should be advised to pass up that cycle for fear of a multiple gestation. The next course of clomiphene should be readjusted downward. The risk of hyperstimulation syndrome and multiple pregnancies with the use of clomiphene is quite low: approximately 5 to 10 percent in most series. Should ovulation not be achieved by clomiphene alone, this agent can be tried in combination with hCG, the latter being given 1 week later as a single dose of 10,000 iu intramuscularly.

Patients who do not ovulate after clomiphene or clomiphene and hCG can be considered as candidates for HMG in combination with hCG. This combination is given to stimulate normal ovarian follicular growth and maturation leading to ovulation. HMG should be started at a minimal dosage (that is, 2 ampules i.m. daily) with close monitoring of serum estrogen levels for signs of response. Once serum estrogens show an increase (500–1000 pg/ml) then hCG is given as a single dose of 10,000 i.m. and sexual exposure is advised on a q.o.d. basis. The use of HMG plus hCG is associated with a somewhat higher incidence of the hyperstimulation syndrome and multiple pregnancies, and therefore close monitoring of serum estrogens is more critical here. If no response of the serum estrogens is noted after two ampules of HMG, the dosage regimen of HMG is increased in a stepwise manner every second day until serum estrogen levels show a sign of response. hCG should be administered at that point, as described above. If pregnancy does not occur despite an adequate estrogen response and subsequent progesterone elevation (indicating ovulation had occurred), the same dosage should be recommended for next one to two months in the hope of achieving fertilization. If, however, serum estrogens show an unexpectedly great increase in response to the administration of HMG, then hyperstimulation and superovulation are distinct possibilities and the couple should be advised to pass up that cycle for fear of multiple gestation. The infertile couple should be cautioned to temper their anxiety to obtain a pregnancy at all costs in order to minimize the chance of multiple pregnancies with their associated risks.

Recent data from several fertility centers suggest that the combination of clomiphene citrate and HMG and hCG may help in decreasing the dosage of HMG required to bring about an estrogen rise, thereby cutting the costs of such therapy.

Most recently the use of gonadotropin-releasing hormone (GnRH) has been used for ovulation induction. The success rates with GnRH are approximately the same as reported above with clomiphene plus hCG. Administration of GnRH appears to be effective in producing proper elevations of FSH and LH leading to follicle growth and subsequent ovulation. At this writing GnRH is not available except on an experimental basis.

A pregnancy resulting from the use of clomiphene, HMG, hCG, or varying combinations of these drugs carries the same favorable prognosis as naturally occurring pregnancies, with no evidence of increased fetal wastage or teratogenicity by the polycystic ovary syndrome. Further, the course of hirsutism in PCO patients does not appear to be significantly altered by a pregnancy.

In a small percentage of women with polycystic ovaries associated with hyperprolactinemia (10 to 15 percent), treatment of the prolactin elevation by means of bromocriptine can be tried in an attempt to lower the elevated prolactin and to bring about normal ovulatory cycles. In such women, a minimal dose of 2.5 mg bromocriptine can be started and gradually raised in increments of 2.5 mg. In over 80 percent of such patients, prolactin levels are quickly normalized and menses ensue.

Ovarian wedge resection formerly was widely used for the treatment of anovulation and infertility associated with the polycystic ovary syndrome. This modality has largely been superseded by pharmacologic agents and is rarely used today to achieve fertility. The major drawback in the use of ovarian wedge resection is the risk of subsequent abdominal adhesions resulting from the surgical manipulation of pelvic structures.

TREATMENT OF HIRSUTISM

Excessive coarse (terminal) hair growth in facial regions, chest, breast, or other areas of the body is generally the most difficult component of the polycystic ovary syndrome from a treatment point of view. Treatment schemes include (1) suppression of hyperandrogenism in the hope of preventing new hair growth and (2) removal of existing unwanted hair. In most cases a combination of both approaches is necessary, with neither method (if used alone) being entirely effective. For additional information on the treatment of hirsutism see Chapter 33.

Suppression of Hyperandrogenism

Oral Contraception. In the author's experience, oral contraceptives appear to be the most effective therapy available in the United States for suppression of the hyperandrogenism of the polycystic ovary syndrome. In Europe, effective antiandrogens are available but they are unavailable in the United States. The author's reference is Ortho-Novum, 2 mg for 21-day cycles beginning on day 5 following the onset of menses. This regimen usually results in regularization of menstrual flow and promotes anovulatory cycles for those women desiring contraception. It is useful to obtain baseline and repeat measurements of serum testosterone at about $1\frac{1}{2}$ months into the therapy scheme to determine if the hyperandrogenic parameters are suppressed by the therapy. If androgen measurements are normalized in this period of time, one can be encouraged to proceed for the lengthy time (12 months or more) usually needed to see improvement. The woman may first observe no new areas of facial hair growth, followed by softening or thinning of the terminal hairs, and finally less frequent need to remove unwanted hair. This sequence of events will occur in approximately 50 percent of women treated; however, only one-third of women treated with oral contraceptives will eventually achieve sufficient improvement to enable them to discontinue their depilatory efforts.

Although androgen suppression by oral contraceptives or other means may occur within days, the major effects of androgen suppression on terminal hair growth occur slowly, and the patient should be told in advance not to expect significant results for approximately 9 to 12 months. In general, 12 months of cyclic therapy followed by a 3-month rest period is recommended.

Patients should not be offered oral contraceptives as therapy if there is a family history of breast cancer, previous history of breast nodules, if the woman is over 40 years of age, or if the woman has major doubts or fears about oral contraceptives. Further, periodic visits are useful to be certain that the oral contraceptives are not resulting in hypertension, diabetes mellitus, or other untoward effects.

Occasionally patients will claim that the 2 mg dosage of Ortho-Novum is "too strong," causing nausea, vomiting, or both. In these circumstances it may be desirable to use a less potent agent, such as Ovulin-21. For additional discussion about oral contraceptives see Chapter 85.

Glucocorticoids. Exogenous glucocorticoids may be useful in suppressing hyperandrogenism, particularly in milder cases of androgen excess. If a test regimen of dexamethasone in a dose of 2 mg daily for 3 to 4 days suppresses testosterone or free testosterone parameters into the "normal" range, this regimen may be tried on a long-term basis. Prednisone, 5–7.5 mg, is given h.s. to suppress the nocturnal increase of adrenal steroid output. This dosage schedule rarely produces any of the undesirable side effects of high doses of steroids. In the author's experience, glucocorticoid therapy frequently results in normalization of menses and often clears up androgen-related acne, but it results in diminution of hair growth in only approximately 25 percent of hirsute women.

Antiandrogens

Spironolactone. This agent, given in a dosage of 25 mg t.i.d. or q.i.d., had been reported by some investigators to improve hirsutism. In the author's limited experience, spironolactone seems to be more effective in decreasing growth of body hair rather than facial hair. Certainly this regimen has fewer potential side effects than oral contraceptives and may be useful in women who do not want oral contraceptives or in whom such agents are contraindicated.

Cimetidine. The histamine blocker has been reported to reduce hair growth by acting as an inhibitor of androgen receptor activity. Cimetidine, in a dosage of 300 mg q.i.d., may be beneficial if given for a period of months. Unfortunately, the cost of such therapy is almost prohibitive.

Cyproterone Acetate. This antiandrogen has been used extensively in European clinics with favorable results in 75 percent of women, far better than those achieved with any of the above regimens. Unfortunately, this drug is not approved for use in the United States.

Removal of Existing Hair

Although most hirsute women have already explored various methods of treating unwanted hair by the time they seek medical advice, it is nevertheless useful to review these methods with the patient so that the proper guidance can be offered and misconceptions or superstitions as to these various methods can be openly discussed at a professional level.

Bleaching. In some cases excessive hair growth in the mustache and sideburn areas can be cosmetically controlled by bleaching. Commercial preparations using a 6 percent hydrogen peroxide solution, along with ammonia and a few soap chips to form a simple paste, can be applied by dabbing with a swab-stick for a period of 15 to 30 minutes, depending on skin tolerance. In women with sensitive skin, shorter exposure times are advised. This procedure can be repeated on a daily basis provided that no extensive skin irritation is caused by the depilatory mixture. Should skin sensitivity develop, shorter times of exposure or a weaker concentration of ammonia can also be tried. In patients with very sensitive skin a mild steroid cream may also be used under a physician's guidance. Bleaching preparations using potassium persulfate are best avoided in view of the anaphylactoid reactions that have been reported.

Tweezing. This seems to be the most commonly used and cosmetically acceptable method for removal of individual long terminal hairs on the chin, chest, and even breast areas. Whereas infrequent tweezing is generally without risk, a folliculitis may develop at the exposed pore. The patient should be advised to prepare the skin with a mild antiseptic in an attempt to prevent such secondary folliculitis. In women with a tendency to keloid formation, this method of depilation should be avoided. It is advisable not to pluck hairs from circumareolar regions as well as from pigmented nevi.

Hot Wax Epilation. This represents a form of mass plucking. Carefully performed, this method can be acceptable to some women; however, ingrown hairs can develop and acute and chronic folliculitis may result from this approach, which in turn may lead to chronic scarring. If inspection of such depilitated regions reveals evidence of multiple ingrown hairs or skin-pitting, alternate methods of depilation should be recommended.

Chemical Depilatories. Chemical keratolytic agents are available at cosmetic counters in the form of cream applications. Whereas such agents (Nair or Neet) are used widely for removing hair from legs and thighs, the use of these agents in the facial regions has generally been less successful. Using chemical depilatories is often time-consuming and is associated with skin irritation in the more sensitive regions. In these regions, such keratolytic agents should be used only if they do not cause undue local skin irritation. Again, a low-potency topical corticosteroid may be required after each application to relieve such skin irritations.

Shaving. Shaving is the safest of the mechanical methods of hair removal, since hairs are clipped at the skin with little or no damage to the hair follicle apparatus and little abrasion of the skin surface. Whereas this method has gained wide acceptance in removal of leg and underarm hair, many women are fearful of shaving regions of the face. There is common belief that shaving of hair results in stimulation of the hair follicle and more rapid regrowth. Shaving does not accelerate the rate of hair regrowth, although the early "stubble" during the initial days following shaving appears thicker and unacceptable to many women. Such women need to be reassured that shaving does not promote rapid hair regrowth and that shaving in combination with antiandrogen drug therapy may lessen the need for depilation with time.

Electrolysis. This is by far the most satisfactory method of permanent hair removal. After careful antiseptic preparation of the skin, a thin electronic needle is inserted along the hair shaft to a point below the skin, presumably to the level of the hair follicle. An electric current of predetermined voltage is introduced, which coagulates the hair root. Older methods using galvanic currents are time-consuming and have largely been replaced by short-wave radio-frequency thermolysis units, which generate local temperatures of 170–200° F. and produce electrocoagulation of the hair root. When properly performed in the hands of a qualified electrologist, who must adjust the amplitude and timing of the electrical current, the procedure is safe and relatively painless. The treated hair is easily removed with no resistance or discomfort. The technique of electrolytic removal of the hair follicle at the root is largely an empiric one. The electrologist arrives at a decision to use a particular amplitude and duration of electrical current based upon factors such as skin sensitivity, thickness of the follicle to be electrocoagulated, and so on. After electrolysis, a temporary blanching of the hair follicle is generally followed by a mild erythema lasting 15 to 20 minutes. Under optimal conditions, electrolysis is an effective procedure for hair removal and probably the most effective method currently available. However, the field of electrolysis is largely unlicensed and medically unsupervised in most states and the technical skills of electrologists vary greatly. Referral to a skilled electrologist (if available in your area) is frequently the most important advice that the physician can provide. In the absence of such direct information, an electrologist who is licensed or who carries "degrees" by self-policing organizations should be sought out.

In recent years several products have been marketed which utilize the principle of an electrified tweezer. These have been widely advertised for home use; however, this approach seems unsound, since the hair shaft is a poor electrical conductor with little chance of transferring sufficient current to the hair roots for electrocoagulation. The use of such do-it-yourself apparatuses should be discouraged, since their effectiveness is probably equal only to that of simple plucking.

TREATMENT OF OBESITY

Although obesity may not be part of the patient's complaint, it is seen in 50 to 60 percent of women who present for evaluation and therapy of polcystic ovary syndrome. Successful management of obesity in such women may have a beneficial effect on their menstrual irregularities and infertility as well as on their hirsutism. Certainly PCO patients with morbid obesity (50 lb above ideal body weight or greater) can be expected to have more complications from a pregnancy, and it appears that pharmacologic management of hirsutism is made more difficult by coexisting obesity. Thus, in devising a treatment regimen for the woman with polycystic ovary syndrome, management of the obesity component becomes as important in the overall plan as treatment of any of the other complaints.

In women with lesser degrees of obesity (40 lb overweight or less), a program of calorie restriction can be offered. A well-balanced, 1000-calorie diet such as offered by self-help groups (for example, Weight Watchers, Lean Line, and so on) can be an effective method for weight control. Such approaches generally offer the possibility of 8 to 10 lb of weight loss per month for the not too obese woman.

In women whose PCO syndrome is complicated by major obesity, simple calorie restriction methods are not very effective for normalization of body weight, since they take too long to accomplish their goals and have an unacceptable rate of dropping-out along the way. We have found that a well-organized weight loss program using supplemented starvation is effective in over 50 percent of well-motivated patients. We use a 300-calorie protein-sparing supplement (Optifast) for this purpose. Patients are withdrawn from food, put on the protein supplement 5 times a day, along with 25 mEq of potassium and multivitamins, and are seen on a weekly basis for intensive medical-psychologic-dietary counseling. In PCO patients with major obesity, weight loss per se may result in normalization of menses. Patients undergoing major weight loss are advised to defer any desire to become pregnant during the period of weight loss. Management of the hirsutism by means of pharmacologic agents, use of local hair-removing agents, or both can be started along with the weight reduction program.

It is apparent that in the obese woman with PCO syndrome, major weight loss by itself will go a long way toward improving self-image. In addition, it appears that pregnancy induction and treatment of hirsutism are considerably facilitated after normalization of body weight. For additional discussion on the treatment of obesity, see Chapter 47.

OVARIAN TUMORS WITH ENDOCRINE MANIFESTATIONS

PETER E. SCHWARTZ, M.D. and
FREDERICK NAFTOLIN, M.D., Ph.D.

Ovarian neoplasms that have endocrine manifestations are predominantly of sex cord-stromal origin. These tumors include the granulosa-theca cell tumors, which most often are associated with estrogenic effects, and Sertoli-Leydig cell tumors, which tend to be associated with virilization. Lipid (lipoid) tumors also may have endocrine manifestations, usually virilization. Human chorionic gonadotropin levels may be elevated in the rare germ cell malignancies of the ovary, including pure choriocarcinomas and embryonal carcinomas, as well as mixed germ cell tumors. Struma ovarii may produce thyroglobulin and triiodothyronine. The common epithelial cancers may infrequently be associated with excessive estrogen production, resulting in proliferation and hyperplasia of the endometrium. Paraendocrine syndromes, in particular hypercalcemia, have been associated with epithelial and germ cell tumors of the ovary. This chapter focuses on the clinical management of patients with ovarian neoplasms causing endocrine manifestations.

SEX CORD-STROMAL TUMORS

Sex cord-stromal tumors (Table 1) may cause feminization or virilization and they are an infrequent cause of precocious puberty. Patients with excessive estrogen production from these tumors may present with amenorrhea when in the active menstruating years, or with bleeding if they are postmenopausal. These patients usually have granulosa cell tumors or thecomas, which are ovarian neoplasms arising from the gonadal stroma. Thecomas often have estrogenic manifestations, including endometrial hyperplasia and occasionally carcinoma. In contrast to granulosa cell tumors, they tend to occur in women over age 30. These tumors are usually diagnosed at the time of laparotomy and are treated with surgical resection only. It is debatable whether the few patients reported to have malignant thecomas truly had thecomas. We tend to think of thecomas as benign lesions.

In our experience, most patients with early stage granulosa cell tumors are found to have asymptomatic tumors on routine pelvic examination, whereas those with advanced malignancies present with symptoms compatible with rapidly advancing epithelial ovarian cancers, that is, abdominal bloating and discomfort. The diagnosis of a sex cord-stromal tumor often may not be made preoperatively. For example, an endometrial carcinoma patient may have a clinically nondetectable granulosa cell tumor found at the time of hysterectomy and bilateral salpingo-oophorectomy as part of the routine treatment for endometrial cancer. The level of concern on the physician's part probably is the major deciding factor in making an early diagnosis. While the outcome of such cases is generally good, timely consultation with a gynecologist or endocrinologist may have a significant effect on any single patient's course and outcome.

Prompt surgery is required in the management of a patient with an adnexal mass suspected of being a malignancy. At the time of the surgical procedure there must be careful intra-abdominal inspection to delineate the extent of disease. The involved ovary should be removed, and frozen section diagnosis is needed. A young woman found to have a unilateral granulosa cell tumor may be quite satisfactorily treated with a unilateral oophorectomy. The opposite ovary should be sampled as well as the omentum. Cytologic washings should be obtained from the pelvis and each lateral paracolic space. This is accomplished by instilling approximately 100 cc of normal saline into each of these spaces and aspirating the irrigant. The samples are sent for cytologic and cell block assessment. The retroperitoneal spaces should be very carefully palpated for enlarged pelvic and para-aortic lymph nodes. Any nodules present in the retroperitoneum are removed. Frozen section examination can establish the presence of metastatic granulosa cell tumor. If the tumor is confirmed as being confined to one ovary, that is, stage Ia disease (Table 2), the patient should be carefully followed for the rest of her life, as granulosa cell tumors are the classic late recurring tumors of the female pelvic reproductive organs. Recurrent granulosa cell tumors have been reported as late as 33 years following the original diagnosis.

A small subgroup of young women with stage Ia granulosa cell tumors have symptoms compatible with a ruptured ectopic pregnancy. At laparotomy, the hemoperitoneum is found to be secondary to a ruptured granulosa cell tumor. These tumors are quite friable, and even if initially they appear to be intact, they may rupture in the process of resection. It would appear that rupture of a granulosa cell tumor in a young woman does not compromise her survival. However, the number of patients who have been found to have ruptured stage Ia tumors in any series is extremely limited.

Advanced stage granulosa cell tumors are most often diagnosed in peri- and postmenopausal women. They present with the same manifestations as seen in the common epithelial cancers. Patients suspected of having epithelial cancers are routinely evaluated with diagnostic radiologic techniques to be certain that the bowel, ureters, and bladder are not involved, and they then undergo bowel preparation prior to an exploratory laparotomy. Following modern concepts of the importance of "debulking" at the time of surgery, a major effort is made to remove all gross tumor. This includes resecting the primary cancer by performing a bilateral salpingo-oophorectomy and total hysterectomy, removing the most common sites to which these tumors may spread microscopically or grossly. The procedure should include a total omentectomy and resection of any implants greater than 2 cm, preferably removing all implants if pos-

TABLE 1 Histologic Classification of Ovarian Neoplasms*

Sex Cord-Stromal Tumors	Common Epithelia Tumors
Granulosa Cell Tumor	Serous Tumors
Tumors in the Thecoma-Fibroma Group	Benign
Thecoma	Borderline malignancy
Fibroma	Malignant
Unclassified	Mucinous Tumors
Sertoli-Leydig Cell Tumors	Benign
Gynandroblastoma	Borderline malignancy
	Malignant
Lipid (Lipoid) Cell Tumor	Endometrioid Tumors
	Benign
Germ Cell Tumors	Borderline malignancy
Dysgerminoma	Malignant
Endodermal Sinus Tumor	Clear Cell (Mesonephroid) Tumors
Embryonal Carcinoma	Benign
Teratomas	Borderline malignancy
Immature	Malignant
Mature	Brenner Tumors
Solid	Benign
Cystic	Borderline malignancy (proliferating)
Monodermal	Malignant
Struma Ovarii	Mixed Epithelial Tumors
Carcinoid	Benign
Mixed Germ Cell Tumors	Borderline malignancy
	Malignant
Mixed Germ Cell and Sex Cord-Stromal Tumors	Undifferentiated Carcinoma
Gonadoblastoma	Unclassified Epithelial Tumors
Pure	
Mixed with Dysgerminoma or other form of Germ Cell	Secondary (Metastatic) Tumors
Tumor	

*Adapted from the World Health Organization histologic classification of ovarian neoplasms. Scully RE: Tumors of the ovary and maldeveloped gonads. *Atlas of Tumor Pathology*, second series, Fascicle 16. Washington, DC: Armed Forces Institute of Pathology, 1978, pp 32–33

TABLE 2 International Federation of Gynecology and Obstetrics Stage-Grouping for Primary Carcinoma of the Ovary

Stage	Description
Stage I	Growth limited to the ovaries
Stage Ia	Growth limited to one ovary; no ascites*
(i)	No tumor on the external surface; capsule intact
(ii)	Tumor present on the external surface, capsule ruptured, or both
Stage Ib	Growth limited to both ovaries; no ascites
(i)	No tumor on the external surface; capsule intact
(ii)	Tumor present on the external surface, capsule ruptured, or both
Stage Ic	Tumor either stage Ia or stage Ib, but with ascites present or positive peritoneal washings
Stage II	Growth involves one or both ovaries with pelvic extension
Stage IIa	Extension and/or metastases to the uterus and/or tubes
Stage IIb	Extension to other pelvic tissues
Stage IIc	Tumor either stage IIa or stage IIb, but with ascites present or positive peritoneal washings
Stage III	Growth involves one or both ovaries with intraperitoneal metastases outside the pelvis, positive retroperitoneal nodes, or both. Tumor limited to the true pelvis with histologically proven malignant extension to small bowel or omentum
Stage IV	Growth involves one or both ovaries with distant metastases. If pleural effusion is present, there must be positive cytology to allot a case to stage IV. Parenchymal liver metastases
Special Category	Unexplored cases that are thought to be ovarian carcinoma

*Ascites is peritoneal effusion that in the surgeon's opinion is pathologic, clearly exceeds normal amounts, or both.

sible. Granulosa cell tumors spread by peritoneal seeding in a fashion exactly analogous to the common epithelial cancers of the ovary. Aggressive tumor reduction surgery is appropriate, because these tumors respond to surgery alone for prolonged periods of time before clinical recurrence is obvious. They have been reported to be sensitive to radiation therapy and, more recently, have been shown to be sensitive to combination chemotherapy. Again, a basic principle for response to radiation therapy or chemotherapy is that those patients who have the least volume of tumor left behind respond best.

One should carefully assess the material obtained for histologic examination prior to initiating postoperative therapy, as the granulosa cell tumor is probably the most frequently overdiagnosed tumor of the pelvic reproductive organs. It is quite common for patients to be referred with a diagnosis that is not substantiated by pathologists who are knowledgeable regarding gynecologic malignancies. Adjuvant therapy postoperatively is recommended on a routine basis for patients who are over age 40, as our experience would indicate that those patients who initially are diagnosed at age 40 or older seem to have a much greater likelihood of developing recurrent cancer. Naturally, if a stage Ia granulosa cell tumor is found in a woman who has completed child bearing, it would be in her best interest to undergo a total abdominal hysterectomy and bilateral salpingo-oophorectomy despite the fact that these tumors most often occur unilaterally.

We routinely recommend whole abdominal irradiation with additional radiation to the pelvis as prophylactic treatment for patients over age 40 who have stage I granulosa cell tumors. The experience using this approach remains quite limited owing to the infrequent presentation of these tumors, and it is difficult to substantiate whether this approach really reduces the likelihood of recurrence in the future. We treat patients with VAC (vincristine, actinomycin D, cyclophosphamide) combination chemotherapy for advanced disease when the residual tumor is greater than 2 cm (Table 3). This treatment consists of weekly vincristine, 1.5 mg/m^2 i.v. for a minimum of 10 and a maximum of 12 courses. The maximum dose of vincristine for any course is 2.5 mg. Actinomycin D, 0.5 mg, is given intravenously daily for 5 days every 4 weeks, and cyclophosphamide, 6 mg/kg i.v. is given for 5 days every 4 weeks. Patients are re-evaluated every four weeks by physical examination, including a pelvic examination, prior to

TABLE 3   Chemotherapy Used for Ovarian Cancer

VAC Chemotherapy	
Vincristine:	1.5 mg/m^2 i.v. weekly for 10 to 12 weeks
Actinomycin D:	0.5 mg i.v. q.d. × 5, repeat every 28 days
Cyclophosphamide:	6 mg/kg i.v. q.d. × 5, repeat every 28 days
MAC Chemotherapy*	
Methotrexate:	15 mg i.v. q.d. × 5
Actinomycin D:	0.5 mg i.v. q.d. × 5
Cyclophosphamide:	5 mg/kg i.v. q.d. × 5
CVB Chemotherapy	
Cis-diamminedichloro-platinum	20 mg/m^2 i.v. q.d. × 5, repeat every 21 days
Vinblastine	0.15 mg/kg i.v. q.d. × 2. repeat every 21 days
Bleomycin	30 units i.v. weekly for 12 treatments

*Repeat each course following bone marrow recovery, that is, WBC > 3000, platelets > 150,000 per ccm.

initiating the next course of combination chemotherapy. The actinomycin D and cyclophosphamide are continued for a total of 18 courses. Experience using this regimen, although limited, has been extremely satisfactory.

VAC chemotherapy is extremely toxic. Vincristine is associated with neuropathy at about the time of the fourth weekly course. Patients initially complain about tingling in their fingers, then tingling in their toes. The neuropathy progresses to a point at which there is a loss of fine motor coordination and subsequently the loss of deep tendon reflexes and foot drop. The development of foot drop requires discontinuation of the vincristine regardless of the number of treatments administered. Young women tend to tolerate vincristine far better than older women. The most severe neuropathy we have observed was in a 58-year-old patient with an advanced granulosa cell tumor who was unable to lift her legs against gravity following the seventh weekly course of vincristine. Following discontinuation of the treatment the neuropathy spontaneously resolved, as will all vincristine related neuropathies. This patient went on to receive 18 courses of actinomycin D and cyclophosphamide, underwent a negative second look operation, and remains free of disease 3 1/2 years later.

Actinomycin D and cyclophosphamide are associated with alopecia and bone marrow suppression, which are spontaneously reversible. Most patients will require hospitalization following the initial course of the actinomycin D and cyclophosphamide in order to receive broad-spectrum antibiotics during a four- to five- day period when they have fever associated with bone marrow suppression. We usually recommend a 20 percent daily dosage reduction in subsequent courses of treatment and reduction of the actinomycin D and cyclophosphamide course from five to four days. Although this regimen is very toxic there is no call for initial dose reduction, because results observed with VAC chemotherapy appear best when it is administered in the intense form recommended above.

Sertoli-Leydig tumors (arrhenoblastomas) occur much less frequently than granulosa cell tumors and represent about 1 percent of malignant ovarian neoplasms. They tend to occur most often in women in the second and third decades of life, although we have seen them in children and in women over age 50. This neoplasm is reported to be associated with virilization in 70 to 80 percent of patients. In our experience, only about 20 percent of patients presented with virilization. In most teenagers, this lesion presents as an asymptomatic mass involving one ovary. Like granulosa cell tumors, Sertoli-Leydig cell tumors may be friable and occasionally cause symptoms compatible with either ectopic pregnancy or a ruptured corpus hemorrhagicum. The routine management of unilateral adnexal masses is exactly the same as for granulosa cell tumors. At surgery one should stage the disease by confirming the nature of the mass by frozen section diagnosis and biopsies made of the opposite ovary, omentum, and any peritoneal or retroperitoneal nodule.

If the tumor is confined to one ovary in a young woman, no further therapy is recommended except for careful, long-term follow-up. Most Sertoli-Leydig tumors that recur tend to do so within a three-year period from the original diagnosis, and aggressive surgery at the time of reoperation is most appropriate. Advanced Sertoli-Leydig cell tumors should be treated with aggressive debulking surgery at the initial operation, as these tumors also tend to spread in a fashion analagous to the common epithelial cancers. It is appropriate to perform bilateral salpingo-oophorectomy, hysterectomy, omentectomy, and bulk tumor reductive surgery. Postoperatively, we routinely use VAC chemotherapy for the management of this disease. Once again we are dealing with very small numbers of patients, but it would appear that VAC is extremely effective in managing advanced Sertoli-Leydig tumors.

Following the completion of a planned program of combination chemotherapy for either granulosa cell or Sertoli-Leydig tumors, we recommend a second look operation. The purpose of this is to assess the tumor response as well as to remove any cancer that may be present at this time. Treatment is discontinued for those patients found to be both clinically and surgically free of disease. Patients who are found to have persistent cancer go on to alternative cytotoxic chemotherapy regimens unless the lesion is localized to one area. There does appear to be a role for dubulking surgery and small field irradiation in the management of recurrent sex cord-stromal tumors. Alternative chemotherapy includes adriamycin, cis-diamminedichloroplatinum, and DTIC (immidazole carboxamide) for widespread disease.

The histologic appearance of sex cord-stromal tumors does not necessarily reflect the endocrine manifestation. Granulosa cell tumors have occasionally been associated with virilization, and Sertoli-Leydig cell tumors have been associated infrequently with estrogenic manifestations, such as endometrial hyperplasia and, in one of our patients, adenocarcinoma of the endometrium.

Attempts have been made to follow patients postoperatively with serum assays for estrogen and progesterone levels. The experience is anecdotal and is usually inconsistent. Our attempts to use serum steroid levels have not resulted in identification of consistent levels to influence management.

GYNANDROBLASTOMA

This is an extremely rare tumor that histologically contains both granulosa-theca cell elements and Sertoli-Leydig cell elements. Clinical management would be the same as that for either granulosa cell tumors or Sertoli-Leydig cell tumors and would depend on the stage of the disease when the patient is first seen and on the presence of residual tumor.

LIPID (LIPOID) CELL TUMORS

Lipid (lipoid) cell tumors of the ovary are extremely uncommon and cause hirsutism or virilization. These tumors usually present as stage I lesions and have infrequently been reported to metastasize. They may produce a variety of androgens and occasionally have been associated with ACTH production. We recently had the experience of treating a patient with a lipid cell tumor who presented with Cushing's syndrome secondary to ovarian tumor corticosteroid production. She was unsuccessfully treated with VAC chemotherapy and received a variety of other combination chemotherapies, as well as antiestrogen therapy, but was unresponsive to any of these regimens. At postmortem examination the patient was found to have massive metastases confined to the peritoneal cavity in a fashion compatible with that of an advanced epithelial cancer of the ovary. The adrenal glands were atrophic and the pituitary gland was normal. Our recommendation for this rare malignant disease remains the use of VAC chemotherapy following aggressive debulking surgery.

GERM CELL TUMORS

Human chorionic gonadotropin may be secreted by germ cell tumors of the ovary, including choriocarcinomas—either pure or as one element of a mixed germ cell tumor—and embryonal carcinomas. The management for patients with a primary ovarian choriocarcinoma, that is, nongestational trophoblastic disease, is to remove the tumor and debulk any tumor metastases present. Postoperatively patients are treated with MAC combination chemotherapy (methotrexate, actinomycin D, and cyclophosphamide) (Table 3). Beta chorionic gonadotropin titers (β-hCG) are obtained on a weekly basis thereafter, and combination chemotherapy treatment is continued as long as the titers are elevated. One should treat the patient for at least one course past the first normal β-hCG titer. MAC chemotherapy is extremely toxic and is associated with severe bone marrow suppression requiring hospitalization. In our experience this is the most toxic regimen routinely used in the management of gynecologic malignancies, and granulocyte transfusions as well as platelet transfusions may be required to manage the associated bone marrow suppression.

Patients who have choriocarcinoma as one element of a mixed germ cell tumor, that is, a tumor that may contain focal choriocarcinoma in association with dysgerminoma, endodermal sinus tumor, or immature teratoma, are usually treated with VAC chemotherapy. In our experience it is more common to have choriocarcinoma as a focal area in a mixed germ cell tumor than to find a pure ovarian choriocarcinoma. We recently treated a patient with a hydatidiform mole of the ovary, an event estimated to occur once in six million pregnancies. This patient underwent a unilateral oophorectomy to remove the hydatidiform mole, was followed with β-hCG titers, and has remained alive and free of disease without further treatment for more than one year following her first negative titer. However, choriocarcinoma cannot be managed in this fashion, as it is a highly virulent disease. It must be treated with appropriate combination chemotherapy.

Patients with stage I embryonal carcinomas of the ovary have been reported to have a 50 percent five-year survival rate, and the overall survival rate for all stages of disease is about 30 percent. As is the case with most germ cell tumors, the majority of patients present with stage I lesions. It is a routine at Yale-New Haven Hospital to treat these patients with VAC chemotherapy and follow the progress of the disease using β-hCG titers in addition to alpha-fetoprotein (α-FP) determinations, because embryonal carcinomas of the ovary have been associated with elevations of both these oncofetal proteins. Stage I embryonal carcinomas are now being treated prophylactically for six months with VAC chemotherapy, and patients then undergo second look operations. Advanced embryonal carcinomas are treated with cis-diamminedichloroplatinum, vinblastine, and bleomycin (Table 3) for at least one course beyond the first normal α-FP and β-hCG titers. Cis-diamminedichloroplatinum toxicity includes nephropathy, neuropathy, and severe nausea and vomiting. Vinblastine is associated with severe bone marrow suppression, and bleomycin has cutaneous (rash) and pulmonary (interstitial fibrosis) complications.

Struma ovarii is a benign lesion of germ cell origin which may infrequently be associated with symptoms of hyperthyroidism. Its treatment is simply the removal of the involved ovary. Malignant struma ovarii is rarely reported and its treatment is the same as for the other germ cell tumors; debulking surgery followed by VAC chemotherapy.

EPITHELIAL CANCERS OF THE OVARY

The common epithelial tumors of the ovary (Table 1) occasionally have been associated with endometrial proliferation/hyperplasia and less frequently with virilization. Cancers associated with stromal hyperplasia of the ovary are most likely to have endocrine manifestations, and these include mucinous and Brenner tumors. A third category of tumors associated with endocrine manifestations is the Kruckenberg tumor, which is a particular form of metastatic cancer in the ovary.

The management of the common epithelial tumors of the ovary depends predominantly on the stage of the disease and in part on the patient's age. Patients with benign cystadenomas are treated with unilateral oophorectomy if the disease is confined to one ovary, and bilateral salpingo-oophorectomy and hysterectomy if both ovaries are involved. If only one ovary is involved and the patient wishes to preserve reproductive function, this is acceptable. Patients with borderline malignant tumors proven to be confined to one ovary may also be treated with a unilateral salpingo-oophorectomy, provided the opposite ovary and omentum have been sampled and washings have been performed in the pelvis and paracolic spaces. Patients with invasive carcinomas of the ovary are treated aggressively with bilateral salpingo-oophorectomy, hysterectomy, and omentectomy. Metastatic disease should be treated with aggressive debulking surgery.

It is our routine to use postoperative adjuvant chemotherapy in the form of melphalan for low grade ovarian cancers confined to the ovaries. Melphalan is an oral alkylating agent that has been demonstrated to be as effective as whole abdominal irradiation using the moving strip technique for the management of stage I and II disease and stage III disease when no residual gross tumor is present. Estimated five-year survival rates for patients treated with melphalan alone are approximately 85 to 90 percent for stage I cancer. The standard dosage is 0.2 mg/kg orally for 5 days every 4 weeks, provided the total white blood cell count is greater than 3000 and the platelet count is greater than 150,000 per mm^3. Patients are re-evaluated every four weeks by routine physical examination including pelvic examination, prior to initiating the next course of treatment. Side effects are usually mild and include minimal nausea while taking the drug and lethargy at the time of bone marrow suppression. Mild thrombocytopenia and granulocytopenia are noted and may delay the onset of the next course of treatment one to four extra weeks after four to eight courses are administered. Dosage reduction is not usually necessary. A maximum dosage of 80 mg is used for any 5-day course. Second look surgery is recommended at the completion of 12 courses of treatment or 18 months of therapy, whichever comes first. An in-

frequent, long-term complication of alkylating agent therapy is acute nonlymphocytic leukemia. This most often occurs in patients treated for two or more years with alkylating agents and it may be exacerbated by combining radiation therapy with alkylating agents. Treatment of patients found to be free of gross and microscopic disease at second look operations is discontinued and they are followed clinically. Patients found to have cancer at second look operations receive combination chemotherapy; in our experience such patients respond better to these agents than to radiation therapy.

Patients with high grade (poorly differentiated) epithelial cancers or advanced stage lesions are treated with combination chemotherapy consisting of adriamycin (50 mg/m^2 i.v.) and cis-diamminedichloroplatinum (50 mg/m^2 i.v.). These agents are extremely toxic. Adriamycin side effects include nausea, vomiting, and total alopecia in addition to substantial granulocytopenia and mild thrombocytopenia; it has also been associated with congestive heart failure when given in dosages greater than 450–550 mg/m^2. We have found serial left ventricular ejection fractions (LVEF) to be extremely effective in predicting which patients may develop congestive heart failure if they continue to receive adriamycin. Routine use of serial LVEF successfully avoids this complication while affording safe administration of this agent for higher cumulative doses than usually recommended.

Cis-diamminedichloroplatinum has been associated with severe nausea and vomiting, high-pitch hearing loss, serum magnesium depletion, and nephropathy. Nephropathy can be avoided by hydrating the patients vigorously before and after treatment. We routinely give 4 l of intravenous fluid in a 4-hour period along with mannitol diuresis to avoid renal injury (Table 4).

TABLE 4   Cis-Diamminedichloroplatinum Hydrate and Diuresis Schedule for Outpatients

1000 cc D5 0.9 NS with $MgSO_4$ 2 gm over 1 hour
1000 cc D5 0.9 NS with mannitol 25 gm over 1 hour
500 cc D5 0.9 NS over 30 minutes
500 cc D5 0.9 NS and cis-diamminedichloroplatinum (patient should have voided 500 cc prior to cis-diamminedichloroplatinum administration)
1000 cc D5 0.9 NS with 10 mEq KCl over 1 hour
The patient should be instructed to drink 8 oz of fluid every hour for 8 hours following chemotherapy infusion

These agents are administered every 28 days for a maximum of 18 courses prior to second look operations. Patients are evaluated by physical examination, including pelvic examination, every four weeks prior to initiating the next course of treatment. Adriamycin is discontinued when the absolute LVEF drops 15 percent or to levels of 45 percent or less. Cis-diamminedichloroplatinum is administered for the entire 18 courses unless renal function deteriorates.

Alternative chemotherapy includes the addition of cyclophosphamide, hexamethylmelamine, or both to the adriamycin–cis-diamminedichloroplatinum combination. Excellent results have been reported with the combination of hexamethylmelamine, cyclophosphamide, methotrexate, and 5-fluorouracil.

We have recently identified steroid receptor proteins for estrogen and progestins in the common epithelial cancers of the ovary and, using the anti-estrogen tamoxifen, have successfully controlled these cancers for periods of three to seven months in patients who have had advanced epithelial cancers unresponsive to standard therapy. Our most recent protocol compares adriamycin and cis-diamminedichloroplatinum chemotherapy with the combination of tamoxifen, adriamycin, and cis-diamminedichloroplatinum. Tamoxifen in a dose of 10 mg twice daily has few side effects and allows us to administer the adriamycin and cis-diamminedichloroplatinum without reducing the dosage of these active agents.

We have also identified the presence of aromatase activity in the common epithelial cancers of the ovary. It is possible that these cancers are capable of converting androgens to estrogens, which may then act as growth factors for the cancer. Much basic research needs to be done before anti-aromatase agents, such as aminoglutethemide, are used.

METASTATIC CANCER

Kruckenberg tumors are metastatic cancers involving both ovaries; characteristically, the ovaries retain their general shape and are mobile, and histologically, these tumors contain signet ring cells and hyperplasia of the stroma. They have been associated with endometrial hyperplasia and are treated by resection to prevent bowel or urinary tract obstruction. Subsequent treatment is based on identifying the site of the primary cancer.

PARAENDOCRINE SYNDROME

Paraendocrine syndromes have been defined as endocrine disorders produced by tumors whose cells are structurally unlike those of the endocrine gland they mimic functionally. We have recently reported on nine patients on the Gynecologic Oncology Service at Yale-New Haven Hospital who have been found to be hypercalcemic. Three of these patients had ovarian cancers. Two had epithelial carcinomas with clear cell features and one had a dysgerminoma. It would appear that ovarian cancers as well as squamous cell carcinomas of the reproductive organs are capable of secreting a humoral factor(s) that resembles parathyroid hormone in its ability to stimulate bone resorption and renal adenylate cyclase and to inhibit proximal tubular phosphate resorption. Management of the hypercalcemia consists of the management of the malignancy itself, which is to attempt to remove it and treat it appropriately with combination chemotherapy.

Adrenocorticotropic hormone production has been associated with cases of poorly differentiated ovarian adenocarcinomas, as has carcinoid syndrome. Ectopic chorionic gonadotropin production has been verified from a variety of ovarian tumors, as has placental lactogen. Hypoglycemia has rarely been associated with ovarian tumors and tumorlike conditions. At least one gastrin secreting ovarian tumor has been reported. Management of these tumors requires resection of the primary tumor, debulking metastases when present, and adjuvant chemotherapy based on the histologic appearance of the primary lesion.

TUMORLIKE CONDITIONS

There are many tumorlike conditions of the ovary which may be associated with endocrine manifestations (Table 5). These changes occur most often in young women and may be associated with virilization, although conditions such as solitary follicle cysts may infrequently be associated with precocity. Menstrual abnormalities may occur when follicle and corpus luteum cysts are present. Endometrial hyperplasia and endometrial cancers

TABLE 5 Ovarian Tumorlike Conditions That May Be Associated with Endocrine Manifestations

Solitary follicle cyst
Polycystic ovarian disease (Stein-Leventhal syndrome)
Stromal hyperplasia
Stromal hyperthecosis
Massive edema
Theca-lutein cysts (hyperreactio luteinalis)
Pregnancy luteoma
Hilus cell hyperplasia

TABLE 1 Use Effectiveness of Various Contraceptive Methods (Pregnancies/100 Women-years)

Method	Range
Pill	1–2
IUD	1–6
Diaphragm	2–20
Condom	3–36
Spermicides	2–36
Rhythm	1–47

have been associated with polycystic ovarian disease. The management of these tumorlike conditions is based on the histologic confirmation of the lesion to rule out the presence of a malignancy. Castration is usually unnecessary except for the management of polycystic ovarian disease found in association with invasive endometrial cancer. In cases of endometrial hyperplasia, progestin treatment or ovulation induction is often employed following endometrial curettage or biopsy to rule out the presence of a malignancy.

HORMONAL CONTRACEPTION: ORAL CONTRACEPTIVES

SUBIR ROY, M.D.

This chapter reviews why combination oral contraceptives (OCs) are desirable in terms of effectiveness as compared with other methods of contraception; the benefits and adverse effects of their use; the effects of estrogens and gestagens in producing these changes; the absolute and relative contraindictions; when to begin therapy with respect to pregnancy termination; how long to employ therapy; which combination of estrogen and gestragen to employ; and how to proceed in order to use hormonal contraception safely. This review does not deal with gestagen-only therapy, which is associated with unacceptable failure rates as well

as excessive bleeding problems and hence is not recommended as a contraceptive modality. Depomedroxyprogesterone acetate (DMPA), although widely used outside the United States, is not recommended for contraceptive purposes by the USFDA. In addition, the resumption of normal ovulatory function upon cessation of therapy is variable. The progesterone or norgestrel containing intrauterine devices have variable effect on preventing ovulation while uniformly reducing endometrial growth. Their place in hormonal contraception is not covered in this chapter.

Silastic devices containing contraceptive steroids for continuous delivery, such as the subcutaneous implants (containing levonorgestrel) or contraceptive vaginal rings (containing levonorgestrel or norethindrone alone or in combination with estradiol) are research tools and are not yet available for commercial use. Therefore, no further mention is made of them.

WHY USE ORAL CONTRACEPTIVES?

Oral contraceptives are the most effective reversible method of contraception available today. Failures related to patient use are given in Table 1. It is important to realize that failures are inversely correlated with patient age, education, and socioeconomic class, and directly correlated with patient motivation. The desire to delay rather than to prevent pregnancy may strongly influence the outcome of using OCs, as well as other methods. One of the major advantages of the OC, like the IUD, is that it is a coitally independent method of contraception, allowing for greater freedom and spontaneity in sexual relations than coitally dependent methods. Finally, there may be certain benefits to the women's health which may be directly attributed to OC use. Those effects (summarized in Table 2) have not been emphasized in the past.

TABLE 2   Benefits of Oral Contraceptives

Regular Cyclic Menses
  Reduced menstrual blood loss
  Reduced dysfunctional bleeding
  Reduced iron deficiency anemia

Inhibition of Ovulation
  Reduced dysmenorrhea
  Reduced functional ovarian cysts
  Reduced premenstrual tension
  Reduced ovarian cancer

Miscellaneous
  Reduced benign breast disease
  Reduced endometrial cancer
  Reduced rheumatoid arthritis
  Reduced salpingitis

TABLE 4   Mild Adverse Effects of Oral Contraceptives

Estrogenic Effects
  Nausea
  Breast tenderness
  Fluid retention (up to 3–4 lbs)
  Hypertension
  Mood change and depression

Gestagenic Effects
  Weight gain (>10 lbs)
  Acne
  Nervousness
  Amenorrhea

Combination Effect
  Breakthrough bleeding
  Chloasma

WHY NOT USE ORAL CONTRACEPTIVES?

Uncommon, serious adverse effects may occur with OC usage (Table 3). Their incidence and risk rates are based on usage of OCs containing estrogen and gestagen dosages generally higher than the "low-dose" OCs currently being used. Therefore, these conditions may occur less frequently with the newer formulations.

More commonly, mild adverse effects may occur. The estrogenic component alone produces about half of these, while the gestagenic component alone, or in combination with the estrogenic component, may produce the remainder of the symptoms (Table 4). Because of these side effects, there are both absolute and relative contraindications to OC usage. These are summarized in Table 5.

In insulin-requiring or diet-controlled DM patients, the use of OCs of the low-dose variety [30–35 μg ethinyl estradiol (EE2) with 0.4 or 0.5 mg norethindrone (NET)] has not been associated with altered requirements for insulin.

BEGINNING ORAL CONTRACEPTIVE USE

Provided the subject has none of the absolute contraindications to OC usage or has acceptable relative contraindications, OC usage may be initiated.

Adolescent

The sexually active teenager should have at least 3 regular cyclic menses with intervals between 21 and 35 days prior to starting OCs unless she has oligomenorrhea in association with polycystic ovarian disease (PCO) and hirsutism. In individuals with PCO, OC use reduces the LH which

TABLE 3   Serious Adverse Effects

Condition	Increased Risk	Incidence
Cholelithiasis	2x	1/1250
Thrombophlebitis	3x	1/10,000
Thromboembolism	4x	1/30,000
CVA (thrombotic or hemorrhagic)	3x	1/30,000
Liver adenomas		1/50,000
MI in smokers >35 years old	3x	1/50,000

TABLE 5   Contraindications to Oral Contraceptives

Absolute
  Vascular disease
  Hypertension
  Hyperlipidemia
  Cancer of breast or endometrium
  Pregnancy
  Heart disease
  Liver disease
  Kidney disease
  Breast feeding

Relative
  Diabetes mellitus-gestational
  Smoking
  Migrane headaches
  Undiagnosed amenorrhea
  Depression
  Varicose veins

is associated with improvement in this condition. Initiation of OC usage prior to regular menses following menarche may lead to a greater incidence of postpill amenorrhea than the usual 1 percent rate one year after stopping OCs.

Following Pregnancy

Since the first menses following abortion is usually preceded by ovulation, while that following a term delivery is usually not, it is important to initiate OCs earlier in the former than in the latter circumstance. OCs should be started immediately if pregnancy lasts less than 12 weeks; after 1 week if 12 to 28 weeks; and after 2 weeks if 28 weeks to term and the woman is not nursing. This schedule allows the postpregnancy hypercoagulable state to regress prior to initiation of OCs, which may stimulate the liver to increase the production of factors responsible for the hypercoagulable condition.

WHEN TO START ORAL CONTRACEPTIVES

OCs should be started on the fifth day following the onset of menses. The steroid-containing pills are 21 in number, and for patient compliance it is better to use a 28-day regimen (with 7 additional placebo pills) so that a pill is ingested daily. Breast-feeding women should not take OCs because there is a reduction of protein and fat in milk as well as in the amount of milk that is produced. Additionally, the milk contains small amounts of the synthetic hormones contained in the OCs which may be deleterious to the newborn.

WHEN TO STOP ORAL CONTRACEPTIVES

There is no need to stop OCs every few years to rest the suppressed hypothalamic-pituitary-gonadal axis. Pregnancy may occur during such interruptions of therapy.

Pills may be taken until the patient is 40 years of age provided she does not smoke or 35 years of age if she smokes. Beyond 40 years, the risk of serious adverse effects (see Table 3) outweighs the benefits of OCs (see Table 2). In the perimenopausal or menopausal period, OC administration may provide more hormones than are required to relieve menopausal symptoms. Much lower amounts of hormones are needed at this time in a woman's life and can be provided with conjugated estrogen in combination with cyclic 21 carbon gestagens, such as medroxyprogesterone acetate.

WHICH ORAL CONTRACEPTIVE?

Patients should use 30–35 μg EE2 preparations with the lowest gestagen dosage consistent with clinical efficacy. Worldwide, the OC most widely prescribed is probably Lo-Ovral, which contains 30 μg EE2 and 300 μg dl-norgestrel, or Nordette, containing 30 μg EE2 and 150 μg levnorgestrel (l-Ng). These formulations are associated with very low rates of pregnancy, breakthrough bleeding, and failure of withdrawal bleeding. Despite these encouraging clinical experiences, these formulations containing norgestrel do produce significant changes in carbohydrate metabolism and lipid parameters. The use of 75 μg dl-Ng alone without estrogen for 18 months has been shown to alter carbohydrate metabolism by elevating both glucose and insulin at all time periods of an oral glucose tolerance test. These formulations have been reported to reduce high-density lipoprotein-cholesterol (HDL-C), the lipid component thought to be "protective" against the development of cardiovascular disease.

Another low-dose formulation contains 35 μg EE2 and 0.4 mg norethindrone (NET). Formulations with less than 0.5 mg NET alone have not been associated with alterations of carbohydrate metabolism. Oral GTT tests of 35 μg EE2 with 0.4 mg NET compounds have shown no deterioration of glucose tolerance with this formulation. Effects of this formulation on lipids appear to be balanced or distributed uniformly among the lipid fractions so that no significant alteration of lipid metabolism is noted. Whether increasing the dosage of NET to 1 mg would produce similar changes in carbohydrate and lipids as occur with OCs containing norgestrel is unknown, but one would expect changes in carbohydrate metabolism with this dosage of NET based on earlier studies.

Women with a predisposition to acne should use NET formulations, since norgestrel reduces sex-hormone binding globulin (SHBG) and produces increased amounts of non-SHBG bound testosterone and norgestrel, which may enhance androgenic effects such as acne.

Based on the above considerations, it is recommended empirically to use formulations containing 30–35 μg EE2 with less than 1 mg NET on the basis of the theoretic advantage of their production of fewer metabolic alterations. Even if the changes in carbohydrate and lipid metabolism by norgestrel-containing OCs are subclinical, their long-range effects are not known at this time.

HOW TO USE ORAL CONTRACEPTIVES

The pretreatment evaluation of a candidate for OCs includes a thorough screening history to assess absolute or relative contraindications to OC usage (see Table 5). A thorough history and physical examination are required to establish that there are no baseline reasons to exclude OCs. Baseline laboratory assessment is routine except that GC cultures should be restricted to those less than 25 years of age unless the patient warrants it based on history or physical examination.

An informed consent must be obtained prior to therapy which provides the subject with sufficient information to make a decision whether the benefits outweigh the risks of using OCs. An example of an informed consent used at LAC/USC Medical Center is given at the end of this chapter.

The subject must be alerted to signs of potential adverse effects of OC usage. These include pain in the legs, chest, head, or abdomen, or headaches. The subject should be told to contact her physician immediately if any of these signs or symptoms occurs. The physician must assess these findings and should stop therapy during this assessment.

The schedule of return visits should be after 3 months of use and then annually, unless there are side effects, in which case they would be sooner.

COMMON PROBLEMS (P) AND WAYS TO TREAT (T) THEM

P: Patient forgot to take a pill:
T: Take it as soon as she remembers.

P: Patient forgot to take two or more pills:
T: Stop using OCs for that cycle. Use alternate method of birth control. May begin another cycle of OCs 5th day after onset of withdrawal bleeding or after seven days of being off the pill.

P: Patient started pills too late (for example, more than seven days between active pills):
T: Inform the patient that she may not be protected from pregnancy during this cycle and that she should use some form of contraception during the first 10 to 14 days of this cycle.

P: Breakthrough bleeding and spotting (BTB/BTS) during first three cycles of OC use:

T: Provide reassurance: It takes a few months for the body to adjust to the synthetic steroids. With low-dose OCs, BTB/BTS may occur more often, but the metabolic advantages of their use probably warrant accepting BTB/BTS for a few cycles if it resolves.

P: BTB/BTS just before expected menses after many cycles of pill use:
T: Stop OCs and restart in seven days.

P: BTB/BTS occurring any other time of cycle after many cycles of pill use:
T: Add conjugated estrogens, 2.5 mg, or ethinyl estradiol, 20 µg, to her usual pill regimen. If two courses of such therapy do not eliminate the problem, stop OC use and investigate further. This type of bleeding is usually secondary to gestagen dominance, so doubling the number of pills would not alter the estrogen:gestagen ratio.

P: Patient complains of withdrawal amenorrhea:
T: About 1 percent of low-dose OC users will have withdrawal amenorrhea. Although expensive, pregnancy tests with a βhCG sensitivity of 100 mIU/ml can be performed on either serum or urine at the time of the expected menses to rule out a pregnancy. Concern about developmental anomalies should preclude use of OCs during early pregnancy.

Usually, two consecutive cycles of withdrawal amenorrhea do not occur, so a patient can be instructed to continue on the same low-dose OC for another cycle.

If amenorrhea persists and the patient is not pregnant, she can be switched to a pill with no more than 50 µg estrogen. In order not to be confused about the relative potency of ethinyl estradiol being two times that of mestranol, it is probably better to use formulations with ethinyl estradiol (EE2), since all low-dose OCs use EE2. Unfortunately, there are no OCs that have more EE2 with the same gestagen dosage.

P: Patient wants to delay the onset of her menses:
T: Have the patient continue taking the active pills (from another pill pack) for the required period of days, but not more than seven days. Beyond this period, it may not be possible to prevent the onset of bleeding.

Reprinted below is the text of the informed consent form used at the Los Angeles County-University of Southern California Medical Center.

After receiving information from the film, booklet, or class on birth control methods such as the pill, the IUD, foam, condoms, diaphragm, surgical sterilization, natural methods (rhythm), and experimental research methods, I request oral contraceptives (birth control pills) to prevent pregnancy. I understand the pills are very effective (more than 99%) if I take them correctly. As with every medication, there may be side effects or risks for taking the birth control pill.

Minor side effects that are common and annoying, but not usually serious, include nausea or vomiting, weight gain or loss, mild headaches, breast tenderness, spotting between periods or light or missed periods, mood changes, or acne. I should not be discouraged if I have these side effects because they usually go away after taking the pills for a while or after the doctor prescribes a different pill. Spotty darkening of the skin, particularly on the face, like the "mask of pregnancy," can occur and may persist even after stopping the pill.

I should not take the pill if I have high blood pressure, sugar diabetes, heart or kidney disease, or active liver disease because these conditions can get worse with the pill. I also should not take the pill if I have had a stroke, heart attack, or blood clots in the veins or lung (thrombophlebitis).

If I smoke, I should stop smoking if I want to take the pill because of the increased risk of heart attack or stroke in smoking women who take the pill. There is an increased risk in nonsmokers, although much lower than smokers, of getting a heart attack in women over 35. In all pill users, there is an increased risk of getting a stroke or blood clots in legs (thrombophlebitis) or lungs (pulmonary embolus), all of which may be fatal. At age 40 I should stop the pill and use a different method. I should stop the pill and see the doctor at once if I get severe leg pain, sudden chest pain and shortness of breath, sudden severe headache, sudden loss of vision, severe abdominal pain, or jaundice (yellow skin). Although these conditions are very serious, the chance of getting them is small and the mortality risk is less than that of pregnancy. I should not use the pill if I could be pregnant or am breast-feeding. If I have epilepsy, migraine headaches, or severe depression, the pill may make these conditions worse.

Along with my prescription, the pharmacist will give me a booklet, "What You Should Know About Oral Contraceptives," which I agree to read before taking the pills. I agree to remain under medical care and keep my appointments while taking the pill.

MENOPAUSE

HOWARD L. JUDD, M.D.

According to the Bureau of Census figures for 1979 there were 113 million women in the United States, of whom 32 million were 50 years of age or older. Statistics indicate that the average woman experiences her menopause at age 50 and can expect to live another 28 years. There are also younger women who are without ovarian function

because of spontaneous cessation or surgical removal. Thus a large minority of our population is without ovarian function, and these women live approximately one-third of their lives following ovarian failure.

After the menopause, most women sustain a marked decrease of endogenous estrogen production, which can result in a variety of symptoms. Estrogen replacement therapy can correct many of these symptoms, but its use is associated with a number of potentially harmful side effects. Consequently, it is essential that physicians caring for women understand the potential benefits and risks of this type of therapy. This chapter contains a brief review of indications as well as potential complications and contraindications of estrogen replacement. Specific recommendations also are made regarding methods of administering estrogen replacement as well as alternative forms of therapy.

INDICATIONS FOR ESTROGEN REPLACEMENT

Hot Flashes. The hot flash or flush is the most common symptom compelling postmenopausal women to seek medical attention. Approximately three-quarters of women will experience flashes at the time of the menopause. Eighty percent of those having flashes will complain of them for more than one year and 25 to 50 percent for longer than five years. The symptom is real and changes of skin temperature, skin resistance, core temperature, and pulse rate have been measured at the time of the flash. Hot flashes are triggered by a hypothalamic mechanism. At night, hot flashes are associated with episodes of wakefulness, which contribute to the insomnia seen in older women. Estrogen therapy effectively decreases the frequency and severity of the symptoms and improves sleep patterns. Treatment may only postpone flashes, with the symptom recurring after cessation of therapy. So-called "weaning" of the patient by gradually reducing the dose of estrogen frequently minimizes this problem.

Genitourinary. Following the menopause, atrophic changes of the vagina occur, accompanied by symptoms of vaginal dryness, burning, itching, dyspareunia, discharge, and occasionally bleeding. Patients may also experience dysuria and urinary frequency in the absence of positive urine cultures. These urinary symptoms can result from estrogen deficiency, as the urethra and vagina possess a common embryonic origin. It is well recognized that estrogens are effective in overcoming atrophy of the vaginal epithelium and the associated symptoms. Urinary tract symptoms can also respond to estrogen replacement. Relief of vaginal and urinary symptoms occurs with either systemic or vaginally applied estrogen.

Bone. Osteoporosis is the most important health hazard associated with the climacteric. It is a disorder characterized by a reduction in the quantity of bone without changes in its chemical composition. This process is accelerated by the loss of ovarian function, resulting in a greater prevalence of osteoporosis in women than men. This is a particular problem with early castration and in patients with gonadal dysgenesis. Several other factors, including immobilization, Caucasian race, slender body size, excessive alcohol consumption, low calcium uptake, and cigarette smoking may also increase the risk of this disorder.

Of itself, the loss of bone mass produces minimal symptoms but does lead to reduced skeletal strength and fractures. The vertebral body is the most common site of fracture, but fractures of the humerus, distal radius, and upper femur are also enhanced. This last fracture is of particular concern, because it results in an appreciable mortality rate and profound morbidity. Approximately 125,000 hip fractures occurred in older women in the United States in 1979, and this fracture continues to be associated with a mortality rate of approximately 15 percent.

Several studies indicate low dose estrogen therapy can arrest or retard bone loss if begun shortly after the menopause. This effect will continue for at least eight years. Studies of longer duration have not been published to date. Doses of conjugated equine estrogens-CE (0.625 mg q.d.) and mestranol (25 μg q.d.) have been shown to be effective. Smaller doses of mestranol (10 μg q.d.) also may be protective but this is not established. Estrogen therapy also reduces the incidence of fracture.

Cardiovascular. The possible relationship of the loss of ovarian function and estrogen replacement therapy with the development of heart disease has not been clearly defined. Three lines of investigation have addressed the question of loss of ovarian function and heart disease and findings have not been consistent. First, the mortality rates in women in the United States reveal a linear progression from the third to the ninth decades of life with no demonstrable deviation from this linear increase at the time of the menopause. Second, the Framingham study of 2873 women who had bian-

nual examinations for 24 years revealed there was an increase of heart disease immediately after the menopause. Third, case control studies have compared the degree of coronary heart disease or the incidence of myocardial infarction in women who had undergone early castration with age-matched women with intact ovarian function. Although some of these studies have shown increased risk of cardiovascular disease, all reports have been criticized for deficiencies in design and a clear relationship has not been established. Several studies have addressed the issue of heart disease and estrogen replacement and have shown its use to be associated with either an increased, decreased, or unchanged incidence of heart disease. Since heart disease is the number one cause of death in this country, clarification of the role of estrogen replacement in its occurrence is anxiously awaited.

Other Indications. Aging changes of the skin and psychologic problems may be related to the menopause and beneficial effects of estrogen may occur, but these issues are not defined.

TREATMENT OF THE MENOPAUSE

As long as ovarian function is sufficient to maintain some uterine bleeding, no treatment is usually required. As the menstrual pattern alters and symptoms commence, patients begin to seek help and the needs for treatment must then be addressed.

Every woman with climacteric symptoms deserves an adequate explanation of the physiologic event she is experiencing in order to dispel her fears and minimize such symptoms such as anxiety, depression, sleep disturbances, and so on. Reassurance should emphasize what the climacteric is not—that, contrary to anything the patient may have heard, she need not expect sudden aging or personal disasters of any sort. Specific reassurance about continued sexual activity is important.

Estrogen replacement is the hallmark of treatment of the menopause. Before administering this form of therapy, a discussion of the advantages as well as complications and contraindications of estrogen replacement therapy should be conducted with each patient. The following is a brief review of complications.

Complications

Endometrial Cancer. Several recent reports have suggested that prolonged use of estrogens by postmenopausal women may be associated with an increased risk of the development of endometrial carcinoma. Current concerns are based on two types of data: (1) data reporting a possible increase in the incidence of endometrial carcinoma, and (2) epidemiologic studies showing a possible association between estrogen usage and endometrial cancer.

Several investigative teams have reported an increased incidence of endometrial cancer occurring in the early 1970s. The rise was most marked among middle-aged women but was also noted to a lesser extent among premenopausal women, aged 35 years and above, and elderly subjects over 75 years of age. This increase paralleled the rise in sales of estrogens in the United States from $15,422,000 in 1962 to $82,777,000 in 1975, an increase of 437 percent. Inflation accounted for only a small part of this increase, since the price of the most commonly prescribed estrogen increased only 25 percent during that period. Since 1975 there has been a decrease in the incidence of endometrial cancer. This has paralleled a decline in the national sales of estrogens. Reports have also indicated a rise in the incidence of endometrial carcinoma in other countries, such as Finland and Czechoslovakia. In the latter country there has not been a parallel increase in the use of estrogens.

There also have been numerous recently published reports showing an association between estrogen replacement and endometrial carcinoma. These reports claim that estrogen replacement therapy may be associated with three- to eightfold increase in the likelihood of developing endometrial carcinoma. Questions have been raised as to whether these epidemiologic studies were adequately conducted. Of particular concern has been the selection of control subjects. Despite these concerns, the agreement of general risk factors and observed relationships in the numerous studies reported to date suggest that the relationship between postmenopausal estrogen intake and endometrial carcinoma is real.

In several reports implicating estrogen usage as a factor in endometrial cancer, there was substantial evidence that the association is dose- and duration-related. The cyclic administration of estrogen has not been conclusively shown to be a protective factor. The apparent increase in cancer incidence, and indeed those cases associated with estrogen intake, appear to be confined to localized disease. Among patients with localized disease, the five-year survival rates are approximately 95 percent. This may explain the observation that

there has been made no demonstrable increase in the mortality rate for endometrial carcinoma despite the presumed impact of estrogen usage.

Breast Cancer. The breast cancer risk factors of early age at menarche and delayed age at menopause indicate that ovarian activity is an important determinant of risk in this cancer and suggest a critical role for estrogens. This is strongly supported by findings in the extensive studies of the role of estrogens in the occurrence of mammary tumors of rodents.

Early studies of the possible effects of estrogen replacement therapy on the risk of breast cancer were largely uncontrolled follow-up studies, which suffered from methodologic problems making interpretation difficult. Recently, five case-control studies have been reported which have overcome many of the methodologic difficulties of earlier studies. Three of these studies used healthy population control subjects and found a mild increase in breast cancer risk. One of these studies found a dose relationship. A fourth study used a self-referring healthy population as a control and found an increased overall risk only among women with a previous history of oophorectomy. The investigators also reported an increased risk for women with intact ovaries who received high doses of estrogen. A fifth study, using hospitalized subjects as controls, found no evidence of an increased risk.

Thus there is growing evidence that estrogen replacement therapy may possibly be associated with an increased risk of breast cancer. If so, the magnitude of the elevated risk appear to be small and has not been consistently found. Nevertheless, with a common disease such as breast cancer, even a small increase in risk could potentially result in a substantial number of cases.

Liver. Sex steroids have profound effects on hepatic function. Alterations of hepatic protein and lipid metabolism can lead to various other side effects. These include the following:

Hypertension. Hypertension may occur or be exacerbated in women receiving estrogen replacement therapy. The elevation of blood pressure is usually reversible when the medication is discontinued. The problem is seen less frequently with estrogen replacement therapy then with use of oral contraceptives. Although increases of blood pressure have been reported, estrogen replacement therapy has not been associated with an enhanced risk of cerebrovascular accidents.

The mechanism responsible for this increase in blood pressure is believed to be related to the renin-angiotensin-aldosterone system. Renin substrate is the rate-limiting step of the renin reaction under physiologic conditions. Estrogen administration stimulates the hepatic synthesis of this protein. Associated with this are increases of angiotensin I, and aldosterone secretion.

Thromboembolic Disease. It has been observed that the administration of oral contraceptives increases the risk of overt venous thromboembolic disease and the occurrence of subclinical thrombosis that is extensive enough to be detected by laboratory procedures, such as ^{125}I fibrinogen uptake and plasma fibrinogen chromatography. In uncontrolled studies, thrombophlebitis has been reported with estrogen replacement therapy, whereas this association has not been found in controlled studies.

Lipids. Estrogen replacement therapy also influences hepatic lipid metabolism. An increased incidence of gallbladder disease has been reported with oral contraceptive usage and estrogen replacement therapy. Because cholesterol saturation of bile is between 75 and 90 percent, small increases of cholesterol can produce precipitation leading to stone formation. Increased amounts of cholesterol in bile is a common finding in gallbladder disease. Estrogen replacement therapy increases the cholesterol fraction of bile. Proposed mechanisms for this include increased turnover of body cholesterol and increased hepatic synthesis.

Circulating lipids are also influenced by estrogen replacement therapy. Lipids are mostly bound to proteins in the circulation, and the concentration of the various types of lipoproteins correlate with risk of heart disease. Low density and very low density lipoprotein levels correlate positively, while high density lipoprotein concentration correlates negatively with the risk of heart disease. Estrogen replacement therapy decreases low density and very low density lipoproteins plus cholesterol, and increases high density lipoproteins and triglycerides. In patients with familial defects of lipoprotein metabolism, estrogen replacement therapy has been associated with massive elevations of plasma triglycerides, which has led to pancreatitis and other complications. The effects of estrogen on circulating lipids are also believed to be related to changes in hepatic synthesis, although altered clearance of these substances may be involved.

Contradictions and Precautions

Contraindications to estrogen replacement therapy include undiagnosed vaginal bleeding, acute liver disease, chronic impaired liver function, acute vascular thrombosis (with or without emboli), neuro-ophthalmologic vascular disease, and breast carcinoma. Estrogens may have adverse effects on some patients with pre-existing hypertension, fibrocystic disease of the breast, uterine leiomyoma, familial hyperlipidemias, migrainous headaches, chronic thrombophlebitis, endometriosis, and gallbladder disease. Although estrogen administration has not been shown to have adverse effects on patients who have been treated for endometrial cancer, many physicians continue to be reluctant to administer the medication to these women.

Principles of Estrogen Replacement

Generalized guidelines for hormonal replacement for all postmenopausal patients cannot be outlined. Each patient needs to be evaluated individually and her symptoms and risk factors must be considered.

Current replacement therapy should be directed toward the relief of hot flashes and atrophic vaginitis and the prevention of osteoporosis. Its use for other indications should be approached with caution until further research establishes beneficial effects.

In patients with hot flashes and vaginal atrophy, the severity of the symptom is important. If disabling, replacement should be considered. If minimal or absent, the need for treatment is reduced. About one-third of older women will develop osteoporotic fractures. Since the majority of women will not, I do not recommend estrogen replacement to all women. For the prevention of osteoporosis, other clinical criteria should be considered. Reduced body size, Caucasian race, history of smoking, and early castration are all factors that have been associated with an increased incidence of this disorder. Patients with these risk factors should be encouraged to consider preventive therapy.

The purpose of therapy will also dictate how replacement should be given. Hot flashes can be treated for finite periods of time with progressive reduction in dosage. Prevention of osteoporosis with estrogen requires long-term therapy.

If estrogens are given, certain factors seem to influence the incidence of complications. It does not appear to make any difference which preparation is prescribed. All have been incriminated in the genesis of side effects, particularly endometrial cancer. High dosage and prolonged use are associated with increased risk. Although results have been inconclusive concerning the benefits of interrupted versus continuous therapy, it is recommended that interrupted therapy be administered with at least a four-day medication-free interval. Combination estrogen-progestin (E + P) therapy has certain advantages over estrogen administration alone. This form of therapy reduces the incidence of endometrial cancer and hyperplasia formation but results in periodic vaginal bleeding, an unacceptable condition to some postmenopausal patients. This is helpful, since it appears that progesterone provides protection without regular endometrial shedding. If estrogen is given in a continuous fashion, the use of progesterone for 10 to 13 days each month provides the most complete protection.

When considering E + P administration, it must be remembered that complications of estrogen therapy are not limited just to the effects on the endometrium. For some of the other side effects, the combined use of E + P does not prevent the action of estrogen. The complications associated with oral contraceptives are examples of this. Thus the use of combination replacement has potential advantages but does not prevent all adverse effects of estrogen therapy.

Management of Estrogen Therapy

Prior to the institution of estrogen replacement therapy, a complete and thorough evaluation of the patient should be performed. This examination should include (1) a history, with specific reference to contraindications and precautions; and (2) a physical examination, including blood pressure, breast, and pelvic examinations (including cervical/vaginal smears) for cancer detection.

Following this, a careful analysis of the potential benefits and risks of estrogen replacement must be undertaken, individualized for each patient. If, on the basis of this information, the patient wishes to receive estrogen replacement therapy, the following recommendations should be followed:

1. Estrogen therapy should be given utilizing the lowest dosage compatible with effective treatment of the indicated symptom (such as hot flashes, atrophic vaginitis, or osteoporosis). For hot flashes, daily dosages of .625–1.25 mg of CE for 21 or 25 days each month are usually necessary. In some cases higher dosages may be required. For treatment of vaginal atrophy, .625 mg is usually effective. For prevention of osteoporosis, the lowest daily dosage that provides protection is 0.625 mg. Relative potencies of other estrogens with CE have not been worked out, with the exception of ethinyl estradiol, which is approximately 125 times as potent on a per weight basis.

2. In women with a uterus, sequential addition of a progestin, such as medroxyprogesterone acetate, 10 mg during the last 10 days of estrogen administration, is recommended. Lower doses of medroxyprogesterone acetate may be protective, but this has not been established. The use of 19 nortestosterone agents is not recommended, since these block the estrogen stimulated rise of high-density lipoprotein cholesterol. There are no data available which substantiate that progestin therapy is beneficial to women without a uterus.

3. If treatment with sequential E + P therapy is instituted, it is my view that endometrial biopsy is not required prior to institution of therapy (unless other indications exist, such as postmenopausal bleeding). This recommendation is based on several observations. First, the use of cyclic progesterone will treat hyperplastic lesions of the endometrium. Second, the average yearly incidence of endometrial cancer in women not taking estrogens is 0.7 per thousand. Based on routine endometrial sampling of postmenopausal subjects, 50 to 75 per cent of discovered endometrial cancers are symptomatic, that is, associated with abnormal vaginal bleeding. Thus it would require over 2900 endometrial biopsies to uncover a single lesion in an asymptomatic woman. Conservative estimates of the charges by a physician to perform the biopsy and the pathology laboratory to process the sample would be $40 or greater. Based on these estimates, it would cost in excess of $100,000 to identify each patient with asymptomatic endometrial cancer. These figures indicate that the routine use of pretreatment endometrial biopsy in asymptomatic patients who are to receive E + P therapy is not cost effective.

It is recognized that E + P therapy may result in some scheduled withdrawal vaginal bleeding (that is, during the pill-free interval of one week). The patient should be alerted to this probability and counseled concerning the benign nature of this event. However, if breakthrough bleeding occurs at an unscheduled time (during drug therapy), endometrial biopsy should be performed to exclude the development of abnormal histology. Prudence suggests a biopsy be performed in all E + P recipients after two years of treatment even in the absence of unscheduled bleeding. The timing of further biopsies, should any be needed, is a clinical decision based on the results of the histologic examination of the endometrium obtained. The presence of endometrial hyperplasia dictates discontinuation of E + P therapy or more prolonged use of progestin.

4. Some patients may not accept the addition of progestin to their estrogen replacement regimen; others may experience adverse reactions to this combination and request removal of the progestin component. In the absence of progestin, estrogen replacement therapy carries markedly increased risks of development of endometrial hyperplasia, and with time the possibility of endometrial carcinoma. With this in mind, the physician should observe the following guidelines carefully:

—Estrogen only therapy (0.625 mg CE or equivalent) is given cyclically for 21 or 25 days each calendar month.

—A pretreatment endometrial biopsy should be performed before initiating estrogen only therapy. If hyperplasia is present, then estrogen only therapy should not be instituted.

—Endometrial biopsy must be performed on all patients who have *any* vaginal bleeding, whether scheduled or unscheduled.

—Prudent management recommends annual endometrial biopsy in patients who do not experience bleeding.

The presence of endometrial hyperplasia requires discontinuation of estrogen only therapy. At the present time, no firm conclusions can be made regarding the carcinogenicity of estrogens. However, the continuing accumulation of data suggesting a relationship cannot be ignored. Prudent physicians now recognize the possibility and advise their patients accordingly.

5. All patients on estrongen replacement should be seen regularly, usually at six- to twelve-month intervals. At these examinations, blood pressure should be taken, a breast and pelvic examination performed, and an evaluation of the effectiveness of treatment noted (that is, relief of symptoms). It is also wise to measure the triglyceride level at the time of the first visit following institution of therapy.

6. Treatment programs for hot flashes should be discontinued and re-evaluated every 12 to 18 months. The prophylaxis and treatment of osteoporosis, if successful, will require more prolonged therapy. The exact length of time estrogen should be administered for this purpose has not been defined. Atrophic vaginitis may require treatment for several years and may recur anytime after cessation of therapy.

7. At the present time, the preferred route of administration of cyclic E + P therapy is oral, despite misgivings over portal absorption and liver metabolism. Studies are awaited to define other routes. Injectable therapy, while effective, is *not* recommended on the basis of cost, dose effectiveness, and the hazards of prolonged action. Vaginal placement is effective for relieving symptoms of atrophy. On gm of CE vaginal cream given every other day is sufficient to return the vaginal epithelium to premenopausal values in most patients. Application of this amount of hormone vaginally has a limited effect, if any, on systemic markers of its action, particularly hepatic markers. Thus it may be safe to utilize vaginally administered estrogens in women with hepatic contraindications to estrogen replacement, such as chronic impaired liver function, a history of vascular thrombosis, hypertension, familial hyperlipidemia, and gallbladder disease. Larger doses of vaginally administered CE have been associated with proliferative changes of the endometrium, so progesterone administration should be considered if the patient has a uterus.

8. Women may have severe menopausal symptoms but have contraindications to estrogen replacement therapy. Other medications can be utilized and may be helpful. Ten to 20 mg of medroxyprogesterone acetate and 20–80 mg of megestrol acetate have been shown to reduce the incidence of hot flashes. Clonidine, an antihypertensive agent, in doses of 0.2–0.4 mg may also be effective, but its use is associated with side effects. Sedatives and psychopharmacologic agents have been used to reduce this symptom but their effectiveness has not been studied critically. A variety of nonestrogenic therapeutic modalities, including exercise, calcium, calcitonin, vitamin D, and fluorides, have been recommended for the prevention of osteoporosis, but to date only calcium supplements have been studied prospectively in a double-blind manner and have been shown to be effective. The use of calcium is discussed extensively in Chapter 52. There is no good substitute therapy for vaginal atrophy. Dyspareunia may be partially relieved by the use of lubricants.

It should be clear to the reader that all the important questions have not been answered concerning the problems related to cessation of ovarian function and estrogen replacement. However, if physicians follow the general guidelines reviewed in this chapter, therapy for climacteric symptoms can be expected to be beneficial in most cases.

DISEASES OF THE BREAST

GALACTORRHEA

GEORGE TOLIS, M.Sc., M.D.

Galactorrhea is milk secretion from the breast. If present in a nonpuerperal subject, it may indicate a neuroendocrine derangement. Galactorrhea is graded from I to IV. In grade IV, milk secretion is copious, whereas in grade I, the patient is unaware of it and it is usually demonstrated by the physician.

The galactorrhea syndrome can be subdivided into normoprolactinemic and hyperprolactinemic instances. The current belief is that even in the former cases, there had been a period of hyperprolactinemia.

NORMOPROLACTINEMIC GALACTORRHEA

Chest trauma, infectious process, such as herpes zoster, or breast stimulation can lead to normoprolactinemic galactorrhea. We also have seen women with burns who developed inappropriate milk secretion in the presence of normoprolactinemia. In such patients we usually treat the underlying disorder, that is, nerve infiltration for herpetic pain or suggested avoidance of continual stimulus, such as nipple suckling or breast manipulation. If such measures are ineffective, we then administer bromocriptine instead of estrogens. Although it is established that estrogens (such as Tace) or even androgens may suppress nonpuerperal and puerperal galactorrhea, we believe that the associated morbidity and the lactotrope stimulating capacity of estrogens are reasons not to administer them for the treatment of normoprolactinemic galactorrhea. We believe that suppression of prolactin may further modify the status of lactogenic receptors in the breast and result in suppression of inappropriate lactation. Even if bromocriptine is not effective in the presence of normoprolactinemic galactorrhea, we avoid the use of estrogens. Some have suggested that pyridoxine, 600 mg daily, may be effective in suppressing galactorrhea.

The galactorrhea associated with endocrine disease usually involves normal or only slightly elevated levels of prolactin. The treatment of galactorrhea associated with hypothyroidism necessitates attaining a state of euthyroidism as evidenced not only by normal serum T_4 and T_3 values but by normalization of suppression of the enhanced TSH response to TRH. In some patients with hypothyroidism, galactorrhea may be present with serum prolactin levels of only 12 ng/ml; galactorrhea may disappear with thyroxine treatment at a time when prolactin levels have been lowered by only 30 percent. In these instances, although basal serum prolactin levels are within the normal range and do not change significantly with the achievement of euthyroid status, this may decrease the enhanced prolactin release characteristic of the hypothyroid state.

Galactorrhea may also be seen in polycystic ovarian syndrome, feminizing adrenal carcinoma, and Cushing's disease; in these instances there is only a modest elevation of prolactin levels at most. There appears to be considerable individual variation in the level of prolactin associated with galactorrhea, both prior to and subsequent to treatment. The treatment of galactorrhea associated with these endocrinopathies is directed at the underlying disease.

Galactorrhea may also be associated with neuroleptic drug treatment; in these instances there is usually moderate elevation of prolactin levels. If this is the case, we suggest that drugs be used in minimal quantities or in combination with others that have fewer antidopaminergic properties. If either course is not feasible and the galactorrhea, and associated amenorrhea, are matters of concern, the recommended treatment is 1.25 mg bromocriptine every night for a 4-week period, followed by the addition of 1.25 mg each morning, for a total of 3 months. In unpublished studies, the above dosage does not seem to interfere with the action of the neuroleptics on thought processes, illusions, and so on.

Galactorrhea may also be seen with modest hyperprolactinemia in renal failure. In this instance the dosage of bromocriptine is gradually increased at monthly intervals, that is, for the first month, 1.25 mg bromocriptine are administered each evening; for the second month, 1.25 mg each morning and each evening: for the third month, 1.25 mg each morning and 2.5 mg each evening: and for the fourth month, 2.5 mg b.i.d.

IDIOPATHIC HYPERPROLACTINEMIA AND GALACTORRHEA

This is defined as galactorrhea and hyperprolactinemia in patients without radiologic evidence of an adenoma (see Chapter 10), even though it may well be that current roentgenographic methodologies are still not refined enough to demonstrate such microadenomas. In this condition, therapy is begun with 1.25 mg bromocriptine each evening and the dosage increased by 1.25 mg at weekly intervals, so that by the fourth week the patient receives 2.5 mg twice daily. If side effects of hypotension or gastrointestinal upset occur, the dosage is increased more slowly. If such a patient wishes to become pregnant, we usually advise her to have protected intercourse until the second vaginal bleeding ensues following the initiation of therapy. Therafter, we recommend discontinuation of bromocriptine therapy ten days after the onset of menses in order to permit conception while the patient is off bromocriptine. A beta-subunit assay is obtained if menstruation is delayed by one week. If it is felt that the patient is unreliable with regard to drug compliance, bromocriptine therapy is maintained and discontinued once pregnancy is diagnosed within a week of delayed menstrual flow.

For treatment of micro- or macroadenoma, see Chapter 9.

HORMONAL THERAPY OF BENIGN BREAST DISEASE

PIERRE MAUVAIS-JARVIS, M.D.

A study of estradiol and progesterone receptors in benign breast disease emphasized the fact that only breast lesions with high epithelial cellularity contain significant levels of steroid receptors. This is the case of breast fibroadenomas in particular, but it may also be true for mastodynia and early breast lesions with intense cellular hyperplasia. In other words, the younger the woman and the more recent the breast lesion, the greater the chances that progesterone receptors will be present and the disease will be hormone responsive.

THERAPEUTIC ALTERNATIVES

From a pathophysiologic point of view, several approaches have been proposed for the hormonal treatment of benign breast disease. These are summarized as follows:

Prolactin Lowering Agents

Based upon the fact that prolactin is involved in the genesis of breast cancer in rodents, extensive studies have been carried out on prolactin secretion in humans with benign breast disease. It appears likely that basal plasma prolactin levels are normal in patients with breast disease. However, in some cases plasma prolactin may increase to levels higher than in normal women either during sleep or under TRH stimulation. Therefore, the use of a well-known dopamine agonist, bromocriptine (Parlodel), has been proposed for the treatment of benign breast disease, particularly in the case of mastodynia. Results obtained are contradictory and in my view are not convincing. In addition, the side effects of bromocriptine make its long-term utilization uncomfortable. I believe that no beneficial effect of this treatment has been objectively observed either clinically or with mammography or thermography, at least in patients having an authentic benign breast disease as opposed to galactorrhea due to a pituitary prolactinoma.

Antigonadotropic Agents

Danazol, a derivative of 17α-ethyltestosterone, has been proposed as an antigonadotropic alternative for the treatment of benign breast disease. It is claimed that during experimental studies using Danazol for the treatment of endometriosis, many patients manifested subjective and objective improvement of coincidental benign breast disturbances. Danazol was therefore proposed for the treatment of various benign breast disorders, including fibrocystic disease. The treatment is based upon the negative feedback effect that danazol might exert on gonadotropin secretion. Such an action may lead to a decrease in estrogen production by the ovaries. It has also been suggested that danazol might act directly on target organs as an antiestrogen and also that it might inhibit ovarian steroidogenesis directly. However, no formal proof of any such effects has been demonstrated. Since the aim of danazol treatment is to obtain a low estrogenic activity in the mammary gland, it was interesting to compare it to progestin treatment (see below). The clinical results obtained in my experience with danazol were no more successful than those obtained with progestins. In addition, the side effects of danazol treatment given in a dosage of 200–400 mg daily are those of a mild anabolic and androgenic agent. In my experience, at least, these side effects have been worse than those observed in patients treated with progestins.

Antiestrogens

The use of Tamoxifen has been proposed in the treatment of benign breast disease, specifically for fibrocystic disease. Only two studies have claimed that good results were obtained with daily doses of 10 mg of this antiestrogen. However, the group of patients treated was not large enough and the survey too short (approximately four months) to evaluate the published results readily. In my opinion the rationale for the use of antiestrogens in premenopausal women is not clear. Antiestrogens, such as clomiphene citrate and Tamoxifen, increase pituitary gonadotropin secretion and then estradiol secretion by the ovaries.

Progesterone and Progestins

This treatment is based upon the fact that benign breast disease usually arises in a hormonal milieu of unopposed estrogen. Indeed, patients with severe mastodynia and breast tenderness often have inadequate corpus luteum function characterized by luteal phase plasma progesterone levels which are lower than normal and plasma estradiol levels that are not significantly different from those in normal women.

The fact that progestins can have a biologic effect on the breasts of these patients is derived from observations that progestin treatment of patients with fibroadenomas leads to translocation of progesterone receptor from the cytosol to the nucleus. More recently it has been observed that systemic administration of progestins or local administration of progesterone (by percutaneous absorption) to patients with fibroadenomas increases the 17β-hydroxysteroid dehydrogenase activity in these tumors. This enzyme activity is responsible for the transformation of estradiol, the active estrogen, into estrone, a less active one. In addition, the latter is more rapidly cleared from mammary cells than the former.

PROGESTATIONAL THERAPY

This therapeutic approach to benign breast disease is based on the use of two hormonal agents, namely progesterone and synthetic progestins.

Progesterone

It is difficult to utilize progesterone orally because of its rapid metabolism by the liver. However, it has recently been made available in France in micronized form. At the rate of 300 mg per day given every 12 hours, plasma progesterone levels of 10–20 ng/ml can be obtained 1 to 2 hours after oral absorption. Twelve hours following administration, plasma progesterone remains higher than 3 ng/ml. The main metabolites of progesterone, that is, 20α-dihydroprogesterone and 5α-dihydroprogesterone, remain in physiologic proportion in the plasma. Following administration of 300 mg of micronized progesterone to menopausal women, urinary excretion of pregnanediol can be as much as 20 mg per day.

Progesterone may be given by routes other than oral, particularly in vaginal suppositories. When administered at a dose of 50 mg per day, plasma levels of progesterone similar to those of a normal luteal phase are obtained. However, because of its lack of high antigonadotropic potency, treatment of benign breast disease by systematically administered progesterone does not seem to be an illegible therapeutic method.

On the other hand, progesterone may be used topically by way of percutaneous administration. The percutaneous application of progesterone consists of an alcohol water gel in which the steroid is dissolved. Fifty milligrams of progesterone are applied to the breast daily.

It has been previously demonstrated that topically applied radioactive progesterone can be absorbed through the skin. Labeled metabolites (pregnanediol and allopregnanediol) were recovered in urine tested 48 hours after percutaneous administration of the precursor. I also calculated that percutaneous absorption of the steroid was low, only 10 percent.

Recent in vitro studies confirm the presence of significantly higher levels of progesterone in breasts than in peripheral blood after percutaneous administration of this steroid. In addition, the high fat solubility of progesterone is responsible for a prolonged local retention of the steroid. There is no systemic effect of the steroid, in addition, owing to an extensive in situ metabolism of progesterone in the breast. In particular, no significant modification in endometrial histology and no breakthrough bleeding were observed. For this reason, percutaneous progesterone can be administered every day, including during the menstrual period. Indeed, the fact that progesterone is continuously present inside the breast might result in a permanent antiestrogenic effect, which competes with the possible presence of a high local estradiol concentration.

Progestins

The most effective derivatives in the treatment of benign breast disease are estrane derivatives. Progestins in this series are derived from 19-nortestosterone. Numerous compounds originate from this precursor, but from a practical point of view, it would appear that there are two in widespread use: norethisterone and norgestrel. In vivo, norethisterone acetate, ethynodiol diacetate, lynestrenol, norethynodrel, dimethisterone, and quinestranol are mainly converted into norethisterone, which appears to be the active form of these different molecules. Only norethisterone binds to the cytosolic receptor for progesterone.

Oral absorption of estrane-derived progestins is very rapid and complete. Their urinary and fecal excretion is slower than that of pregnane derivatives, partly because of their binding to plasma proteins, such as TeBG. Their half-life can exceed 24 hours and may induce an accumulation of the steroid in the bloodstream in the case of twice daily administration. Their androgenic activity is relatively high and is probably responsible for their very pronounced antigonadotropic potency, which is much greater than that of pregnane derivatives.

The antiestrogen activity of estrane derivatives is very strong. It has been postulated that

norethisterone and its derivatives might partially inhibit the binding of estradiol to its specific receptor. In addition, certain estrane derivatives have a strong antigonadotropic activity; this is particularly true of lynestrenol. Administered from day 10 to day 25 of the menstrual cycle in normal women, lynestrenol not only suppresses the ovulatory peak of LH, but also results in estradiol levels less than or equal to 50 pg/ml.

In practice, the combined treatment with lynestrenol given orally 25 days per cycle and progesterone percutaneously administered every day provides both therapeutic action in benign breast disease and effective contraception.

There are no side effects from percutaneous administration of progesterone. However, the sequential administration of lynestrenol is not without side effects, mainly related to the androgenic potency of estrane derivative progestins: weight increase and sometimes seborrhea. Owing to the possibility of deterioration of carbohydrate tolerance with an increase in insulin secretion, this treatment cannot be considered for diabetic or prediabetic patients.

Results of Treatment

Percutaneous Progesterone Alone. The therapeutic results obtained with percutaneous progesterone were verified using clinical, radiographic, and thermographic criteria. Good clinical results included complete disappearance of breast pain and tenderness, in particular during the premenstrual period. The mammary gland became supple and nodularity disappeared. Total improvement was observed in 73.8 percent of cases of mastodynia, and some improvement was also obtained in 10 percent of the patients with increased nodularity of the breast. In all the other groups percutaneous progesterone alone was almost ineffective, and only the addition of oral progestogen yielded significant results (Table 1). In a double-blind study, 92 percent of the women greatly improved with progesterone, while only 24 percent improved with the placebo (Table 2).

The mammography results were less clear-cut and there was often a disparity between clinical improvement and radiologic findings, especially as it was difficult to obtain comparable films at two consecutive examinations. Moreover, edema is not easily visualized on mammography, whereas intralobular sclerosis and thickening of glandular tissue can be seen, and masks the eventual modification of glandular tissue after hormonal treatment. However, the radiologist can, with

Editor's Note: Progesterone cream is not available in some countries, including the United States. As an alternative approach, many physicians recommend a progestin-dominant birth control pill containing 300 mg dl-norgestrel and 30 μg ethinyl estradiol. If this is unacceptable, medroxyprogesterone acetate, 10 mg per day on the last 10 days of the cycle, may be imposed since progestins of the estrone series are not available in the U.S.A.

TABLE 1   Clinical Results Obtained in Various Benign Breast Diseases*

	Number	Percutaneous Progesterone (6 months) (%)	Number	Percutaneous Progesterone plus Progestins (9 months) (%)
Masodynia	355	73.8	249	96
Increased nodularity	19	10.5	115	85
Fibroadenomas	37	0	71	50
Cysts	125	0	122	50
Fibrocystic disease	138	0	63	10

*After six months of treatment with percutaneously administered progesterone or nine months of treatment with daily administration of percutaneous progesterone plus lynestrenol

Note: These data were taken from Sitruk-Ware R. L., et al, in Mauvais-Jarvis P, Vikers CFH, Wepierre J (eds): *Percutaneous Absorption of Steroids*. London: Academic Press, 1979

care, obtain two comparable films wherein the disappearance of edema after treatment can be seen. In spite of this, there is often a clear improvement of vascular pictures obtained at thermography.

In normal conditions, the lowest mammary temperature is observed at the beginning of the cycle when the vascular pattern is less marked. Thereafter, breast temperature increases and at the end of the cycle is 1–2°C higher. At this premenstrual period, superficial vessels are larger and more numerous.

In patients with mastodynia, the mammary temperature is higher throughout the cycle, and the range between the beginning and the end of the cycle may be as great as 3°C. The vascular pictures are characterized by very large vessels even in the postmenstrual period.

In one study, after treatment with percutaneous progestins a clear improvement was observed in 50 percent of patients, with normalization of the mammary temperature and the vascular pattern. In 20 percent of the cases thermography showed a less clear-cut improvement. In the remaining 30 percent of cases, thermography was unchanged, with an asymmetric vascular pattern, even when clinical improvement was observed (Table 1).

TABLE 2   Results of Treatment for Mastodynia*

	Percutaneous Progesterone (%)	Placebo (%)
Good results	92	24
Failure	8	76

*After three months of treatment in a double-blind study of 97 patients

In another study, 78 percent of the patients with mastodynia showed normal pictures after treatment. A high percentage of cases of increased nodularity of the breasts (80 percent) and fibrocystic disease (75 percent) also showed improvement. In the latter cases, the best results were obtained when mastodynia was also present.

In the cases of fibroadenoma or cysts, no changes were observed. In fact, the percutaneous treatment was conducted alone for no more than three months. The percutaneous progesterone treatment was more effective when the women were younger (less than 40 years of age) and when mastodynia had appeared recently and was not associated with a lump. Thermographic improvement correlated well with the clinical results.

Since mastodynia is considered the first symptom of benign breast disease and reflects the predominant effect of estrogen on breast tissue (particularly edema), the fact that progesterone is continuously present in the breast might permit a permanent antiestrogenic effect and prevent further development of cellular hyperplasia and fibrosis.

For all these reasons, treatment of mastodynia with percutaneously applied progesterone seems to be the most effective for isolated mastodynia without organized breast lumps and without important menstrual disorders. In addition, when mastodynia appears during oral contraceptive therapy, percutaneous progesterone treatment given concomitantly with birth control pills makes the breast pain and tenderness disappear. In cases studied by thermography the picture was fairly well improved after the first month of topical progesterone application.

Combined Treatment with Percutaneous Progesterone and Oral Lynestrenol. Results obtained by combined progesterone-lynestrenol treatment of diverse mastopathies are also given in Table 1. The therapeutic results of hormonal treatment of benign breast disease were expressed as above (see the section on treatment with percutaneous progesterone).

Complete improvement in breast pain and tenderness was observed from the very beginning of the treatment in 96 percent of the 249 cases of mastodynia.

The 4 percent failure rate was observed when this symptom was associated with fibrocystic disease or cysts. In fact, in the patients with fibrocystic disease, only 10 percent improved with the treatment. In these cases, microcysts disappeared and did not develop again during the course of the treatment. The cysts treated first by needle aspiration did not reappear during the hormonal treatment in 50 percent of the cases. The fibroadenomas were greatly reduced or disappeared in 50 percent of the cases. Lesions completely disappeared in 85 percent of the patients with increased nodularity of the breasts, and in the remaining 15 percent no improvement was observed. In the latter cases the lesions had been present for many years and were far larger than in the cases in which treatment was effective.

It appears clear that the higher percentage of positive results with this treatment occurred in cases with symptoms ascribable to recent lesions, in particular, the cases of isolated mastodynia in which treatment was also invariably effective. The results of this treatment were also remarkable in the cases in which increased nodularity of the breasts had recently appeared and in which sclerosis was either absent or minimal.

Some positive results were also obtained in "young" fibroadenomas. This confirms in vitro data showing that estradiol and progesterone receptors were found only in fibroadenomas with considerable cellularity and no fibrosis. A correlation was found between the presence of progesterone receptors in "young" fibroadenomas and the response to hormonal treatment.

In contrast, "old" fibroadenomas with marked fibrosis and poor cellularity did not respond to treatment with progesterone and progestins. This is also the case in chronic fibrocystic disease in which sclerosis is the main histologic component. The presence of estradiol or progesterone receptors was not assayed in this type of disease. However, indirectly, the negative results obtained by the progestational treatment might indicate that in this sort of chronic disease hormone dependence had disappeared a long time before.

The above observations lead to the following therapeutic considerations:

The hormonal treatment of benign breast disease is effective if it is begun very early in the course of the disease, particularly in the cases in which unopposed estrogen action is responsible for edema and reversible glandular hyperplasia. For these reasons, I believe that mastodynia is not a physiologic event but is probably the first symptom of a hyperestrogenic milieu inside the breast. The presence of estradiol and progesterone receptors in lesions with epithelial cell proliferation gives additional support to such a hypothesis. Thus recent lesions may be successfully treated by the administration of progesterone and progestins to correct the systemic and local hormonal insufficiencies.

There is no direct proof that the same hormonal environment plays a major role in the development of breast cancer. However, indirect evidence links human breast cancer to luteal insufficiency. Thus it is possible that the lack of progesterone secretion is a common risk factor for development of both benign breast diseases and cancer. Only early and lengthy treatment of a large group of patients, either with benign breast disease or with a high risk of developing breast cancer, can confirm that speculation.

INDEX

Note: Page numbers followed by *t* indicate tables; those followed by *f* indicate figures.

433